Escherichia coli
RECENT ADVANCES ON PHYSIOLOGY, PATHOGENESIS AND BIOTECHNOLOGICAL APPLICATIONS

Edited by **Amidou Samie**

Escherichia coli **- Recent Advances on Physiology, Pathogenesis and Biotechnological Applications**
http://dx.doi.org/10.5772/63146
Edited by Amidou Samie

Contributors

Wanda Reygaert, Swee Hua Erin Lim, Polly Soo Xi Yap, Shun Kai Yang, Kok Song Lai, Inés Arana, Maite Orruño, Claudia Parada, Vladimir Kaberdin, Athumani Msalale Lupindu, Noel Pabalan, Eloisa Singian, Lani Tabangay, Hamdi Jarjanazi, harshini mukundan, Loreen Stromberg, Heather Mendez, Mana Oloomi, Saeid Bouzari, Maryam Javadi, Slaven Jozić, Mladen Šolić, Rodica Elena Ionescu, Robert Price, Mehmet Berkmen, Mamoru Yamada, William R. McCleary, Juana V. Villegas, Rodrigo Boguen, Pamela Uribe, Stéphanie Blanquet-Diot, Charlène Roussel, Charlotte Cordonnier, Tom Van De Wiele, Valérie Livrelli, Barbara Kot, Bernardo Franco, Naurú Idalia Vargas-Maya, Tsuyoshi Imai, Thanh-Loc Thi Dang, Cristina Paiva De Sousa, Henrique Cezar Alves, Jose Dalton Cruz Pessoa, Luis Carlos Trevelin, Angela Merici De Oliveira Leal, Felipe de Paula Nogueira Cruz, Pamela Carla Pereira De Assis, Timothy Kudinha

Published by InTech
Janeza Trdine 9, 51000 Rijeka, Croatia

Publishing Process Manager Martina Usljebrka
Technical Editor SPi Global
Cover InTech Design team

First published July, 2017
Printed in Croatia
Legal deposit, Croatia: National and University Library in Zagreb

Additional hard copies can be obtained from orders@intechopen.com

Escherichia coli - Recent Advances on Physiology, Pathogenesis and Biotechnological Applications,
Edited by Amidou Samie
p. cm.
Print ISBN 978-953-51-3329-2
Online ISBN 978-953-51-3330-8

For EU product safety concerns:
IN TECH d.o.o., Prolaz Marije Krucifikse Kozulić 3, 51000 Rijeka, Croatia,
info@intechopen.com or visit our website at intechopen.com.

Meet the editor

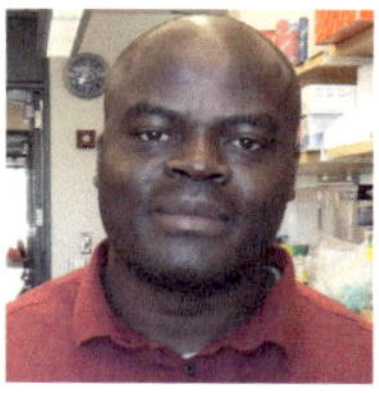

Dr. Amidou Samie is an associate professor of Microbiology at the University of Venda, in South Africa, where he graduated for his PhD in May 2008. He joined the Department of Microbiology the same year and has been giving lectures on topics covering parasitology, immunology, molecular biology and industrial microbiology. He is currently a rated researcher by the National Research Foundation of South Africa at the category C2 and has published widely in the field of infectious diseases and graduated several MSc and PhD students. His research activities cover mostly topics in infectious diseases from epidemiology to control. His particular interest lies in the study of intestinal protozoan parasites and opportunistic infections among HIV patients as well as the potential impact of childhood diarrhea on growth and child development. He also conducts research on water-borne diseases and water quality and is involved in the evaluation of point of use water treatment technologies using nanoparticles from silver and copper in collaboration with the University of Virginia in the USA. He also studies the use of medicinal plants for the control of infectious diseases as well as antimicrobial drug resistance.

Contents

Preface

Escherichia coli also known as *E. coli* is a rod-shaped Gram-negative bacterium. It grows freely in the intestine of all humans and most animals. It is one of the most studied organisms and serves as the prokaryotic model of organisms. In spite of the fact that this organism is the most studied, it continues to generate many discussions in the academic and industrial sectors and is used for several purposes particularly in the study and application of microbiology and biotechnology. A simple search of the major databases like PubMed, Google scholar, and others will generate hundreds of publications every day. This therefore further emphasizes the importance of this organism.

E. coli is a versatile organism that plays a role in different sectors of human life. Though mostly a commensal organism living in the intestines of humans and animals, *E. coli* can be responsible for both intestinal and extraintestinal infections. *E. coli* for example is an important cause of urinary tract infections with severe consequences including male infertility, which is a topic not often discussed in many books debating the pathogenesis of this organism. *E. coli* also plays an important role as a model organism due to its ability to grow easily in simple culture media, its short generation time, and the ease with which its genetic material can be manipulated just to cite but a few. Furthermore, many molecular processes have been discovered by studying *E. coli*, and many of these have been extended to other bacterial organisms. Such issues include, for example, the adaptation of cells in difficult environments, genetic processes, and the production of specific enzymes through different biochemical pathways.

The present book is therefore a good mix of pathogenesis, cell biology, biotechnology, and molecular applications of *E. coli*. The book does not intend to give an exhaustive study of the organism but focuses on specific topics of interest such as pathogenesis and antibiotic resistance mechanisms, innovative methods in bacterial detection, environmental water disinfections, and cell biology. A special attention was given to urinary tract infections that represent important diseases in both males and females, as well as its implication in male fertility/sterility and the mechanism thereof. This is especially important as many cases of infertility are often misdiagnosed and the index of suspicion might be actually very far away from *E. coli*. The development of antibiotic resistance is another important stumbling block to the control of infectious diseases with the recent emergence of multiple antibiotic resistance (MAR) among different bacterial organisms including *E. coli*.

As a contaminant and often used as an indicator of contamination of environmental waters, there is a need for the design of simple methods that are effective in the removal of microbial contaminants from water sources. In this book, a number of chapters have been dedicated to development of innovative methods for environmental water disinfection using substances such as pressurized carbon dioxide, the use of nanoparticles, and the use of essential oils for the control of this organism. Further topics discussed in the book include physiology, micronutrient utilization in the form of phosphate homeostasis, and mechanisms of survival in stressful conditions such as in salty environment in the case of increased temperature with global warming or just in nutrient-deprived conditions and provide a good start for further discussions for future research. The different chapters also raise several questions in terms of the identification of issues that need further attention for the development of knowledge.

The book therefore discusses recent advances in all the topics cited above and presents an interesting reading particularly sharpened toward application compared to just basic science. Here we present different aspects of this marvelous organism from its pathogenic capacity both at the intestinal and extraintestinal infections; its use as a model organism has been discussed as well. For those working in the laboratory, methods for the detection, isolation, and characterization of *E. coli* have been discussed including innovative methods for the detection of lipopolysaccharides, which can be used as markers of infections or even contamination. The use of biosensor instruments for the detection of *E. coli* in different types of samples including humans, animals, and environmental samples has also been discussed. With the recent advances in cell phone technology, it is appropriate to adapt such useful tool for application in the detection of water contamination, for example, as discussed in the book.

Professor Amidou Samie
Department of Microbiology,
University of Venda,
Limpopo Province,
South Africa

Section 1

E. coli in Disease

Chapter 1

Enterotoxigenic and Enterohemorrhagic *Escherichia coli*: Survival and Modulation of Virulence in the Human Gastrointestinal Tract

Charlène Roussel, Charlotte Cordonnier,
Valérie Livrelli, Tom Van de Wiele and
Stéphanie Blanquet-Diot

Additional information is available at the end of the chapter

http://dx.doi.org/10.5772/intechopen.68309

Abstract

Enterotoxigenic *Escherichia coli* (ETEC) and Enterohemorrhagic *Escherichia coli* (EHEC) are major food- and water-borne pathogens that constitute a serious public health threat in low-income and developed countries, respectively. Survival and expression of virulence genes in the human digestive tract are key features in bacterial pathogenesis, but the mechanisms behind these processes remain largely unknown due to obvious prohibition of human studies. Use of well-controlled and multi-parametric *in vitro* models can aid in addressing knowledge gaps in ETEC and EHEC pathogenesis. After a general description of the physiopathology of ETEC and EHEC infections, this chapter will give an overview of all the *in vitro* studies that have investigated the effect of the main physicochemical and biotic parameters of the human gut on pathogen survival and expression of virulence factors. We bring a picture of how ETEC and EHEC are able to adapt to each of the successive environments of the human gastrointestinal tract by reading many cues provided by both the host and the gut microbiota.

Keywords: enterotoxigenic *Escherichia coli* (ETEC), enterohemorrhagic *Escherichia coli* (EHEC), survival, virulence genes expression, human gastrointestinal tract, *in vitro* models

1. Introduction

Since its identification in 1885, *Escherichia coli* (*E. coli*) has become one of the most comprehensively studied bacterial species. While *E. coli* is widely found in the environment and foods and is an important member of the commensal microbiota of mammals, some strains have evolved to include pathogenic mechanisms that cause significant diseases in humans and animals. In humans, *E. coli* strains can cause diverse enteric/diarrheagenic or extra-intestinal infections by means of virulence factors that affect a wide range of cellular processes. Pathogenic *E. coli* associated with gastrointestinal illness have been divided into eight pathotypes based on their virulence profiles: (i) enteropathogenic *E. coli* (EPEC), (ii) enterohaemorrhagic *E. coli* (EHEC), (iii) enterotoxigenic *E. coli* (ETEC), (iv) enteroinvasive *E. coli* (EIEC), (v) enteroaggregative *E. coli* (EAEC), (vi) diffusely adherent *E. coli* (DAEC), (vii) adherent invasive *E. coli* (AIEC) and (viii) Shiga toxin-producing enteroaggregative *E. coli* (STEAEC) [1]. This chapter will cover only two of them: ETEC and EHEC, which show opposite trends during their pathogenic processes. Even if in both cases human infections are primarily acquired through consumption of contaminated food products or drinking water, ETEC is a major cause of infantile diarrhea in developing countries, while EHEC is one of the main *E. coli* pathotypes associated with food poisoning outbreaks in the developed world.

To cause human illness, pathogenic enteric *E. coli* must not only survive the passage through the human gastrointestinal (GI) tract but also accomplish their pathogenic process by a complex and coordinated multistage strategy, including adherence to the host intestine and toxin/virulence protein production. The current chapter will provide a state of the art of ETEC and EHEC physiopathology, then focus on pathogen survival in the human digestive tract and regulation of virulence determinants by GI cues. As studies on humans are ethically inconceivable and small animal models do not recapitulate human pathogenesis, we will introduce the potential of dynamic *in vitro* digestion systems for increasing our understanding of ETEC and EHEC pathogenesis in a physiologically relevant GI environment.

2. Physiopathology of ETEC and EHEC infections

2.1. Epidemiological data

ETEC are a significant cause of watery diarrhea in developing countries where sanitation and clean water remain scarce and a main cause of traveler's diarrhea [2]. In contrast, EHEC are a major public health concern of developed countries [3] (**Figure 1**). Hence, ETEC are among the top four pathogens causing moderate to severe diarrhea among children in Africa and South Asia, while EHEC are the third most common zoonotic pathogen in Europe associated with large food poisoning outbreaks in EU, the USA, Canada, and Japan. The most common serogroups implicated in outbreaks and sporadic cases are O6, O78, O8, O128, and O153 for ETEC and O157:H7, O26:H11, O45:H2, O103:H2, O111:H8, O121:H19, and O145:H28 for EHEC.

http://dx.doi.org/10.5772/intechopen.68309

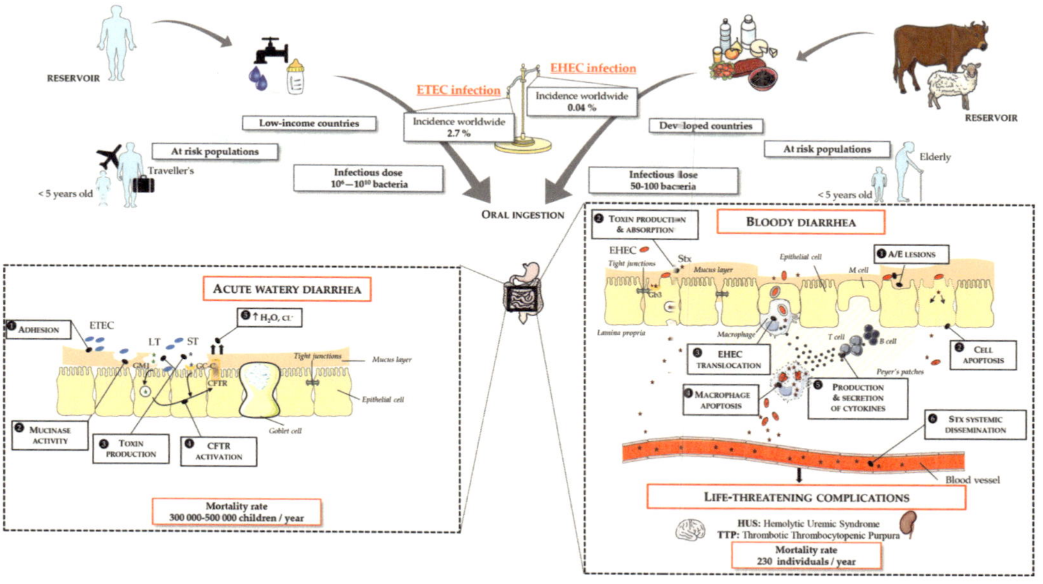

Figure 1. ETEC and EHEC pathogenesis including epidemiological data on the infections and at-risk populations, reservoir, mode of transmission and virulence factors of the pathogen, and clinical signs are described. A/E: Attaching and effacing; CFTR: cystic fibrosis transmembrane regulator; GC-C: guanylyl cyclase C; GM1: monosialoganglioside receptor; LT: heat-labile enterotoxins; ST: heat-stable enterotoxins; Stx: Shiga toxin.

ETEC cause approximately 280 million episodes of diarrhea worldwide, leading to hundreds of thousands of deaths per year [4]. With regard to EHEC, it is estimated that the pathogen is responsible for 2,801,000 acute illnesses, 3890 cases of haemolytic and uremic syndrome (HUS), 270 cases of permanent end-stage renal disease, and 230 deaths worldwide [3]. For both pathogens, infants less than 5 years old are a high-risk population. ETEC are responsible for 20–25% of diarrhea in young children, mostly in low-income countries, and up to 40% of traveler's diarrhea [5]. In developing countries, children suffer from diarrhea attacks 7–8 times a year, with a peak incidence occurring between 6 and 18 months, and ETEC strains are responsible for one of each three attacks [6, 7]. In such countries, ETEC infections have then shown to play a significant part in the complex association between malnutrition and repeated bouts of diarrheal illness among young children. The impact of EHEC is also greater in infants and children, compared to other ages with 42% of cases of HUS and 29% of deaths occurring in children between the ages of 0 and 4 years [3].

While the lack of ongoing monitoring systems makes it difficult to understand ETEC pathogenesis worldwide, dedicated surveillance systems of human EHEC infections have been developed in most of the industrialized areas of the world [8]. In Europe, the surveillance of EHEC infections is embedded in the Food and Waterborne Diseases and Zoonoses (FWD) surveillance system coordinated by the European Center for Disease Prevention and Control (ECDC). FWD is a passive surveillance system, collecting data on EHEC infections including laboratory-confirmed cases, probable cases, and possible cases. Cases of HUS are specifically recorded through a network of pediatric nephrologists and infection-control practitioners on the basis of clinical diagnosis.

2.2. Reservoir and route of transmission

Both ETEC and EHEC infections are typically acquired through the ingestion of contaminated food or water (**Figure 1**). However, a major difference between ETEC and EHEC is that ETEC only have a human reservoir of infection while EHEC are zoonotic pathogens [2, 9]. The main source of ETEC infection is contaminated water, such as surface water and drinking water (especially for weaning food) suffering from a lack of adequate sanitation and sewage facilities [2]. Nevertheless, a variety of food items including vegetables and herbs imported from endemic countries have also been recently implicated in uncommon sporadic cases or outbreaks in industrialized countries. Ruminants, especially cattle, are a natural reservoir of EHEC, and hence entry into the food chain through fecal contamination. Food (mainly undercooked beef products, unpasteurized milk, and vegetable) and water are the principal sources of human contamination with EHEC. Person-to-person transmission of EHEC may significantly contribute to outbreaks from a primary source, whereas this mode of transmission is not likely under most circumstances for ETEC infection.

The infective dose widely differs between ETEC and EHEC. It fluctuates between 10^8 and 10^{10} cells for ETEC in adults, but vulnerable populations such as infants may be susceptible to infection at lower doses [7, 10]. The infective dose for EHEC is recognized to be much lower: less than 50 to a few hundred organisms are usually sufficient to lead to the clinical signs [11].

2.3. Clinics and treatments

ETEC or EHEC show similar clinical pictures at the beginning of infections: watery diarrhea leading to rapid dehydration, usually associated with nausea, vomiting, and abdominal cramps [2, 11]. With regard to ETEC, following an incubation period of 10–72 hours, the duration of illness is typically 3–5 days, and resolved usually without antimicrobial treatment, even though symptoms can persist for 2–3 weeks. ETEC infections are generally self-limited and cannot be distinguished from Cholera on clinical grounds. Symptoms are much more severe in children from developing countries where diarrhea and malnutrition combine to form a vicious cycle leading to declining health status and death. Unlike ETEC, EHEC infections may evolve toward extra-digestive complications. EHEC infections typically progress from watery to bloody diarrhea and resolve within a week or 10 days in the majority of infected individuals. Nevertheless, in 5–7% of cases, the infection may lead to life-threatening complications, namely HUS and thrombotic thrombocytopenic purpura (TTP), and death [11, 12]. HUS is characterized as a triad of acute kidney failure, microangiopathic hemolytic anemia, and thrombocytopenia, and remains the most common cause of acute renal failure in children in the EU and US. The elderly mostly develop TTP, which differs from HUS because of neurological symptoms including lethargy, severe headache, convulsions, and encephalopathy.

Currently, treatment for ETEC and EHEC infections consists primarily of supportive therapy, with oral rehydration to prevent dehydration and loss of electrolytes. For EHEC, general supportive measures also include peritoneal dialysis or hemodialysis and management of anemia with transfusion of whole blood or packed red cells [13]. Conventional antibiotic treatment is generally not recommended for EHEC-infected patients as it increases HUS or neurological complications [14]. The use of antimicrobials is also problematic during ETEC infection since an etiologic diagnosis cannot be made rapidly, mainly in childhood diarrhea [2]. Fluoroquinolones are shown to be effective during ETEC traveler's diarrhea [15] but should be used with caution due to the rise of antimicrobial resistance worldwide and the risk of side effects. For both pathogens, antimotility agents can be prescribed but need to be carefully administered as they can prolong the residence time of bacteria or their toxins in the intestine.

In this context, alternative prophylactic or therapeutic strategies are currently under development for ETEC and EHEC. Vaccines against the pathogens are still not commercially available, although vaccine strategies have been developed and used with variable success in animal models and/or humans [16, 17]. However, Dukoral®, a vaccine commercialized for *Vibrio cholerae*, can be prescribed to prevent traveler's diarrhea due to ETEC. Global alternative approaches involving dietary supplementation or probiotics have also been considered for both ETEC [18, 19] and EHEC [20, 21], with various levels of evidence from *in vitro* and *in vivo* studies. Other therapeutic options targeting a specific step in bacterial pathogenesis have been developed, mainly for EHEC, such as the use of agents that link toxins or block their binding at the cell surface [13] or antibodies that inhibit the terminal complement complex formation [22].

2.4. Virulence factors

After ingestion by humans, ETEC and EHEC pursue a strategy of infection involving colonization of the intestinal mucosal surface and production of toxins. The main sites of colonization differ between the two pathogens: from the upper jejunum to the ileum for ETEC [23, 24] and terminal ileum and colon for EHEC [25–27]. Notably, EHEC show a preferential tropism to the follicle-associated epithelium (FAE) of small intestinal Peyer's patches [25, 28], which has not been described for ETEC. Even if for both pathogens toxins are clearly identified as their main virulence factor, bacterial pathogenesis is not limited to toxin-mediated effects, and a combination of virulence traits is required to make ETEC and EHEC strains fully pathogenic to humans. This part describes the main virulence factors that have been identified for ETEC and EHEC.

2.4.1. Acid resistance

After being ingested, the pathogens must first breach the acidic barrier of the human stomach to reach their intestinal niche. It is well described that *E. coli* strains have intricate acid resistance (AR) systems that enable their survival in the harsh gastric environment, the glutamate-dependent AR system providing the highest level of acid protection [29]. Such acid resistance is a critical virulence trait of the infection, especially for EHEC for which the infectious dose is typically very low.

2.4.2. Colonization factors

ETEC adhere to the intestinal epithelium by means of several colonization factors (CFs). More than 25 CFs that are antigenically and structurally diverse, have been identified in ETEC and include fimbrial and fimbrillar structures. Among them, seven are generally more prevalent than others: CFA/I (colonization factor antigen) and CS1 to CS6 (*coli* surface antigen) [30]. Most CF receptors have not been yet identified, but CFs are thought to bind to glycoprotein conjugates in mucus fraction from the small intestine and on the surface of host cells. Non-fimbrial adhesins such as TibA, a glycosylated autotransporter; Tia, an outer membrane protein; and EtpA, which acts as a molecular bridge binding host cell receptors to the tips of ETEC flagella, have also been implicated in the pathogenesis [31].

EHEC colonization involves attaching and effacing (A/E) lesions on the enterocytes, which are characterized by ultra-structural changes, including loss of microvilli and intimate attachment of the bacterium to the cell surface [32]. Genes encoding A/E lesion formation are localized on a pathogenicity island, the locus for enterocyte effacement (LEE), which encodes a bacterial type III secretion system (T3SS). Colonization is mainly mediated by the primary adhesin, namely intimin (encoded by *eae* gene), but other putative adherence factors have been described, such as long polar fimbriae—Lpf—or curli [33]. A number of other non-fimbrial EHEC adhesins have been implicated in adhesion including the plasmid-encoded *toxB*, the chromosomally encoded adhesins Iha, Cah, and OmpA [32, 33].

Mucin-degrading enzymes, which allow temporary access to intestinal cell membrane and promote bacterial adhesion have been recently identified in both ETEC and EHEC. In ETEC, YghJ, a mucin-binding metalloprotease [34] and EatA, a member of serine protease autotransporters of the Enterobacteriaceae (SPATE) family [35] have been described. In EHEC, one protein has been shown to have mucinase activity: StcE, an extracellular zinc metalloprotease which specifically recognizes α-O-glycan-containing substrates [36].

2.4.3. Secretion of toxins

Toxins are considered as the main virulence factor for both ETEC and EHEC as they are responsible for the main clinical symptoms and/or systemic complications. In ETEC, secretory diarrheas are mediated through the action of heat-stable (ST) and/or heat-labile (LT) enterotoxins.

ETEC strains are able to secrete either one or two toxins (LT and/or ST), but it has been shown that LT toxin is less likely to cause disease than ST or LT/ST ETEC toxins [7]. LT toxins encoded by the *eltAB* gene are similar in structure and function to Cholera toxin by sharing 80% homology. LT shows an AB_5 configuration with a catalytically active LT_A subunit and a pentameric ring of LT_B subunits responsible for binding and internalization [37]. LT are mainly secreted associated with outer membrane vesicles (OMVs) and bind irreversibly to monoganglioside (GM1) on the host cell. LT leads to an increase in cAMP that induces cystic fibrosis transmembrane regulator (CFTR) phosphorylation, eliciting massive fluid loss and watery diarrhea. In addition to causing diarrhea, LT plays multiple roles in modulating host cell function and providing a competitive advantage for ETEC adherence to cultured intestinal epithelial cells. ST toxins encoded by the *estAB* gene are small cysteine-rich peptides which mimic the human hormone guanylin. They are divided into two structural and antigenically distinct groups: STa and STb which reversibly bind to guanylyl cyclase C (GC-C) and sulphatide, respectively [37], leading to CFTR activation and diarrhea.

Shiga toxins (Stx) are produced by EHEC in the lumen of the intestine, and then cross the epithelial barrier by poorly described mechanisms to eventually reach their target organs [38]. Two toxin families encoded in the genomes of lysogenic lambdoid phages are produced by the bacteria, namely Stx1 and Stx2, the latter being associated with the most severe complications [39]. Stx contain two major structural subunits, A and B [40]. The B subunit binds to the toxin cellular receptor, globotriaosylceramide-3 (Gb3), expressed on host microvascular endothelial cell surfaces (kidney, intestine, and brain). This explains the life-threatening complications associated with EHEC infections. The A subunit exhibits an RNA N-glycosidase activity against the 28S rRNA, resulting in inhibition of protein synthesis and cell death.

3. Bacterial survival in the human digestive tract

Bacterial survival in the human GI tract is a key parameter in ETEC and EHEC physiopathology. Nevertheless, how pathogens can survive in the human digestive environment remains largely unknown as studies in humans are impossible. For regulatory, ethical, technical, and cost reasons, artificial digestive systems are increasingly used as an alternative to *in vivo* studies in humans. Until now, almost no data are available for ETEC under human digestive simulated conditions while a number of studies have assessed the survival of EHEC during human *in vitro* digestion.

Masters et al. [41] have shown that after exposure to pH 2, ETEC became undetectable by plate counting after 2 hours. A recent study using flow cytometry analysis indicated that there was no significant difference in the percentage of live bacteria when ETEC were subjected to pH 5 or pH 7 [42]. Only one study has investigated the impact of 30 g/L bile on the survival of ETEC *in vitro*. Despite the known bactericidal effect of bile in the intestine, growth curves for ETEC in Luria Bertani (LB) media and LB-bile showed similar slopes during the exponential growth phase [43].

With regard to EHEC, most of the studies have been carried out, like for ETEC, using simplified *in vitro* approaches integrating a limited number of digestive parameters, such as acid pH or bile salts [44, 45]. Even if the pathogen is considered as acid resistant, large variations in survival rates have been obtained for *E. coli* O157:H7 in acidified culture media or in simulated gastric fluid [45, 46]. This wide range of response may be explained by differences in culture conditions, bacterial strains, and pH values used to simulate the gastric phase. Other more recent studies have evaluated the survival of EHEC strains by using dynamic multicompartmental *in vitro* models that closely mimic the gastric, small intestinal, and colonic human digestive conditions. In the TNO GastroIntestinal model (TIM), which simulates the stomach and the three segments of the human small intestine, it has been shown that EHEC survival was affected in the stomach and duodenum (when ingested within a food matrix but not with a glass of water), while bacterial growth was observed at the end of digestion in the jejunum and ileum [47–49]. This growth renewal in the distal parts of the small intestine was probably linked to the occurrence of less stringent conditions, such as neutral pH and lower concentrations of bile salts due to their reabsorption (as occurred *in vivo*). EHEC survival in the TIM model was found to be strain/serotype dependent [48] and influenced by food matrices [47–49] and age conditions [48]. In particular, thanks to the potential of the TIM model, Roussel et al. [49] have shown that differences in digestive physicochemical parameters related to age conditions may partly explain the higher susceptibility of children (compared to adults) to EHEC infections and HUS. Additional studies performed under human-simulated colonic conditions (including colonic microbiota) have shown that EHEC strains were not able to colonize [50], probably due to the barrier effect of gut microbiota or to the high short-chain fatty acid (SCFAs) concentrations found in the colon and known to inhibit EHEC growth [51, 52]. Taken together, these data suggest that the ability of EHEC to colonize the human gut would be rather linked to growth renewal of the pathogen in the distal parts of the small intestine than the ability to maintain in the colon.

4. Regulation of virulence genes by gastrointestinal cues

To be fully pathogenic, bacteria must not only survive in the human GI tract but also coordinate expression of virulence determinants in response to localized gut microenvironments. An increased number of *in vitro* or *in vivo* studies have shown that both ETEC and EHEC are able to respond to various GI cues and employ these cues to modulate the expression of their virulence factors [33, 53], as described below (**Figure 2**). Compared to ETEC, where all

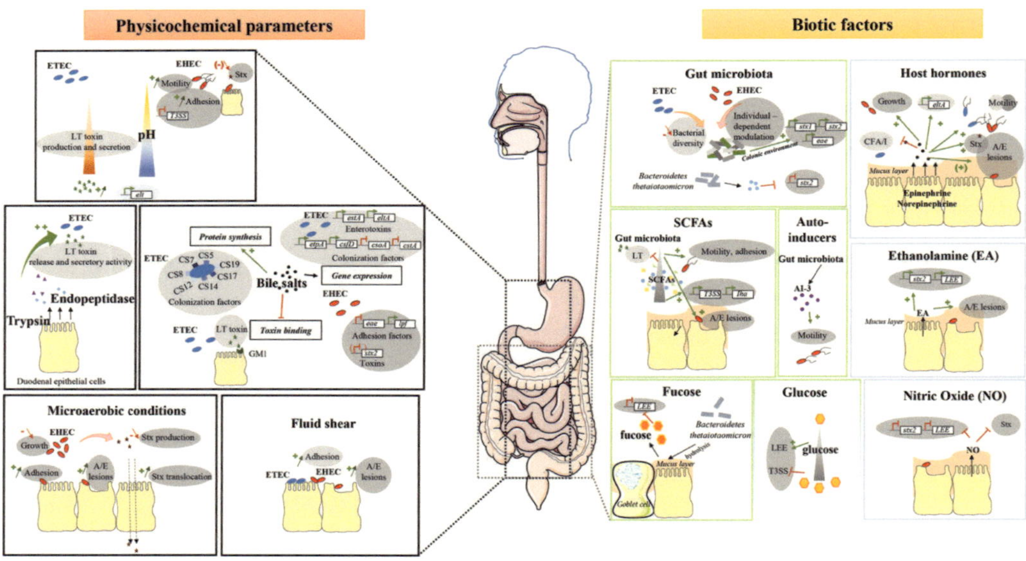

Figure 2. The figure provides a state of the art on the effects of biotic and abiotic parameters of the human gut on ETEC and EHEC virulence, as assessed by *in vitro* studies. Data related to ETEC and EHEC are surrounded by light grey and dark grey, respectively. A/E: Attaching and effacing; AI: autoinducer; CFA: colonization factor antigen; CS: *coli* surface; EA: ethanolamine; *elt*: heat-labile enterotoxin encoding gene; *est*: heat-stable enterotoxin encoding gene; *etpA*: ETEC two-partner protein A encoding gene; GM1: monosialoganglioside receptor; *IhA*: IrgA homologe adhesion encoding gene; LEE: locus for enterocyte effacement; *lpf*: long polar fimbriae encoding gene; LT: heat-labile enterotoxins; NO: nitric oxide; SCFA: short-chain fatty acids; Stx: Shiga toxin; T3SS: type 3 secretion system.

http://dx.doi.org/10.5772/intechopen.68309

the available studies have been performed in simple *in vitro* digestive conditions, recent data have been obtained for EHEC in more physiological conditions simulated by dynamic multi-compartmental models.

4.1. Regulation by physicochemical parameters of the human gut

4.1.1. pH

Once ingested, pathogens are exposed to the host digestive tract characterized by acid conditions in the stomach where pH gradually decreases during digestion from around 6 to 2, followed by pH close to neutrality in the small intestine.

For ETEC, the release of ST seems to be not pH-dependent [54], while it is acknowledged that extracellular pH has an influence on the release of LT toxin which increases with alkalinity [55, 56]. ETEC seems to use the pH gradient in the GI tract to modulate LT toxin production and secretion: when bacteria reach the small intestine, alkaline pH induces both transcription and maximal release of LT [42].

For EHEC, House et al. [57] have examined, using DNA microarrays, the gene expression profiles of EHEC O157 that had been acid stressed and then neutralized relative to the same unstressed strain. Virulence factors associated with adhesion, motility, and type III secretion were significantly modulated leading to enhancement of motility and host cell adhesion. The T3SS genes encoding proteins that mediate colonization and infection in the large intestine were downregulated following acid stress [33, 57]. Impact of low pH on Stx gene expression and production is not yet fully understood: House et al. [57] have shown no change whereas other studies have revealed that acid pH decreases Stx production [58, 59]. In the gastric and small intestinal TIM model, Roussel et al. [49] have shown that *stx1* and *stx2* genes were upregulated in the gastric compartment even if Stx-mediated cytotoxicity is generally associated with distal parts of the small intestine or large intestine. Higher expression levels were observed under child digestive conditions compared to adult ones where less acidic conditions are found, which is in accordance with the results of Yuk et al. [58] and Huang et al. [59].

4.1.2. Bile

Once the small intestine is reached, bile salts form a major challenge to pathogens, with bile concentrations sequentially decreasing from duodenum to colon due to reabsorption.

Chatterjee and Chowdhury [60] have shown *in vitro* that 2 g/L crude bile can prevent the binding of LT toxin to GM1 and that this effect was associated to arachidonic, linoleic, and oleic unsaturated fatty acids detected in crude bile. The same authors demonstrated *in vivo* in rabbit ileal loops that linoleic acid prevented LT-mediated fluid accumulation in a dose-dependent manner [60]. In another study by Nicklasson et al. [61], 1.5 g/L crude bile and 2 g/L bile salts sodium deoxycholate and sodium glycocholate-induced *in vitro* the expression of CS5-encoding gene *csfD*. A global transcriptional analysis of two ETEC strains showed that bile salts at a concentration of 30 g/L in LB medium upregulated *estA*, *eltA*, or *etpA* (encoding for STa, LTa enterotoxins, and EtpA, respectively) while *csoA* and *cstA* (encoding for CS1 and

CS3 colonization factors) were downregulated [43]. In this study, the transcriptional response to bile salts was strain-dependent, suggesting that the results should not be extrapolated to the entire pathovar without further investigation. Finally, at the protein level, 1.5 g/L bile salts were required for surface expression of at least CS5, CS7, CS8, CS12, CS14, CS17, and CS19 [62–64]. Haines et al. [62] have shown that bile salts seem not to be required for the expression of CS1, CS2, and CS3, while the opposite was demonstrated by Sjoling et al. [63]. These results suggest that both interaction of LT toxin with its receptor and expression of ETEC colonization factors may be differentially induced along the human intestine where bile acid concentrations range from 2 to 20 g/L.

Studies have also shown that bile may serve as an environmental cue for EHEC by modulating the expression of specific virulence factors [33]. DNA microarray analysis of EHEC O157:H7 treated with 1.5 g/L bile salts showed upregulation of *acrA* and *acrB* genes encoding a bile salts efflux pump [65]. Expression of several other well-known virulence factors including those encoded on the LEE pathogenicity island, was not altered by bile salt treatment. On the contrary, a significant decrease in *eae* gene transcripts was observed *in vitro* by other authors when 5–8 g/L bile salts were added [66, 67]. Bile salts also modulate the expression of other adhesins, such as Lpf: Arenas-Hernández et al. [68] and Yin et al. [66] found that concentrations of 1.5–5 g/L led to an upregulation of *lpf* genes. In the TIM system, *eae* and *lpf* overexpression occurred under child digestive conditions at the end of *in vitro* digestion, when most of the bacterial cells have reached the distal parts of the small intestine [49]. This might suggest a higher ability of EHEC to colonize the terminal ileum or colon in children compared to adults. Lastly, there is no consensus for the effect of bile salts on *stx* gene expression. Kus et al. [65] reported that 1.5 g/L bile salt downregulated *stx2* genes, whereas no influence was observed by Hamner et al. [67] with concentrations of 8 g/L.

4.1.3. Digestive enzymes

Very few studies have investigated how human digestive enzymes may influence the expression of virulence genes in pathogens, none in EHEC and only two in ETEC. In the latter, *in vitro* studies have shown that trypsin, an endopeptidase secreted by duodenal epithelial cells, is able to increase LT release [55] and its secretory activity [69].

4.1.4. Oxygen levels

Various oxygen levels can be found in the human GI tract with concentrations decreasing from the upper to the lower digestive tract and from mucosal surfaces to gut lumen. Up to date, the effect of various oxygen concentrations on pathogen virulence has been studied only in EHEC.

In an *in vitro* cell culture model, James and Keevil [70] have shown that the presence of oxygen enhanced EHEC ability to adhere to epithelial cells. In other recent studies, polarized human colon carcinoma cells in a vertical diffusion chamber system were used to investigate the influence of reduced apical oxygen levels on EHEC colonization [38] and Stx production [71]. The authors demonstrated that both EHEC-host adhesion and expression and translocation of T3SS effector proteins were increased under microaerobic conditions (1–2% oxygen). Microaerobiosis also significantly reduced bacterial growth as well as Stx production and release into the medium, while Stx translocation across the epithelial monolayer was enhanced. The role of oxygen levels on modulation of EHEC virulence was further confirmed by Lewis et al. [27] who showed in *in vitro* organ culture (IVOC) of human colonic biopsy samples that A/E lesion formation was dependent on oxygen levels. These lesions were suppressed under oxygen-rich culture conditions routinely used for IVOC. Taken together, these results suggest that the microaerobic environment adjacent to the intestinal microvilli may upregulate the expression of EHEC virulence factors that promote successful colonization of the large intestine.

4.1.5. Fluid shear

Fluid shear can be defined as distribution of frictional forces due to the hydrodynamic flow generated by GI peristaltic activity against the surface of intestinal epithelial cells. In the human gut, there is a decreasing gradient of fluid shear stress from mucosa to gut lumen. It has been generally assumed that shear stress inhibits pathogen adhesion, thereby serving as a non-specific host defense against bacterial colonization [72]. For both ETEC and EHEC, this concept has been very poorly described in the literature.

Tchesnokova et al. [72] have shown, using *in vitro* erythrocytes and Caco-2 cell models, a shear-enhanced binding of intestinal CfaE, the tip-localized minor subunit of CFA/I, in both prototypical and clinical ETEC strains. EHEC attachment to host cells is also enhanced by levels of shear force similar to peristaltic forces in the intestinal tract, which are required to fully activate LEE-encoded virulence mechanisms [73]. These preliminary data suggest that, in addition to a range of chemical environmental signals, ETEC and EHEC are capable of sensing and responding to mechanical cues in the human GI tract.

4.2. Regulation by biotic factors of the human gut

4.2.1. Gut microbiota and their metabolites

4.2.1.1. Gut microbiota

During passage through the human gut, enteric pathogenic bacteria such as ETEC and EHEC also have to face a high number of commensal bacteria that compete with them for nutrients and space. There is scarce data on the interactions of EHEC, but even more so for ETEC, with human gut microbiota.

For ETEC, only two studies have investigated gut microbiota changes during ETEC challenge [74, 75]. The authors conclude that ETEC infections are associated with a rapid and reversible change in gut microbial community structure as well as a significant decrease in overall bacteria diversity. However, there is no available data on how gut microbiota may influence ETEC virulence.

With regard to EHEC, Thévenot et al. [50] have recently shown in an *in vitro* model of the human colon, that *E. coli* O157:H7 has an individual dependent effect on the colonic microbiota, as assessed by qPCR analysis on major phyla and genus. The same authors also showed that EHEC infection led in the *in vitro* colonic environment to a significant increase in *stx1*, *stx2*, and *eae* expression 9–12 h post-administration. Besides, it has been also proposed that EHEC was sensing autoinducers produced by the GI microbiota, such as the quorum signaling molecule AI-3. EHEC respond to AI-3 by increasing flagellar synthesis and motility that allow the pathogen to more closely approach the mucosal epithelium at the site of colonization [76]. On the contrary, other soluble factors secreted by the normal gut microbiota may protect the host against EHEC infection. De Sablet et al. [77] have shown, in cecal contents of gnotobiotic rats colonized with human microbiota, that small molecules produced in part by *Bacteroides thetaiotaomicron*, a predominant species of the normal human intestinal microbiota, repressed *stx2* mRNA expression. Mutants of *B. thetaiotaomicron* with impaired production of a specific transporter of vitamin B12 were no longer able to inhibit the production of Stx2 [78]. This work suggests that concentration of vitamin B12 in the gut and by extension, activities of commensal bacterial species producing and/or consuming vitamin B12, may modulate the production of the main virulence factor of EHEC. Other studies have also demonstrated that the interplay between the nutrient requirements of normal flora and EHEC is important in determining pathogen virulence [76]. Njoroge et al. [79] uncovered the importance of glucose availability in regulating T3SS by EHEC: high-glucose growth media suppressed type III secretion while low-glucose conditions induced LEE expression. EHEC also use fucose that is made available from mucus by the microbiota (especially by *Bacteroides thetaiotaomicron*) to modulate their own metabolism and virulence. Pacheco et al. [80] described a novel two-component system that enables regulation of virulence gene expression and carbon-source choice by EHEC upon sensing fucose, resulting in a decrease in LEE transcript levels. All these results tend to indicate that differential microbiota composition may contribute to host resistance or susceptibility to EHEC infections. Then, differences in diet and antibiotic regimens, which cause shifts in the composition of the GI microbiota may also influence the outcome of the disease.

4.2.1.2. Short-chain fatty acids

Several studies have investigated how ETEC and EHEC may respond to gut microbiota metabolites such as SCFAs. The three main SCFAs present in the intestine are acetate, propionate, and butyrate and their concentrations vary from the small intestine to the colon.

A single study with ETEC has shown that addition of SCFAs from C-2 to C-7 at a concentration of 2 mg/mL in the culture medium significantly reduced or even abolished LT production [81]. A higher number of studies have evaluated how EHEC may sense SCFAs. Acetate (10–40 mM) and propionate (2–10 mM) had no effect on Stx2 production levels *in vitro* [78] while acetate production by *Bifidobacterium* strains was associated with an anti-infectious activity through the inhibition of Stx production and translocation [82]. Low SCFA concentrations (particularly of butyrate—from 6.25 to 25 mM), more typical of the distal ileum, enhanced the expression of EHEC virulence genes involved in motility, adhesion, and induction of A/E lesion formation [51, 52]. Other studies reported that high concentrations of SCFAs (above 50 mM), typically found in the distal colon, were associated with increased expression of T3SS [83] and Iha adhesin [84]. Very recently, Lackraj et al. [85] have investigated how EHEC modulate flagella expression and motility in response to SCFA mixes typical in compositions and concentrations of the small and large intestines.

They showed that when EHEC were exposed to SCFA mixes representative of the small intestine, there was a significant upregulation of flagellar genes, flagellar protein FliC, and motility, while the opposite was observed with SCFA mixes representative of the large intestine. Lastly, a high-fiber diet, via enhanced butyrate levels, increased host's expression of Gb3 and susceptibility of mice to disease [86]. Conversely, increased levels of microbiota-derived acetate protected animals from disease that is caused by the toxin. Collectively, these data suggest that molecular cues secreted by commensal microbiota such as SCFAs may modulate EHEC motility, adhesion, and toxin production, differently in the small and large intestines.

4.2.2. Host hormones

Microbial endocrinology is a newly recognized microbiology research area investigating the interactions of bacteria with stress-associated hormones, such as catecholamine. Among these hormones, only epinephrine and norepinephrine have been investigated as environmental cues for ETEC and EHEC.

Lyte et al. [87] demonstrated that physiological concentrations of norepinephrine increased the *in vitro* growth of an ETEC strain isolated from calf, as well as the expression of the virulence factor F5 fimbrial adhesin. On the contrary, Sturbelle et al. [88] did not observe any effect of norepinephrine or epinephrine on the *in vitro* growth of a piglet ETEC strain, and Haines et al. [62] found a significant inhibition of porcine ETEC growth by norepinephrine. However, a significant increase in motility and expression of F4 fimbriae and LT toxin-encoding genes was shown in the ETEC culture supplemented with conditioned medium (containing autoinducers) and epinephrine [88]. Lastly, Haines et al. [62] found that norepinephrine inhibited CFA/I expression in an ETEC strain isolated from humans.

As described for ETEC, Lyte et al. [89] found that norepinephrine increased *in vitro* EHEC growth. EHEC also use norepinephrine as a signal for differential regulation of virulence factors mediating invasion, motility, and A/E lesion formation [90]. Regulation of EHEC virulence by epinephrine and norepinephrine is still not fully understood but it has been shown that the pathogen uses the histidine sensor kinases QseC and QseE as sensors of the two hormones [33, 76]. So, host-derived hormones epinephrine and/or norepinephrine seem to assist ETEC and EHEC in cueing their site of colonization and enhance approach to the epithelial layer through increased motility and adhesion.

4.2.3. Other factors

The influence of other GI factors, such as ethanolamine (EA) and nitric oxide (NO), has been studied on EHEC virulence, but not on ETEC. However, the nature of the associated regulations is still not fully understood.

EA comes from the turnover of intestinal epithelial cells and commensal microbiota and is generated from the breakdown of phosphatidylethanolamine. EHEC cultured in minimal media containing EA showed increased expression of both *stx2* and genes encoded on the LEE pathogenicity island, as well as a higher number of attaching and effacing (A/E) lesions on host epithelial cells [91].

NO is an essential mediator of the innate immune response of infected colonic mucosa. Chemical or cellular sources of NO have been shown to inhibit *stx*- and LEE-encoded genes mRNA expression and Stx synthesis, without altering EHEC viability [92, 93].

5. Conclusion

This chapter shows that we get clearer evidence that the food- and water-borne pathogens ETEC and EHEC are able to adapt to each of the successive environments of the human GI tract by reading many cues provided by both the host and the gut microbiota. Exposure to different environmental cues may impact pathogen survival but also alter the expression of virulence genes. Nevertheless, the data obtained until now show many gaps and inconsistencies. In particular, most of the current studies have been carried out using oversimplified *in vitro* approaches, and what is still missing is the integration of signals delivered in a sequential but not in an isolated fashion. Relevant alternatives to better understand how ETEC and EHEC respond to these various cues in a temporal-spatial fashion may imply relevant animal models (e.g., human microbiota-associated animals) [94] or digestion models closely mimicking the human digestive tract, such as the TIM or the SHIME (Simulator of the Human Intestinal Microbial Ecosystem) [95]. In particular, TIM and SHIME would be of high interest to (i) assess how the modalities of ingestion (e.g., infectious dose, growth phase, and food vehicle) and age conditions (adult, infant, and elderly) may influence pathogen survival and virulence in the human GI tract, (ii) investigate how ETEC and EHEC interact with luminal and mucosal gut microbiota under physiological fluid shear stresses and microaerobic conditions, and (iii) study host-microbiota-pathogen interactions by using intestinal cells in culture coupled with TIM or SHIME models, like in the HMI (host microbe interactions) module [96]. For an in-depth understanding of pathogen behavior in the human GI tract, these models should be used in combination with new technologies such as -omics or quantitative imaging technologies.

Author details

Charlène Roussel[1,2†], Charlotte Cordonnier[1,3†], Valérie Livrelli[3,4], Tom Van de Wiele[2] and Stéphanie Blanquet-Diot[1*]

*Address all correspondence to: stephanie.blanquet@udamail.fr

1 CIDAM, Conception, Engineering and Development of Food and Drug, Faculty of Pharmacy, University of Auvergne, Clermont-Ferrand, France

2 Cmet, Center for Microbial Ecology and Technology, Faculty of Bioscience Engineering, Ghent University, Ghent, Belgium

3 M2iSH, Microbes, Intestine, Inflammation and Host Susceptibility, UMR INSERM/University of Auvergne, Faculty of Pharmacy, University of Auvergne, Clermont-Ferrand, France

4 Bacteriology Department, CHU Clermont-Ferrand, France

† Co-first authors

References

[1] Clements A, Young JC, Constantinou N, Frankel G. Infection strategies of enteric pathogenic Escherichia coli. Gut Microbes. 2012;**3**(2):71-87. DOI: 10.4161/gmic.19182

[2] Qadri F, Svennerholm A-M, Faruque ASG, Sack RB. Enterotoxigenic Escherichia coli in developing countries: Epidemiology, microbiology, clinical features, treatment, and prevention. Clinical Microbiology Reviews. 2005;**18**(3):465-483. DOI: 10.1128/CMR.18.3.465-483.2005

[3] Majowicz SE, Scallan E, Jones-Bitton A, Sargeant JM, Stapleton J, Angulo FJ, Yeung DH, Kirk MD. Global incidence of human Shiga toxin–producing Escherichia coli infections and deaths: A systematic review and knowledge synthesis. Foodborne Pathogens and Disease. 2014;**11**(6):447-455. DOI: 10.1089/fpd.2013.1704

[4] Liu LJH, Johnson HL, Cousens S, Perin J, Scott S, Lawn JE, et al. Child Health Epidemiology Reference Group of WHO and UNICEF. Global, regional, and national causes of child mortality: An updated systematic analysis for 2010 with time trends since 2000. Lancet. 2012;**379**:2151-2161. DOI: 10.1016/S0140-6736(12)60560-1

[5] Boschi-Pinto C, Velebit L, Shibuya K. Estimating child mortality due to diarrhea in developing countries. Bulletin of the World Health Organization. 2008;**86**:710-717

[6] Iseri L, Zafer Apan T, Aksoy A, Koç F, Sedef Göçmen J, Nuristani D. The prevalence of enterotoxigenic E. coli isolated from the stools of children aged 0-10 years with diarrhea in mid-anatolia region, Turkey. Brazilian Journal of Microbiology. 2011;**42**(1):243-247. DOI: 10.1590/S1517-83822011000100030

[7] Gupta SK, Keck J, Ram PK, Crump JA, Miller MA, Mintz ED. Part III. Analysis of data gaps pertaining to enterotoxigenic Escherichia coli infections in low and medium human development index countries, 1984-2005. Epidemiological Infections. 2008;**136**(6):721-738. DOI: 10.1017/S095026880700934X

[8] Caprioli A, Gaia S, Morabito S. Public health microbiology of Shiga toxin-producing Escherichia coli. Microbiology Spectrum. 2014;**2**(6). DOI: 10.1128/microbiolspec.EHEC-0014-2013

[9] Gyles CL. Shiga toxin-producing Escherichia coli: An overview. Journal of Animal Sciences. 2007;**82**(13 suppl):E45-62. DOI: 10.2527/jas.2006-508

[10] Levine MM, Nalin DR, Hoover DL, Bergquist EJ, Hornick RB, Young CR. Immunity to enterotoxigenic Escherichia coli. Infections and Immunity. 1979;**23**(3):729-736

[11] Smith JL, Fratamico PM, Gunther NWT. Shiga-toxin-producing Escherichia coli. Advances in Applied Microbiology. 2014;**86**:145-197. DOI: 10.1016/B978-0-12-800262-9.00003-2

[12] Bryan A, Youngster I, McAdam AJ. Shiga toxin producing Escherichia coli. Clinical Laboratory Medicine. 2015;**35**(2):247-272. DOI: 10.1016/j.cll.2015.02.004

[13] Goldwater PN, Bettelheim KA. Treatment of enterohemorrhagic Escherichia coli (EHEC) infection and hemolytic uremic syndrome (HUS). BMC Medicine. 2012;**10**(12). DOI: 10.1186/1741-7015-10-12

[14] Agger M, Scheutz F, Villumsen S, Mølbak K, Petersen AM. Antibiotic treatment of verocytotoxin-producing *Escherichia coli* (VTEC) infection: A systematic review and a proposal. Journal of Antimicrobiology and Chemotherapy. 2015;**70**(9):2440-2446. DOI: 10.1093/jac/dkv162

[15] CDC [internet]. 2014. Available from: http://www.cdc.gov/ecoli/etec.html [accessed: 2016-08-26]

[16] Ahmed T, Bhuiyan TR, Zaman K, Sinclair D, Qadri F. Vaccines for preventing enterotoxigenic Escherichia coli (ETEC) diarrhoea. Cochrane Database Systemic Review. 2013;**7**:CD009029. DOI: 10.1002/14651858.CD009029.pub2

[17] Garcia-Angulo VA, Kalita A, Torres AG. Advances in the development of enterohemorrhagic Escherichia coli vaccines using murine models of infection. Vaccine. 2013;**31**(32):3229-3235. DOI: 10.1016/j.vaccine.2013.05.013

[18] Roussel C, Sivignon A, Van de Wiele T, Blanquet-Diot S. Foodborne enterotoxigenic *Escherichia coli*: From gut pathogenesis to new preventive strategies involving probiotics. Future Microbiology. 2017;12:73-93. DOI: 10.2217/fmb-2016-0101.

[19] Sheikh A, Shamsuzzaman S, Ahmad SM et al. Zinc influences innate immune responses in children with enterotoxigenic Escherichia coli-induced diarrhea. Journal of Nutrition. 2010;**140**(5):1049-1056. DOI: 10.3945/jn.109.111492

[20] Cordonnier C, Thévenot J, Etienne-Mesmin L, Alric M, Livrelli V, Blanquet-Diot S. Probiotic and enterohemorrhagic Escherichia coli: An effective strategy against a deadly enemy? Critical Reviews in Microbiology. DOI: 10.1080/1040841X.2016.1185602

[21] Connolly JP, Finlay BB, Roe AJ. From ingestion to colonization: The influence of the host environment on regulation of the LEE encoded type III secretion system in enterohaemorrhagic Escherichia coli. Frontiers in Microbiology. 2015;**5**(6):568. DOI: 10.3389/fmicb.2015.00568

[22] Lapeyraque AL, Malina M, Fremeaux-Bacchi V, Boppel T, Kirschfink M, Oualha M, Proulx F, et al. Eculizumab in severe Shiga-toxin-associated HUS. New England Journal of Medicine. 2011;**364**(26):2561-2563. DOI:10.1056/NEJMc1100859

[23] Stintzing G, Möllby R. Colonization of the upper jejunum by enteropathogenic and enterotoxigenic Escherichia coli in paediatric diarrhoea. Acta Paediatrica Scandinavia. 1982;**71**(3):457-465

[24] Allen KP, Randolph MM, Fleckenstein JM. Importance of heat-labile enterotoxin in colonization of the adult mouse small intestine by human enterotoxigenic Escherichia coli strains. Infections and Immunity. 2006;**74**(2):869-875. DOI: 10.1128/IAI.74.2.869-875.2006

[25] Phillips AD, Navabpour S, Hicks S, Dougan G, Wallis T, Frankel G. Enterohaemorrhagic Escherichia coli O157:H7 target Peyer's patches in humans and cause attaching/effacing lesions in both human and bovine intestine. Gut. 2000;**47**(3):377-381. DOI: 10.1136/gut.47.3.377

[26] Chong Y, Fitzhenry R, Heuschkel R, Torrente F, Frankel G, Phillips AD. Human intestinal tissue tropism in Escherichia coli O157: H7-initial colonization of terminal ileum and Peyer's patches and minimal colonic adhesion ex vivo. Microbiology. 2007;**153**(3):794-802. DOI: 10.1099/mic.0.2006/003178-0

[27] Lewis SB, Cook V, Tighe R, Schüller S. Enterohemorrhagic Escherichia coli colonization of human colonic epithelium in vitro and ex vivo. Infections and Immunity. 2015;**83**(3):942-949. DOI: 10.1128/IAI.02928-14

[28] Etienne-Mesmin L, Chassaing B, Sauvanet P, Denizot J, Blanquet-Diot S, Darfeuille-Michaud A, et al. Interactions with M cells and macrophages as key steps in the pathogenesis of enterohemorrhagic Escherichia coli infections. PLoS One. 2011;**6**(8):e23594. DOI: 10.1371/journal.pone.0023594

[29] Zhao B, Houry WA. Acid stress response in enteropathogenic gammaproteobacteria: An aptitude for survival. Biochemistry and Cell Biology. 2010;**88**(2):301-314. DOI: 10.1139/O09-182

[30] Fleckenstein JM, Hardwidge PR, Munson GP, Rasko DA, Sommerfelt H, Steinsland H. Molecular mechanisms of enterotoxigenic Escherichia coli infection. Microbes and Infection. 2010;**12**(2):89-98. DOI: 10.1016/j.micinf.2009.10.002

[31] Stevens MP, Frankel GM. The locus of enterocyte effacement and associated virulence factors of enterohemorrhagic Escherichia coli. Microbiology Spectrum. 2014;**2**(4):EHEC-0007-2013. DOI: 10.1128/microbiolspec.EHEC-0007-2013

[32] Mcwilliams BD, Torres AG. Enterohemorrhagic Escherichia coli adhesins. Microbiology Spectrum. 2014;**2**(3). DOI: 10.1128/microbiolspec.EHEC-0003-2013

[33] Barnett Foster D. Modulation of the enterohemorrhagic E. coli virulence program through the human gastrointestinal tract. Virulence. 2013;**4**(4):315-323. DOI: 10.4161/viru.24318

[34] Luo Q, Kumar P, Vickers TJ, Sheikh A, Lewis WG, Rasko DA, et al. Enterotoxigenic Escherichia coli secretes a highly conserved mucin-degrading metalloprotease to effectively engage intestinal epithelial cells. Infections and Immunity. 2014;**82**(2):509-521. DOI: 10.1128/IAI.01106-13

[35] Kumar P, Luo Q, Vickers TJ, Sheikh A, Lewis WG, Fleckenstein JM. EatA, an immunogenic protective antigen of enterotoxigenic Escherichia coli, degrades intestinal mucin. Infections and Immunity. 2014;**82**(2):500-508. DOI: 10.1128/IAI.01078-13

[36] Yu AC, Worrall LJ, Strynadka NC. Structural insight into the bacterial mucinase StcE essential to adhesion and immune evasion during enterohemorrhagic E. coli infection. Structure. 2012;**20**(4):707-717. DOI: 10.1016/j.str.2012.02.015

[37] Dubreuil JD. The whole Shebang: The gastrointestinal tract, Escherichia coli enterotoxins and secretion. Current Issues in Molecular Biology. 2012;**14**(2):71-82

[38] Schüller S. Shiga toxin interaction with human intestinal epithelium. Toxins. 2011;**3**(6):626-639. DOI: 10.3390/toxins3060626

[39] Siegler RL, Obrig TG, Pysher TJ, Tesh VL, Denkers ND, Taylor FB. Response to Shiga toxin 1 and 2 in a baboon model of hemolytic uremic syndrome. Pediatric Nephrology. 2007;**18**(2):92-96. DOI: 10.1007/s00467-002-1035-7

[40] Bergan J, Lingelem ABD, Simm R, Skotland T, Sandvig K. Shiga toxins. Toxicon. 2012;**60**(6):1085-1107. DOI: 10.1016/j.toxicon.2012.07.016

[41] Masters CI, Shallcross JA, Mackey BM. Effect of stress treatments on the detection of Listeria monocytogenes and enterotoxigenic Escherichia coli by the polymerase chain reaction. Journal of Applied Bacteriology. 1994;**77**(1): 73-79

[42] Gonzales L, Ali ZB, Nygren E, et al. Alkaline pH is a signal for optimal production and secretion of the heat labile toxin, LT in enterotoxigenic Escherichia coli (ETEC). PLoS One. 2013;**8**(9):e74069. DOI: 10.1371/journal.pone.0074069

[43] Sahl JW, Rasko DA. Analysis of global transcriptional profiles of enterotoxigenic Escherichia coli isolate E24377A. Infections and Immunity. 2012;**80**(3):1232-1242. DOI: 10.1128/IAI.06138-11

[44] Tamplin ML. Inactivation of Escherichia coli O157:H7 in simulated human gastric fluid. Applied Environmental Microbiology. 2005;**71**(1):20-25. DOI: 10.1128/AEM.71.1.320-325.2005

[45] Bergholz TM, Whittam TS. Variation in acid resistance among enterohaemorrhagic Escherichia coli in a simulated gastric environment. Journal of Applied Microbiology. 2007;**102**(2):352-362. DOI: 10.1111/j.1365-2672.2006.03099.x

[46] Takumi K, de Jonge R, Havelaar A. Modelling inactivation of Escherichia coli by low pH: Application to passage through the stomach of young and elderly people. Journal of Applied Microbiology. 2000;**89**(6):935-943.

[47] Etienne-Mesmin L, Livrelli V, Privat M, Denis S, Cardot JM, Alric M, Blanquet-Diot S. Effect of a new probiotic Saccharomyces cerevisiae strain on survival of Escherichia coli O157:H7 in a dynamic gastrointestinal model. Applied Environmental Microbiology. 2011;**77**(3):1127-1131. DOI: 10.1128/AEM.02130-10

[48] Miszczycha SD, Thévenot J, Denis S, Callon C, Livrelli V, Alric M, Montel MC, Blanquet-Diot S, Thevenot-Sergentet D. Survival of Escherichia coli O26:H11 exceeds that of Escherichia coli O157:H7 as assessed by simulated human digestion of contaminated raw milk cheeses. International Journal of Food Microbiology. 2014;**172**:40-48. DOI: 10.1016/j.ijfoodmicro.2013.11.029

[49] Roussel C, Cordonnier C, Galia W, Le Goff O, Thévenot J, Chalancon S et al. Increased EHEC survival and virulence gene expression indicate an enhanced pathogenicity upon simulated pediatric gastrointestinal conditions. Pediatric Research. 2016;**80**(5):734-743. DOI: 10.1038/pr.2016.144

[50] Thévenot J, Cordonnier C, Rougeron A, Le Goff O, Nguyen HTT, Denis S et al. Enterohemorrhagic Escherichia coli infection has donor-dependent effect on human gut

microbiota and may be antagonized by probiotic yeast during interaction with Peyer's patches. Applied Microbiology and Biotechnology. 2015;**99**(21):9097-9110. DOI: 10.1007/s00253-015-6704-0

[51] Nakanishi N, Tashiro K, Kuhara S, Hayashi T, Sugimoto N, Tobe T. Regulation of virulence by butyrate sensing in enterohaemorrhagic Escherichia coli. Microbiology. 2009;**155**(2): 521-530. DOI: 10.1099/mic.0.023499-0

[52] Tobe T, Nakanishi N, Sugimoto N. Activation of motility by sensing short-chain fatty acids via two steps in a flagellar gene regulatory cascade in enterohemorrhagic Escherichia coli. Infections and Immunity. 2011;**79**(3):1016-24. DOI: 10.1128/IAI.00927-10

[53] Gonzales-Siles L, Sjöling A. The different ecological niches of enterotoxigenic Escherichia coli. Environmental Microbiology. 2016;**18**:741-751. DOI: 10.1111/1462-2920.13106

[54] Johnson WM, Lior H, Johnson KG. Heat-stable enterotoxin from Escherichia coli: factors involved in growth and toxin production. Infections and Immunity. 1978;**20**(2):352-359

[55] Kunkel SL, Robertson DC. Factors affecting release of heat-labile enterotoxin by enterotoxigenic Escherichia coli. Infections and Immunity. 1979;**23**(3):652-659

[56] Hegde A, Bhat KG, Mallya S. Effect of stress on production of heat-labile enterotoxin by Escherichia coli. Indian Journal of Medical Microbiology. 2009;**27**:325-328. DOI: 10.4103/0255-0857.55446

[57] House B, Kus JV, Prayitno N, Mair R, Que L, Chingcuanco F, Gannon V, Cvitkovitch DG, Barnett Foster D. Acid-stress-induced changes in enterohaemorrhagic Escherichia coli O157:H7 virulence. Microbiology. 2009;**155**(9):2907-2918. DOI: 10.1099/mic.0.025171-0

[58] Yuk HG, Marshall DL. Adaptation of Escherichia coli O157:H7 to pH alters membrane lipid composition, verotoxin secretion, and resistance to simulated gastric fluid acid. Applied Environmental Microbiology. 2004;70(6):3500-3505. DOI: 10.1128/AEM.70.6.3500-3505.2004

[59] Huang YJ, Tsai TY, Pan TM. Physiological response and protein expression under acid stress of Escherichia coli O157:H7 TWC01 isolated from Taiwan. Journal of Agricultural and Food Chemistry. 2007;**55**(17):7182-7191. DOI: 10.1021/jf071014s

[60] Chatterjee A, Chowdhury R. Bile and unsaturated fatty acids inhibit the binding of cholera toxin and Escherichia coli heat-labile enterotoxin to GM1 receptor. Antimicrobial Agents and Chemotherapy. 2008;**52**(1):220-224. DOI: 10.1128/AAC.01009-07

[61] Nicklasson M, Sjöling Å, Von Mentzer A, Qadri F, Svennerholm AM. Expression of colonization factor CS5 of enterotoxigenic Escherichia coli (ETEC) is enhanced in vivo and by the bile component Na glycocholate hydrate. PLoS One. 2012;**7**(4):e35827. DOI: 10.1371/journal.pone.0035827

[62] Haines S, Gautheron S, Nasser W, Renauld-Mongénie G. Identification of novel components influencing colonization factor antigen I expression in enterotoxigenic Escherichia coli. PLoS One. 2015;**10**(10):e0141469. DOI: 10.1371/journal.pone.0141469

[63] Sjoling A, Wiklund G, Savarino SJ, Cohen DI, Svennerholm AM. Comparative analyses of phenotypic and genotypic methods for detection of enterotoxigenic Escherichia coli toxins and colonization factors. Journal of Clinical Microbiology. 2007;**45**(10):3295-3301. DOI: 10.1128/JCM.00471-07

[64] Grewal HMS, Valvatne H, Bhan MK, Van Dijk L, Gaastra W, Sommerfelt H. A new putative fimbrial colonization factor, CS19, of human enterotoxigenic Escherichia coli. Infections and Immunity. 1997;**65**(2):507-513

[65] Kus JV, Gebremedhin A, Dang V, Tran SL, Serbanescu A, Barnett Foster D. Bile salts induce resistance to polymyxin in enterohemorrhagic Escherichia coli O157:H7. Journal of Bacteriology. 2011;**193**(17):4509-4515. DOI: 10.1128/JB.00200-11

[66] Yin X, Zhu J, Feng Y, Chambers JR, Gong J, Gyles CL. Differential gene expression and adherence of Escherichia coli O157:H7 in vitro and in ligated pig intestines. PLoS One. 2011;**6**(2):e17424. DOI: 10.1371/journal.pone.0017424 DOI:10.1371%2Fjournal.pone.0017424#pmc_ext

[67] Hamner S, McInnerney K, Williamson K, Franklin MJ, Ford TE. Bile salts affect expression of Escherichia coli O157:H7 genes for virulence and iron acquisition, and promote growth under iron limiting conditions. PLoS One. 2013;**8**(9):e74647. DOI: 10.1371/journal.pone.0074647

[68] Arenas-Hernández MMP, Rojas-López M, Medrano-López A, Nuñez-Reza KJ, Puente JL, Martínez-Laguna Y. Environmental regulation of the long polar fimbriae 2 of enterohemorrhagic Escherichia coli O157:H7. FEMS Microbiology Letters. 2014;**357**(2):105-114. DOI: 10.1111/1574-6968.12513

[69] Rappaport RS, Sagin JF, Pierzchala WA, Bonde G, Rubin BA, Tint H. Activation of heat-labile Escherichia coli enterotoxin by trypsin. The Journal of Infectious Diseases. 1976;**133**(Suppl):41-54

[70] James BW, Keevil CW. Influence of oxygen availability on physiology, verocytotoxin expression and adherence of Escherichia coli O157. Journal of Applied Microbiology. 1999;**86**(1):117-124

[71] Tran SL, Billoud L, Lewis SB, Phillips AD, Schüller S. Shiga toxin production and translocation during microaerobic human colonic infection with Shiga toxin-producing E. coli O157:H7 and O104:H4. Cell Microbiology. 2014;**16**(8):1255-1266. DOI: 10.1111/cmi.12281

[72] Tchesnokova V, McVeigh AL, Kidd B, Yakovenko O, Thomas WE, Sokurenko EV, Savarino SJ. Shear-enhanced binding of intestinal colonization factor antigen I of enterotoxigenic Escherichia coli. Molecular Microbiology. 2010;**76**(2):489-502. DOI: 10.1111/j.1365-2958.2010.07116.x

[73] Alsharif G, Ahmad S, Islam MdS, Shah R, Busby SJ Krachler AM. Host attachment and fluid shear are integrated into a mechanical signal regulating virulence in Escherichia coli O157:H7. Proceedings of the National Academy of Sciences of the United States of America. 2015;**112**(17):5503-5508. DOI: 10.1073/pnas.1422986112

[74] David LA, Weil A, Ryan ET et al. Gut microbial succession follows acute secretory diarrhea in humans. MBio. 2015; **6**(3):e00381-00315. DOI: 10.1128/mBio.00381-15

[75] Pop M, Paulson JN, Chakraborty S, Astrovskaya I, Lindsay BR, Li S et al. Individual-specific changes in the human gut microbiota after challenge with enterotoxigenic Escherichia coli and subsequent ciprofloxacin treatment. BMC Genomics. 2016;**17**:440. DOI: 10.1186/s12864-016-2777-0

[76] Baumler J, Sperandio V. Interactions between the microbiota and pathogenic bacteria in the gut. Nature. 2016;**535**:85-93. DOI: 10.1038/nature18849

[77] de Sablet T, Chassard C, Bernalier-Donadille A, Vareille M, Gobert AP, Martin C. Human microbiota-secreted factors inhibit Shiga toxin synthesis by enterohemorrhagic Escherichia coli O157:H7. Infections and Immunity. 2013;**77**(2):783-790. DOI : 10.1128/IAI.01048-08

[78] Cordonnier C, Le Bihan G, Emond-Rheault JG, Garrivier A, Harel J, Jubelin G. Vitamin B12 uptake by the gut commensal bacteria bacteroides thetaiotaomicron limits the production of Shiga toxin by enterohemorrhagic Escherichia coli. Toxins. 2016;**8**(1). DOI: 10.3390/toxins8010014

[79] Njoroge JW, Nguyen Y, Curtis MM, Moreira CG, Sperandio V. Virulence meets metabolism: Cra and KdpE gene regulation in enterohemorrhagic Escherichia coli. MBio. 2012;3(5):e00280-12. DOI: 10.1128/mBio.00280-12

[80] Pacheco AR, Curtis MM, Ritchie JM, Munera D, Waldor MK, Moreira CG et al. Fucose sensing regulates bacterial intestinal colonization. Nature. 2012;**492**(7427):113-117. DOI: 10.1038/nature11623

[81] Takashi K, Fujita I, Kobari K. Effects of short chain fatty acids on the production of heat-labile enterotoxin from enterotoxigenic Escherichia coli. The Japanese Journal of Pharmacology. 1989;**50**(4):495-498

[82] Fukuda S, Toh H, Hase K, Oshima K, Nakanishi Y, Yoshimura K, et al. Bifidobacteria can protect from enteropathogenic infection through production of acetate. Nature. 2011;**469**(7331):543-547. DOI: 10.1038/nature09646

[83] Takao M, Yen H, Tobe T. LeuO enhances butyrate-induced virulence expression through a positive regulatory loop in enterohaemorrhagic Escherichia coli. Molecular Microbiology. 2014;**93**(6):1302-1313. DOI: 10.1111/mmi 12737

[84] Herold S, Paton JC, Srimanote P, Paton AW. Differential effects of short-chain fatty acids and iron on expression of Iha in Shiga-toxigenic Escherichia coli. Microbiology. 2009;**155**(11): 3554-3563. DOI: 10.1099/mic.0.029454-0

[85] Lackraj T, Kim JI, Tran SLL, Barnett Foster D. Differential modulation of flagella expression in enterohemorrhagic Escherichia coli O157:H7 by intestinal short chain fatty acid mixes. Microbiology. 2016;**162**(10):1761-1772. DOI: 10.1099/mic.0.000357

[86] Zumbrun SD, Melton-Celsa AR, Smith MA, Gilbreath JJ, Merrell DS, O' Brien AD. Dietary choice affects Shiga toxin-producing Escherichia coli (STEC) O157:H7 colonization and

disease. Proceedings of the National Academy of Sciences of the United States of America. 2013;**110**:E2126–E2133. DOI: 10.1073/pnas.1222014110

[87] Lyte M, Erickson AK, Arulanandam BP, Frank CD, Crawford MA, Francis DH. Norepinephrine-induces expression of the K99 pilus adhesion of enterotoxigenic Escherichia coli. Biochemical and Biophysical Research Communications. 1997;**323**:682-686. DOI : 10.1006/bbrc.1997.6356

[88] Sturbelle RT, de Avila LF da C, Roos TB, Borchardt JL, da Conceição R de C dos S, Dellagostin OA, et al. The role of quorum sensing in Escherichia coli (ETEC) virulence factors. Veterinary Microbiology. 2015;**180**(3-4):245-252. DOI: 10.1016/j.vetmic.2015.08.015

[89] Lyte M, Arulanandam B, Nguyen K, Frank C, Erickson A, Francis D. Norepinephrine induced growth and expression of virulence associated factors in enterotoxigenic and enterohemorrhagic strains of Escherichia coli. Advances in Experimental Medicine and Biology. 1997;**412**:331-339

[90] Njoroge J, Sperandio V. Enterohemorrhagic Escherichia coli virulence regulation by two bacterial adrenergic kinases, QseC and QseE. Infections and Immunity. 2012;**80**(2):688-703. DOI: 10.1128/IAI.05921-11

[91] Kendall MM, Gruber CC, Parker CT, Sperandio V. Ethanolamine controls expression of genes encoding components involved in interkingdom signaling and virulence in enterohemorrhagic Escherichia coli O157:H7. MBio. 2012;**3**(3). DOI: 10.1128/mBio.00050-12

[92] Vareille M, de Sablet T, Hindré t, Martin C, Gobert AP. Nitric oxide inhibits Shiga-toxin synthesis by enterohemorrhagic Escherichia coli. Proceedings of the National Academy of Sciences of the United States of America. 2007;**104**(24):10199-10204. DOI: 10.1073/pnas.0702589104

[93] Branchu P, Matrat S, Vareille M, Garrivier A, Durand A, Crépin S, Harel J, Jubelin G, Gobert AP. NsrR, GadE, and GadX interplay in repressing expression of the Escherichia coli O157:H7 LEE pathogenicity island in response to nitric oxide. PLoS Pathogens. 2014;**10**(1):e1003874. DOI: 10.1371/journal.ppat.1003874

[94] Ritchie JM. Animal models of enterohemorrhagic Escherichia coli infection. Microbiology Spectrum. 2014;**2**(4):EHEC-0022-2013. DOI: 10.1128/microbiolspec.EHEC-0022-2013.

[95] Van den Abeele P, Roos S, Eeckhaut V, MacKenzie DA, Derde M, Verstraete W, et al. Incorporating a mucosal environment in a dynamic gut model results in a more representative colonization by lactobacilli. Microbial Biotechnology. 2012;**5**(1):106-115. DOI: 10.1111/j.1751-7915.2011.00308.x

[96] Marzorati M, Vanhoecke B, De Ryck T, Sadaghian Sadabad M, Pinheiro I, Possemiers S, et al. The HMI™ module: A new tool to study the host-microbiota interaction in the human gastrointestinal tract in vitro. BMC Microbiology. 2014;**14**:133. DOI: 10.1186/1471-2180-14-13

Chapter 2

Virulence Factors and Innovative Strategies for the Treatment and Control of Uropathogenic *Escherichia coli*

Barbara Kot

Additional information is available at the end of the chapter

http://dx.doi.org/10.5772/67778

Abstract

Urinary tract infections (UTIs) are considered to be the most frequent bacterial infections. *Escherichia coli* is the major factor of community-acquired UTI (80–90%) and a large part of nosocomial UTI (30%), including cystitis, pyelonephritis, prostatitis, and asymptomatic bacteriuria. Uropathogenic *E. coli* (UPEC) shows a variety of virulence factors that allow their transition from the intestinal tract to the urinary tract and causing infection. The virulence factors responsible for pathogenesis outside the gastrointestinal tract belong to various functional groups. Antimicrobial resistance among *E. coli* causing UTIs is increasing in many countries around the world. This paper presents key virulence factors of UPEC such as adhesins, toxins, iron acquisition systems, and biofilm formation by UPEC, which are major problems in patients with long-term catheterization. The resistance of UPEC to antibiotics and innovative strategies of treatment and control of UPEC including drug therapy, preventive vaccines, probiotics, cranberry as source of antimicrobial metabolites, bacteriophages, new therapeutic antibiofilm treatment such as engineered phages, nanoparticles, and plant-derived antibacterial agents are also presented.

Keywords: UPEC, UTI, virulence factors, biofilm, antimicrobial resistance, treatment of UPEC, prevention

1. Introduction

Urinary tract infections (UTIs) are considered the most frequent bacterial infections in humans usually caused by *Enterobacteriaceae*. Among them, *Escherichia coli* is a predominant etiological factor of UTI [1]. The pathogenic *E. coli* strains belong to different pathotypes including enteric *E. coli* and extraintestinal *E. coli* (ExPEC). Seven major pathotypes of enteric *E. coli* cause mainly gastroenteritis but sometimes are responsible for diseases outside the intestinal tract [2]. Three pathotypes of the ExPEC are able to exist in the gut but do not cause diseases in this place. Whereas, colonization by the ExPEC strains of other host niches including the central nervous system, blood, and the urinary tract leads to illness in human [3]. Among ExPEC, uropathogenic *E. coli* (UPEC) is the most frequently associated with human diseases. UPEC strains cause 80–90% of community-acquired UTIs and more than 30% of hospital-acquired UTIs [4]. Development of UTIs depends on anatomical factors of host, defense mechanisms, and virulence factors of infecting microorganism. Bacterial infections of the urinary tract are important problem, because about 60% of women in the United States will have at least one UTI during their life. About 8 million physician visits per year are related to these often chronic infections, making UTIs a problem of economic and medical significance [5]. UPEC can colonize the bladder and cause cystitis or may ascend into the kidneys, causing pyelonephritis [3]. *E. coli* may also spread from the urinary tract to the bloodstream causing bacteremia in above 30% of cases and the potential sepsis [6]. The presence of high numbers of *E. coli* in the urine without the clinical symptoms is referred as asymptomatic bacteriuria (ABU) and such infection in healthy, nonpregnant women is generally not treated [7]. Infections of the urinary tract occur when *E. coli* enter through the urethra and effectively colonize the bladder. *E. coli* is the most common pathogen causing cystitis, pyelonephritis with the possibility of causing kidney damage and death. This microorganism can induce acute renal failure and in case of complications after renal transplantation, *E. coli* is the most common clinical isolate [8]. It is considered that human intestinal tract is a primary reservoir of UPEC strains, although in some cases, clonal group of UPEC strains can be transmitted by contaminated food [9]. Host inflammatory responses on the breach of the sterile urinary tract by UPEC consist of the production of cytokines and chemokines, neutrophil influx, the exfoliation of infected bladder epithelial cells, and the generation of reactive nitrogen and oxygen species [5]. Genomic differences among UPEC and other *E. coli* show evolutionary adaptations, which enable UPEC to colonize environmental niches within the urinary tract such as epithelia lining the lumenal walls of the urethra, bladder, renal pelvis, and collecting ducts of the kidneys [10].

UPEC strains have different virulence factors that enable the bacteria to adhere and colonize the uroepithelial cells and to establish the UTIs. UPEC harbor more genes encoding adhesins, iron acquisition systems, and toxins than K12 strains and commensal *E. coli* isolates. These virulence genes are often encoded on mobile genetic elements called pathogenicity islands [11, 12].

This paper describes key virulence factors of UPEC, the role of biofilm formation by UPEC in development of UTIs and in catheter-associated UTIs. The resistance to antibiotics and new therapeutic approaches of treatment and control of UPEC will be also discussed.

2. Virulence factors of UPEC

2.1. Adhesins

Adhesive proteins as the most important determinants of pathogenicity of UPEC strains are arguable [13], but based on many observations of ABU strains, it was found that these strains are nonadherent and nonhemolytic [14]. UPEC adhesins activate host signaling

http://dx.doi.org/10.5772/67778

pathways that promote bacterial invasion [15]. Bacterial adherence to urothelium is important in the development of UTI because it allows the bacteria to persist in the urinary tract against flushing by urine flow. Function of type 1 fimbriae as virulence factors in human pathology remains unclear because they are expressed in both commensal and pathogenic *E. coli* strains [16, 17]. The type 1 fimbriae are heteropolymeric surface organelles that consist of several subunits. These fimbriae bind *E. coli* cells to the urothelial mannosylated glycoproteins uroplakin by subunit FimH, which is located at the distal tip of the type 1 fimbriae. UPEC commonly expresses FimH that efficiently bind monomannose- and trimannose-containing glycoprotein receptors. Whereas, commensal *E. coli* strains usually bind to trimannose residues [18]. Binding of FimH to uroplakins that are expressed in the differentiated urothelium of the bladder and urethers causes adhesion and cellular invasion of *E. coli* and promotes formation of intracellular bacterial communities which leads to the acute stage of infection [19, 20]. FimH adhesin enables UPEC to escape before the immune response by internalization within urothelial cells. Inside infected urothelial cells, *E. coli* is harbored within vesicles [21, 22]. Blocking of FimH adhesin with antibodies or inactivity of the *fimH* gene has a negative effect on the ability of UPEC to colonize the bladder epithelium [5]. *fimH* gene is the most commonly identified virulence gene in the isolates causing UTI [17].

About 80% of UPECs express P fimbriae that are frequently associated with acute pyelonephritis [23]. P fimbriae are encoded by *pap*A-K gene operon which can be localized on one or more pathogenic-associated islands [24]. The P-fimbrial–tip adhesins (PapG adhesins) bind to Gal α (1–4) Gal in glycosphingolipids of the membrane of urothelial cells localized in the kidney. The PapG adhesins are encoded by four classes of *papG* genes but only two of them are associated with uropathogenicity. Class II adhesin genes are predominant among the isolates from pyelonephritis and from renal transplant patients, while class III genes are found more frequently among cystitis isolates [25–27]. Attachment of P fimbriae to receptors leads to activation of the immune cell response and to the development of inflammation- and pain-associated with UTIs. P fimbriae improve bacterial colonization of the tubular epithelium that can adversely affect renal filtration leading to total obstruction of the nephron and consequently contributes to the full pathophysiology of pyelonephritis [14].

S fimbriae of *E. coli* bind to sialyl galactosides occurring in the receptors of erythrocytes and renal tubular epithelium cells, and are also involved in UTIs development. S fimbriae show binding to epithelial cells of lower urinary tract and kidney and may facilitate bacterial dissemination within host tissues [15, 28].

E. coli strains harboring operons coding fimbrial Dr and afimbrial Afa adhesins are also associated with UTIs. Dr adhesins bind to decay-accelerating factor (DAF) which is widely distributed along the urinary tract and plays an important role in colonization of urinary tract by Dr adhesin-producing *E. coli* [29]. UPECs with Afa adhesins have a tropism to renal tissue and have the ability to induce chronic or recurrent infection [30]. The research recently conducted by Muenzner et al. [31] showed that uropathogenic *E. coli* strains, which express the Dra/AfaE adhesins, bind to CEACAMs (carcinoembryonic antigen-related cell adhesin molecules) present on epithelial cells. The interaction of CEACAMs with Dra/AfaE adhesins causes increase of integrin activity, promote matrix adhesion, and suppress epithelial exfoliation, which promotes host infection.

Curli are highly adhesive extracellular amyloid fibers produced by UPEC and other *Enterobacteriaceae* [32]. The major subunit of curli is the CsgA [33]. Curli promote adherence to epithelial cells and resistance against the human antimicrobial peptide LL-37, and also cause induction of the proinflammatory cytokine IL-8. They exhibit exclusive role in promoting UPEC biofilms and represent one of the major biofilm components [34]. Curli are produced at limitation of nutrients and salts, at reduced oxygen tension and at temperature below 30°C. However, it is believed that many pathogenic bacteria and commensal strains can also express curli at 37°C during infection in humans [35]. Curli fimbriae interact with serum proteins and this might promote bacterial dissemination in host. UPEC strains-producing curli are more likely to cause urosepticaemia than strains which do not produce curli [36].

2.2. Toxins

Production of toxins by UPEC is an important virulence factor because they may induce an inflammatory response and lead to symptoms of urinary tract infections. The most important virulence factor of UPEC is α-hemolysin (HlyA). This toxin is strongly proinflammatory and leads to secretion of IL-6, IL-8, and chemotaxins that increase clinical severity in UTI patients [27, 37]. HlyA belongs to the family of RTX (repeats in toxin) [38]. HlyA is a lipoprotein of 110 kDa that forms pores in host cells, leading at high concentrations of HlyA to cell lysis, that enable UPEC to defeat mucosal barriers, damage effector immune cells, and gain access to nutrients and iron [39]. At sublytic concentrations, HlyA implicates the inhibition of chemotaxis and bacterial killing by phagocytes and induces apoptosis of neutrophils and renal cells, and also promotes the exfoliation of bladder epithelial cells [40]. Hilbert et al. [41] found that cytotoxicity, cytokine suppression, and HlyA production were tightly linked in clinical strains, and that *E. coli* utilizes HlyA to inhibit epithelial cytokine production *in vitro*. HlyA is responsible for about 50% of UTIs cases which leads to renal complications [27].

Cytotoxic necrotizing factor 1 (CNF1) is produced by approximately one third of UPEC [14]. The toxicity of this protein is linked with its ability to constitutive activation of the Rho GTPases that affect numerous cellular functions such as the formation of actin stress fibers and membrane ruffle formation. The result is the entry of *E. coli* into urothelial cells [42]. CNF1 promote apoptosis of bladder epithelial cells, probably stimulating their exfoliation and increasing bacterial entry to underlying tissue [43]. Besides, CNF1 inhibits activities of neutrophils, reducing phagocytosis and antimicrobial activity [44].

Secreted autotransporter toxin (Sat) is referred to as serine protease autotransporter and is associated with pyelonephritic *E. coli* strains. Sat is considered a virulence factor because it has toxic activity against cell lines of bladder or kidney origin. Sat induces elongation of cells and loosening of cellular junctions in cell lines of kidney. Furthermore, Sat triggers vacuolation within the cytoplasm of both human bladder and kidney cell lines [45]. Another secreted toxin called Vat (vacuolating autotransporter toxin), often expressed by UPEC strains, shows the ability to induce a variety of cytopathic effects in target host cells, including swelling and vacuolation. However, the role of Vat in UTI pathogenesis has not been thoroughly studied [46].

2.3. Iron acquisition systems

Limiting iron availability in the urinary tract is an important host defense against bacterial pathogens. For growth and metabolic activity, bacteria require a cytoplasmic iron concentration of about 10^{-6} M, while free iron concentrations in the mammalian host are extremely low (10^{-25} M in the blood and lower at other sites of organism) [47]. Consequently, pathogenic bacteria have to be equipped with systems for acquisition of iron from the host. Bacteria produce siderophores, low-molecular-weight molecules that bind and transport iron (Fe^{3+}) through the bacterial membrane into cytosol where the iron is released. Iron bound siderophores are transported through (with) specific receptors at the outer membrane that facilitate carrying of siderophore-iron complexes through the bacterial membrane. Common siderophore system is enterobactin and its receptor FebA, which is expressed by both pathogenic and K12 *E. coli* strains, although in the context of infection and also other siderophore systems (salmochelin and IroN, aerobactin and IutA, and yersiniabactin and FyuA) have been observed in UPEC [3]. The occurrence of these systems in UPEC strains difficult to identify certain systems as virulence factors of UPEC [48].

3. Biofilm formation by UPEC

Currently biofilm is defined as a structured bacterial community embedded in a self-produced matrix and attached to an abiotic or living surface [49].

The biofilm matrix is composed with exopolysaccharides, which form a hydrated viscous layer and protects enclosed bacterial cells against dehydration, toxic molecules such as antibiotics, and from immune system of host [50]. Bacteria within the biofilm differ in gene expression resulting in a phenotype different from the planktonic bacteria. The slow growth of pathogens in biofilms is the major factor conferring resistance to antibiotics [51]. The ability of bacteria to form biofilm is associated with pathogenesis of numerous diseases. Biofilm formation results in chronic, persistent infections that are difficult to eradicate with antimicrobial treatment. It is believed that biofilms occur in up to 60% of human infections [52]. UPEC can persist within the bladder tissue in underlying epithelial cells or create biofilm-like pods in the recurrent cystitis [53]. Biofilm of *E. coli* may form on the urothelium and is involved in infections associated with biomaterials such as catheters or prostheses. UPEC strains are frequently isolated from biofilms formed in the lumen of catheters and showing resistance to antibiotic treatment [54]. Catheter-associated urinary tract infection (CAUTI) is the most common nosocomial infection, and approximately 80% of UTIs acquired in the hospital are associated with catheterization [55]. The insertion of indwelling catheter into the bladder increases the susceptibility of patients to UTIs, because these devices are the initiation site of infection by introducing opportunistic organisms into the urinary tract [56]. UPEC strains are capable of colonizing the intestinal and vaginal tracts, and these sites are potential reservoirs of microorganisms for UTIs and CAUTIs [57]. The urinary catheter connects the colonized perineum with the sterile bladder providing a route for bacterial entry along the catheter lumen or the external surface of the catheter [58]. CAUTI is related to the susceptibility of catheter material to microbial colonization. The initial stage of biofilm formation on a urinary catheter includes deposition of conditioning film of host urinary components, such as proteins, electrolytes, and other organic molecules [59]. These molecules on the surface of the urinary catheter may change its surface and neutralize any antiadhesive properties [60]. Planktonic bacteria are attached to the surface of the urinary catheter through hydrophobic and electrostatic interaction [61]. Development of biofilm on surface of the catheter occurs through the division of binding bacterial cells, appending additional planktonic bacteria and secretion of extracellular matrix. Detachment of single cell or group of bacterial cells from the biofilm may result in the passage of pathogens into the urine [51]. For this reason, biofilm formation on the urinary catheters is critical for initiating and maintaining of CAUTIs and is a reservoir of resistant pathogenic bacteria [62]. Several factors contribute to the formation of biofilm by *E. coli*, e.g. fimbriae, curli, and flagella. Type 1 fimbriae involved in biofilm formation may also support the colonization of urinary catheter surface [15]. The risk of CAUTI depends on the duration of catheterization, the quality of catheter care, and host susceptibility. Prolonged catheterization is the most important risk factor associated with CAUTI [62]. Long-term urinary catheter use (more than 30 days) causes permanent bacterial colonization of the urine in 100% cases [63]. Examination of people in a nursing home showed that long-term catheterization was significantly related with bacteriuria, pyelonephritis, and renal inflammation [58]. Forming of biofilm on the urinary catheters is a public health problem for patients who need these medical devices. It is recommended that patients who are chronically catheterized were treated with 5–10 days of targeted antibiotic therapy [64].

4. Antimicrobial resistance of UPEC

Antimicrobial resistance in UPEC is a clinical problem in patients with UTIs, in particular in women with recurrent UTI. The empirical antimicrobial treatment in case of recurrent UTIs exerts significant resistance pressure on the uropathogens and the fecal flora, which serves as resistance reservoirs for potential uropathogens [65–67]. Antimicrobial resistance among *E. coli* causing UTI is increasing in many countries around the world and shows considerable variations during different time periods and in different areas [68, 69].

The level of resistance of UPEC strains from hospitalized patients in Poland and Turkey to ampicillin was 56% [70, 71], while above 85% of UPEC strains from patients in India were resistant to this antibiotic [68]. High percentage (67.3%) of *E. coli* strains resistant to tetracycline was isolated from people with UTI from different parts of India [68].

Sanchez et al. [72] suggested that the increase of resistance of UPEC to ciprofloxacin is a result of widespread use of this antibiotic in the treatment of uncomplicated UTIs in the early 2000s. The most recent published data suggested that the level of resistance to trimethoprim-sulfamethoxazole increased and in different countries was over 21–24.2% [71–73]. This trend has continued for decades and the increasing resistance of *E. coli* to trimethoprim-sulfamethoxazole can be explained by frequent use of this antimicrobial agent because it is recommended as the second-line drug in treating acute uncomplicated cystitis in women. Authors reported low resistance of *E. coli* to nitrofurantoin (0.85–1.6%) and no increase in resistance in the last decade was observed [71, 72].

http://dx.doi.org/10.5772/67778

The extended spectrum of β-lactamases (ESBLs) produced by *Enterobacteriaceae* is responsible for resistance of amino and ureido penicillin, oxyimino cephalosporin, and monobactams, but not to 7-α-substituted β-lactam [74]. The production of ESBLs by UPEC strains complicates treatment because these strains are resistant not only to β-lactam antibiotics but often are also resistant to other classes of antibiotics-like aminoglycosides, quinolones, and cotrimoxazole, such as gentamicin, ciprofloxacin, and trimethoprim-sulfamethoxazole, respectively [75–77]. This reduces the treatment options to a limited number of antibiotics and empirical therapy with cephalosporins and fluoroquinolones often fail in patients with UTI [78]. Hoban et al. [79] found that these resistant microorganisms are more susceptible to the carbapenems, imipenem, and ertapenem, than to other antibiotics. ESBL-producing microorganisms were primarily considered multiresistant organisms originating in hospitals, but in recent years, the number of ESBL producers increased also among outpatients, especially related with UTIs. The authors reported 21 and 21.4% ESBL-producing *E. coli* found in community-acquired UTIs in Turkey [80] and in North India [81], respectively, while in Mexico, 31% of uropathogenic *E. coli* isolated from hospitalized patients [77] and 17.6% *E. coli* from hospitalized European UTI patients [79] were producers of ESBLs. UTIs complicated by ESBL producers tend to lead to uncertain outcomes and prolong hospitalization, especially that these organisms tend to be multidrug resistant [74]. Among ESBLs, the CTX-M enzymes are the most prevalent among isolates of UPE from inpatients and outpatients leading to serious problems for the antimicrobial management of these infections [82, 83]. There is a need for new therapy of UTI caused by multiresistant ESBL-producing UPEC.

5. Treatment and control of UPEC

Currently, the antibiotic therapy is an important part of the therapeutic strategy for UTI. The increased antibiotic resistance in recent years suggests that the choice of antibiotic should be guided by the results of sensitivity assay, although in cases of community-acquired UTI, an empirical therapy is often used [23]. The drugs of first-line choice for empirical treatment of uncomplicated UTI in all European countries are fosfomycin trometamol, pivmecillinam, or nitrofurantoin macrocrystals [84]. Trimethoprim-sulfamethoxazole is also used in countries where resistance to this chemotherapeutic is low. Higher rates of side effects in comparison with other drugs limit the use of quinolones as second-line therapy. Moreover, in many countries in Europe, high resistance rates of *E. coli* strains to nalidixic acid were observed [85], and thus aminoglycosides and carbapenem are the drugs of choice. In patients with recurrent infections of the urinary tract, the antibiotics may be recommended prophylactically. It is believed that two recurrences of UTI within 6 months after therapy or three episodes per year could be considered an indication to establish prophylaxis after treatment. The drugs for this purpose are nitrofurantoin, trimethoprin-sulfamethoxazole, fosfomycin trometamol, and cotrimoxazole at lower doses than therapeutic [86]. However, repeated antibiotic treatment of UTI and prophylactic use of antibiotics frequently results in a rise in resistance to antibiotics and adversely affects microbiota of patients which may lead to secondary infections posttreatment, such as gastrointestinal infection and vaginal yeast infection [87, 88].

For this reason, alternative or additional prophylactic strategies have been investigated. One of them is improving the management of UTI by the development of preventive vaccines. Effective vaccine for UTI will need to generate a strong mucosal immune response in the urinary tract. Designing a UTI vaccine that would be effective against UPEC is difficult due to heterogeneous nature of the UPEC population. UTI vaccine should be designed based on more than one antigen because not all strains express the exact set of virulence genes during infections. A vaccine based on the multiple virulence factors, such as fimbrial adhesins or iron receptors, could be clinically effective against UTI [89]. The vaccine with whole or lysed fractions of inactivated bacteria can be effective to generate protective immunity. Urovac® is one of such vaccines (Solco Basel AG, Birsfelden, Switzerland, and Protein Express, Cincinnati, OH, USA) containing ten heat-killed uropathogens, including six UPEC strains. The UPEC strains in the Urovac® show different virulence factors, such as hemolysin, type 1, P, and S fimbrial adhesins, CNF-1, siderophores, and the *E. coli* CFT073 pathogenicity island marker and many different O and H antigens. Evaluating the efficacy of vaginally administrated Urovac® found that the immunization did not ensure significant long-term protection from UTI or an increase in mean levels of UPEC antibodies in serum, vagina, or urine [90]. However, among the women receiving Urovac, 72% were free from UTIs, while only 30% of women given placebo remained free from UTIs caused by *E. coli*. Moreover, in the Urovac vaccinated group, the number of *E. coli* caused UTIs was significantly lower compared to the control group [91]. Another vaccine which is used in Switzerland since 1988 and sold in other countries worldwide is OM-89/Uro-Vaxom® (OM Pharma, Myerlin, Switzerland). Uro-Vaxom is an oral capsule containing a lyophilized mix of membrane proteins from 18 UPEC strains. The clinical studies showed that Uro-Vaxom was significantly more effective than placebo in preventing recurrent UTI [92].

Other prophylaxis method is use of different *Lactobacillus* species in the form of probiotics which reduced the risk of UTI and vaginal infections. Use of *Lactobacillus* species maintains low pH and produces hydrogen peroxide that inhibits growth of *E. coli* in urinary tract but also activates Toll-like receptor-2 and therefore leads to reduced inflammatory reaction [93]. Beerepoot et al. [94] conducted study in which postmenopausal women with recurrent UTI prophylactically received trimethoprim-sulfamethoxazole or oral capsules containing *L. rhamnosus* GR-1 and *L. reuteri* RC-14. After 12 months of treatment, the reduction in recurrence was more than 50% in both groups. However, in group that received trimethoprim-sulfamethoxazole, the two-fold increase in resistance was observed.

Research on dietary supplementation showed that cranberry juice and its extracts reduced UTI recurrences. The active metabolite of cranberry, proanthocyanidin A prevents bacterial adhesion to the urothelial layer by inhibiting P fimbriae expression [95]. The minimum daily dose of proanthocyanidin A, which is able to reduce significantly the number of urinary *E. coli* to be 36 mg [96]. The study conducted by Wojnicz et al. [97] showed that cranberry extract Żuravit S.O.S.® reduced motility and adhesion to epithelial cells in *E. coli* strains isolated from urine of patients with pyelonephritis and also limited the ability of these strains to form biofilm.

Bacteriophages are highly specific and very effective in lysing bacteria. The use of lytic phages that are able to pass through the extracellular matrix against *E. coli* biofilm causes a reduction of bacteria number in biofilm and also prevents biofilm formation on catheter coated with hydrogel containing bacteriophages [98, 99]. Biofilm-associated UTIs are difficult to treat due to the high level of antimicrobial resistance showed by biofilm structures. Many authors recommend macrolides (erythromycin, clarithromycin, and azithromycin) as the treatment of choice in biofilm-associated infections because these antibiotics inhibit the production of primary component of the matrix, alginate [100, 101]. Ciprofloxacin, norfloxacin, gentamicin, or nitrofurazone are often used as components in coating and impregnating the catheters in the aim to inhibit bacterial attachment and development of biofilm [55, 102]. New therapeutic antibiofilm treatments are studied as alternative to antibiotics in order to inhibit biofilm formation and also to avoid the emergence of resistant bacterial populations. The silver showed antimicrobial activity by interacting with bacterial cell membrane and is used to coat catheters. The study showed a statistically significantly lower frequency of bacterial infection in patients treated with a silver alloy-coated catheter compared to those treated with uncoated catheter. Schaeffer et al. [103] reported that bacteriuria was present in 27% of patients with the silver-coated silicone catheter and in 55% of group with uncoated silicone catheter. It was also demonstrated that silver alloy used in hydrogel-coated urinary catheter reduced of up 45% of CAUTI [104]. However, the study conducted by Desai et al. [105] showed that *E. coli* adherence was not significantly lower on silver-impregnated silicone or latex catheters compared to adherence of *E. coli* on catheters without silver.

The new antibiofilm strategy is phage therapy using engineered bacteriophages that have biofilm-degrading enzymatic activity. It was demonstrated that engineered phages that express biofilm-degrading enzymes are more efficient in removing bacterial biofilms than nonenzymatic phage alone. Lu and Collins [106] generated bacteriophage which expressed biofilm-degrading enzyme (DspB) during infection. The DspB showed simultaneous action against both bacterial cells in the biofilm and the biofilm matrix. The engineered enzymatic phage reduced bacterial biofilm cell in 99.9%. One of the new ways of eliminating biofilm is the use of nanoparticles. Water-based synthesis of yttrium fluoride (YF_3) nanoparticles that showed antibacterial properties against *E. coli* was described. The minimal inhibitory concentration was observed at 0.01 mg/mL. In addition, YF3 nanoparticles-coated catheters were able to significantly reduce bacterial colonization compared to the uncoated surface, which provides the potential to develop the concept of utilizing yttrium fluoride nanoparticles as novel antimicrobial and antibiofilm agents [107].

The alternative strategies to decrease UPEC infection include the use of plant-derived antibacterial agents containing different functional groups in their structure and development of resistance in bacteria to these antimicrobials is less frequent [108]. Borges et al. [109] showed that phenolic acids such as gallic and ferulic acid have prevented biofilm formation and show potential to reduce the mass of biofilms formed by the Gram-negative bacteria including *E. coli*. The antibiofilm effect of trans-cinnamaldehyde (TC) on UPEC was reported by Amalaradjou et al. [110]. These authors showed that TC was effective against UPEC biofilm on polystyrene or latex, and the expression of *E. coli* genes encoding attachment and invasion of bladder cells was significantly decreased by TC [111]. Phytochemicals as alternative antimicrobials in preventing and inactivating *E. coli* biofilm on urinary catheters were also assessed. It was demonstrated that TC at the concentration of 0.5% was highly effective for preventing *E. coli* biofilm formation in the lumen of urinary catheter and after 1 day of completely inhibited biofilm formation. Whereas, completely inactivated biofilm after 1 day was observed at 1.25%

and 1.5% TC solution. *p*-Coumaric and ferulic acids have preventive action on *E. coli* biofilm formation on urinary catheter but complete inactivation of the biofilm formed at presence of these phytochemicals was not observed [112]. Recently showed that two alkaloids, piperine from black pepper and reserpine from Indian snakeroot, decreased swarming and swimming motilities of the uropathogenic *E. coli* CFT073. Additionally, piperine increased penetration of ciprofloxacin and azithromycin in to biofilm of *E. coli* CFT073. Authors suggest that these substances can affect on bacterial colonization by inhibition bacterial motility and also may help in treatment of infection by strengthening the penetration of antibiotic in biofilms [113].

One of the other strategies to prevent colonization, invasion, and biofilm formation by UPEC is inhibition of the assembly of pili by family of bicyclic 2-pyridones, termed pilicides.

The activity of pilicides was evaluated in two different pilus biogenesis systems in UPEC. Hemagglutination mediated by either type 1 or P pili, adherence to bladder cells, and biofilm formation mediated by type 1 pili were all reduced by 90% in laboratory and clinical *E. coli* strains [114]. Pilicide ec240 was found to disrupt type 1 pili, P pili, S pili, and flagellar motility [115]. Other pilicides also inhibit the production of Dr pili that are important in pyelonephritis [116]. Mannosides are FimH receptor analogues and bind to this pilus with high affinity, which results in blocking FimH binding to mannosylated receptors. The use of mannosides is considered a new strategy in treating and preventing UTIs because they prevent bladder colonization and invasion and are effective against multidrug-resistant UPEC and against established UTIs [117].

6. Conclusions

UTIs belong to the most common bacterial infections. *E. coli* is the major factor of community-acquired UTIs and a large part of nosocomial UTIs is also caused by this microorganism. UPECs have a wide range of virulence factors and spread of antimicrobial resistance that threaten effective treatment of UTIs using antibiotics. Intensive research that can identify essential virulence mechanisms of UPEC can lead to the development of UTI treatments and prophylactics. The identification of virulence determinants, especially responsible for initial attachment and adhesion of bacterial cells to receptors can be the basis for the development of targeted therapy that prevents the development of UTI. New strategies of UTIs treatment and prevention include chemical compounds such as pilicides and mannosides that block UPEC adhesion or vaccines against siderophores, pili, and UPEC toxins. However, they are still at the preclinical stage of development. These novel antivirulence therapies for treatment of UTIs still require substantial effort associated with future clinical trials.

Author details

Barbara Kot

Address all correspondence to: barbara.kot@uph.edu.pl

Department of Microbiology, Institute of Biology, Siedlce University of Natural Sciences and Humanities, Siedlce, Poland

References

[1] Kaper JB, Nataro JP, Mobley HL. Pathogenic *Escherichia coli*. Nat Rev Microbiol. 2004;**2**:123-140. DOI:10.1038/nrmicro818

[2] Allocati N, Masulli M, Alexeyev MF, Di Ilio C. *Escherichia coli* in Europe: An overview. Int J Environ Res Public Health. 2013;**10**:6235-6254. DOI:10.3390/ijerph10126235

[3] Wiles TJ, Kulesus RR, Mulvey MA. Origins and virulence mechanisms of uropathogenic *Escherichia coli*. Exp Mol Pathol. 2008;**85**:11-19. DOI:10.1016/j.yexmp.2008.03.007

[4] Samet M, Ghaemi E, Nejad MH, Jamali A. Prevalence of different virulence factors and biofilm production ability of urinary *Escherichia coli* isolates. Int J Biol Med Res. 2014;**5**: 4546-4549.

[5] Bower JM, Eto DS, Mulvey MA. Covert operations of uropathogenic *Escherichia coli* within the urinary tract. Traffic. 2005;**6**:18-31. DOI: 10.1111/j.1600-0854.2004.00251.x

[6] Siegman-Igra Y, Fourer B, Orni-Wasserlauf R, Golan Y, Noy A, Schwartz D, Giladi M. Reappraisal of community-acquired bacteremia: A proposal of a new classification for the spectrum of acquisition of bacteremia. Clin Infect Dis. 2002;**34**:1431-1439. DOI:10.1086/339809

[7] Schneeberger C, Kazemier BM, Geerlings SE. Asymptomatic bacteriuria and urinary tract infections in special patient groups: Women with diabetes mellitus and pregnant women. Curr Opin Infect Dis. 2014;**27**:108-114. DOI: 10.1097/QCO.0000000000000028

[8] Abbott KC, Oliver JD, Hypolite I, Lepler LL, Kirk AD, Ko CW, Hawkes CA, Jones CA, Agodoa LY. Hospitalizations for bacterial septicemia after renal transplantation in the United States. Am J Nephrol. 2001;**21**:120-127. DOI:10 1159/000046234

[9] Manges AR, Johnson JR, Foxman B, O'Bryan TT, Fullerton KE, Riley LW. Widespread distribution of urinary tract infections caused by a multidrug-resistant *Escherichia coli* clonal group. N Engl J Med. 2001;**345**:1007-1013. DOI:10.1056/NEJMoa011265

[10] Welch RA, Burland V, Plunkett G 3rd, Redford P, Roesch P, Rasko D, Buckles EL, Liou SR, Boutin A, Hackett J, Stroud D, Mayhew GF, Rose DJ, Zhou S, Schwartz DC, Perna NT, Mobley HL, Donnenberg MS, Blattner FR. Extensive mosaic structure revealed by the complete genome sequence of uropathogenic *Escherichia coli*. Proc Natl Acad Sci U S A. 2002;**99**:17020-17024. DOI:10.1073/pnas.252529799

[11] Gal-Mor O, Finlay BB. Pathogenicity islands: A molecular toolbox for bacterial virulence. Cell Microbiol. 2006;**8**:1707-1719. DOI:10.1111/j.1462-5822.2006.00794.x

[12] Oelschlaeger TA, Dobrindt U, Hacker J. Pathogenicity islands of uropathogenic *E. coli* and the evolution of virulence. Int J Antimicrob Agents. 2002;**19**:517-521. DOI:10.1016/S0924-8579(02)00092-4

[13] Martinez JJ, Mulvey MA, Schilling JD, Pinkner JS, Hultgren SJ. Type 1 pilus-mediated bacterial invasion of bladder epithelial cells. EMBO J. 2000;**19**:2803-2812. DOI: 10.1093/emboj/19.12.2803

[14] Bien J, Sokolova O, Bozko P. Role of uropathogenic *Escherichia coli* virulence factors in development of urinary tract infection and kidney damage. Int J Nephrol. 2012;**2012**:681473. DOI: 10.1155/2012/681473

[15] Mulvey MA. Adhesion and entry of uropathogenic *Escherichia coli*. Cell Microbiol. 2002; **4**:257-271.

[16] Bergsten G, Wullt B, Schembri MA, Leijonhufvud I, Svanborg C. Do type 1 fimbriae promote inflammation in the human urinary tract? Cell Microbiol. 2007;**9**:1766-1781. DOI: 10.1111/j.1462-5822.2007.00912.x

[17] Yun KW, Kim HY, Park HK, Kim W, Lim IS. Virulence factors of uropathogenic *Escherichia coli* of urinary tract infections and asymptomatic bacteriuria in children. J Microbiol Immunol Infect. 2014;**47**:455-461. DOI:10.1016/j.jmii.2013.07.010

[18] Sokurenko EV, Courtney HS, Maslow J, Siitonen A, Hasty DL. Quantitative differences in adhesiveness of type 1 fimbriated *Escherichia coli* due to structural differences in fimH genes. J Bacteriol. 1995;**177**:3680-3686.

[19] Justice SS, Hung C, Theriot JA, Fletcher DA, Anderson GG, Footer MJ, Hultgren SJ. Differentiation and developmental pathways of uropathogenic *Escherichia coli* in urinary tract pathogenesis. Proc Natl Acad Sci U S A. 2004;**101**:1333-1338. DOI: 10.1128/IAI.73.11.7657-7668.2005

[20] Eto DS, Jones TA, Sundsbak JL, Mulvey MA. Integrin-mediated host cell invasion by type 1-piliated uropathogenic *Escherichia coli*. PLoS Pathog. 2007;**3**:e100. DOI:10.1371/journal.ppat.0030100

[21] Mulvey MA, Schilling JD, Martinez JJ, Hultgren SJ. Bad bugs and beleaguered bladders: Interplay between uropathogenic *Escherichia coli* and innate host defenses. Proc Natl Acad Sci U S A. 2000;**97**:8829-8835.

[22] Bishop BL, Duncan MJ, Song J, Li G, Zaas D, Abraham SN. Cyclic AMP-regulated exocytosis of *Escherichia coli* from infected bladder epithelial cells. Nat Med. 2007;**13**:625-630. DOI: 10.1038/nm1572

[23] Minardi D, d'Anzeo G, Cantoro D, Conti A, Muzzonigro G. Urinary tract infections in women: Etiology and treatment options. Int J Gen Med. 2011;**4**:333-343. DOI:10.2147/IJGM.S11767

[24] Rasko DA, Phillips JA, Li X, Mobley HL. Identification of DNA sequences from a second pathogenicity island of uropathogenic *Escherichia coli* CFT073: Probes specific for uropathogenic populations. J Infect Dis. 2001;**184**:1041-1049. DOI:10.1086/323602

[25] Manning SD, Zhang L, Foxman B, Spindler A, Tallman P, Marrs CF. Prevalence of known P-fimbrial G alleles in *Escherichia coli* and identification of a new adhesin class. Clin Diagn Lab Immunol. 2001;**8**:637-640. DOI: 10.1128/CDLI.8.3.637-640.2001

[26] Marrs CF, Zhang L, Tallman P, Manning SD, Somsel P, Raz P, Colodner R, Jantunen ME, Siitonen A, Saxen H, Foxman B. Variations in 10 putative uropathogen virulence genes

among urinary, faecal and peri-urethral *Escherichia coli* J Med Microbiol. 2002;**51**:138-142. DOI:10.1099/0022-1317-51-2-138

[27] Marrs CF, Zhang L, Foxman B. *Escherichia coli* mediated urinary tract infections: are there distinct uropathogenic *E. coli* (UPEC) pathotypes? FEMS Microbiol Lett. 2005;**252**:183-190. DOI: 10.1016/j.femsle.2005.08.028

[28] Marre R, Kreft B, Hacker J. Genetically engineered S and F1C fimbriae differ in their contribution to adherence of *Escherichia coli* to cultured renal tubular cells. Infect Immun. 1990;**58**:3434-3437.

[29] Nowicki B, Selvarangan R, Nowicki S. Family of *Escherichia coli* Dr adhesins: decay-accelerating factor receptor recognition and invasiveness. J Infect Dis. 2001;**183**, Suppl 1:S24–S27. DOI:10.1086/318846

[30] Le Bouguénec C. Adhesins and invasins of pathogenic *Escherichia coli*. Int J Med Microbiol. 2005;**295**:471-478.

[31] Muenzner P, Kengmo Tchoupa A, Klauser B, Brunner T, Putze J, Dobrindt U, Hauck CR. Uropathogenic *E. coli* exploit CEA to promote colonization of the urogenital tract mucosa. PLoS Pathog. 2016;**12**:e1005608. DOI:10.1371/journal.ppat.1005608

[32] Cegelski L, Pinkner JS, Hammer ND, Cusumano CK, Hung CS, Chorell E, Åberg V, Walker JN, Seed PC, Almqvist F, Chapman MR, Hultgr SJ. Small-molecule inhibitors target *Escherichia coli* amyloid biogenesis and biofilm formation. Nat Chem Biol. 2009; **5**:913-919. DOI:10.1038/nchembio.242

[33] Barnhart MM, Chapman MR. Curli biogenesis and function. Annu Rev Microbiol. 2006;**60**:131-147. DOI:10.1146/annurev.micro.60.080805.142106

[34] Römling U Characterization of the rdar morphotype, a multicellular behaviour in *Enterobacteriaceae*. Cell Mol Life Sci. 2005;**62**:1234-1246. DOI:10.1007/s00018-005-4557-x

[35] Kai-Larsen Y, Lüthje P, Chromek M, Peters V, Wang X, Holm A, Kádas L, Hedlund KO, Johansson J, Chapman MR, Jacobson SH, Römling U, Agerberth B, Brauner A. Uropathogenic *Escherichia coli* modulates immune responses and its curli fimbriae interact with the antimicrobial peptide LL-37. PLoS Pathog. 2010;**6**:e1001010. DOI: 10.1371/journal.ppat.1001010

[36] Hung C, Marschall J, Burnham CA, Byun AS, Henderson JP. The bacterial amyloid curli is associated with urinary source bloodstream infection. PLoS One. 2014;**9**:e86009. DOI: 10.1371/journal.pone.0086009

[37] Fatima N, Agrawal M, Shukla I, Khan PA. Characterization of uropathogenic *E. coli* in relation to virulence factors. Sci Rep. 2012;1:342. DOI:10.4172/scientificreports.342

[38] Bhakdi S, Mackman N, Nicaud JM, Holland IB. *Escherichia coli* hemolysin may damage target cell membranes by generating transmembrane pores. Infect Immun. 1986;**52**:63-69.

[39] Keane WF, Welch R, Gekker G, Peterson PK. Mechanism of *Escherichia coli* alpha-hemolysin-induced injury to isolated renal tubular cells. Am J Pathol. 1987;**126**:350-357.

[40] Smith YC, Grande KK, Rasmussen SB, O'Brien AD. Novel three-dimensional organoid model for evaluation of the interaction of uropathogenic *Escherichia coli* with terminally differentiated human urothelial cells. Infect Immun. 2006;**74**:750-757. DOI:10.1128/IAI.74.1.750-757.2006

[41] Hilbert DW, Paulish-Miller TE, Tan CK, Carey AJ, Ulett GC, Mordechai E, Adelson ME, Gygax SE, Trama JP. Clinical *Escherichia coli* isolates utilize alpha-hemolysin to inhibit in vitro epithelial cytokine production. Microbes Infect. 2012;**14**:628-638. DOI:10.1016/j.micinf.2012.01.010

[42] Hertting O, Chromek M, Slamova Z, Kadas L, Soderkvist M, Vainumäe I, Tallvik T, Jacobson SH, Brauner A. Cytotoxic necrotizing factor 1 (CNF1) induces an inflammatory response in the urinary tract in vitro but not in vivo. Toxicon. 2008;**51**:1544-1547. DOI: 10.1016/j.toxicon.2008.03.019

[43] Mills M, Meysick KC, O'Brien AD. Cytotoxic necrotizing factor type 1 of uropathogenic *Escherichia coli* kills cultured human uroepithelial 5637 cells by an apoptotic mechanism. Infect Immun. 2000;**68**:5869-5880.

[44] Davis JM, Carvalho HM, Rasmussen SB, O'Brien AD. Cytotoxic necrotizing factor type 1 delivered by outer membrane vesicles of uropathogenic *Escherichia coli* attenuates polymorphonuclear leukocyte antimicrobial activity and chemotaxis. Infect Immun. 2006;**74**:4401-4408. DOI:10.1128/IAI.00637-06

[45] Guyer DM, Radulovic S, Jones FE, Mobley HL. Sat, the secreted autotransporter toxin of uropathogenic *Escherichia coli*, is a vacuolating cytotoxin for bladder and kidney epithelial cells. Infect Immun. 2002;**70**:4539-4546. DOI: 10.1128/IAI.70.8.4539-4546.2002

[46] Ewers C, Li G, Wilking H, Kieβling S, Alt K, Antáo EM, Laturnus C, Diehl I, Glodde S, Homeier T, Böhnke U, Steinrück H, Philipp HC, Wieler LH. Avian pathogenic, uropathogenic, and newborn meningitis-causing *Escherichia coli*: How closely related are they? Int J Med Microbiol. 2007;**297**:163-176. DOI:10.1016/j.ijmm.2007.01.003

[47] Andrews SC, Robinson AK, Rodríguez-Quiñones F. Bacterial iron homeostasis. FEMS Microbiol Rev. 2003;**27**:215-237. DOI: http://dx.doi.org/10.1016/S0168-6445(03)00055-X

[48] Garcia EC, Brumbaugh AR, Mobley HL. Redundancy and specificity of *Escherichia coli* iron acquisition systems during urinary tract infection. Infect Immun. 2011;**79**:1225-1235. DOI:10.1128/IAI.01222-10

[49] Costerton JW, Stewart PS, Greenberg EP. Bacterial biofilms: A common cause of persistent infections. Science. 1999; **284**:1318-1322. DOI: 10.1126/science.284.5418.1318

[50] Soto SM, Marco F, Guiral E, Vila J. Biofilm formation in uropathogenic *Escherichia coli* strains: Relationship with urovirulence factors and antimicrobial resistance. In: Nikibakhsh A, editor. Clinical Management of Complicated Urinary Tract Infection. InTech; 2011. http://www.intechopen.com/books/clinical-management-of-complicated-urinary-tractinfection/biofilm-formation-in-uropathogenic-escherichia-coli-strains-relationship-with-urovirulence-factors-a

[51] Trautner BW, Darouiche RO. Role of biofilm in catheter-associated urinary tract infection. Am J Infect Control. 2004;**32**:177-183. DOI:10.1016/j.ajic.2003.08.005

[52] Ponnusamy P, Natarajan V, Sevanan M. In vitro biofilm formation by uropathogenic *Escherichia coli* and their antimicrobial susceptibility pattern. Asian Pac J Trop Med. 2012;**5**:210-213. DOI:10.1016/S1995-7645(12)60026-1

[53] Anderson GG, Palermo JJ, Schilling JD, Roth R, Heuser J, Hultgren SJ. Intracellular bacterial biofilm-like pods in urinary tract infections. Science. 2003;**301**:105-107. DOI:10.1126/science.1084550

[54] Nicolle LE. Catheter-related urinary tract infections. Drugs Aging. 2005;**22**:627-639.

[55] Ha US, Cho YH. Catheter-associated urinary tract infections: new aspects of novel urinary catheters. Int J Antimicrob Agents. 2006;**28**:485-490. DOI 10.1016/j.ijantimicag.2006.08.020

[56] Jacobsen SM, Stickler DJ, Mobley HL, Shirtliff ME. Complicated catheter-associated urinary tract infections due to *Escherichia coli* and *Proteus mirabilis*. Clin Microbiol Rev. 2008;**21**:26-59. DOI: 10.1128/CMR.00019-07.

[57] Johnson JR. Virulence factors in *Escherichia coli* urinary tract infection. Clin Microbiol Rev. 1991;**4**:80-128.

[58] Warren JW, Muncie HL Jr, Hebel JR, Hall-Craggs M. Long-term urethral catheterization increases risk of chronic pyelonephritis and renal inflammation. J Am Geriatr Soc. 1994;**42**:1286-1290.

[59] Denstedt JD, Wollin TA, Reid G. Biomaterials used in urology: Current issues of biocompatibility, infection, and encrustation. J Endourol. 1998;**12**:493-500. DOI:10.1089/end.1998.12.493

[60] Gristina AG. Biomaterial-centered infection: Microbial adhesion versus tissue integration. Science. 1987;**237**:1588-1595. DOI: 10.1126/science.3629258

[61] Pratt LA, Kolter R. Genetic analysis of *Escherichia coli* biofilm formation: roles of flagella, motility, chemotaxis and type I pili. Mol Microbiol. 1998;**30**:285-293. DOI: 10.1046/j.1365-2958.1998.01061.x

[62] Tambyah PA. Catheter-associated urinary tract infections: diagnosis and prophylaxis. Int J Antimicrob Agents. 2004;**24** Suppl 1:S44–S48. DOI:10.1016/j.ijantimicag.2004.02.008

[63] Djeribi R, Bouchloukh W, Jouenne T, Menaa B. Characterization of bacterial biofilms formed on urinary catheters. Am J Infect Control. 2012;**40**:854-859. DOI:10.1016/j.ajic.2011.10.009

[64] Nicolle LE. The chronic indwelling catheter and urinary infection in long-term-care facility residents. Infect Control Hosp Epidemiol. 2001;**22**:316-321. DOI:10.1086/501908

[65] Raum E, Lietzau S, von Baum H, Marre R, Brenner H. Changes in *Escherichia coli* resistance patterns during and after antibiotic therapy: A longitudinal study among outpatients in Germany. Clin Microbiol Infect. 2008;**14**:41-48. DOI:10.1111/j.1469-0691.2007.01841.x

[66] de Lastours V, Chau F, Tubach F, Pasquet B, Ruppé E, Fantin B. Independent behavior of commensal flora for carriage of fluoroquinolone-resistant bacteria in patients at admission. Antimicrob Agents Chemother. 2010;**54**:5193-5200. DOI:10.1128/IAI.73.9.5301-5310.2005

[67] Lichtenberger P, Hooton TM. Antimicrobial prophylaxis in women with recurrent urinary tract infections. Int J Antimicrob Agents. 2011;**38**:Suppl:36-41. DOI: 10.1016/j.ijantimicag.2011.09.005

[68] Kumar Y, Sood S, Sharma A, Mani KR. Antibiogram and characterization of resistance markers among *Escherichia coli* isolates from urinary tract infections. J Infect Dev Ctries. 2013;**7**:513-519. DOI: 10.3855/jidc.2706

[69] Niranjan V, Malini A. Antimicrobial resistance pattern in *Escherichia coli* causing urinary tract infection among inpatients. Indian J Med Res. 2014;**139**:945-948.

[70] Kot B, Wicha J., Żak-Puławska Z. Susceptibility of *Escherichia coli* strains isolated from persons with urinary tract infections in 2007-2008 to antimicrobial agents. Przegl Epidemiol. 2010;**64**:307-312.

[71] Eryılmaz M, Bozkurt ME, Yildiz MM, Akin A. Antimicrobial resistance of urinary *Escherichia coli* isolates. Trop J Pharm Res. 2010;**9**:205-209.

[72] Sanchez GV, Master RN, Karlowsky JA, Bordon JM. *In vitro* antimicrobial resistance of urinary *Escherichia coli* isolates among U.S. outpatients from 2000 to 2010. Antimicrob Agents Chemother. 2012;**56**:2181-2183. DOI: 10.1128/AAC.06060-11

[73] Ferjani S, Saidani M, Ennigrou S, Hsairi M, Ben Redjeb S. Virulence determinants, phylogenetic groups and fluoroquinolone resistance in *Escherichia coli* isolated from cystitis and pyelonephritis. Pathol Biol. 2012;**60**:270-274. DOI:10.1016/j.patbio.2011.07.006

[74] Calbo E, Romani V, Xercavins M, Gomez L, Vidal CG, Quintana S, Vila J, Garau J. Risk factors for community-onset urinary tract infections due to *Escherichia coli* harbouring extended-spectrum beta-lactamases. J Antimicrob Chemother. 2006;**57**:780-783. DOI:10.1093/jac/dkl035

[75] Machado ETM, Coque R, Canton F, Baquero JC, Peixe L. Dissemination in Portugal of CTX-M-15-, OYA-1-, and TEM-1-producing *Enterobacteriaceae* strains containing the aac(6')-Ib-cr gene, which encodes an aminoglycoside- and fluoroquinolone-modifying enzyme. Antimicrob Agents Chemother. 2006;**50**:3220-3221. DOI:10.1128/AAC.00473-06

[76] Oteo J, Pérez-Vázquez M, Campos J. Extended-spectrum [beta]-lactamase producing *Escherichia coli*: changing epidemiology and clinical impact. Curr Opin Infect Dis. 2010;**23**:320-326.

[77] Alcántar-Curiel MD, Alpuche-Aranda CM, Varona-Bobadilla HJ, Gayosso-Vázquez C, Jarillo-Quijada MD, Frías-Mendivil M, Sanjuan-Padrón L, Santos-Preciado JI. Risk factors for extended-spectrum β-lactamases-producing *Escherichia coli* urinary tract infections in a tertiary hospital. Salud Publica Mex. 2015;**57**:412-418.

[78] Chaudhary U, Aggarwal R. Extended-spectrum lactamases (ESBL) – An emerging threat to clinical therapeutics. Indian J Med Microbiol. 2004;**22**:75-80.

[79] Hoban DJ, Lascols C, Nicolle LE, Badal R, Bouchillon S, Hackel M, Hawser S. Antimicrobial susceptibility of *Enterobacteriaceae*, including molecular characterization of extended-spectrum beta-lactamase-producing species, in urinary tract isolates from hospitalized patients in North America and Europe: results from the SMART study 2009-2010. Diagn Microbiol Infect Dis. 2012;**74**:62-67. DOI: 10.1016/j.diagmicrobio.2012.05.024

[80] Yumuk Z, Afacan G, Nicolas-Chanoine MH, Sotto A, Lavigne JP. Turkey: A further country concerned by community-acquired *Escherichia coli* clone O25-ST131 producing CTX-M-15. J Antimicrob Chemother. 2008;**62**:284-288. DOI:10.1093/jac/dkn181

[81] Datta P, Gupta V, Sidhu S. Extended spectrum beta lactamase positive uropathogenic *E. coli* – Epidemiological factors and resistance. BJMP 2014;**7**:a718.

[82] Canton R, Coque TM. The CTX-M b-lactamase pandemic. Curr Opin Microbiol. 2006;**9**: 466-475. DOI: 10.1016/j.mib.2006.08.011

[83] Ho PL, Poon WW, Loke SL, Leung MS, Chow KH, Wong RC, Yip KS, Lai EL, Tsang KW; COMBAT study group. Community emergence of CTX-M type extended-spectrum beta-lactamases among urinary *Escherichia coli* from women. J Antimicrob Chemother. 2007;**60**:140-144. DOI:10.1093/jac/dkm144

[84] Schito GC, Gualco L, Naber KG, Botto H, Palou J, Mazzei T, Marchese A. Do different susceptibility breakpoints affect the selection of antimicrobials for treatment of uncomplicated cystitis? J Chemother. 2010;**22**:345-354. DOI:10.1179/joc.2010.22.5.345

[85] Schito GC, Naber KG, Botto H, Palou J, Mazzei T, Gualco L, Marchese A. The ARESC study: An international survey on the antimicrobial resistance of pathogens involved in uncomplicated urinary tract infections. Int J Antimicrob Agents. 2009;**34**:407-413. DOI:10.1016/j.ijantimicag.2009.04.012

[86] Ludwig M, Hoyme U, Weidner W. Recurrent urinary tract infection in women. Long-term antibiotic prophylaxis. Urologe A. 2006;**45**:436-442. DOI:10.1007/s00120-006-1023-9

[87] MacDonald TM, Beardon PH, McGilchrist MM, Duncan ID, McKendrick AD, McDevitt DG. The risks of symptomatic vaginal candidiasis after oral antibiotic therapy. Q J Med. 1993;**86**:419-424. DOI: http://dx.doi.org/419-424

[88] Dethlefsen L, Huse S, Sogin ML, Relman DA. The pervasive effects of an antibiotic on the human gut microbiota, as revealed by deep 16S rRNA sequencing. PLoS Biol. 2008; **6**:e280. DOI: 10.1371/journal.pbio.0060280

[89] Wieser A, Romann E, Magistro G, Hoffmann C, Nörenberg D, Weinert K, Schubert S. A multiepitope subunit vaccine conveys protection against extraintestinal pathogenic *Escherichia coli* in mice. Infect Immun. 2010;**78**:3432-3442. DOI: 10.1128/IAI.00174-10

[90] Uehling DT, Hopkins WJ, Elkahwaji JE, Schmidt DM, Leverson GE. Phase 2 clinical trial of a vaginal mucosal vaccine for urinary tract infections. J Urol. 2003;**170**:867-869. DOI:10.1097/01.ju.0000075094.54767.6e

[91] Hopkins WJ, Elkahwaji J, Beierle LM, Leverson GE, Uehling DT. Vaginal mucosal vaccine for recurrent urinary tract infections in women: Results of a phase 2 clinical trial. J Urol 2007;**177**:1349-1353. DOI:10.1016/j.juro.2006.11.093

[92] Bauer HW, Rahlfs VW, Lauener PA, Blessmann GS. Prevention of recurrent urinary tract infections with immuno-active *E. coli* fractions: A meta-analysis of five placebo-controlled double-blind studies. Int J Antimicrob Agents. 2002;**19**:451-456. DOI:10.1016/S0924-8579(02)00106-1

[93] Amdekar S, Singh V, Singh DD. Probiotic therapy: Immunomodulating approach toward urinary tract infection. Curr Microbiol. 2011;**63**:484-490. DOI:10.1007/s00284-011-0006-2

[94] Beerepoot MAJ, Riet G, Nys S, van der Wal WM, de Borgie CAJM, de Reijke TM, Prins JM, Koeijers J, Verbon A, Stobberingh E, Geerlings SE. Lactobacilli vs antibiotics to prevent urinary tract infections: A randomized, double-blind, noninferiority trial in postmenopausal women. Arch Intern Med. 2012;**172**:704-712. DOI: 10.1001/archinternmed.2012.777

[95] Howell AB. Bioactive compounds in cranberries and their role in prevention of urinary tract infections. Mol Nutr Food Res. 2007;**51**:732-737. DOI:10.1002/mnfr.200700038

[96] Howell AB, Botto H, Combescure C, Blanc-Potard AB, Gausa L, Matsumoto T, Tenke P, Sotto A, Lavigne JP. Dosage effect on uropathogenic *Escherichia coli* anti-adhesion activity in urine following consumption of cranberry powder standardized for proanthocyanidin content: A multicentric randomized double blind study. BMC Infect Dis. 2010;**10**:94. DOI: 10.1186/1471-2334-10-94

[97] Wojnicz D, Sycz Z, Walkowski S, Gabrielska J, Włoch A, Kucharska A, Sokół-Łętowska A, Hendrich AB. Study on the influence of cranberry extract Żuravit S·O·S® on the properties of uropathogenic *Escherichia coli* strains, their ability to form biofilm and its antioxidant properties. Phytomedicine. 2012;**19**:506-514. DOI:10.1016/j.phymed.2011.12.013

[98] Carson L, Gorman SP, Gilmore BF. The use of lytic bacteriophages in the prevention and eradication of biofilms of *Proteus mirabilis* and *Escherichia coli*. FEMS Immunol Med Microbiol. 2010;**59**:447-455. DOI: 10.1111/j.1574-695X.2010.00696.x

[99] Chibeu A, Lingohr EJ, Masson L, Manges A, Harel J, Ackermann HW, Kropinski AM, Boerlin P. Bacteriophages with the ability to degrade uropathogenic *Escherichia coli* biofilms. Viruses. 2012;**4**:471-487. DOI: 10.3390/v4040471

[100] Ichimiya T, Takeoka K, Hiramatsu K, Hirai K, Yamasaki T, Nasu M. The influence of azithromycin on the biofilm formation of *Pseudomonas aeruginosa* in vitro. Chemotherapy. 1996;**42**:186-191.

[101] Soto SM. Importance of biofilms in urinary tract infections: new therapeutic approaches. Adv Biol. 2014; ID 543974, 13 pages. DOI:10.1155/2014/543974

[102] Hamill TM, Gilmore BF, Jones DS, Gorman SP. Strategies for the development of the urinary catheter. Expert Rev Med Devices. 2007;**4**:215-225. DOI:10.1586/17434440.4.2.215

[103] Schaeffer AJ, Story KO, Johnson SM. Effect of silver oxide/trichloroisocyanuric acid antimicrobial urinary drainage system on catheter-associated bacteriuria. J Urol. 1988;**139**:69-73.

[104] Rupp ME, Fitzgerald T, Marion N, Helget V, Puumala S, Anderson JR, Fey PD. Effect of silver-coated urinary catheters: Efficacy, cost-effectiveness, and antimicrobial resistance. Am J Infect Control. 2004;**32**:445-450. DOI:10.1016/S0196655304004742

[105] Desai DG, Liao KS, Cevallos ME, Trautner BW. Silver or nitrofurazone impregnation of urinary catheters has a minimal effect on uropathogen adherence. J Urol. 2010;**184**:2565-2571. DOI: 10.1016/j.juro.2010.07.036

[106] Lu TK, Collins JJ. Dispersing biofilms with engineered enzymatic bacteriophage. Proc Natl Acad Sci U S A. 2007;**104**:11197-11202. DOI: 10.1073/pnas.0704624104

[107] Lellouche J, Friedman A, Gedanken A, Banin E. Antibacterial and antibiofilm properties of yttrium fluoride nanoparticles. Int J Nanomed. 2012;**7**:5611-5624. DOI: 10.2147/IJN.S37075

[108] Domadia P, Swarup S, Bhunia A, Sivaraman J, Dasgupta D. Inhibition of bacterial cell division protein FtsZ by cinnamaldehyde. Biochem Pharmacol. 2007;**832**:831-840. DOI: 10.1016/j.bcp.2007.06.029

[109] Borges A, Saavedra MJ, Simões M. The activity of ferulic and gallic acids in biofilm prevention and control of pathogenic bacteria. Biofouling 2012;**28**:755-767. DOI: 10.1080/08927014.2012.706751

[110] Amalaradjou MAR, Narayanan A, Baskaran SA, Venkitanarayanan K. Antibiofilm effect of trans-cinnamaldehyde on uropathogenic *Escherichia coli*. J Urol. 2010;**184**:358-363. DOI: 10.1016/j.juro.2010.03.006

[111] Amalaradjou MAR, Narayanan A, Venkitanarayanan K. Trans-cinnamaldehyde decreases attachment and invasion of uropathogenic *Escherichia coli* in urinary tract epithelial cells by modulating virulence gene exptression. J Urol. 2011;**185**:1526-1531. DOI: 10.1016/j.juro.2010.11.078

[112] Kot B, Wicha J, Piechota M, Wolska K, Grużewska A. Antibiofilm activity of trans-cinnamaldehyde, p-coumaric, and ferulic acids on uropathogenic *Escherichia coli*. Turk J Med Sci. 2015;**45**:919-924. DOI:10.3906/sag-1406-112

[113] Dusane DH, Hosseinidoust Z, Asadishad B, Tufenkji N. Alkaloids modulate motility, biofilm formation and antibiotic susceptibility of uropathogenic *Escherichia coli*. PLoS One. 2014;**9**:e112093. DOI: 10.1371/journal.pone.0112093

[114] Pinkner JS, Remaut H, Buelens F, Miller E, Aberg V, Pemberton N, Hedenström M, Larsson A, Seed P, Waksman G, Hultgren SJ, Almqvist F. Rationally designed small compounds inhibit pilus biogenesis in uropathogenic bacteria. Proc Natl Acad Sci U S A. 2006;**103**:17897-17902. DOI: 10.1073/pnas.0606795103

[115] Greene SE, Pinkner JS, Chorell E, Dodson KW, Shaffer CL, Conover MS, Livny J, Hadjifrangiskou M, Almqvist F, Hultgrenet SJ. Pilicide ec240 disrupts virulence circuits in uropathogenic *Escherichia coli*. mBio. 2014;**5**:e02038-14. DOI:10.1128/mBio.02038-14

[116] Piatek R, Zalewska-Piatek B, Dzierzbicka K, Makowiec S, Pilipczuk J, Szemiako K, Cyranka-Czaja A, Wojciechowski M. Pilicides inhibit the FGL chaperone/usher assisted biogenesis of the Dr fimbrial polyadhesin from uropathogenic *Escherichia coli*. BMC Microbiol. 2013 Jun 12;**13**:131. DOI: 10.1186/1471-2180-13-131.

[117] Totsika M, Kostakioti M, Hannan TJ, Upton M, Beatson SA, Janetka JW, Hultgren SJ, Schembri MA. A FimH inhibitor prevents acute bladder infection and treats chronic cystitis caused by multidrug-resistant uropathogenic *Escherichia coli* ST131. J Infect Dis. 2013;**15**; 208: 921-928. DOI: 10.1093/infdis/jit245

Chapter 3

The Pathogenesis of *Escherichia Coli* Urinary Tract Infection

Timothy Kudinha

Additional information is available at the end of the chapter

http://dx.doi.org/10.5772/intechopen.69030

Abstract

Urinary tract infections (UTIs) are the commonest human bacterial infections and are responsible for substantial morbidity and mortality, resulting in increased healthcare costs. Most UTIs are caused by specialized *Escherichia coli* (*E. coli*) strains referred to as uropathogenic *E. coli* (UPEC). UPEC possess a variety of virulence factors (VFs), which the organism uses to attach, invade, and injure the host. These VFs include adhesins, toxins, iron acquisition factors, lipopolysacharide capsules, and other invasins. Most studies on UTI pathogenesis have targeted VFs. The source of UPEC is the host's fecal flora. According to the pathogenicity theory, UPEC strains with special VFs move from the host's fecal flora to the urogenital tract and cause UTI. However, another theory states that the numerically abundant strain is responsible for UTI. Effective UTI management is hampered by the recent rise in antibiotic resistance, specifically, the recent emergence of multidrug-resistant *E. coli* sequence type 131. The distribution of VFs and other bacterial characteristics among different patient groups and UTI syndromes, is crucial understanding UTI pathogenesis, which would guide clinical decision making. For ST131 clonal group, further epidemiological studies are needed to clarify transmission pathways, risk factors for spread, and reservoirs, so that effective control measures can be devised.

Keywords: *Escherichia coli*, urinary tract infections, virulence factors, multidrug resistance

1. Introduction

Urinary tract infections (UTIs) are an important medical problem, being the second most common bacterial infection of humans after respiratory tract infection. They are often recurrent, frequently difficult to treat, and can cause parenchymal damage to the kidney, leading to renal insufficiency and further complications [1–3]. UTIs impose a substantial burden on society and the health care system in relation to diagnosis, management, lost productivity, morbidity, and sometimes death [4–6]. Furthermore, increasing resistance to therapeutically important antimicrobial agents and the recent emergence of the virulent and multidrug-resistant ST131 clonal group have made UTI management progressively more costly and challenging [7, 8]. Several studies suggest that a greater array of VFs is generally needed to cause more invasive UTIs, although the extent appears to differ according to age and gender. Thus, further studies targeting VFs, which have been proposed as the best target for vaccine development, are needed. A better understanding of UTI pathogenesis, especially for the most common cause of UTI, namely *Escherichia coli,* is crucial for treatment and prevention of UTIs.

2. Etiology of UTI

UTIs are mainly caused by bacteria, although fungi and some viruses have also been implicated. Among bacteria, Gram-negative bacteria of the *Enterobacteriaceae* family, including *E. coli, Klebsiella, Enterobacter, Proteus* species, *etc.*, are mostly involved. However, some Gram-positive organisms, principally *Staphylococcus aureus, Staphylococcus saprophyticus* and *Streptococcus agalactiae,* also play a role especially among young women. *E. coli* is the dominant causative agent in all patient groups, causing 80–90% of all UTIs [5]. Consequently, *E. coli* serves as a model pathogen for studying UTI pathogenesis.

Escherichia coli is a normal constituent of the intestinal microbiota of humans and animals [9, 10]. The distinctive *E. coli* strains that cause most UTIs have been designated uropathogenic *E. coli* (UPEC). They possess diverse virulence-associated factors (VFs) that assist them in attaching to, invading, and injuring the host, and include adhesins, toxins, siderophores, protective polysaccharide coatings, invasins, and serum resistance-associated proteins. The presence and numbers of such VFs predicts *in vivo* virulence [11].

3. Epidemiology and risk factors for *E. coli* UTI

Overall, UTI is more prevalent among females than males, attributable to the close proximity of the urogenital tract to the anus in females, the greater length of the male urethra, and the antibacterial activity of prostatic fluid in men [12, 13]. Functional, hormonal, and anatomical changes that occur during pregnancy predispose pregnant women to UTI [14]. UTI during pregnancy can result in devastating maternal and neonatal complications, including maternal sepsis, preterm labor, and premature delivery [14]. Thirty percent of patients with untreated asymptomatic bacteriuria (ASB) develop symptomatic cystitis and up to 50% develop pyelonephritis [13]. ASB is also associated with intrauterine growth retardation and low-birth-weight infants [13]. Up to 27% of preterm births have been associated with UTI in pregnancy [14].

Among bacterial infections in children, UTI ranks highly, even outnumbering bacterial meningitis, pneumonia, and bacteremia [15]. About 1% of infants < 3 months old develop UTI, with more males affected than females. Proper and urgent UTI management is crucial in children as an estimated 10–15% of children with UTI will develop permanent kidney damage, leading to other chronic diseases such as hypertension and renal insufficiency [16, 17].

The propensity of UTIs to recur, often within a few weeks or months after an initial acute infection, is a problem in UTI management. Approximately 20–30% of women will have a recurrent bladder infection within 6 months after an initial episode, and an additional 3% will experience a third infection [18, 19].

4. *E. coli* UTI pathogenesis

UTI pathogenesis is a complex process that is influenced by various host biological and behavioral factors, and by properties of the infecting pathogen, including VFs. This presents a challenge in epidemiological studies regarding the role of specific VFs in UTI pathogenesis because of the confounding effect of host factors.

In most noncompromised individuals, the urinary tract is normally sterile, and the entry of exogenous microorganisms is prevented by urine flow, secreted and tissue-associated antibacterial factors, and the bactericidal activities of effector immune cells. In most cases, the host fecal flora is the source of the infecting *E. coli* strain, and spreads via the perineal, vaginal, and periurethral areas to the lower urinary tract (i.e., urethra and bladder) where they may establish colonization [20]. Two hypotheses have been proposed to explain the movement of the organism from the fecal flora to the urinary tract. The prevalence hypothesis holds that the numerically most prevalent *E. coli* clones in the feces will be involved, whilst the pathogenicity theory holds that *E. coli* strains with enhanced virulence potential will be selected [20]. These two mechanisms may not be mutually exclusive, but instead may jointly contribute to UTI pathogenesis [21].

Although the host's fecal flora is the major source of the *E. coli* infecting strain, other proximal external reservoirs of the organism have been described. Community outbreaks of UTI have been reported [22–24], but without any evidence of person-to-person transmission. Foods and water have been proposed as possible vehicles of such outbreaks [22–24]. Specifically, extensive molecular similarities between *E. coli* from retail meat products and healthy or infected humans have been described [22]. Within-household spread of *E. coli* among co-habitating humans and their pets, including between sexual partners, have been confirmed [4, 10, 11]. The VFs of the invading bacteria and the host's defense mechanisms determine the outcome of the infection [25]. A variety of host factors, such as age, gender, pregnancy, or immunological status, may predispose to UTI and allow less virulent pathogens to cause the disease [20]. If the infection is confined to the lower urinary tract, with symptoms such as dysuria and frequency of urination, the infection is referred to as acute cystitis. If the infection spreads to the upper urinary tract with symptoms such as flank pain, fever, and malaise, the infection is defined as an acute pyelonephritis.

5. Uropathogenic *E. coli* (UPEC) and virulence factors (VFs)

Virulence refers to the ability of an organism to cause disease, and is a function of the presence of distinct accessory traits, referred to as virulence factors (VFs). VFs are specific properties that enable organisms to overcome host defenses and cause disease [26]. However, although several VFs have been identified in UPEC, experimental and epidemiological data have shown that none uniquely defines these pathogens.

UPEC VFs are grouped by functional categories as adhesins, toxins, iron acquisition systems, and protectins. VFs are encoded by genes located on chromosomes or plasmids, with some being exclusively chromosomal (e.g., *pap* and *hly*), others exclusively or principally plasmid-associated, e.g., *iss* and *traT*, and some either chromosomal or plasmid-associated (*afa*). Consequently, VFs may be vertically or horizontally transmitted, further contributing to the complexity of understanding the role played by specific VF genes in UTI pathogenesis.

6. Structure of adhesins

Adhesins, which appear as hair-like fibers called fimbriae (or pili), facilitate the colonization with *E. coli* in the urinary tract by attaching to host epithelial cells. This attachment promotes the persistence of the organism in the bladder, and serves as a reservoir for ascending infection in the urinary tract [27].

Various adhesins have been identified and are classified mainly according to receptor specificity, with some being mannose resistant and others sensitive. P fimbriae (or pili), the best-described group of mannose-resistant adhesins of UPEC, are so named because they specifically bind to the Gal(α1–4) Gal disaccharide galabiose, which is an antigen within the human P blood group system [26]. Different components of the P fimbriae have been described, including four different units that are at the tip of the fibrillum, including PapG, PapE, PapF, and PapK [28–30]. These fimbrial proteins and other accessory proteins are encoded by a chromosomal multicistronic gene cluster termed *pap* (pilus associated with pyelonephritis), which can be carried on large chromosomal insertions called pathogenicity associated islands (PAIs) [31].

Actual attachment of the organism to host epithelial cells is effected through PapG by recognition of glycolipid receptors expressed on host kidney cells and red blood cells [32]. Three variants of PapG, encoded by distinct alleles of the corresponding gene, *pap*, have been identified, namely PapGI, PapGII, and PapGIII [32–34]. Most studies indicate that allele II is the main PapG variant in *E. coli* bacteremia (regardless of primary source), acute pyelonephritis, and acute prostatitis, whilst allele III predominates in acute cystitis [33, 9]. Other studies found statistically significant associations between allele III and several compromising host conditions, such as urinary anatomical abnormalities, diabetes [33, 35].

Type 1 fimbriae are the commonest adhesive organelles of *E. coli*. They mediate adhesion of the organism to secreted and cell-bound mannosylated glycoproteins and exhibit mannose sensitive hemagglutination of guinea pig erythrocytes [36]. The ubiquitous distribution of these fimbriae in *E. coli* makes it difficult to show an association with UTI outside an experimental setting. However, type 1 fimbriae exhibit several different phenotypes due to allelic variation of the gene for the lectin subunit, fimH, and these phenotypes have been shown to be distributed differentially among fecal and UTI isolates [37–39]. Type 1 fimbriae are encoded by a chromosomal fim gene cluster that contains genes for a structural subunit, an adhesin, several accessory proteins, and regulatory proteins (fimACDFGH) [30, 39].

Phase variation controls the expression of type 1 fimbriae by site specific recombination. A 314-bp phase-variable invertible element, that contains the promoter, controls the transcription of the fimbrial genes fimACDFGH. The promoter drives the expression of type 1 fimbriae when the switch is in the ON orientation but not when it is in the OFF orientation [40]. It has been shown that the expression of type 1 fimbriae coordinately affects the expression of P fimbriae in an inverse manner, providing evidence of a direct communication between genes related to pathogenesis [41, 42].

Although most studies have confirmed that type 1 fimbriae are particularly important in bladder colonization [43, 44], the proportions of UPEC strains from urine and feces expressing type 1 fimbriae appear to be similar [26], ranging from a high of 71% among isolates from cystitis patients to a low of 58% among those from patients with ASB, with fecal strains in the mid-range at 60% [26]. However, in contrast, the level of expression of type 1 fimbriae among UPEC blood isolates (81%) is significantly different from that of fecal strains [45, 46].

Another adhesin family is the Afa/Dr family, which consists of adhesins that include the uropathogen-associated fimbrial adhesin Dr, along with other nonfimbrial adhesins, including Afa-1, Afa-2, Afa-3, Afa 4, NFu1, and Dr-11. These adhesins have a different structure from other *E. coli* fimbrial adhesins in that they appear as fine mesh, a coil-like structure or as a filamentous capsule coating on the cell surface [45, 47, 48]. Epidemiological studies show that *E. coli* strains that express adhesins of the Afa/Dr family are involved in 25–50% of cases of cystitis in children, and 30% of cases of pyelonephritis in pregnant women [49]. Moreover, *E. coli* strains expressing Dr adhesins have been associated with a two-fold increase in the risk of a second UTI. It has also been shown that UPEC encoding the Dr adhesin could survive for more than 1 year within renal tissue [49, 50]. These findings suggest a possible role for Dr/Afa adhesins in recurrent or chronic UTI.

Finally, the closely-related S fimbriae and F1C (fimbriae of serotype 1C), so named because of their binding specificity for terminal sialyl-galactoside residues, mediate X-type mannose resistant hemagglutination of human erythrocytes [51–53]. They agglutinate human and bovine red cells [54, 55]. S fimbriae have a similar, but less well defined, structure to both type 1 and P fimbriae. Just like type 1 and P fimbriae, expression of S fimbriae exhibits phase variation [51]. Binding sites for S fimbriae are located on epithelial cells of the proximal and distal tubules, collecting ducts and glomerulus [55]. In humans, S-fimbriated *E. coli* strains are more closely associated with meningitis and bacteremia than with UTI [56]. They could therefore be important in the movement of the organism from the urinary tract to the blood stream. Few studies have been carried out on the role played by these two types of fimbriae in UTI pathogenesis. FIC fimbriae are expressed by about 14% of UPEC and 7% of *E. coli* fecal isolates [53].

7. Iron acquisition systems for UPEC

Bacteria and the host compete for available iron, which is needed for oxygen transport and storage, DNA synthesis, electron transport, and metabolism of peroxides [57, 58]. Pathogenic bacteria, including UPEC, have devised ways of accessing iron by producing siderophore-mediated iron transport systems. UPEC exhibit multiple mechanisms for extracting iron from the host, mainly siderophore-siderophore receptor systems, but also heme uptake [59–62]. Siderophores, which are secreted low molecular weight molecules, have a high affinity for ferric (Fe^{3+}) iron, which is insoluble as a free cation. UPEC retrieve iron-bound siderophores through receptors that facilitate the transportation of siderophore-iron complexes through the bacterial membrane and into the cytosol where the iron is concentrated and utilized. While all *E. coli* can produce the siderophore enterobactin, production of alternative siderophores has been shown to increase virulence of strains causing bacteremia [10].

Several enterobacteria contain a gene cluster called the high pathogenicity island (HPI), which encodes proteins for biosynthesis of the yersiniabactin siderophore and its uptake system [63, 64]. The HPI is widespread among members of the *Enterobacteriaceae* family, and is essential for virulence in *Yersinia* and certain pathotypes of *E. coli* [63]. One of the important genes residing on the HPI is *fyuA* encoding the 71 kDa outer membrane protein *FyuA* (ferric siderophore uptake), which act as a receptor for Fe-yersiniabactin uptake [65]. FyuA, which was first described in *Yersinia species*, is associated with virulence in many members of the *Enterobacteriaceae* family [65]. Studies by Hancock and Klemm have confirmed that the ferric yersiniabactin receptor (FyuA) is required by UPEC for efficient biofilm formation [66].

Aerobactin is another important hydroxamate siderophore synthesized from the condensation of two lysine and one citrate molecules. In UPEC, the aerobactin system is encoded by a five-gene operon with four genes encoding the enzymes needed for aerobactin synthesis and a fifth encoding the outer membrane receptor protein [67, 68]. The synthesis genes are designated *iuc*, for iron uptake and chelation and the receptor gene is *iut*, for iron uptake and transport [69]. Successive steps in the biosynthesis of aerobactin are catalyzed by the iuc genes and involve hydroxylation of lysine and acetylation of the hydroxyl group to form hydroxamic acid molecules which react with citrate to form aerobactin [69].

Previous studies have shown that the aerobactin system and P fimbriae are commonly found together in UPEC isolates from patients with UTI and urosepsis [70, 71]. However, among urosepsis patient isolates, this association is only true for chromosomally encoded aerobactin [71]. An association of chromosomally encoded aerobactin with hemolysin among urosepsis or UTI patient isolates has also been confirmed [71]. These observations suggest that the association of aerobactin with other VFs differs between plasmid and chromosomal aerobactin. Plasmids carrying the aerobactin region sometimes also carry antimicrobial resistance genes [71–73]. The aerobactin system is found more commonly among UPEC strains from patients with pyelonephritis (73%), cystitis (49%), or bacteremia (58%) than among ASB patient isolates (38%) or fecal strains (41%), which suggest that aerobactin contributes to virulence both within and outside of the urinary tract. The association of aerobactin with more serious forms of UTI is seen specifically in infants, girls, and women [26, 9].

Finally, UPEC produce salmochelins in order to access iron during invasion of the host. The salmochelin siderophore system, so named because it was first shown to be characteristic of *Salmonella* strains [74], is also present in UPEC. This siderophore system is encoded by *iroA* gene cluster, which is made up of five genes, *iroB, iroC, iroD, iroE,* and *iroN*. *iroN* gene encodes an outer membrane siderophore receptor which transports different catechol siderophores, including N-(2,3-dihydroxybenzoy)-L-serine and enterochelin. *iroB* encodes a glucosyltransferase that glucosylates enterobactin, *iroC* encodes an ABC transporter required for transport of salmochelins, whilst *iroD* and *iroE* encode a cytoplasmic esterase, and a periplasmic hydrolase, respectively [75]. The salmochelin receptor iroN may play a dual role as an iron uptake receptor as well as an internalization factor [10]. Using a neonatal rat model, it was shown that *iroN* plays a major role during the bacteremic step of the disease [76]. These findings suggest that *iroN* is associated with increased virulence. Studies by Bauer et al. showed that *iroN* occurred 2.1–4 times more frequently in UTI isolates than in rectal isolates [77].

8. Toxins produced by UPEC

Most hemolytic UPEC strains secrete a heat-labile cytolytic protein toxin known as alpha hemolysin [78], which is encoded by a polycistronic operon, consisting of four genes arranged in the order of hly-CADB [79]. The product of hlyC is important in the activation of the hemolytic toxin, which is the product of the *hlyA* gene. The gene products of *hlyB* and *hlyD* together with TolC are involved in secretion of the hemolysin through the bacterial cell wall [80]. The hemolysin determinants are located on the bacterial chromosome in human isolates of *E. coli*, in contrast to the plasmid location among animal strains [32].

Alpha hemolysin lyses red cells of all mammals and even of fish [81], and is toxic to host cells resulting in inflammation, tissue injury, and impaired host defenses. Hemolysin stimulates super-oxide anion and hydrogen peroxide release from and oxygen consumption by renal tubular cells, including histamine release from mast cells and basophils [82, 83]. Hemolytic uropathogenic strains almost always also express P fimbriae [84]. Hemolysin production is found most commonly in UPEC strains from patients with pyelonephritis (49%), followed by cystitis isolates and ASB [85]. These data demonstrate an association of hemolysin production with invasive uropathogenic strains. UPEC strains that produce increased amounts of alpha hemolysin are also more resistant to the complement action of human serum when compared to strains that are nonhemolytic or produce reduced amounts of hemolysin [81].

UPEC also produce a toxin referred to as cytotoxic necrotising factor type 1 (CNF-1). CNF-1 is a chromosomally encoded UPEC toxin that catalyzes the glutamine deamination of the small GTPases RhoA, Rac, and Cdc 42 [86], leading to the disturbance of numerous eukaryotic cellular functions including formation of actin stress fibers, lamellipodia, filopodia, and modulation of inflammatory signaling pathways [87, 88].

Yamamoto et al. showed that 61% of UTI isolates and 38% of bacteremia isolates produced CNF-1 as opposed to only 10% of commensal fecal isolates [89]. Of these isolates, approximately 98% that produced CNF-1 also produced hemolysin. Studies by Mitsumori et al. showed a

CNF-1 prevalence of 64% among UPEC isolates from prostatitis and 36% from pyelonephritis. These results suggest that CNF-1 is associated with increased virulence in UTI pathogenesis. CNF-1 production may also increase the inflammatory response of the host [90]. Specifically, Elliott et al. reported that CNF-1 evokes edema and necrosis and is associated with inflammation in the intestines of rabbits in a diarrhea model of infection [90]. Human neutrophils have been observed to be less effective at killing CNF-1 positive, than CNF-1 negative bacteria.

9. Protectins

UPEC also express outer membrane proteins, such as traT and Iss, which may enhance serum resistance through avoidance of complement killing [26]. Bacteria are killed by normal human serum through the lytic activity of the complement system [91]. The alternative pathway is activated by bacteria in the absence of specific antibody and plays a more important role in serum killing than the classic pathway [92]. Resistance of *E. coli* to killing by serum results from the individual or combined effects of capsular polysaccharide, O-polysaccharide side chains, and surface proteins [93].

Although the K1 capsule is important in certain strains, other mechanisms appear to be more significant determinants of serum resistance in some populations of *E. coli* isolates. On the whole, smooth strains are more serum resistant than rough strains [94] and the degree of serum resistance is proportional to the amount of lipopolysaccharide (O antigen) the strain contains [95]. Serum-resistant strains are usually more nephropathogenic than comparable serum-sensitive strains in a variety of models of UTI [96, 97] even though these resistant strains may not be associated with increased lethality [96].

9.1. Outer membrane protease T

Outer membrane protease T (OmpT) of *E. coli* is a surface membrane serine protease and is the prototypical member of the omptin family of Gram-negative bacteria [98]. OmpT is an enzyme that catalyzes the activation of plasminogen to plasmin [99, 100], a function that is physiologically relevant for the virulence of *Yersinia pestis* and for clinical *E. coli* isolates [101, 102]. OmpT also plays a role in virulence by cleavage of protamine and other cation peptides with antibiotic activity [103, 104]. Studies by Hui et al. indicated that OmpT promotes *E. coli* persistence in the urinary tract by interfering with the antimicrobial activity of urinary cationic peptides [100].

9.2. Uropathogenic specific protein

Uropathogenic specific protein (Usp) in *E. coli*, which was discovered by chance, is encoded by *usp* located on PAIs [105]. Usp, which is homologous to the *Vibrio cholerae* zonula occludens toxin gene [106], is significantly more prevalent among UPEC isolates than fecal *E. coli* isolates from healthy individuals. Several studies have shown various roles for Usp in UTI pathogenesis in different UTI syndromes and patient groups. Studies by Rijavec et al. showed a strong association between Usp and bacteremia of urinary tract origin, suggesting that Usp is important in the migration of UPEC from the urogenital tract to the blood stream [107]. Other studies have shown comparable prevalences of Usp in cystitis, pyelonephritis, and prostatitis isolates [108]. Furthermore, Usp has (frequently) been associated with all common serotypes of UPEC [109].

10. Biofilm production by UPEC

Biofilm production by *E. coli* is an important VF which may also protect bacteria from antibiotic action and so contribute to resistance [110–113]. Recent studies have shown that biofilm production in *E. coli*, mediated by co-expression of curli and cellulose, supports long-term survival of UPEC in the urinary tract by surrounding the organism with an inert, hydrophobic extracellular matrix [110, 113, 114]. Most studies of biofilm formation in UTI have addressed its role in recurrences.

Curli belong to a class of fibers known as amyloids and are involved in adhesion to surfaces, cell aggregation and, finally, biofilm development. Curli fibers are encoded in the curling subunit gene (*csg*) gene cluster, made up of two differently transcribed operons. One operon codes for *csgB*, *csgA*, and *csgC*, and the other one for *csgD*, *csgE*, and *csgG* [115]. Expression of both curli operons is important for curli fiber assembly. Curli fibers are also essential for internalization of bacteria during an infection [30].

Co-expression of curli and cellulose tends to decrease in prevalence from more severe to less severe UTI, then to commensal isolates, suggesting that biofilm may facilitate progression from the lower to upper urinary tract [110]. Furthermore, co-expression of both biofilm components is associated with a high prevalence of individual VF genes, high VF scores, and phylogenetic group B2, consistent with heightened urovirulence of such strains. Notably, there may be an interaction between classic VFs and biofilm formation. For example, in one study, all isolates that co-expressed both biofilm components also harbored fyuA, implying that iron uptake via the yersiniabactin system may play a significant role in biofilm growth [64]. Additionally, recent studies have shown that the biofilm components, curli fimbriae and cellulose, also play important roles in adhesion, invasion, and long-term survival of UPEC within the host urinary tract [110, 111].

11. Phylogenetic group and VF distribution among patient groups and clinical syndromes

E. coli is commonly classified into four main phylogenetic groups namely A, B1, B2, and D [116] as defined by multilocus enzyme electrophoresis and multilocus sequence typing [117]. Several studies have shown that *E. coli* pathogenic strains from extraintestinal infections mostly derive from group B2, and to a less extent group D [21, 118, 119]. Most studies quote prevalence rates around 63–65% for group B2 in pathogenic strains, and 10–15% for group D [21]. Commensal

E. coli are mainly associated with phylogenetic groups A or B1, and are mainly devoid of virulence determinants [118, 120, 121]. The overlapping associations of VFs and phylogeny with clinical virulence makes it difficult to understand which directly determines virulence. However, some studies in children showed that pyelonephritis isolates more often belonged to group B2, contained on average higher prevalences of individual VF genes, and consequently had higher VF scores than did cystitis or fecal isolates, suggesting that both VF repertoire and phylogenetic background play important roles in UTI pathogenesis.

UTI syndrome-specific differences among *E. coli* clinical and fecal isolates from men are consistent with findings from women, which have shown a gradient of virulence from *E. coli* strains causing more invasive UTI syndromes, such as pyelonephritis and febrile UTI, through those causing cystitis, to fecal strains [9, 122]. However, men are less likely than women or girls, to develop cystitis due to low-virulence strains, which is consistent with a previous observation that isolates from men with febrile UTI appeared relatively virulent, even in the presence of host compromise [122].

In most patient groups, pyelonephritis isolates tend to exhibit the highest prevalences of many individual VFs, have the highest VF scores, and are the most likely to belong to phylogenetic group B2, ST131, and a UTI-associated O type. The reported higher prevalence of pap operon genes (encoding P fimbriae) in pyelonephritis than cystitis isolates correlates with increased tropism for the kidney of P fimbriated strains [121, 123]. papGII has been shown, experimentally, to contribute to pathogenesis of pyelonephritis [124, 125], and OmpT is strongly associated with febrile UTI in men [122, 126]. However, it is not clear whether these VFs act individually or in concert with other known or unknown VFs in causing pyelonephritis.

In men and women, although cystitis and pyelonephritis isolates differ in inferred molecular virulence, phylogenetic group distribution is similar between the two clinical syndromes. However, within each phylogenetic group, VF scores exhibit a gradient across source groups (fecal < cystitis < pyelonephritis), suggesting the presence of different virulence strata within each phylogenetic group, with more virulent strains selectively causing pyelonephritis and less virulent strains being associated with cystitis and fecal isolates in that order. This suggests that VF repertoire is as, or more, important than phylogenetic background for predicting pathogenic behavior in UPEC [122, 127].

Although cystitis and pyelonephritis isolates differ significantly in inferred virulence in various patient groups, no single VF profile is unique to any clinical syndrome or patient group, implying that UTI pathogenesis is multiply determined, as suggested by several previous studies [122, 128]. Thus, intervention strategies based on VF genes might have to involve multiple targets, which would offer the extra advantage of protection against a wide range of UTI syndromes.

12. Transmission of VFs

The genes encoding specific UPEC VFs can be exclusively chromosomal (e.g., *pap* and *hly*); exclusively or principally plasmid-associated (e.g., *iss* and *traT*); or can occur in either location (e.g., the aerobactin operon and afa/drab). Plasmid-borne VFs have an obvious vehicle for horizontal transmission among *E. coli* lineages. Such VFs tend to be distributed more broadly but more sporadically within the species than are chromosomal VFs [129]. Studies have demonstrated that certain VFs commonly occur together, in a way that suggests co-selection or direct genetic linkage [130, 131]. Direct genetic linkage of VFs has been shown on PAIs and plasmids [132–134].

13. Antimicrobial drugs and uropathogenic *Escherichia coli*

Managing UTI caused by UPEC has become challenging over the years due to increasing resistance to the commonly used antibiotics [135–139], which poses a great threat to future capacity to treat UTI caused by UPEC. Although TMP-SMX has traditionally been used as a first-line treatment for UTI [140], there are reports of increased resistance to this antibiotic, which in some countries is in the range 15–20% [137]. Many UPEC strains resistant to TMP-SMZ are also resistant to amoxicillin and cephalexin. Nitrofurantoin remains highly effective against UPEC, but is mainly used for cystitis treatment due to its inability to attain sufficient serum levels to treat invasive or systemic infections [137], and all have excellent bioavailability and achieve high urinary concentrations. However, increased FQ use has resulted in a rise in the prevalence of resistance, and FQ-resistant *E. coli* has become a major problem in several countries [141].

14. Relationship between antibiotic resistance and virulence or phylogenetic background in UPEC

Previous studies show that in *E. coli* isolates from patients with urosepsis, resistance to antimicrobial agents such as ampicillin, sulfonamides, tetracycline, chloramphenicol, and streptomycin is negatively associated with virulence and a phylogenetic group B2, but positively associated with host compromise (immune deficiency, diabetes, and other urinary anatomical abnormalities) [26]. There is a similar negative association between FQ resistance and VFs and group B2 [142–144]. This suggests that, resistance may provide a greater fitness advantage to *E. coli* than traditional VFs or a group B2 background, allowing them to cause infections in compromised hosts with weakened defenses who are frequently exposed to antibiotics.

15. *E. coli* sequence type 131 (ST131)

Determining the clonal types of UPEC is crucial for understanding the role of clonal spread to emerging antimicrobial resistance, which is important for defining and interrupting transmission pathways. Multidrug-resistant *E. coli* sequence type 131 (ST131) has emerged over the past decade as a globally disseminated cause of extraintestinal infections in humans and animals [145–147]. The recent emergence of this clone has coincided with an increase in antibiotic resistance among *E. coli* generally, suggesting a contributing role for ST131 in resistance.

In contrast to traditional antimicrobial resistant *E. coli*, which mostly derive from low virulence phylogenetic groups A and B1, ST131 derives exclusively from phylogenetic group B2, which is traditionally known to be enriched for VF genes. This, plus limited experimental evidence of virulence and several case reports of unusually severe or fatal extraintestinal infections due to ST131, suggests that the emergence of ST131 may be due to a high virulence potential (in addition to antibiotic resistance) compared with other *E. coli* types. However, despite this, some studies have reported absence of traits commonly associated with B2 phylogeny, particularly adhesins (e.g., P, S, and FIC fimbriae) and toxins (e.g., hemolysin and cnf1).

Most ST131 clinical isolates are FQ resistant, and many are also co-resistant to aminoglycosides and/or trimethoprim-sulfamethoxazole (TMP-SMZ). A minority produces extended-spectrum beta-lactamases (ESBLs) that confer resistance to extended-spectrum cephalosporins. *E. coli* clonal group ST131 may be associated with other beta-lactamases but some isolates are cephalosporin susceptible [148, 149].

Despite limited epidemiological evidence of increased virulence of ST131, a recent study revealed that ST131 exhibits a marked prevalence gradient across source groups, from pyelonephritis to cystitis isolates, and finally to fecal isolates [126]. This is consistent with increased urovirulence, and provides epidemiological evidence of increased virulence for ST131, which has been presumed but without evidence from experimental animal models [8, 150]. The antibiotic resistance advantage, in combination with the possible presence of enhanced virulence, could explain the recent worldwide emergence of ST131. The increasing prevalence of ESBL-producing *E. coli* has been associated with the emergence of CTX-M-ST131 pandemic clonal group [151]. Available evidence supports that ST131 is an important contributor to the spread of ESBLs among reproductive-age women in some regions, albeit limited research in many parts worldwide [141, 152].

Four VF genes (*iutA, ompT, usp,* and *traT*) are associated with ST131 isolates, and so could represent potential targets for vaccines or other interventions, particularly if a functional role in virulence or dissemination can be demonstrated for them. Most of the ST131 isolates (85%) are of the O25b variant, and the remainder are type O16 [153, 154].

Resistance of ST131 to extended-spectrum cephalosporins is often due to production of ESBLs. The initial descriptions of ST131 emphasized its association with CTX-M-15, but subsequent studies have shown that it is more commonly ESBL-negative but FQ-resistant [154–156]. Previous studies in Australia and Japan showed that ST131-O25b, ST131-O16, and group D-ST405 clonal groups contribute to the spread of ESBL-producing *E. coli* [151, 152]. The dominant ESBL, in *E. coli*, globally and in Australia [157] is CTX-M-15, which is frequently encoded on plasmids carried by the ST131 pandemic clonal group.

16. Conclusions

A wide range of UPEC VFs have been established epidemiologically or experimentally (*in vivo*) as being important in UTI pathogenesis. No single VF profile has been proven to be important in causing any particular UTI syndrome. Indeed, studies have suggested that

UTI pathogenesis is multiply determined. Thus, intervention strategies based on VF genes might have to involve multiple targets, which would offer the extra advantage of protection against a wide range of UTI syndromes. This observation, which is in agreement with previous studies, provides evidence that VF repertoire is as, or more, important than phylogenetic background for predicting pathogenic behavior in UPEC.

The prevalence of antibiotic resistance among human urine *E. coli* isolates has risen substantially in recent years, especially to first line agents such as fluoroquinolones and trimethoprim-sulphamethoxazole. Furthermore, multidrug-resistant *E. coli* ST131 has shown rapid global dissemination among humans and animals, which has coincided with the general increase in resistance among *E. coli* clinical isolates. A better understanding of the microbiological basis for the emergence of UPEC antibiotic resistance is necessary for guiding efforts aimed at interrupting this process. Further studies on ST131 are clearly needed to explain its impressive emergence so that control measures can be devised and implemented.

Author details

Timothy Kudinha

Address all correspondence to: tkudinha@yahoo.com

Charles Sturt University, Orange, NSW, Australia

References

[1] Draghijeva E. Virulence factors in *Escherichia coli* from children with pyelonephritis. Clinical Microbiology and Infection. 1999;**6**:328-333

[2] Leroy S, Chalumeau T, Ulinski T, et al. Impressive renal damage after acute pyelonephritis in a child. Pediatric Nephrology. 2010;**25**:1365-1368

[3] Prakash Kalra OM, Raizada A. Approach to a patient with urosepsis. Journal of Global Infectious Diseases. 2009;**1**:57-63

[4] Foxman B, Barlow R, D'Arcy H, Gillespie B, Solbel J. Urinary tract infection: Self-reported incidence and associated costs. Annals of Epidemiology. 2000;**10**:509-515

[5] Foxman B, Brown P. Epidemiology of urinary tract infections: Transmission and risk factors, incidence, and costs. Infectious Disease Clinics of North America. 2003;**17**:227-241

[6] Griebling TL. Urologic diseases in America project: Trends in resource use for urinary tract infections in men. Journal of Urology. 2005;**173**:1288-1294

[7] Ikram R, Rebecca Psutka R, Carter A, Priest P. An outbreak of multi-drug resistant *Escherichia coli* urinary tract infection in an elderly population: A case-control study of risk factors. BMC Infectious Diseases. 2015;**15**:224

[8] Johnson JR, Porter SB, Zhanel G, Kuskowski MA, Denamur E. Virulence of *Escherichia coli* clinical isolates in a murine sepsis model in relation to sequence type ST131 status, fluoroquinolone resistance, and virulence genotype. Infection and Immunity. 2012;**80**:1554-1562

[9] Ruiz J, Simon K, Horcajada JP, Velasco M, Barranco M, Roig G, Moreno-Martinez A, Martinez JA, Jimenez de Anta T, Mensa J, Vila J. Differences in virulence factors among clinical isolates of *Escherichia coli* causing cystitis and pyelonephritis in women and prostatitis in men. Journal of Clinical Microbiology. 2002;**40**:4445-4449

[10] Zhang L, Foxman B. Molecular epidemiology of *Escherichia coli* mediated urinary tract infections. Frontiers in Bioscience. 2003;**8**:e235–e244

[11] Johnson JR, Kuskowski MA, O'Bryan TT, Colodner R, Raz R. Virulence genotype and phylogenetic origin in relation to antibiotic resistance profile among *Escherichia coli* urine sample isolates from Israeli women with acute uncomplicated cystitis. Antimicrobial Agents and Chemotherapy. 2005;**49**:26-31

[12] Lipsky BA. Urinary tract infections in men. Epidemiology, pathophysiology, diagnosis, and treatment. Annals of Internal Medicine. 1989;**110**:138-150

[13] Gupta K, Stamm WE. Urinary tract infections. In: Dale DC, Federman DD, editors. ACP Medicine. New York: WebMD; 2005. Section 7, chap. 23

[14] Ovalle A, Levancini M. Urinary tract infections in pregnancy. Current Opinion in Urology. 2001;**11**:55-59

[15] Wald E. Urinary tract infections in infants and children: A comprehensive overview. Current Opinion in Pediatrics. 2004;**16**:85-88

[16] Schlager TA. Urinary tract infections in children younger than 5 years of age: Epidemiology, diagnosis, treatment, outcomes and prevention. Paediatrics Drugs. 2001;**3**: 219-227

[17] Chen M, Jahnukainen T, Bao W, Dare E, Ceccatelli S, Celsi G. Uropathogenic *Escherichia coli* toxins induce caspase-independent apoptosis in renal proximal tubules via ERK signaling. American Journal of Nephrology. 2003;**23**:140-151

[18] Scholes D, Hooton TM, Roberts PL, Stapleton AE, Gupta K, Stamm WE. Risk factors for recurrent urinary tract infection in young women. The Journal of Infectious Diseases. 2000;**182**:1177-1182

[19] Eto DS, Jones TA, Sundsbak JL, Mulvey MA. Integrin-mediated host cell invasion by type-1piliated uropathogenic *E. coli*. PLos Pathogens. 2007;**3**:e100, 0949-0960

[20] Moreno E, Andreu A, Perez T, Sabate M, Johnson JR, Prats G. Relationship between *Escherichia coli* strains causing urinary tract infection in women and the dominant faecal flora of the same hosts. Epidemiology and Infection. 2006;**134**:1015-1023

[21] Moreno E, Andreu A, Pigrau C, Kuskowski MA, Johnson JR, Prats G. Relationship between *Escherichia coli* strains causing acute cystitis in women and the fecal *E. coli* population of the host. Journal of Clinical Microbiology. 2008;**46**:2529-2534

[22] Manges AR, Johnson JR, Foxman B, O'Bryan TT, Fullerton KE, Riley LW. Widespread distribution of urinary tract infections caused by a multidrug-resistant *Escherichia coli* clonal group. The New England Journal of Medicine. 2001;**345**:1007-1013

[23] Manges AR, Tabar H, Tellis P, Vincent C, Tellier PP. Endemic and epidemic lineages of *Escherichia coli* that cause urinary tract infections. Emerging Infectious Diseases. 2008;**14**:1575-1583

[24] Pitout JD, Gregson DB, Church DL, Elsayed S, Laupland KB. Community-wide outbreaks of clonally related CTX-M-14 beta-lactamase-producing *Escherichia coli* strains in the Calgary health region. Journal of Clinical Microbiology. 2005;**43**:2844-2849

[25] Svanborg C, Bergsten G, Fischer H, et al. Uropathogenic *Escherichia coli* as a model of host-parasite interaction. Current Opinion in Microbiology. 2005;**9**:33-39

[26] Johnson JR. Virulence factors in *Escherichia coli* urinary tract infection. Clinical Microbiology Reviews. 1991;**4**:80-128

[27] Mobley HL, Island MD, Massad G. Virulence determinants of uropathogenic *Escherichia coli* and *Proteus mirabilis*. Kidney International Supplements. 1994;**47**:S129-S136

[28] Kuehn MJ, Heuser J, Normark S, Hultgren SJ. P pili in uropathogenic *E. coli* are composite fibres with distinct fibrillar adhesive tips. Nature. 1992;**356**:252-255

[29] Xiang-Qi Mu, Bullitt E. PNAS. Structure and assembly of P-pili: A protruding hinge region used for assembly of a bacterial adhesion filament. 2006;**26**:9861-9866. DOI: 10.1073_pnas.0509620103

[30] Antao E, Wieler LH, Ewers C. Adhesive threads of extraintestinal pathogenic *Escherichia coli*. A review. Gut Pathogens. 2009;**1**:22

[31] Lane MC, Mobley HL. Role of P-fimbrial-mediated adherence in pyelonephritis and persistence of uropathogenic *Escherichia coli* (UPEC) in the mammalian kidney. Kidney International. 2007;**72**:19-25

[32] Johnson JR. *papG* alleles among *Escherichia coli* strains causing urosepsis: Associations with other bacterial characteristics and host compromise. Infection and Immunity. 1998;**66**:4568-4571

[33] Johnson JR, Brown JJ, Maslow JN. Clonal distribution of the three alleles of the Gal (α1-4) Gal-specific adhesin gene *papG* among *Escherichia coli* strains from patients with bacteremia. The Journal of Infectious Diseases. 1998;**177**:651-661

[34] Manning SD, Zhang L, Foxman B, Spindler A, Tallman P, Marrs CF. Prevalence of known P-fimbrial G alleles in *Escherichia coli* and identification of a new adhesin class. Clinical and Diagnostic Laboratory Immunology. 2001;**8**:637-640

[35] Flores-Mireles AL, Walker JN, Caparon M, and Hultgren SJ. Urinary tract infections: Epidemiology, mechanisms of infection and treatment options. Nature Reviews Microbiology. 2015;**13**:269-284

[36] O'Hanley P, Low D, Romero I, Lark D, Vosti K, Falkow S, et al. Gal-Gal binding and haemolysin phenotypes and genotypes associated with uropathogenic *Escherichia coli*. The New England Journal of Medicine. 1985;**313**:414-420

[37] Sokurenko EV, Chesnokova V, Doyle RJ, Hasty DL. Diversity of the *Escherichia coli* type 1 fibrial lectin. Journal of Biological Chemistry. 1997;**272**:17880-17886

[38] Sokurenko EV, Chesnokova V, Dykhuizen DE, Ofek I, Wu XR, Krogfelt KA, Struve C, Schembri MA, Hasty DL. Pathogenic adaptation of *Escherichia coli* by natural variation of the FimH adhesion. Proceedings of the National Academy of Sciences of the United States of America. 1998;**95**:8922-8926

[39] Schembri MA, Klemm P. Coordinate gene regulation by fimbriae induced signal transduction. EMBO Journal. 2001;**20**:3074-3081

[40] Simms AN, Mobley HLT. Multiple genes repress motility in uropathogenic *Escherichia coli* constitutively expressing type 1 fimbriae. Journal of Bacteriology. 2008;**190**:3747-3756

[41] Snyder JA, Hagen BJ, Lockatell CV, Maroncle N, Hagan EC, Johnson DE, Welch RA, Mobley HLT. Coordinate expression of fimbriae in uropathogenic *E. coli*. Infection and Immunity. 2005;**73**:7588-7596

[42] Schwan WR, Lee JL, Lenard FA, Matthews BT, Beck MT. Osmolarity and pH growth conditions regulate fim gene transcription and type 1 pilus expression in uropathogenic *Escherichia coli*. Infection and Immunity. 2002;**70**:1391-1402

[43] Hull RA, Donovan WH, Del Terzo M, Stewart C, Rogers M, and Darouiche RO. Role of Type 1 fimbria- and P fimbria-specific adherence in colonization of the neurogenic human bladder by *Escherichia coli*. Infection and Immunity. 2002;**70**:6481-6484

[44] Staerk K, Khandige S, Kolmos HJ, Moeller-Jensen J, Anderson TE. Uropathogenic *Escherichia coli* express type 1 fimbriae only in surface adherent populations under physiological growth conditions. The Journal of Infectious Diseases. 2016;**213**:386-394

[45] Opal SM, Gemski AS, Lyhte LW. Aerobactin and alpha-hemolysin as virulence determinants in *Escherichia coli* isolated from human blood, urine and stool. The Journal of Infectious Diseases. 1990;**161**:794-796

[46] Johnson JR, Roberts PL, Stamm WE. P fimbriae and other virulence factors in *Escherichia coli* urosepsis: Association with patients' characteristics. The Journal of Infectious Diseases. 1987;**156**:225-229

[47] Arthur M, Johnson CE, Rubin RH, Arbeit RD, Campanelli C, Kim C, Steinbach S, Agarwal M, Wilkinson R, Goldstein R. Molecular epidemiology of adhesin and hemolysin virulence factors among uropathogenic *Escherichia coli*. Infection and Immunity. 1989;**57**:303-313

[48] Orskov I, Orskov F. Serologic classification of fimbriae. Current Topics in Microbiology and Immunology. 1990;**151**:71-90

[49] Nowicki B, Selavarangan R, Nowicki S. Family of *Escherichia coli* Dr adhesins: Decay-accelerating factor recognition and invasiveness. The Journal of Infectious Diseases. 2001;**183**:524-527

[50] Servin, AL. Pathogenesis of Afa/Dr diffusely adhering *Escherichia coli*. Clinical Microbiology Reviews. 2005;**18**:264-292

[51] Mulvey MA. Adhesion and entry of uropathogenic *Escherichia coli*. A mini review. Cell Microbiology. 2002;**4**:257-271

[52] Mitsumori K, Terai A, Yamamoto S, Yoshid O. Identification of S, F1C and three PapG fimbrial adhesins in uropathogenic *Escherichia coli* by polymerase chain reaction. FEMS Immunology and Medical Microbiology. 1998;**21**:261-268

[53] Khan SA, Kniep B, Oelschlaeger TA, Van Die I, Korhonen T, Hacker J. Receptor structure for F1C fimbriae of uropathogemic *Escherichia coli*. Infection and Immunity. 2000; **68**:3541-3547

[54] Virkola R, Parkkinen J, Hacker J, Korhonen TK. Sialyloligosaccharide chains of laminin as an extracellular matrix target for S fimbriae of *Escherichia coli*. Infection and Immunity. 1993;**61**:4480-4484

[55] Korhonen TK, Virkola R, Holthofer H. Localization of binding sites for purified *Escherichia coli* P fimbriae in the human kidney. Infection and Immunity. 1986;**54**:328-332

[56] Ott M, Hacker J, Schmoll T, Jarchau T, Korhonen TK, Goebel W. Analysis of the genetic determinants coding for the S-fimbrial adhesion (*sfa*) in different *Escherichia coli* strains causing meningitis or urinary tract infections. Infection and Immunity. 1986;**54**:646-653

[57] Andrews SC, Robinson AK, Rodríguez-Quiñones F. Bacterial iron homeostasis. FEMS Microbiology Reviews. 2003;**27**:215-237

[58] Bagg A, Neilands JB. Ferric uptake regulation protein acts as a repressor, employing iron (II) as a cofactor to bind the operator of an iron transport operon in *Escherichia coli*. Biochemistry. 1987;**26**:5471-5477

[59] Russo TA, Carlino UB, Johnson JR. Identification of *ireA*, a novel iron regulated virulence gene in an extraintestinal pathogenic isolate of *Escherichia coli*. Infection and Immunity. 2001;**69**:6209-6216

[60] Torres AG, Redford P, Welch RA, Payne SM. TonB-dependent systems of uropathogenic *Escherichia coli*: Aerobactin and heme transport and TonB are required for virulence in the mouse. Infection and Immunity. 2001;**69**:6179-6185

[61] Watts RE, Totsika M, Challinor VL, Mabbett AN, Ulett GC, De Voss JJ, Schembri MA. Contribution of siderophore systems to growth and urinary tract colonization of asymptomatic bacteriuria *Escherichia coli*. Infection and Immunity. 2011;**80**:333-3434

[62] Garcia EC, Brumbaugh AR, Mobley HLT. Redundancy and specificity of *Escherichia coli* iron acquisition systems during urinary tract infection. Infection and Immunity. 2011;**79**:1225-1235

[63] Schubert S, Rakin A, Heesenman J. The Yersinia high-pathogenicity island (HPI). Evolutionary and functional aspects. International Journal of Medical Microbiology. 2004;**274**:883-894

[64] Hancock V, Ferrieres L, Klemm P. The ferric yersiniabactin uptake receptor *fyuA* is required for efficient biofilm formation by urinary tract infections *Escherichia coli* in human urine. Microbiology. 2008;**154**:167-175

[65] Schubert S, Picard B, Gouriou AS, Heesemann J, Denamur E. Yersinia high-pathogenicity island contributes to virulence in *Escherichia coli* causing extraintestinal infections. Infection and Immunity. 2002;**70**:5335-5337

[66] Hancock V, Klemm P. Global gene expression profiling of asymptomatic bacteriuria *Escherichia coli* during biofilm growth in human urine. Infection and Immunity. 2007;**75**:966-976

[67] Carbonetti NH, Boonchai S, Parry SH, Väisänen-Rhen V, Korhonen TK, Williams PH. Aerobactin-mediated iron uptake by *Escherichia coli* isolates from human extraintestinal infections. Infection and Immunity. 1986;**51**:966-968

[68] Crosa JH. Genetics and molecular biology of siderophore-mediated iron transport in bacteria. Microbiological Reviews. 1989;**53**:517-530

[69] De Lorenzo V, Bindereif A, Paw BH, Neilands JB. Aerobactin biosynthesis and transport genes of plasmid Co1V-K30 in *Escherichia coli* K-1. Journal of Bacteriology. 1986;**165**:570-578

[70] Jacobson SH, Hammarlind M, Lidefeldt KJ, Osterberg E, Tullus K, Brauner A. Incidence of aerobactin-positive *Escherichia coli* strains in patients with symptomatic urinary tract infection. European Journal of Clinical Microbiology and Infectious Diseases. 1988;**7**:630-634

[71] Colonna B, Nicoletti M, Visca P, Casalino M, Valenti P, Maimone F. Composite IS1 elements encoding hydroxamate-mediated iron uptake in FIme plasmids from epidemic *Salmonella* spp. Journal of Bacteriology. 1985;**162**:307-316

[72] Bennett PM. Plasmid encoded antibiotic resistance: Acquisition and transfer of antibiotic resistance genes in bacteria. British Journal of Pharmacology. 2008;**153**:S347-S357

[73] Phillips I, Eykyn S, King A, Gransden WR, Rowe B, Frost JA, Gross RJ. Epidemic multiresistant *Escherichia coli* infection in West Lambeth Health District. Lancet. 1988;**7**:1038-1041

[74] Hantke K, Nicholson G, Rabsch W, Winkelmann G. Salmochelins, siderophores of *Salmonella enterica* and uropathogenic *Escherichia coli* strains, are recognized by the outer membrane receptor *iroN*. Proceedings of the National Academy of Sciences of the United States of America. 2002;**100**:3677-3682

[75] Caza M, Lepine F, Milot S, Dozois CM. Specific roles of the *iroBCDEN* genes in virulence of an avian pathogenic *Escherichia coli* O78 strain and in production of salmochelins. Infection and Immunity. 2008;**76**:3539-3549

[76] Negre VL, Bonacorsi S, Schubert S, Bidet P, Nassif X, Bingen E. The siderophore receptor iroN but not the high-pathogenicity island or the hemin receptor chuA contributes to the bacteremic step of *Escherichia coli* neonatal meningitis. Infection and Immunity. 2004;**72**:1216-1220

[77] Bauer R, Zhang L, Foxman B, Siitonen A, Jantunen M, Saxen H, Marrs C. Molecular epidemiology of 3 putative virulence genes for *Escherichia coli* urinary tract infection-*usp, iha, and* $iroN_{(E.\ coli)}$. Journal of Infectious Diseases. 2002;**185**:1521-1524

[78] Kucheria R, Dasgupta P, Sacks SH, Khan MS, Sheerin NS. Urinary tract infections: New insights into a common problem. Postgraduate Medical Journal. 2005;**81**:83-86

[79] Burgos Y, Benton L. Common origin of plasmid encoded alpha-hemolysin genes in *Escherichia coli*. BMC Microbiology. 2010;**193**:1-13

[80] Holland IB, Schimdt L, Young J. Type I protein secretion in bacteria, the ABC-transport dependent pathway (review). Molecular Membrane Biology. 2005;**22**:29-39

[81] Birosova E, Siegfried L, Kmetova M, et al. Detection and virulence factors in alpha-haemolytic *Escherichia coli* strains isolated from various clinical materials. CMI. 2004;**10**:569-573

[82] König B, König W, Scheffer J, Hacker J, Goebel W. Role of *Escherichia coli* alpha-hemolysin and bacterial adherence in infection: Requirement for release of inflammatory mediators from granulocytes and mast cells. Infection and Immunity. 1986;**54**:886-892

[83] Scheffer J, König W, Hacker J, Goebel W. Bacterial adherence and hemolysin production from *Escherichia coli* induces histamine and leukotriene release from various cells. Infection and Immunity. 1985;**50**:271-278

[84] Czirók E, Milch H, Csiszár K, Csik M. Virulence factors of *Escherichia coli*. Correlation with *Escherichia coli* pathogenicity of haemolysin production, haemagglutinating capacity, antigens K1, K5, and colicinogenicity. Acta Microbiologica Hungarica. 1986;**33**:69-83

[85] Marrs C, Zhang L, Foxman B. *Escherichia coli* mediated urinary tract infections: Are there distinct uropathogenic *E.coli* (UPEC) pathotypes? FEMS Microbiology Letters. 2005;**252**:183-190

[86] Lemonnier M, Landraud L, Lemichez E. Rho GTPase-activating bacterial toxins: From bacterial virulence regulation to eukaryotic cell biology. FEMS Microbiology Review. 2007;**31**:515-534

[87] Etienne-Manneville S, Hall A. Rho GTPases in cell biology. Nature. 2002;**420**:629-635

[88] Bower JM, Eto DS, Mulvey MA. Covert operations of uropathogenic *Escherichia coli* within the urinary tract. Traffic. 2005;**6**:18-31

[89] Yamamoto S, Terai A, Yuri K, Kurazono H, Takeda Y, Yoshida O. Detection of uro-virulence factors in *Escherichia coli* by multiplex polymerase chain reaction. FEMS Immunology & Medical Microbiology. 1995;**12**:85-90

[90] Rippere-Lampe KE, O'Brien AD, Conrau R, Lockman HA. Mutation of the gene encoding cytotoxic necrotizing factor type 1 (cnf1) attenuates the virulence of uropathogenic *Escherichia coli*. Infection and Immunity. 2001;**69**:3954-3964

[91] Elliott SJ, Srinivas S, Albert MJ, et al. Characterization of the roles of hemolysin and other toxins in enteropathy caused by alpha-hemolytic *Escherichia coli* linked to human diarrhea. Infection and Immunity. 1998;**66**:2040-2051

[92] Taylor PW. Bactericidal and bacteriolytic activity of serum against gram-negative bacteria. Microbiological Reviews. 1983;**47**:46-83

[93] Montenegro MA, Bitter-Suermann D, Timmis JK, et al. *traT* gene sequences, serum resistance and pathogenicity-related factors in clinical isolates of *Escherichia coli* and other gram-negative bacteria. The Journal of General and Applied Microbiology. 1985;**131**:1511-1521

[94] Timmis KN, Boulnois GJ, Bitter-Suermann D, Cabello FC. Surface components of *Escherichia coli* that mediate resistance to the bactericidal activities of serum and phagocytes. Current Topics in Microbiology and Immunology. 1985;**118**:197-218

[95] Goldman RC, Joiner K, Leive L. Serum-resistant mutants of *Escherichia coli* O111 contain increased lipopolysaccharide, lack an O antigen-containing capsule, and cover more of their lipid A core with O antigen. Journal of Bacteriology. 1984;**159**:877-882

[96] Domingue GJ, Laucirica R, Baliga P, Covington S, Robledo JA, Li SC. Virulence of wild-type *E. coli* uroisolates in experimental pyelonephritis. Kidney International. 1998;**34**:761-765

[97] Iwahi T, Abe Y, Tsuchiya K. Virulence of *Escherichia coli* in ascending urinary-tract infection in mice. Journal of Medical Microbiology. 1982;**15**:303-316

[98] Mangel W, Toledo DL, Brown MT, Worzalla K, Lee M, Dunn JJ. Omptin: An *Escherichia coli* outer membrane proteinase that activates plasminogen. Methods in Enzymology. 1994;**244**:384-399

[99] Leytus SP, Bowles LK, Konisky K, Mangel WF. Activation of plasminogen to plasmin by a protease associated with outer membrane of *Escherichia coli*. Proceedings of the National Academy of Sciences of the United States America. 1981;**78**:1485-1489

[100] Hui CY, Guo Y, He QS, et al. *Escherichia coli* outer membrane protease OmpT confers resistance to urinary cationic peptides. Microbiology and Immunology. 2010;**54**:452-459

[101] Lundrigan MD, Webb RM. Prevalence of *ompT* among *Escherichia coli* isolates of human origin. FEMS Microbiology Letters. 1992;**76**:51-56

[102] McCarter JD, Stephens D, Shoemaker K, Rosenberg S, Kirsch JF, Georgiou G. Substrate specificity of *Escherichia coli* outer membrane protease ompT. Journal of Bacteriology. 2004;**186**:5919-5925

[103] Guina T, Yi EC, Wang H, Hackett M, Miller SI. A PhoP-regulated outer membrane protease of *Salmonella enterica* serovar Typhimurium promotes resistance to alpha-helical antimicrobial peptides. Journal of Bacteriology. 2000;**182**:4077-4086

[104] Stumpe S, Schmid R, Stephens DL, Georgiou G, Bakker E. Identification of OmpT as the protease that hydrolyzes the antimicrobial peptide protamine before it enters growing cells of *Escherichia coli*. Journal of Bacteriology. 1998;**180**:4002-4006

[105] Kanamura S, Kurazono H, Ishitoya S, et al. Distribution and genetic association of putative uropathogenic virulence factors *iroN, iha, kpsMT, ompT* and *usp* in *Escherichia coli* isolated from urinary tract infections in Japan. Journal of Urology. 2003;**170**:2490-2493

[106] Nakano M, Yamamoto S, Terai A, Ogawa O, Makino S, Hayashi H, Nair GB, Kurazono H. Structural and sequence diversity of the pathogenicity island of uropathogenic *Escherichia coli* which encodes the USP protein. FEMS. 2001;**205**:71-76

[107] Rijavec M, Muller-Premru M, Zakotnik B, Zgur-Bertok D. Virulence factors and biofilm production among *E. coli* strains causing bacteremia of urinary tract origin. Journal of Medical Microbiology. 2008;**57**:1329-1334

[108] Kanamaru S, Kurazono H, Nakano M, Terai A, Ogawa O, Yamamoto S. Subtyping of uropathogenic *Escherichia coli* according to the pathogenicity island encoding uropathogenic-specific protein: Comparison with phylogenetic groups. International Journal of Urology. 2006;**13**:754-760

[109] Yamamoto S. Molecular epidemiology of uropathogenic *Escherichia coli*. Journal of Infection and Chemotherapy. 2007;**13**:68-73

[110] Kai-Larsen Y, Luthje P, Chromek M, et al. Uropathogenic *Escherichia coli* modulates immune responses and its curli fimbriae interact with the antimicrobial peptide LL-37. PLoS Pathogens. 2010;**6**:e1001010

[111] Luthje P, Brauner A. Ag43 promotes persistence of uropathogenic *Escherichia coli* isolates in the urinary tract. Journal of Clinical Microbiology. 2010;**48**:2316-2317

[112] Schroeder M, Brooks BD and Brooks AE. The complex relationship between virulence and antibiotic resistance. Genes (Basel). 2017;**8**:39

[113] Kostakioti M, Hadjifrangiskou M, Hultgren SL. Bacterial biofilms: Development, dispersal, and therapeutic strategies in the dawn of the post-antibiotic era. Cold Spring Harbor Perspectives in Medicine. 2013;**3**:a010306

[114] De la Fuente-Núñez C, Reffuveille F, Fernández L, Hancock RE. Bacterial biofilm development as a multicellular adaptation: Antibiotic resistance and new therapeutic strategies. Current Opinion in Microbiology. 2013;**16** 580-589

[115] Gophna U, Barlev M, Sejffers R, Oelschlager TA, Hacker J, Ron EZ. Curli fibers mediate internalization of *Escherichia coli* by eukaryotic cells. Infection and Immunity. 2001;**69**:2659-2665

[116] Bailey JK, Pinyon JL, Ananthan S, Hall RM. Distribution of human commensal *Escherichia coli* phylogenetic groups. Journal of Clinical Microbiology. 2010;**48**:3455-3456

[117] Johnson JR, Russo TA. Extraintestinal pathogenic *Escherichia coli*: "The other bad *E. coli*." Journal of Clinical Medicine. 2002;**139**:155-162

[118] Kuntaman K, Lestari ES, Severin JA, Kershof, et al. Fluoroquinolone resistant *Escherichia coli*, Indonesia. Emerging Infectious Diseases. 2005;**11**:1363-1369

[119] Takahashi A, Kanamaru S, Kurazono H, Kunishima Y, Tsukamoto T, Ogawa O, Yamamoto S. *Escherichia coli* isolates associated with uncomplicated and complicated cystitis and asymptomatic bacteriuria possess similar phylogenies, virulence genes, and O-serogroup profiles. Journal of Clinical Medicine. 2006;**44**:4589-4592

[120] Picard B, Garcia JS, Gouriou S, et al. The link between phylogeny and virulence in *Escherichia coli* extra-intestinal infection. Infection and Immunity. 1999;**67**:546-553

[121] Johnson JR, Russo TA. Molecular epidemiology of extra-intestinal pathogenic (uropathogenic) *Escherichia coli*. A review. The Indian Journal of Medical Microbiology. 2005;**295**:383-404

[122] Johnson JR, Kuskowski MA, Gajewski A, et al. Extended virulence genotypes and phylogenetic background of *Escherichia coli* isolates from patients with cystitis, pyelonephritis, or prostatitis. The Journal of Infectious Diseases. 2005;**191**:46-50

[123] Johnson JR. Microbial virulence determinants and the pathogenesis of urinary tract infection. Infectious Disease Clinics of North America. 2003;**17**:261-278

[124] Goluszko P, Moseley SL, Truong LD, et al. Development of experimental model of chronic pyelonephritis with *Escherichia coli* O75:K5:H-bearing Dr fimbriae: Mutation in the *dra* region prevented tubulo-interstitial nephritis. Journal of Clinical Investigation. 1997;**99**:1662-1672

[125] Roberts JA, Marklund B, I Ilver D, et al. The Gal alpha (1-4) Gal-specific tip adhesin of *Escherichia coli* P-fimbriae is needed for pyelonephritis to occur in the normal urinary tract. Proceedings of the National Academy of Sciences of the United States of America. 1994;**91**:11889-11893

[126] Kudinha T, Johnson JR, Andrew SD, Kong F, Anderson P, Gilbert GL. Distribution of phylogenetic groups, sequence type ST131, and virulence associated traits among *Escherichia coli* isolates from men with pyelonephritis or cystitis and healthy controls. Clinical Microbiology and Infection. 2013;**19**:E173-E180

[127] Piatti G, Mannini A, Balistreri M, Schito AM. Virulence factors in urinary *Escherichia coli* strains: Phylogenetic background and quinolone and fluoroquinolone resistance. Journal of Clinical Microbiology. 2008;**46**:480-487

[128] Kudinha T, Johnson JR, Andrew SD, Kong F, Anderson P, Gilbert GL. Genotypic and phenotypic characterization of *Escherichia coli* isolates from children with urinary tract infection and from healthy carriers. The Pediatric Infectious Disease Journal. 2013;**32**:543-548

[129] Johnson JR, Delavari P, Kuskowski MA, Stell AL. Phylogenetic distribution of extra-intestinal virulence-associated traits in *Escherichia coli*. The Journal of Infectious Diseases. 2001;**183**:78-88

[130] Johnson JR, Stell AL. Extended virulence genotypes of *Escherichia coli* strains from patients with urosepsis in relation to phylogeny and host compromise. The Journal of Infectious Diseases. 2000;**181**:261-272

[131] Escobar-Páramo P, Clermont O, Blanc-Potard AB, Bui H, Le Bouguénec C, Denamur E. A specific genetic background is required for acquisition and expression of virulence factors in *Escherichia coli*. Molecular Biology and Evolution. 2004;**21**:1085-1094

[132] Dobrindt U, Blum-Oehler G, Hartsch T, et al. S-fimbria-encoding determinant *sfa1* is located on pathogenicity island III_{536} of uropathogenic *Escherichia coli* strain 536. Infection and Immunity. 2001;**69**:4248-4256

[133] Guyer DM, Kao J-S, Mobley HLT. Genomic analysis of a pathogenicity island in uropathogenic *Escherichia coli* CFT 073: Distribution of homologous sequences among isolates from patients with pyelonephritis, cystitis, and catheter-associated bacteriuria and from fecal samples. Infection and Immunity. 1998;**66**:4411-4417

[134] Hacker J, Kaper JB. Pathogenicity islands and the evolution of microbes. Annual Review of Microbiology. 2000;**54**:641-679

[135] Barber AE, Norton JP, Spivak AM, and Mulvey MA. Urinary tract infections: Current and emerging management strategies. Clinical Infectious Diseases. 2013;**57**:719-724

[136] Goettsch W, van Pelt W, Nagelkerke N, et al. Increasing resistance of fluoroquinolones in *Escherichia coli* from urinary tract infections in The Netherlands. Journal of Antimicrobial Chemotherapy. 2000;**46**:223-228

[137] Gupta K, Hooton TM, Stamm WE. Increasing antimicrobial resistance and the management of uncomplicated community-acquired urinary tract infection. Annals of Internal Medicine. 2001;**135**:41-50

[138] Karlowsky JA, Hoban DJ, DeCorby MR, Liang NM, Zhanel GG. Fluoroquinolone resistant urinary isolates of *Escherichia coli* from outpatients are frequently multidrug resistant: Results from the North American Urinary Tract Infection Collaborative Alliance-Quinolone Resistance Study. Antimicrobial Agents and Chemotherapy. 2006;**50**:2251-2254

[139] Wong-Beringer A, Hindler J, Loeff M, et al. Molecular correlation for the treatment outcomes in bloodstream infections caused by *Escherichia coli* and *Klebsiella pneumoniae* with reduced susceptibility to ceftazidime. Clinical Infectious Diseases. 2002;**34**:135-146

[140] Foxman B. Epidemiology of urinary tract infections: Incidence, morbidity, and economic costs. American Journal of Medicine. 2002;**113**:5S-13S

[141] Drews SJ, Poutanen SM, Mazzulli T, et al. Decreased prevalence of virulence factors among ciprofloxacillin-resistant uropathogenic *Escherichia coli* isolates. Journal of Clinical Microbiology. 2005;**43**:4218-4220

[142] Vila J, Simon K, Ruiz J, et al. Are quinolone-resistant uropathogenic *Escherichia coli* less virulent? Journal of Infectious Diseases. 2002;**186**:1039-1042

[143] Velasco M, Horcajada JP, Mensa J, et al. Decreased invasive capacity of quinolone-resistant *Escherichia coli* in patients with urinary tract infections. Clinical Infectious Diseases. 2001;**33**:1682-1686

[144] Johnson JR, Van der Sche C, Kuskowski MA, Goessens W, Van Belkum A. Phylogenetic background and virulence profiles of fluoroquinolone-resistant clinical *Escherichia coli* isolates from the Netherlands. Journal of Infectious Diseases. 2002;**186**:1852-1856

[145] Platell JL, Cobbold RN, Johnson JR, et al. Commonality among fluoroquinolone-resistant sequence type ST131 extra-intestinal *Escherichia coli* isolates from humans and companion animals in Australia. Antimicrobial Agents and Chemotherapy. 2011;**55**:3782-3787

[146] Platell JL, Johnson JR, Cobbold RN, Trott DJ. Multidrug-resistant extra-intestinal *Escherichia coli* of sequence type ST131 in animals and foods. Veterinary Microbiology. 2011;**153**:99-108

[147] Rogers BA, Sidjabat HE, Paterson DL. *Escherichia coli* O25b-ST131: A pandemic, multi-resistant, community-associated strain. Journal of Antimicrobial Chemotherapy. 2011;**66**:1-14

[148] Johnson JR, Menard M, Johnston B, Kuskowski MA, Nichol K, Zhanel GG. Epidemic clonal groups of *Escherichia coli* as a cause of antimicrobial resistant urinary tract infections in Canada, 2002-2004. Journal of Antimicrobial Chemotherapy. 2009;**53**:2733-2739

[149] Cheng MF, Chen WL, Hung WY, et al. Emergence of extended spectrum-β-lactamase-producing *Escherichia coli* O25b-ST131: A major community-acquired uropathogen in infants. The Pediatric Infectious Disease. 2015;**4**:469-475

[150] Lavigne J-P, Vergunst A, Goret L. Virulence potential and genomic mapping of the worldwide clone *Escherichia coli* ST131. PLoS One. 2012;**7**:e34294

[151] Matsamura Y, Yamamoto M, Nagao M, Hotta H, et al. Emergence and spread of B2-ST131-O25b, B2-ST131-O16 and D-ST405 clonal groups among extended-spectrum-β-lactamase-producing *Escherichia coli* in Japan. Journal of Antimicrobial Chemotherapy. 2012;**67**:2612-2620

[152] Kudinha T, Johnson JR, Andrew SD, Kong F, Anderson P, Gilbert GL. *Escherichia coli* sequence type 131 (ST131) as a prominent cause of antimicrobial resistance among clinical and fecal *Escherichia coli* isolates from reproductive-age women. Journal of Clinical Microbiology. 2013;**51**:3270-3276

[153] Zhong YM, Liu WE, Liang XH, Li YM, Jian ZJ, Hawkey PM. Emergence and spread of O16-ST131 and O25b-ST131 clones among faecal CTX-M-producing *Escherichia coli* in healthy individuals in Hunan Province, China. Journal of Antimicrobial Chemotherapy. 2015;**70**:2223-2227

[154] Johnson JR, Johnston B, Clabots C, Kuskowski MA, Castanheira M. *Escherichia coli* sequence type ST131 as the major cause of serious multidrug-resistant *E. coli* infections in the United States. Clinical Infectious Diseases. 2010;**51**:286-294

[155] Cerquetti M, Giufre M, Garcia-Fernandez A, et al. Ciprofloxacin-resistant, CTX-M-15 producing *Escherichia coli* ST131 clone in extraintestinal infections in Italy. Clinical Microbiology and Infection. 2010;**16**:1555-1558

[156] Uchida Y, Mochiman T, Morokuma Y, et al. Clonal spread in Eastern Asia of ciprofloxacin-resistant *Escherichia coli* serogroup O25 strains, and associated virulence factors. International Journal of Antimicrobial Agents. 2010;**35** 444-450

[157] Zong Z, Partridge SR, Thomas L, Iredell JR. Dominance of *blaCTX-M* within an Australian extended-spectrum beta-lactamase gene pool. Antimicrobial Agents and Chemotherapy. 2008;**52**:4198-4202

Chapter 4

Effect of Uropathogenic *Escherichia coli* on Human Sperm Function and Male Fertility

Juana V. Villegas, Rodrigo Boguen and
Pamela Uribe

Additional information is available at the end of the chapter

http://dx.doi.org/10.5772/intechopen.68312

Abstract

Infections of the reproductive tract represent nearly 15% of male infertility cases. The most frequently isolated bacterium in the ejaculate of infertile men is *Escherichia coli* (*E. coli*), which causes between 60 and 85% of cases of chronic bacterial prostatitis leading to sperm damage. The aim of this chapter is to discuss the negative effects of *E. coli* on sperm quality and male fertility. The *E. coli* isolated from semen is uropathogenic (UPEC) and can damage sperm in different ways. UPEC induces activation of polymorphonuclear leukocytes with the release of cytokines and reactive oxygen species, the latter being harmful due to their ability to induce lipid peroxidation and early sperm capacitation. Also, UPEC decreases sperm motility, vitality and mitochondrial membrane potential through direct contact or mediated by its soluble metabolites. The negative effects are higher with strains with specific characteristics such as hemolytic capacity. *In vivo* studies with mice models have shown that UPEC inoculated into the epididymis induces inflammatory damage with testicular mass decrease and low sperm concentration. Future studies are needed to clarify the molecular mechanisms by which *E. coli* damages sperm. This knowledge will make it possible to take measures to avoid deleterious consequences on the fertilizing potential of men.

Keywords: sperm motility, mitochondrial function, reactive oxygen species, infertility

1. Introduction

Infertility is currently a highly prevalent disease, defined by the failure to achieve a successful pregnancy after 12 months or more of appropriate, unprotected intercourse or therapeutic donor insemination [1]. Approximately 50% of infertility cases are attributed to the male [2, 3] due to conditions such as varicocele, cryptorchidism, obstructive problems, hormonal disorders, ejaculatory dysfunction as well as infectious causes classified under male genital tract infection (MGTI).

MGTI accounts for 15% of male infertility cases [4]. MGTIs are an important problem in male reproductive health because they cause negative changes in semen parameters [5]. A consequence of MGTI is the inflammatory response evidenced by leukocytospermia, where a treatment with antibiotics and anti-inflammatory drugs may be helpful to try to recover the patient's fertilizing potential [6]. Principal causes of MGTI are bacteria such as *Staphylococcus epidermidis*, *Streptococcus viridans*, *Staphylococcus aureus* and *Escherichia coli* (*E. coli*), which have a negative effect on the fertilizing potential of a man and are strongly associated with MGTI [7, 8]. However, *E. coli has* been shown to exert greater damaging effects on human spermatozoa [7, 9–11].

E. coli is the causal agent in 65–80% of cases of chronic bacterial prostatis [12], and these bacteria have been isolated from semen in 69% of the patients with this pathology [13]. Moreover, *E. coli* causes diverse MGTIs such as urethritis, epididymitis and orchitis, and it is the most frequently isolated bacterium [4].

With this background, this chapter discusses the negative effect of *E. coli on* sperm quality and male fertility. The chapter will be developed by first addressing the uropathogenic *E. coli strains* associated with male infertility. Then, the evidence of the *in vitro* effects of *E. coli on* the male gamete will be analyzed. Evidences will be described, obtained after *in vitro* co-incubation of normal human spermatozoa with *E. coli and* with polymorphonuclear leukocytes, emulating infection. Next, the effects of *E. coli* on human sperm functions observed by direct incubation of spermatozoa with bacteria and without leukocytes will be discussed. Also, evidence of the effects of the metabolic and soluble products of *E. coli* on human sperm function will be analyzed. To complete the picture of the evidence of the effects of this bacterium on male fertility, some studies on animal models will be reviewed.

2. Uropathogenic strains of *E. coli* are associated with male infertility

Among the different pathogenic strains of *E. coli*, the uropathogenic strains are mainly associated with urinary tract infections (UTI). The pathogenic *E. coli* is classified according to the O antigens. Some of these have been associated with uropathogenic *E. coli* (UPEC) being the serotypes O1, O2, O4, O6, O7, O8, O16, O18, O25, and O75 preferentially associated with these strains [14]. Similarly, the most frequently O antigens associated among the serotypes isolated from patients with prostatitis are O1, O2, O4, O16, O18, O22, O25 and O75 serotypes [15], which coincide with *E. coli* strains isolated in cases of infections to the urinary tract. Regarding to the strains isolated from semen of infertile men, the described prevalent antigens are O1, O2, O4 and O6 [16]. These data indicate that the *E. coli* that infects the male reproductive tract is uropathogenic strain, which is not surprising considering the proximity of the urinary and reproductive tracts.

3. Effect of *E. coli* on human spermatozoa is induced through seminal leukocytes

One way *E. coli* induces damage in spermatozoa is by mediating seminal leukocyte activation. The increased presence of leukocytes in semen, known as leukocytospermia, is defined by a concentration equal to or greater than 1 x 10^6 leukocytes per ml of semen [17]. Proinflammatory cytokines, which are usually released by leukocytes during the inflammatory response, are able to decrease sperm motility by themselves [5, 18, 19]. This damaging effect seems to be mediated by polymorphonuclear (PMN) leukocytes instead of by other leukocytes such as lymphocytes or monocytes [20]. The decrease in sperm quality is also mediated by reactive oxygen species (ROS) released by PMN after bacteria-induced activation, with *E. coli* being able to induce a higher response of increased ROS production than other bacteria [9]. Other consequences of ROS released by leukocytes are lipid peroxidation, which affects sperm plasma membrane [21, 22], and early induction of sperm capacitation, which should normally occur later in the female reproductive tract [23].

4. *E. coli* directly affects human sperm function

The direct effect of *E. coli* on sperm was demonstrated through *in vitro* studies performed by directly incubating both cells. It has been demonstrated by several authors that *E. coli* coming into contact with spermatozoa causes decreased sperm motility [7, 24–26]. The decrease in sperm motility due to *E. coli* has been attributed for many years to an agglutinating effect on sperm [27]. Sperm agglutination can be caused by bacterial type 1 and P fimbriae; specifically, the type 1 fimbriae of *E. coli* cause a pattern of head-head type agglutination because they bind mannose residues in the head region of sperm. Instead, type P fimbriae of *E. coli* cause a head-tail agglutination pattern because they bind gal-gal receptors present along the sperm [28].

Electron microscopy has revealed that this bacterium causes damage primarily in the head of spermatozoa, such as rupture of the plasma membrane, vesicle formation and rupture of the inner and outer membranes of the acrosome [29].

Consistent with the plasma membrane damages observed, another report showed that *E. coli* per se causes phosphatidylserine translocation, a cell death indicator [9]. From the point of view of sperm cell death, it was observed that *E. coli* endotoxins such as lipopolysaccharide (LPS), peptidoglycan and porins produce loss of sperm viability [30]. Moreover, it has been shown that LPS and porins cause sperm DNA fragmentation [31]. The effects of these endotoxins are mediated by the toll-like receptor (TLR)-2 and TLR-4, both present in sperm. After TLR-2 and TLR-4 stimulation, sperm damage highlighting DNA fragmentation can be observed [32].

Another direct effect of *E. coli* is at the level of mitochondrial membrane potential ($\Delta\Psi m$). The *in vitro* observation that contact with *E. coli* decreases the $\Delta\Psi m$ together with the motility in spermatozoa [33] was followed by another report showing, also *in vitro,* that *E. coli* directly reduces sperm ΔΨm and alters plasma membrane stability [34]. From the point of view of sperm function, it has been observed that ΔΨm is positively correlated with sperm motility *in vivo* [35, 36]. However, after contact with some strains of *E. coli,* which decrease sperm motility *in vitro,* they had no effect on ΔΨm [37]. This study also found that some *E. coli* isolated from different patients was unable to decrease sperm motility, remarkably even an O6, which is thought to be a highly uropathogenic strain in urinary tract infections [38]. These facts contrast with the notion that *E. coli* in general alters sperm function. These differences could be attributed to the fact that different strains bear specific but different characteristics from other *E. coli* strains. Evidence confirming this was observed in our work, when sperm were incubated with a hemolytic strain of *E. coli.* This strain caused a decrease in motility, ΔΨm, vitality and an increase in intracellular ROS in normal spermatozoa. These effects were not observed with other strains non-hemolysis producers [39]. These differences among strains highlight the importance of knowing what kind of toxins are effectively produced by the *E. coli* strain infecting a patient, because it could indicate the level of sperm damage to be expected. As example, hemolytic *E. coli* strains produce the alpha-hemolysin (HlyA) toxin [40], a calcium-dependent pore-forming toxin which has intracellular effects, inactivating pathways related to cell survival [41]. This toxin can be highly relevant, particularly if we consider that between 40 and 50% of *E. coli* strains isolated from patients with epididymitis release this toxin [42].

Evidence of *E. coli* effects on human spermatozoa shows that this bacterium impairs sperm quality, principally causing decreased motility; nevertheless, there are other consequences for sperm quality, specifically the incubation of sperm with *E. coli* decreases the ability of the male gamete to penetrate the oocyte, the most important step in the function of the spermatozoon [43].

5. Soluble products of *E. coli* also affect human sperm function

The effects of *E. coli* soluble products on sperm have been studied using supernatants of *E. coli* culture as a source of bacterial metabolic product. It has been reported that although the direct contact with *E. coli* was able to alter sperm motility, the metabolic products of *E. coli* had no effect on decreasing motility in human spermatozoa [24]. However, after this report, it was shown that incubation with the soluble factors of *E. coli* reduced sperm motility and ΔΨm [33]. Added to this, the ability of *E. coli* soluble factors to decrease motility, viability, ΔΨm and increase ROS in spermatozoa can be prevented by lactobacilli. In an *in vitro* experiment, after adding lactobacilli to simulate the normal condition in the female genital tract, the harmful effects of *E. coli* soluble factors were inhibited [44].

Among the soluble factors of *E. coli,* a component called spermatozoa immobilization factor (SIF) was first described in 1977. The effect of SIF, as the name implies, is to immobilize spermatozoa, and this effect could be reversed by washing the spermatozoa [45]. Years later, an apparently similar SIF of 56 kDa was isolated and purified from supernatants of a strain of *E. coli.* SIF-56 decreases sperm motility completely and almost instantaneously. It was also observed that SIF-56 at very high concentrations can even induce sperm death [46]. Sperm immobilization mediated by SIF-56 has been shown to depend on 115 kDa-receptor present in sperm [47]. Another *E. coli*

http://dx.doi.org/10.5772/intechopen.68312

soluble factor described is the sperm agglutinating factor (SAF) of 71 kDa, which produces sperm agglutination, decreases ATPase activity and can cause sperm death [48]. A toxin candidate to be further investigated is HlyA, because this toxin is produced by *E. coli* strains most pathogenic to sperm both *in vitro* and *in vivo* [42].

6. Animal model research

In vitro investigations have the disadvantage of not necessarily representing what would happen *in vivo*. Hence, *in vivo* studies in animal models allow us to get closer to the reproductive reality of a man with accessory glands infected by *E. coli*. That is how the progressive reduction of testicular size with a consequent decrease in sperm count caused by the necrotic death of the testicular germ cell has been described in rats inoculated with *E. coli* [49]. After three days of injecting rats with HlyA producing *E. coli*, the epididymis had epithelial damage, leukocyte infiltration and edema and the sperm-fertilizing potential was lost, because despite being motile, the spermatozoa had a premature acrosome reaction [50]. The above-mentioned greater pathogenicity of the HlyA-producing *E. coli* strains was reported in the work of Lang [50], where the *E. coli* strains that did not produce HlyA induced only slight damage to the epididymis. As already stated, sperm recognize peptidoglycans and LPS through TLR-2 and TLR-4, and this recognition event induces sperm cell death. This was confirmed by using knockout mice for both TLR-2 and -4 and by observing that in these animals LPS or peptidoglycans did not induce sperm death [32].

Further evidence of the contribution of some *E. coli* strains to infertility was observed after inoculating the vaginal tract of rats with SAF-producing strains. Control rats were inoculated with *E. coli* non-SAF producers. It was observed that the rats inoculated with SAF-producing strains were incapable of pregnancy, demonstrating that these toxin-producing strains affect fertility profoundly [51].

7. Conclusion

It is clear that *E. coli* has an important role in causing male infertility associated with genital tract infections. The main mechanism postulated for male infertility by *E. coli* is the profound damage to different sperm processes and function, either by direct contact and/or through secreted toxins.

While today there is a consensus that *E. coli* is an important causal agent of MGTI that may actually cause infertility, from the latest evidence presented above, it is clear that this would not be completely true for all UPEC. Due to these differences among the various strains, it seems important to develop molecular studies that can clarify what specific features of the *E. coli* strains are associated with the pathogenic effects on sperm or with an aggressive inflammatory response this point should be followed.

To date, there have only been a few studies at the molecular level to try to explain how *E. coli* causes infertility.

Knowledge of the molecular mechanisms by which *E. coli* damages sperm will make it possible to take measures to avoid its consequences on the fertilizing potential of men.

Author details

Juana V. Villegas[1]*, Rodrigo Boguen[1] and Pamela Uribe[2]

*Address all correspondence to: juana.villegas@ufrontera.cl

1 Department of Internal Medicine, Center of Biotechnology on Reproduction (CEBIOR-BIOREN), Medicine Faculty, University of La Frontera, Temuco, Chile

2 Center of Biotechnology on Reproduction (CEBIOR-BIOREN), Medicine Faculty, University of La Frontera, Temuco, Chile

References

[1] Practice Committee of American Society for Reproductive Medicine. Definitions of infertility and recurrent pregnancy loss: A committee opinion. Fertility and Sterility. 2013;**99**(1):63. DOI: 10.1016/j.fertnstert.2012.09.023

[2] Farhi J, Ben-Haroush A. Distribution of causes of infertility in patients attending primary fertility clinics in Israel. Israel Medical Association Journal. 2011;**13**(1):51-54

[3] Miyamoto T, Tsujimura A, Miyagawa Y, Koh E, Namiki M, Sengoku K. Male infertility and its causes in human. Advances in Urology. 2012;**2012**:384520. DOI: 10.1155/2012/384520

[4] Weidner W, Krause W, Ludwig M. Relevance of male accessory gland infection for subsequent fertility with special focus on prostatitis. Human Reproduction Update. 1999;**5**:421-432. DOI: 10.1093/humupd/5.5.421

[5] Diemer T, Ludwig M, Huwe P, Hales DB, Weidner W. Influence of urogenital infection on sperm function. Current Opinion in Urology. 2000;**10**:39-44

[6] Wolf H, Joseph A. Leukocytospermia is associated with poor semen quality. Fertility and Sterility. 1990;**53**:528-536

[7] Huwe P, Diemer T, Ludwig M, Liu J, Schiefer HG, Weidner W. Influence of different uropathogenic microorganisms on human sperm motility parameters in an in vitro experiment. Andrologia. 1998;**30**(Suppl 1):55-59. DOI: 10.1111/j.1439-0272.1998.tb02827.x

[8] Sanocka-Maciejewska D, Ciupinska M, Kurpisz M. Bacterial infection and semen quality. Journal of Reproductive Immunology. 2005;**67**(1-2):51-56. DOI: 10.1016/j.jri.2005.06.003.

[9] Villegas J, Schulz M, Soto L, Sanchez R. Bacteria induce expression of apoptosis in human spermatozoa. Apoptosis. 2005;**10**(1):105-110. DOI: 10.1007/s10495-005-6065-8

[10] Villegas J, Schulz M, Soto L, Iglesias T, Miska W, Sanchez R. Influence of reactive oxygen species produced by activated leukocytes at the level of apoptosis in mature human spermatozoa. Fertility and Sterility. 2005;**83**:808-810. DOI: 10.1016/j.fertnstert.2004.09.022

[11] Merino G, Carranza-Lira S, Murrieta S, Rodriguez L, Cuevas E, Moran C. Bacterial infection and semen characteristic in infertile men. Archives of Andrology. 1995;**35**(1):43-47. DOI: 10.3109/01485019508987852

[12] Weidner W, Jantos C, Schiefer HG, Haidl G, Friedrich HJ. Semen parameters in men with and without proven chronic prostatitis. Archives of Andrology. 1991;**26**(3):173-183. DOI: 10.3109/01485019108987640

[13] Weidner W, Schiefer HG, Krauss H, Jantos C, Friedrich HJ, Altmannsberger M. Chronic prostatitis: A thorough search for etiologically involved microorganisms in 1,461 patients. Infection. 1991;**19**(suppl. 3):119-125. DOI: 10.1007/BF01643680

[14] Lloyd AL, Rasko DA, Mobley HL. Defining genomic islands and uropathogen-specific genes in uropathogenic *Escherichia coli*. Journal of Bacteriology. 2007;**189**(9):3532-3546. DOI: 10.1128/JB.01744-06

[15] Terai A, Yamamoto S, Mitsumori K, Okada Y, Kurazono H, Takeda Y, et al. *Escherichia coli* virulence factors and serotypes in acute bacterial prostatitis. International Journal of Urology. 1997;**4**(3):289-294. DOI: 10.1111/j.1442-2042.1997.tb00192.x

[16] Bartoov B, Ozbonfil D, Maayan MC, Ohad E, Nitzan Y. Virulence characteristics of male genital tract *Escherichia coli* isolated from semen of suspected infertile men. Andrologia. 1991;**23**(5):387-394. DOI: 10.1111/j.1439-0272.1991.tb02586.x

[17] World Health Organization. WHO Laboratory Manual for the Examination and Processing of Human Semen. 5th ed. Geneva, Switzerland: WHO Press; 2010. p. 271

[18] Hill JA, Haimovici F, Politch JA, Anderson DJ. Effects of soluble products of activated lymphocytes and macrophages (lymphokines and monokines) on human sperm motion parameters. Fertility and Sterility. 1987;**47**:460-465

[19] Hill JA, Cohen J, Anderson DJ. The effects of lymphokines and monokines on sperm-fertilizing ability in the zona-free hamster egg penetration test. American Journal of Obstetrics & Gynecology. 1989;**160**:1154-1160

[20] Diemer T, Huwe P, Ludwig M, Schroeder-Printzen I, Michelmann H, Schiefer HG. Influence of autogenous leucocytes and *Escherichia coli* on sperm motility parameters in vitro. Andrologia. 2003;**23**:100-105. DOI: 10.1046/j.1439-0272.2003.00523.x

[21] Fraczek M, Szumala-Kakol A, Jedrzejczak P, Kamieniczna M, Kurpiz M. Bacteria trigger oxygen radical release and sperm lipid peroxidation in in vitro model of semen inflammation. Fertility and Sterility. 2007;**88**:1076-1085. DOI: 10.1016/j.fertnstert.2006.12.025

[22] Twigg J, Fulton N, Gomez E, Irvine DS, Aitken RJ. Analysis of the impact of intracellular reactive oxygen species generation on the structural and functional integrity of human spermatozoa: Lipid peroxidation, DNA fragmentation and effectiveness of antioxidants. Human Reproduction. 1998;**13**(6):1429-1436

[23] Villegas J, Kehr K, Soto L, Henkel R, Miska W, Sanchez R. Reactive oxygen species induce reversible capacitation in human spermatozoa. Andrologia. 2003;**35**(4):227-232. 564 [pii]

[24] Diemer T, Weidner W, Michelmann HW, Schiefer HG, Rovan E, Mayer F. Influence of *Escherichia coli* on motility parameters of human spermatozoa in vitro. International Journal of Andrology. 1996;**19**(5):271-277. DOI: 10.1111/j.1365-2605.1996.tb00475.x

[25] Berkast M, Aydin S, Yilmaz Y, Cecen K, Bozkurt H. Sperm motility changes after coincubation with various uropathogenic microorganisms: An in vitro experimental study. International Urology and Nephrology. 2008;**40**:383-389. DOI: 10.1007/s11255-007-9289-4

[26] Ekhaise FO, Richard FR. Common bacterial isolated associated with semen complaining of infertility in University of Benin Teaching Hospital (U.B.T.H.), Benin City, Nigeria. World Journal of Medical Science. 2008;**3**(1):28-33

[27] Rosenthal L. Agglutinating properties of *Escherichia coli*: Agglutination of erythrocytes, leucocytes, thrombocytes, spermatozoa, spores of molds, and pollen by strains of *E. coli*. Journal of Bacteriology. 1943;**45**(6):545-550

[28] Monga M, Roberts J. Spermagglutination by bacteria: Receptor-specific interactions. Journal of Andrology. 1994;**15**:151-156. DOI: 10.1002/j.1939-4640.1994.tb00423.x

[29] Diemer T, Huwe P, Michelmann HW, Mayer F, Schiefer HG, Weidner W. *Escherichia coli*-induced alterations of human spermatozoa. An electron microscopy analysis. International Journal of Andrology. 2000;**23**:178-186. DOI: 10.1046/j.1365-2605.2000.00224.x

[30] Galdiero F, Gorga F, Bentivoglio C, Mancuso R, Galdiero E, Tufano MA. The action of LPS porins and peptidoglycan fragments on human spermatozoa. Infection. 1988;**16**(6):349-353. DOI: 10.1007/BF01644545

[31] Gorga F, Galdiero M, Buommino E, Galdiero E. Porins and lipopolysaccharide induce apoptosis in human spermatozoa. Clinical and Diagnostic Laboratory Inmunology. 2001;**8**(11):206-208. DOI: 10.1128/CDLI.8.1.206-208.2001

[32] Fujita Y, Mihara T, Okazaki T, Shitanaka M, Kushino R, Ikeda C, et al. Toll-like receptors (TLR) 2 and 4 on human sperm recognize bacterial endotoxins and mediate apoptosis. Human Reproduction. 2011;**26**(10):2799-2806. DOI: 10.1093/humrep/der234

[33] Schulz M, Sanchez R, Soto L, Risopatron J, Villegas J. Effect of *Escherichia coli* and its soluble factors on mitochondrial membrane potential, phosphatidylserine translocation, viability, and motility of human spermatozoa. Fertility and Sterility. 2010;**94**(2):619-623. DOI: 10.1016/j.fertnstert.2009.01.140

[34] Fraczek M, Piasecka M, Gaczarzewicz D, Szumala-Kakol A, Kazienko A, Lenart S, et al. Membrane stability and mitochondrial activity of human-ejaculated spermatozoa during in vitro experimental infection with *Escherichia coli*, *Staphylococcus haemolyticus* and *Bacteroides ureolyticus*. Andrologia. 2012;**44**(5):315-329. DOI: 10.1111/j.1439-0272.2012.01283.x

[35] Espinoza JA, Schulz M, Sanchez R, Villegas J. Integrity of mitochondrial membrane potential reflects human sperm quality. Andrologia. 2009;**41**(1):51-54. DOI: 10.1111/j.1439-0272.2008.00878.x

[36] Marchetti C, Jouy N, Leroy-Martin B, Deffosez A, Formstecher P, Marchetti P. Comparison of four fluorochromes for the detection of the inner mitochondrial membrane potential in human spermatozoa and their correlation with sperm motility. Human Reproduction. 2004;**19**(10):2267-2276. DOI: 10.1093/humrep/deh416

[37] Boguen R, Uribe P, Treulen F, Villegas JV. Distinct isolates of uropathogenic *Escherichia coli* differentially affect human sperm parameters in vitro. Andrologia. 2014;**46**(8):943-947. DOI: 10.1111/and.12167

[38] Wiles TJ, Kulesus RR, Mulvey MA. Origins and virulence mechanisms of uropathogenic *Escherichia coli*. Experimental and Molecular Pathology. 2008;**85**(1):11-19. DOI: 10.1016/j.yexmp.2008.03.007

[39] Boguen R, Treulen F, Uribe P, Villegas JV. Ability of *Escherichia coli* to produce hemolysis leads to a greater pathogenic effect on human sperm. Fertility and Sterility. 2015;**103**(5):1155-1161. DOI: 10.1016/j.fertnstert.2015.01.044

[40] Bhakdi S, Mackman N, Nicaud JM, Holland IB. *Escherichia coli* hemolysin may damage target cell membranes by generating transmembrane pores. Infection and Immunity. 1986;**52**(1):63-69

[41] Wiles TJ, Dhakal BK, Eto DS, Mulvey MA. Inactivation of host Akt/protein kinase B signaling by bacterial pore-forming toxins. Molecular Biology of the Cell. 2008;**19**(4):1427-1438. DOI: 10.1091/mbc.E07-07-0638

[42] Bhushan S, Hossain H, Lu Y, Geisler A, Tchatalbachev S, Mikulski Z, et al. Uropathogenic *E. coli* induce different immune response in testicular and peritoneal macrophages: implications for testicular immune privilege. PLoS One. 2011;**6**(12):e28452. DOI: 10.1371/journal.pone.0028452

[43] Fraczek M, Wiland E, Piasecka M, Boksa M, Gaczarzewicz D, Szumala-Kakol A, et al. Fertilizing potential of ejaculated human spermatozoa during in vitro semen bacterial infection. Fertility and Sterility. 2014;**102**(3):711-719. e1. DOI: 10.1016/j.fertnstert.2014.06.002

[44] Barbonetti A, Vassallo MR, Cinque B, Filipponi S, Mastromarino P, Cifone MG, et al. Soluble products of *Escherichia coli* induce mitochondrial dysfunction-related sperm membrane lipid peroxidation which is prevented by *Lactobacilli*. PLoS One. 2013;**8**(12):e83136. DOI: 10.1371/journal.pone.0083136

[45] Paulson JD, Polakoski KL. Isolation of a spermatozoal immobilization factor from *Escherichia coli* filtrates. Fertility and Sterility. 1977;**28**(2):182-185.

[46] Prabha V, Sandhu R, Kaur S, Kaur K, Sarwal A, Mavuduru RS, et al. Mechanism of sperm immobilization by *Escherichia coli*. Advances in Urology. 2010;**2010**:e240268. DOI: 10.1155/2010/240268

[47] Kumar V, Prabha V, Kaur S, Kaur K, Singh SK. Receptor dependent immobilization of spermatozoa by sperm immobilization factor isolated from *Escherichia coli*: proof of evidence. International Journal of Urology. 2011;**18**(8):597-603. DOI: 10.1111/j.1442-2042.2011.02784.x

[48] Kaur K, Prabha V. Sperm impairment by sperm agglutinating factor isolated from *Escherichia coli*: Receptor specific interactions. BioMed Research International. 2013;**2013**: 548497. DOI: 10.1155/2013/548497

[49] Lu Y, Bhushan S, Tchatalbachev S, Marconi M, Bergmann M, Weidner W, et al. Necrosis is the dominant cell death pathway in uropathogenic *Escherichia coli* elicited epididymo-orchitis and is responsible for damage of rat testis. PLoS One. 2013;**8**(1):e52919. DOI: 10.1371/journal.pone.0052919

[50] Lang T, Dechant M, Sanchez V, Wistuba J, Boiani M, Pilatz A, et al. Structural and functional integrity of spermatozoa is compromised as a consequence of acute uropathogenic *E. coli*-associated epididymitis. Biology of Reproduction. 2013;**89**(3):59. DOI: 10.1095/biolreprod.113.110379

[51] Kaur K, Prabha V. Spermagglutinating *Escherichia coli* and its role in infertility: In vivo study. Microbial Pathogenesis. 2014;**69-70**:33-38. DOI: 10.1016/j.micpath.2014.03.010

Chapter 5

Antimicrobial Mechanisms of *Escherichia coli*

Wanda C. Reygaert

Additional information is available at the end of the chapter

http://dx.doi.org/10.5772/67363

Abstract

Increasing antimicrobial resistance in strains of *Escherichia coli* is having a major impact on the healthcare industry worldwide. The appearance of extended-spectrum β-lactamase (ESBL) and carbapenem-resistant Enterobacteriaceae (CRE) strains has caused clinicians to worry that these strains might become as deadly as methicillin-resistant *Staphylococcus aureus* (MRSA) strains. It is vital that physicians have resources available to help keep them updated on these bacteria and the potential impact on healthcare. This chapter reviews the major strains of *E. coli* (intestinal and urinary), along with a review of the virulence factors, main diseases caused, and pertinent pathogenesis. The chapter then discusses antimicrobial therapy, what drugs are effective against these *E. coli* strains, and the development of resistance to these specific drug classes. Lastly, the molecular aspects of antimicrobial resistance mechanisms in this organism are discussed. This information will be especially helpful for physicians in providing them with a concise review of *E. coli* and an understanding of what is involved in antimicrobial resistance. Hopefully this information can be used to improve the outcomes for patients with *E. coli* infections.

Keywords: *Escherichia coli*, antimicrobial resistance, ESBL, CRE

1. Introduction

Increasing resistance to antimicrobial drugs is of major concern worldwide. For many developing countries, the possibility of having cheap antibiotics available may now be threatened. There are antimicrobial resistance issues with most pathogenic bacteria and in virtually all of the opportunistic bacterial-caused infections. This translates into increased healthcare costs. These costs include extended length of hospital stay and increased costs for medical supplies including more expensive antimicrobial drugs. In addition, antimicrobial drug-resistant infections lead to higher rates of mortality, especially in patients who had recent prior exposure to antibiotics [1].

Antimicrobial drugs are classified into groups according to the type of antimicrobial activity. These groups include drugs that inhibit bacterial cell wall synthesis, depolarize the cell membrane, inhibit bacterial protein synthesis, inhibit bacterial nucleic acid synthesis, and inhibit bacterial metabolic pathways. The improper use of these drugs has helped to create resistant bacterial strains. Factors that contribute to resistance include the increased use of all antimicrobial drugs and improper antimicrobial prescribing. Many of the less expensive drugs that have fewer side effects have been used too commonly. Improper prescribing may be choosing broad spectrum or ineffective drugs [2–4].

Many strains of *Escherichia coli* are not harmful. In fact, these commensal strains in the gut are necessary for the synthesis of vitamin K_2, which is an important clotting factor [5]. However, there are pathogenic strains, and these strains may become a larger threat if they possess or acquire certain antimicrobial mechanisms. The main ones of concern are the extended-spectrum β-lactamase (ESBL)-producing strains and the carbapenem-resistant Enterobacteriaceae (CRE) strains. The ESBL strains are resistant to most β-lactam drugs, and the CRE strains are resistant to most carbapenem drugs. Greatly increased healthcare costs are associated with the ESBL and CRE strains. Various studies have shown a hospital stay of up to twice as long and increased costs of 1.5–2.5 times as much [6–8]. One study in the United States estimated the increased costs to be $16,450 per patient [6].

All of the pathogenic strains of *E. coli* are armed with the same types of potential virulence factors. These factors include a capsule (in some strains), flagella, the lipopolysaccharide (LPS) cell wall, fimbriae, outer membrane proteins (OMPs), a hemolysin, cytolysins, and siderophores. The specific types of some of these virulence factors plus the possession of other toxins and effectors may vary with each individual pathogenic strain [9].

2. Pathogenic strains of *Escherichia coli*

Commensal strains of *E. coli* are the predominant facultative organism in the human gut. Even though greatly outnumbered by the anaerobic organisms, the *E. coli* are vital to human health, playing roles in biofilm communities and subsequent digestion of oligosaccharides and polysaccharides, among other things [10, 11]. Unfortunately, there are also several pathogenic strains of *E. coli*. The classification names of these strains may vary some depending on the source, but for the purposes of this chapter, we will use the following names. There are six strains of potentially pathogenic intestinal-based diarrhea causing *E. coli*: diffusely adherent *E. coli* (DAEC), enteroaggregative *E. coli* (EAEC), enterohemorrhagic *E. coli* (EHEC), enteroinvasive *E. coli* (EIEC), enteropathogenic *E. coli* (EPEC), and enterotoxigenic *E. coli* (ETEC). In addition, there is one extraintestinal pathogenic strain, uropathogenic *E. coli* (UPEC), which causes urinary tract infections. There is some evidence that a second extraintestinal strain exists, the meningitis-associated *E. coli* (MNEC) strain. Findings on MNEC indicate that the infection starts as a blood infection and then gains access to the central nervous system. A majority of MNEC possess the K1 capsular antigen, and there is a high rate of mortality from the meningitis [12]. This chapter will focus on the six intestinal and the UPEC strains.

2.1. Diffusely adherent *Escherichia coli* (DAEC)

These strains are sometimes referred to as enteroadherent *E. coli* (EAEC) (not to be confused with the enteroaggregative strains, which are sometimes referred to as EAggEC). While not known to cause severe diarrheal disease, the DAEC, which are probably a group of related strains, are thought to be responsible for some types of persistent diarrhea in infants. Whether they possess true virulence factors is still under debate, but these bacteria are able to bind to enterocytes (probably via adhesins such as Afa/Dr) and elicit a response in which the microvilli extend and wrap around the bacteria. Diarrhea in association with DAEC has also shown an ability to induce the production of inflammatory cytokines, such as IL-8 [13–15].

2.2. Enteroaggregative *Escherichia coli* (EAEC)

The EAEC strains were so named because of their tendency to adhere to enterocytes in dense clusters. The bacteria attach to the microvilli and also to other EAEC bacteria. The EAEC are also a heterogeneous group of strains with a similar pathogenesis, resulting in non-bloody diarrhea. Infection is established by adhering to the microvilli via fimbriae (the aggregative adherence fimbriae—AAF), inducing increased mucus production and biofilm formation, inducing an inflammatory response and production of toxins. The main toxins of the EAEC strains are the EAEC heat-stable enterotoxin (EAST1), which enters the enterocytes and activates guanine cyclase, resulting in increased levels of cGMP in the cell and loss of fluid into the intestinal lumen; the plasmid-encoded toxin (Pet), which disrupts the enterocyte cytoskeleton, resulting in cell detachment; and a *Shigella*-like enterotoxin (ShET1), a heat-stable toxin which may also result in fluid secretion [16–18].

2.3. Enterohemorrhagic *Escherichia coli* (EHEC)

The most publicized strain of pathogenic *E. coli* is the EHEC strain. EHEC serotype O157:H7 is well known as the causative agent of outbreaks of food-associated severe diarrhea. Infection with O157:H7 results in sever abdominal cramps and bloody diarrhea and may lead to hemolytic-uremic syndrome (HUS) which can be life-threatening. The most common foods associated with transmission of these bacteria are undercooked meat (especially ground beef), raw milk, and raw vegetables. The EHEC strains do not directly invade the enterocytes, but produce toxins that do enter and severely damage these cells. The responsible cytotoxins are verotoxins I and II (designated as Shiga toxins, Stx-1 and Stx-2). The Shiga toxins are capable of inactivating ribosomes, blocking protein synthesis, and emerging through the basolateral membrane into the subepithelial region. Stx-2 is seen most often in the EHEC strains that cause HUS [19–21].

2.4. Enteroinvasive *Escherichia coli* (EIEC)

In infections with EIEC, the bacteria invade by directly entering M cells. The bacteria pass through these cells and then are able to invade the enterocytes via the basolateral membrane, causing severe damage to the intestinal mucosa. The bacteria are also able to spread laterally through the cell side walls to adjacent cells (via actin). This damage results in dysentery (watery diarrhea with pus, mucus, and blood). The EIEC bacteria do not produce toxins, but participate in direct damage and induce production of IL-1 and IL-8. The pathogenic mechanisms and disease symptoms associated with EIEC are so similar to *Shigella* spp. that differential diagnosis can be difficult. Diagnosis is usually based on physiological and biochemical characteristics that can be detected in the clinical laboratory [19, 22, 23].

2.5. Enteropathogenic *Escherichia coli* (EPEC)

The EPEC strains do not directly invade enterocytes. Instead, these bacteria adhere to the microvilli and inject effector proteins into the cell via a type III secretion system (T3SS). One of these effectors is the translocated intimin receptor (Tir), which initiates recruitment of the host cell actin to form a pedestal under the bacteria. The recruitment of actin and formation of the pedestals result in destruction of the rest of the microvilli and also inhibit the transport of Na^+ and Cl^- in the cell, which results in the subsequent exodus of water into the intestinal lumen. Another effector, the *E. coli* secreted proteins (Esps), interacts with the host cell cytoskeleton and results in disruption of the cell tight junctions [24–26].

2.6. Enterotoxigenic *Escherichia coli* (ETEC)

The ETEC strains are a common cause of acute travelers' diarrhea. These strains usually colonize the proximal small intestine, adhering to the microvilli via various colonization factors including fimbrial, nonfimbrial, helical, and fibrillar types. The EPEC strains secrete two types of toxin: a heat-labile toxin (LT) and heat-stable toxins (STs). The LT is an AB toxin, and the B subunits bind to the monosialoganglioside GM1, which induces the cell to take in the toxin. The LT toxin activates adenylyl cyclase, which increases the cAMP in the cell, resulting in hypersecretion of water and electrolytes into the intestinal lumen. The STs bind to guanylyl cyclase receptors on the microvilli, which stimulate guanylate cyclase and activate the cystic fibrosis transmembrane receptor (CFTR). This results in an increase in cGMP in the cell and impaired absorption of Na^+, which causes hypersecretion of water into the intestinal lumen [19, 24, 27].

2.7. Uropathogenic *Escherichia coli* (UPEC)

The UPEC strains are responsible for most uncomplicated urinary tract infections (UTIs). These strains possess a capsule and bind to uroepithelial cells via fimbriae. The interaction of the bacteria with the host cell induces the internalization of the bacteria where the bacteria multiply rapidly and form biofilm-like intercellular bacterial communities (IBCs). The bacteria are shed intermittently from the uroendothelial cells into the lumen of the bladder. UPEC strains produce several types of toxins including hemolysin A (HlyA) which has pore-forming capability and two cytotoxins, cytotoxic necrotizing factor (CNF-1) and secreted auto-transporter toxin (Sat) [19, 28, 29].

http://dx.doi.org/10.5772/67363

3. Antimicrobial therapy

As mentioned above, antimicrobial drugs are often classified in groups based on their mechanism of antimicrobial action. **Table 1** displays those groups along with examples of the antimicrobial drugs included in each group. The β-lactam drugs, which were among the first antimicrobials to be discovered, target the bacterial cell wall (via peptidoglycan synthesis) and are most useful against gram-positive bacteria (having little effect on gram-negative bacteria because of the lipopolysaccharide cell envelope that protects the thin peptidoglycan cell wall in these bacteria). Over the years, because the β-lactam drugs were readily available and inexpensive and caused few side effects, physicians commonly treated their patients initially with these drugs.

Inhibit cell wall synthesis	β-Lactams Carbapenems Cephalosporins Monobactams Penicillins Glycopeptides
Depolarize cell membrane	Lipopeptides
Inhibit protein synthesis	Bind to 30S ribosomal subunit Aminoglycosides Tetracyclines Bind to 50S ribosomal subunit Chloramphenicol Lincosamides Macrolides Oxazolidinones Streptogramins
Inhibit nucleic acid synthesis	Quinolones Fluoroquinolones
Inhibit metabolic pathways	Sulfonamides Trimethoprim

Table 1. Antimicrobial groups based on mechanism of action.

When bacterial resistance to the β-lactam drugs became an issue (very early on), scientists developed synthetic versions of penicillin such as ampicillin, amoxicillin, and methicillin. In addition, scientists discovered the natural cephalosporin β-lactam drugs. The initial cephalosporins (first generation) were most useful against gram-positive cocci, with some activity against a few gram-negative bacilli. Further development of these drugs has produced second generation (less effective against gram-positive cocci, more effective against gram-negative bacilli); third generation (generally with a broad spectrum of activity against gram-negative organisms); fourth generation (extended-spectrum activity against gram-positive cocci and gram-negative bacilli); and recently, fifth generation (hopefully effective against various multidrug-resistant organisms), with more still in development. Other β-lactam drugs developed during this time frame were the carbapenems (broad-spectrum activity) and monopenems (aztreonam—activity against gram-negative aerobic bacteria) [30–32].

Differences in structure, metabolism, virulence factors, etc., between gram-negative and gram-positive bacteria predict which antimicrobial drug groups may be effective. Fewer of the drug groups have good activity against gram-negative bacteria. Those groups include some of the β-lactam drugs (especially second-, third-, and fourth-generation cephalosporins): aminoglycosides, fluoroquinolones, trimethoprim/sulfamethoxazole (TMP/SXT), and nitrofurans (for UTIs) [33]. Intestinal infections with *E. coli* are most commonly self-limiting and require supportive therapy (antiemetics, antidiarrhetics, rehydration) only. Severe or recurring infections (e.g., traveler's diarrhea) may be treated with fluoroquinolone drugs. Acute dysentery caused by EIEC strains may be treated with fluoroquinolones or appropriate cephalosporins. For infections caused by EHEC, antimicrobial therapy is contraindicated as it greatly increases the risk for development of HUS. UTIs caused by UPEC strains are usually treated with antimicrobial drugs and uncomplicated UTIs with nitrofurantoin or TMP/SXT; complicated UTIs may also be treated with fluoroquinolones [34–37]. Infections with ESBL or CRE strains severely limit treatment options. For ESBL strains, carbapenems may still be an option or newer β-lactam/β-lactamase inhibitor drug combinations; for CRE strains, gentamicin, amikacin, colistin, tigecycline, and fosfomycin may be options. Unfortunately, some ESBL and CRE strains may be resistant to even some of these drugs [38–40].

At the beginning of antimicrobial drug resistance, physicians did not realize how the various drugs affected the bacteria. In addition, in an effort to begin antimicrobial therapy as quickly as possible, physicians often ordered a broad-spectrum drug before knowing the causative agent of the infection. These issues (among others) have led to a large amount of resistance to β-lactam drugs, especially among the gram-negative bacteria. Bacteria that produced β-lactamases (enzymes that inactivate β-lactam drugs) were identified as early as the 1940s (around the same time as penicillin was discovered), and the number of different β-lactamases produced has increased over the years to around 1000 [2–4, 41].

The issue of resistance is not just with the β-lactam drugs. Over the 70 plus years that antimicrobial drugs have been in existence, resistance mechanisms have been seen for most of these drugs. It does not seem to take the bacteria very long from initial use of a drug to development of resistance to that drug. Important resistant milestones include resistance to aminoglycosides and tetracycline in the 1960s, vancomycin in the 1980s, fluoroquinolones in the 1990s, and linezolid in the 2000s [42]. In addition, some of the bacteria have become resistant to multiple antimicrobial agents from many of the drug classes. These multidrug-resistant bacteria, such as methicillin-resistant *Staphylococcus aureus* (MRSA), are currently a major cause of morbidity and mortality [43].

Similar to the threat of MRSA, members of the gram-negative Enterobacteriaceae, in particular *E. coli* and *Klebsiella pneumoniae*, include strains that are ESBLs and CREs. These organisms can be resistant to most commonly used antimicrobials, which makes the infections they cause extremely difficult to treat, leading to increased morbidity and mortality (and healthcare costs) [44, 45].

http://dx.doi.org/10.5772/67363

4. Antimicrobial resistance mechanisms

There are four general antimicrobial resistance mechanisms that bacteria use. These are limiting uptake of the drug, modifying the target of the drug, inactivating the drug, and active efflux of the drug. These mechanisms may be located on the bacterial chromosome and occur naturally in all members of a species (intrinsic) or come from other bacteria, usually via a plasmid (acquired). Intrinsic resistance genes may be expressed constitutively (usually at a low level) or be induced by the presence of antimicrobial drugs. Gram-negative bacteria widely use all four of these mechanisms and are very capable of horizontal transfer of resistance elements. **Table 2** shows which resistance mechanisms and genes are associated with resistance to various antimicrobial drugs [43, 46, 47].

Antimicrobial agents	Mechanisms of resistance	Genetic basis
β-lactams Penicillins Cephalosporins Monobactams Carbapenems	β-lactamases—inactivate drugs Active efflux	*ampC* *bla* genes—plasmid (TEM, SHV, CTX-M, NDM) *acrAB(tolC), acrAD(tolC)*
Aminoglycosides Amikacin Gentamicin Tobramycin	Aminoglycoside modifying enzymes Modify target—16S rRNA Active efflux	*aac, ant, aph*—plasmid *amrA, rmtB* *mdtEF(tolC)*
Tetracyclines Tetracycline	Limiting uptake Active efflux	*ompF* *acrAB(tolC)* *tetA, tetB*—plasmid
Chloramphenicol	Limiting uptake Active efflux	*ompF* *acrAB(tolC)*
Fluoroquinolones Ciprofloxacin Norfloxacin	Limiting uptake Modified target—gyrase Modified target—topoisomerase IV Active efflux	*ompF* *gyrA* *parC* *acrAB(tolC), acrEF(tolC),* *mdtABC(tolC)*
Metabolic pathway inhibitors Trimethoprim/Sulfamethoxazole	Target enzyme modification	TMP—*dhfr* SXT—*dhps*

Table 2. Common antimicrobial resistance genes and mechanisms in *Escherichia coli.*

4.1. Limiting drug uptake

Gram-negative bacteria have an advantage in combating drugs because of the structure and functions of the LPS cell wall, which provides a natural barrier to certain molecules. The LPS is generally hydrophobic which limits access to small hydrophilic drugs, such as the β-lactams. These hydrophilic drugs gain access by traveling through the OMPs. The main

OMPs in *E. coli* are OmpF and OmpC. In addition to the β-lactams, other drugs that may use the porin channels are chloramphenicol, fluoroquinolones, and tetracycline. Hydrophobic drugs such as the aminoglycosides and the macrolides gain access by permeating through the LPS layer. There are two main mechanisms that are used to limit access to drugs via porins: a decrease in the number of porins or a change in charge, within the porin channel, which reduces its function or binding properties. In *E. coli* porin production may be reduced dramatically or even stopped, or a different porin may be produced instead [48, 49].

4.2. Modifying drug target

Gram-negative bacteria make use of the modifying of drug targets against several of the antimicrobial groups including β-lactams, aminoglycosides, fluoroquinolones, and the combination drug TMP/SXT. Even though not as widely used as in gram-positive bacteria, the gram-negative bacteria are able to produce penicillin-binding proteins (PBPs) that are resistant to some β-lactam drugs. PBPs are actually peptidases that are involved in the making of the peptidoglycan cell wall. Penicillin drugs that are able to bind to PBPs inhibit the assembly process. There are several different native PBPs produced by *E. coli*, some of which have reduced binding affinity for some of the β-lactam drugs. No acquired modified form of PBP has been shown to be significant in β-lactam resistance in *E. coli* [50, 51].

The aminoglycoside drugs inhibit protein synthesis by binding to the bacterial 30S ribosomal subunit at the A-site of the 16S rRNA. Bacteria are able to modify the ribosomal subunit via acquisition of plasmids carrying 16S rRNA methyltransferases. The methyltransferases are able to modify the structure of the 16S rRNA, which decreases the ability of the drug to bind to it. Several of these methyltransferases have been identified and characterized. The genes involved include *armA* (for aminoglycoside resistance methylase) and several *rmt* (for ribosomal methyltransferase) genes, with *rmtB* being the most common. The bacteria quite often possess several of these genes simultaneously. These genes most often confer clinically significant resistance to amikacin, gentamicin, and tobramycin, among other aminoglycosides [52–56].

The fluoroquinolone drugs interfere with nucleic acid synthesis during DNA replication by inhibiting either DNA gyrase or topoisomerase IV. Resistance to these drugs occurs commonly from mutations in either the chromosomally encoded GyrA subunit of gyrase (*gyrA* gene) or the ParC subunit of topoisomerase IV (*parC* gene). These mutations decrease the binding ability of the drugs, most commonly ciprofloxacin and norfloxacin. There is also some evidence that low-level resistance may be acquired via plasmids carrying quinolone resistance (*qnr*) genes [56–58].

The combination drug TMP/SXT is currently a common choice for treatment of UTIs. Both of these drugs target enzymes in the bacterial folate biosynthesis pathway via competitive inhibition. Trimethoprim is an analog of the natural substrate of the dihydrofolate reductase (DHFR) enzyme, and SXT is an analog of *p*-amino-benzoic acid, the natural substrate of the dihydropteroate synthase (DHPS) enzyme. This competitive binding blocks the binding of the natural substrate and stops the pathway at that point. Since TMP and SXT affect two different enzymes on the same pathway, the combination drug makes an effective treatment. Chromosomal mutations (often single point mutations) in the *dhfr* or *dhps* genes are commonly the cause of resistance to these drugs [59, 60].

4.3. Inactivating the drug

Drug inactivation is accomplished in one of two ways: by actual degradation of the drug or by transfer of a chemical group to the drug. Gram-negative bacteria use drug inactivation against β-lactams and aminoglycosides. The β-lactam drugs are universally inactivated by β-lactamase enzymes, which degrade the drugs, and *E. coli* produces several of these. The aminoglycoside drugs are inactivated fairly universally by enzymes that transfer one of three small chemical groups to the drug. These enzymes include the acetyltransferases (AACs, *aac* genes), nucleotidyltransferases (ANTs, *ant* genes), and the phosphotransferases (APHs, *aph* genes) [43, 49, 61].

4.3.1. *β-lactamases*

The β-lactam drugs all share a specific core structure, which consists of a four-sided β-lactam ring. The β-lactamases (also originally called penicillinases and cephalosporinases) are capable of inactivating β-lactam drugs via hydrolyzation of a specific site in the β-lactam ring structure causing the ring to open. The drugs are then not able to bind to their target proteins, the PBPs. Within the large number of β-lactamases which have been identified, there are enzymes which can inactivate any of the current β-lactam drugs. The production of β-lactamases is the most common resistance mechanism used by gram-negative bacteria against β-lactam drugs [46, 62].

The β-lactamase enzymes can be classified based on their primary structure or functional characteristics. Structurally they are placed into four main categories (A, B, C, or D). There are three functional groupings: the cephalosporinases, the serine β-lactamases, and the metallo-β-lactamases. These enzymes are also commonly referred to by their enzyme family, for example, the TEM (named after the first patient) family, the sulphydryl variable (SHV) family, and the CTX (preferentially hydrolyze cefotaxime) family [56, 63].

The first β-lactamase to be characterized was from *E. coli* and is chromosomally encoded by the *ampC* gene (so named for ampicillin resistance). This gene is constitutively expressed at a low level, but mutations may result in overexpression of the gene. The AmpC β-lactamases are most effective against the penicillins and some first-generation cephalosporins. There are also many plasmid-borne β-lactamases, which carry a variety of *bla* genes (β-lactamase genes). Because these β-lactamases confer resistance to later generation cephalosporins, they were designated as ESBLs and include the TEM, SHV, and CTX-M enzyme families. The most commonly seen of these in *E. coli* are the CTX-Ms. The ESBLs may also be resistant to multiple drug classes but are generally sensitive to β-lactamase inhibitors. The β-lactamase inhibitors are structurally similar to β-lactamases and have weak antimicrobial ability alone but work synergistically in combination with a β-lactam drug [56, 64–67].

Recently, there has been emergence of β-lactamases that are active against the carbapenems (carbapenemases), found primarily in the *Enterobacteriaceae*. Bacterial strains that carry these are known as CRE strains. The carbapenemases are all metallo-β-lactamases (MBLs), and the most widely distributed are the IMP-1 (for imipenem resistance) and VIM-1 (Verona integron-encoded MBL) types. A new MBL has recently been identified, mainly in strains of *E. coli*. It has been designated as New Delhi MBL (NDM-1). The CRE strains are usually resistance to all the β-lactam drugs and are not inactivated by the standard β-lactam/β-lactamase inhibitor combination drugs. There is a newer β-lactamase inhibitor, avibactam, which has been approved for use with ceftazidime against gram-negative bacteria. In addition, avibactam is being tested for use with aztreonam against CREs [62, 66–68].

4.4. Drug efflux

Bacteria possess methods for disposal of toxic substances to the outside of the cell. The most commonly used mechanism is the efflux pump. Most bacteria have chromosomally encoded efflux pump genes. Some of these pumps are expressed constitutively, and expression of others is induced by various environmental stimuli. Many of these pumps are capable of transporting a variety of substances and are also described as multidrug (MDR) efflux pumps. There are five efflux pump family groups: the ATP-binding cassette (ABC) family, the multidrug and toxic compound extrusion (MATE) family, the major facilitator superfamily (MFS), the small multidrug resistance (SMR) family, and the resistance-nodulation-cell division (RND) family. The RND pumps are generally found only in gram-negative bacteria as these pumps are multicomponent pumps that function in association with an OMP [69–72].

There is only one ABC efflux pump in *E. coli* that is known to contribute to antimicrobial resistance. That is the MacAB transporter that confers resistance to some macrolides [73]. There is also only one MATE efflux pump found in *E. coli*, the NorE pump which is able to transport fluoroquinolones. It is still in question if the NorE pump has a clinically significant impact on antimicrobial resistance [74, 75]. There are five known MFS efflux pumps found in *E. coli*. These are capable of transporting macrolides (MefB and MdfA pumps), fluoroquinolones (QepA2, EmrAB-TolC, and MdfA pumps), tetracycline (EmrAB-TolC and MdfA pumps), trimethoprim (Fsr pump), and chloramphenicol (MdfA pump). In addition, there are several MFS pumps that may be acquired by *E. coli* (e.g., via plasmids) that are specific for tetracyclines, with *tetA* and *tetB* being the most common [76, 77]. There are no clinically significant SMR efflux pumps found in *E. coli* [78].

The RND efflux pumps are the most clinically significant pumps found in gram-negative bacteria. These pumps consist of three components (tripartite): an inner membrane transporter, an outer membrane porin, and a periplasmic accessory protein that functions to connect the other two components. In *E. coli*, the OMP that is associated with all of the antimicrobial efflux pumps is TolC. There are five known RND pumps in *E. coli*: AcrAB-TolC, AcrAD-TolC, AcrEF-TolC, MdtABC-TolC, and MdtEF-TolC. AcrAD-TolC has been shown to efflux aminoglycosides and β-lactams. AcrEF-TolC has been shown to efflux quinolones and tigecycline. MdtABE-TolC has been shown to efflux quinolones. MdtEF-TolC has been shown to efflux erythromycin. The level of expression of these four pumps is relatively low, and if operating alone, the amount of antimicrobials effluxed would probably not be significant. Because *E. coli* has five efflux systems plus multiple other types of antimicrobial resistance mechanisms in play, these pumps undoubtedly help out. The other RND efflux pump in *E. coli*, AcrAB-TolC, is the most clinically significant and accounts for major antimicrobial efflux. This pump has been shown to efflux β-lactams, fluoroquinolones, tetracyclines, chloramphenicol, and lincosamides [72, 79, 80].

http://dx.doi.org/10.5772/67363

5. Conclusion

For many strains of pathogenic *E. coli*, the most common course of therapy is supportive and does not require the use of antimicrobial drugs, or in the case of EHEC, antimicrobial therapy is not recommended. For severe intestinal infections and UTIs, antimicrobial therapy may be necessary. Unfortunately with the issue of ever increasing antimicrobial resistance, the antimicrobial options are becoming fewer. With the emergence of ESBL and CRE *E. coli* strains, the options have gotten extremely limited, and antimicrobial development has not been able to keep up with the demand. Hopefully the newer carbapenem/β-lactamase inhibitor combination drugs and other drugs being developed under the tetracycline and aminoglycoside drug classes will prove to be equal to the task or at least keep the bacteria under control until better options become available.

Author details

Wanda C. Reygaert

Address all correspondence to: reygaert@oakland.edu

Oakland University William Beaumont School of Medicine, Rochester, Michigan, USA

References

[1] Micek S, Johnson MT, Reichley R, Kollef MH. An institutional perspective on the impact of recent antibiotic exposure on length of stay and hospital costs for patients with gram-negative sepsis. BMC Infect Dis. 2012;**12**:56. DOI: 10.1186/1471-2334-12-56.

[2] Goossens H. Antibiotic consumption and link to resistance. Clin Microbiol Infect. 2009;**15**(Suppl 3):12-15. DOI: 10.1111/j.1469-0691.2009.02725.x.

[3] Tacconelli E. Antimicrobial use: risk driver of multidrug resistant microorganisms in healthcare settings. Curr Opin Infect Dis. 2009;**22**:352-358. DOI: 10.1097/QCO.0b013e32832d52e0.

[4] Griffith M, Postelnick M, Scheetz M. Antimicrobial stewardship programs: methods of operation and suggested outcomes. Expert Rev Anti Infect Ther. 2012;**10**:63-73. DOI: 10.1586/eri.11.153.

[5] Bentley R, Meganathan R. Biosynthesis of vitamin K (menaquinone) in bacteria. Microbiol Rev. 1982;**46**:241-280.

[6] Lee SY, Kotapati S, Kuti JL, Nightingale CH, Nicolau DP. Impact of extended-spectrum β-lactamase-producing *Escherichia coli* and *Klebsiella* species on clinical outcomes and hospital costs: a matched cohort study. Infect Control Hosp Epidemiol. 2006;**27**:1226-1232. DOI: 10.1086/507962.

[7] Yang YS, Ku CH, Lin JC, Shang ST, Chiu CH, Yeh KM, Lin CC, Chang FY. Impact of extended-spectrum β-lactamase-producing *Escherichia coli* and *Klebsiella pneumoniae* on the outcome of community-onset bacteremic urinary tract infections. J Microbiol Immunol Infect. 2010;**43**:194-199. DOI: 10.1016/S1684-1182(10)60031-X.

[8] Maslikowska JA, Walker SA, Elligsen M, Mittman N, Palmay L, Daneman N, Simor A. Impact of infection with extended-spectrum β-lactamase-producing *Escherichia coli* or *Klebsiella* species on outcome and hospitalization costs. J Hosp Infect. 2016;**92**:33-41. DOI: 10.1016/j.jhin.2015.10.001.

[9] Kaper JB, Nataro JP, Mobley HL. Pathogenic *Escherichia coli*. Nat Rev Microbiol. 2004;**2**:123-140. DOI: 10.1038/nrmicro818.

[10] Macfarlane S, Bahrami B, Macfarlane GT. Mucosal biofilm communities in the human intestinal tract. Adv Appl Microbiol. 2011;**75**:111-143. DOI: 10.1016/B978-0-12-387046-9. 00005-0.

[11] Conway T, Cohen PS. Commensal and pathogenic *Escherichia coli* metabolism in the gut. Microbiol Spectr. 2015;**3**(3). DOI: 10.1128/microbiolspec.MBP-0006-2014.

[12] Kim KS. Human meningitis-associated *Escherichia coli*. EcoSal Plus. 2016;**7**(1). DOI: 10.1128/ecosalplus.ESP-0015-2015.

[13] Le Bouguénec C, Servin AL. Diffusely adherent *Escherichia coli* strains expressing Afa/ Dr adhesins (Afa/Dr ADEC): hitherto unrecognized pathogens. FEMS Microbiol Lett. 2006;**256**:185-194. DOI: 10.1111/j.1574-6968.2006.00144.x.

[14] Meraz IM, Arikawa K, Nakamura H, Ogasawara J, Hase A, Nishikawa Y. Association of IL-8-inducing strains of diffusely adherent *Escherichia coli* with sporadic diarrheal patients with less than 5 years of age. Braz J Infect Dis. 2007;**11**:44-49.

[15] Mansan-Almeida R, Pereira AL, Giugliano LG. Diffusely adherent *Escherichia coli* strains isolated from children and adults constitute two different populations. BMC Microbiol. 2013;**13**:22. DOI: 10.1186/1471-2180-13-22.

[16] Estrada-Garcia T, Navarro-Garcia F. Enteroaggregative *Escherichia coli* pathotype: a genetically heterogeneous emerging foodborne enteropathogen. FEMS Immunol Med Microbiol. 2012;**66**:281-298. DOI: 10.1111/j.1574-695X.2012.01008.x.

[17] Jensen, BH, Olsen KE, Struve C, Krogfelt KA, Petersen AM. Epidemiology and clinical manifestations of enteroaggregative *Escherichia coli*. Clin Microbiol Rev. 2014:**27**:614-630. DOI: 10.1128/CMR.00112-13.

[18] Kong H, Hong X, Li X. Current perspectives in pathogenesis and antimicrobial resistance of enteroaggregative *Escherichia coli*. Microb Pathog. 2015:**85**:44-49. DOI: 10.1016/j. micpath.2015.06.002.

[19] Croxen MA, Finlay BB. Molecular mechanisms of *Escherichia coli* pathogenicity. Nat Rev Microbiol. 2010;**8**:26-38. DOI: 10.1038/nrmicro2265.

[20] Nguyen Y, Sperandio V. Enterohemorrhagic *E. coli* (EHEC) pathogenesis. Front Cell Infect Microbiol. 2012;**2**:90. DOI: 10.3389/fcimb.2012.00090.

[21] Page AV, Liles WC. Enterohemorrhagic *Escherichia coli* infections and the hemolytic-uremic syndrome. Med Clin North Am. 2013;**97**:681-695. DOI: 10.1016/j.mcna.2013.04.001.

[22] van den Beld MJ, Reubsaet FA. Differentiation between *Shigella*, enteroinvasive *Escherichia coli* (EIEC) and noninvasive *Escherichia coli*. Eur J Clin Microbiol Infect Dis. 2012;**31**:899-904. DOI: 10.1007/s10096-011-1395-7.

[23] Ud-Din A, Wahid S. Relationship among *Shigella* spp. and enteroinvasive *Escherichia coli* (EIEC) and their differentiation. Braz J Microbiol. 2014;**45**:1131-1138.

[24] Arenas-Hernández MM, Martinez-Laguna Y, Torres AG. Clinical implications of Enteroadherent *Escherichia coli*. Curr Gastroenterol Rep. 2012;**14**:386-394. DOI: 10.1007/s11894-012-0277-1.

[25] Lai Y, Rosenshine I, Leong JM, Frankel G. Intimate host attachment: enteropathogenic and enterohaemorrhagic *Escherichia coli*. Cell Microbiol 2013;**15**:1796-1808. DOI: 10.1111/cmi.12179.

[26] Wong Fok Lung T, Pearson JS, Schuelein R, Hartland EL. The cell death response to enteropathogenic *Escherichia coli* infection. Cell Microbiol. 2014;**16**:1736-1745. DOI: 10.1111/cmi.12371.

[27] Fleckenstein JM, Hardwidge PR, Munson GP, Rasko DA, Sommerfelt H, Steinsland H. Molecular mechanisms of enterotoxigenic *Escherichia coli* infection. Microbes Infect. 2010;**12**:89-98. DOI: 10.1016/j.micinf.2009.10.002.

[28] Reygaert WC. Innate immune response to urinary tract infections involving *Escherichia coli*. J Clin Cell Immunol. 2014;**5**:6. DOI: 10.4172/2155-9899.1000280.

[29] Subashchandrabose S, Mobley HL. Virulence and fitness determinants of uropathogenic *Escherichia coli*. Microbiol Spectr. 2015;**3**(4). DOI: 10.1128/microbiolspec.UTI-0015-2012.

[30] Muñiz CC, Zelaya TE, Esquivel GR, Fernández FJ. Penicillin and cephalosporin production: a historical perspective. Rev Latinoam Microbiol. 2007;**49**:88-98.

[31] Reygaert WC. Ceftobiprole: an emerging therapeutic option for resistant and complicated infections. Clin Med Insights: Therapeutics. 2011;**3**:57-66. DOI: 10.4137/CMT.S5032.

[32] Gaurav K, Karmakar S, Kundu K, Kundu S. Design, development and synthesis of novel cephalosporin group of antibiotics. In: Pana, M, editor: Antibiotic resistant bacteria – a continuous challenge in the new millennium. InTech;2012. p.487-502. ISBN:978-953-51-0472-8. DOI: 5772/29658. Available from: http://www.intechopen.com/books/antibiotic-resistant-bacteria-a-continuous-challenge-in-the-new-millennium/design-development-synthesis-and-in-vitro-antibacterial-activity-of-some-novel-cephem-antibiotics.

[33] Katzung BG, Trevor AJ, editors. Basic & Clinical Pharmacology, 13th ed. New York. McGraw-Hill Education;2015.1216 p.

[34] Davis TK, McKee R, Schnadower D, Tarr PI. Treatment of shiga toxin-producing *Escherichia coli* infections. Infect Dis Clin N Am. 2013;**27**:577-597. DOI: 10.1016/j.idc.2013.05.010.

[35] Hill DR, Beeching NJ. Traveler's diarrhea. Curr Opin Infect Dis. 2010;**23**:481-487. DOI: 10.1097/QCO.0b013e32833dfca5.

[36] Pfeiffer ML, DuPont HL, Ochoa TJ. The patient presenting with acute dysentery—a systematic review. J Infect. 2012;**64**:374-386. DOI: 10.1016/j.jinf.2012.01.006.

[37] Shepherd AK, Pottinger PS. Management of urinary tract infections in the era of increasing antimicrobial resistance. Med Clin North Am. 2013;**97**:737-757. DOI: 10.1016/j.mcna.2013.03.006.

[38] Nguyen HM, Shier KL, Graber CJ. Determining a clinical framework for use of cefepime and β-lactam/β-lactamase inhibitors in the treatment of infections caused by extended-spectrum-β-lactamase-producing Enterobacteriaceae. J Antimicrob Chemother. 2014;**69**:871-880. DOI: 10.1093/jac/dkt450.

[39] Shaikh S, Fatima J, Shakil S, Rizvi SM, Kamal MA. Antibiotic resistance and extended spectrum beta-lactamases: types, epidemiology and treatment. Saudi J Biol Sci. 2015;**22**:90-101. DOI: 10.1016/j.sjbs.2014.08.002.

[40] Morrill HJ, Pogue JM, Kaye KS, LaPlante KL. Treatment options for carbapenem-resistant *Enterobacteriaceae* infections. Open Forum Infect Dis. 2015;**2**(2):ofv050. DOI: 10.1093/ofid/ofv050.

[41] Davies J, Davies D. Origins and evolution of antibiotic resistance. Microbiol Mol Biol Rev. 2010;**74**:417-433. DOI: 10.1128/MMBR.00016-10.

[42] Center for Disease Control. *Antibiotic Resistance Threats in the United States*, 2013. Available at: www.cdc.gov/drugresistance/about.html.

[43] Reygaert WC. Insight on the antimicrobial resistance mechanisms of bacteria. Adv Clin Med Microbiol. 2016;**2**:1-11.

[44] Adler A, Katz, DE, Marchaim, D. The continuing plague of extended-spectrum β-lactamase-producing Enterobacteriaceae infections. Infect Dis Clin North Am. 2016;**30**:347-375. DOI: 10.1016/j.idc.2016.02.003.

[45] Guh AY, Bulens SN, Mu Y, Jacob JT, Reno J, Scott J, et al. Epidemiology of carbapenem-resistant Enterobacteriaceae in 7 US communities, 2012-2013. JAMA. 2015;**314**:1479-1487. DOI: 10.1001/jama.2015.12480.

[46] Reygaert WC. Antimicrobial resistance mechanisms of *Staphylococcus aureus*. In: Méndez-Vilas A, editor. Microbial pathogens and strategies for combating them: science, technology and education, Vol. 1. Badajoz, Spain: Formatex Research Center; 2013. p. 297-305.

[47] Mehrad B, Clark NM, Zhanel GG, Lynch JP 3rd. Antimicrobial resistance in hospital-acquired gram-negative bacterial infections. Chest. 2015;**147**:1413-1421. DOI: 10.1378/chest.14-2171.

[48] Delcour AH. Outer membrane permeability and antibiotic resistance. Biochim Biophys Acta. 2009;**1794**:808-816. DOI: 10.1016/j.bbapap.2008.11.005.

[49] Blair JM, Webber MA, Baylay AJ, Ogbolu DO, Piddock AJ. Molecular mechanisms of antibiotic resistance. Nat Rev Microbiol. 2015;**13**:42-51. DOI: 10.1038/nrmicro3380.

[50] Georgopapadakou NH. Penicillin-binding proteins and bacterial resistance to β-lactams. Antimicrob Agents Chemother. 1993;**37**:2045-2053.

[51] Sauvage E, Kerff F, Terrak M, Ayala JA, Charlier P. The penicillin-binding proteins: structure and role in peptidoglycan biosynthesis. FEMS Microbiol Rev. 2008;**32**:234-258. DOI: 10.1111/j.1574-6976.2008.00105.x.

[52] Mingeot-Leclercq MP, Glupczynski Y, Tulkens PM. Aminoglycosides: activity and resistance. Antimicrob Agents Chemother. 1999;**43**:727-737.

[53] Sergiev PV, Bogdanov AA, Dontsova OA. Ribosomal RNA guanine-(N2)-methyltransferases and their targets. Nucleic Acids Res. 2007;**35**:2295-2301.

[54] Wachino J, Shibayama K, Kurokawa H, Kimura K, Yamane K, Suzuki S, et al. Novel plasmid-mediated 16S rRNA m[1] A1408 methyltransferase, NpmA, found in a clinically isolated *Escherichia coli* strain resistant to structurally diverse aminoglycosides. Antimicrob Agents Chemother. 2007;**51**:4401-4409. DOI: 10.1128/AAC.00926-07.

[55] Zhou Y, Yu H, Guo Q, Xu X, Ye X, Wu S, Guo Y, Wang M. Distribution of 16S rRNA methylases among different species of Gram-negative bacilli with high-level resistance to aminoglycosides. Eur J Clin Microbiol Infect Dis. 2010;**29**:1349-1353. DOI: 10.1111/j.1365-2125.2009.03592.x.

[56] Schultsz C, Geerlings S. Plasmid-mediated resistance in *Enterobacteriaceae*. Drugs. 2012;**72**:1-16. DOI: 10.2165/11597960-000000000-00000.

[57] von Baum H, Marre R. Antimicrobial resistance of *Escherichia coli* and therapeutic implications. Int J Med Microbiol. 2005;**295**:503-511.

[58] Hooper DC, Jacoby GA. Mechanisms of drug resistance: quinolone resistance. Ann N Y Acad Sci. 2015;**1354**:12-31. DOI: 10.1111/nyas.12830.

[59] Huovinen P, Sundström L, Swedberg G, Sköld O. Trimethoprim and sulfonamide resistance. Antimicrob Agents Chemother. 1995;**39**:279-289.

[60] Vedantam G, Guay G, Austria NE, Doktor SZ, Nichols BP. Characterization of mutations contributing to sulfathiazole resistance in *Escherichia coli*. Antimicrob Agents Chemother. 1998;**42**:88-93.

[61] Ramirez MS, Tolmasky ME. Aminoglycoside modifying enzymes. Drug Resist Updat. 2010;**13**:151-171. DOI: 10.1016/j.drup.2010.08.003.

[62] Bush K, Jacoby GA. Updated functional classification of β-lactamases. Antimicrob Agents Chemother. 2010;**54**:969-976. DOI: 10.1128/AAC.01009-09.

[63] Bush K. Proliferation and significance of clinically relevant β-lactamases. Ann N Y Acad Sci. 2013;**1277**:84-90. DOI: 10.1111/nyas.12023.

[64] Jacoby GA. AmpC β-lactamases. Clin Microbiol Rev. 2009;**22**:161-182. DOI: 10.1128/CMR.00036-08.

[65] Thomson KS. Extended-spectrum-β-lactamase, AmpC, and carbapenemase issues. J Clin Microbiol. 2010;**48**:1019-1025. DOI: 10.1128/JCM.00219-10.

[66] Bush K, Bradford PA. β-Lactams and β-lactamase inhibitors: an overview. Cold Spring Harb Perspect Med. 2016;**6**(8). pii: a025247. DOI: 10.1101/cshperspect.a025247.

[67] Pfeifer Y, Cullik A, Witte W. Resistance to cephalosporins and carbapenems in Gram-negative bacterial pathogens. Int J Med Microbiol. 2010;**300**:371-379. DOI: 10.1016/j.ijmm.2010.04.005.

[68] Bajaj P, Singh NS, Virdi JS. *Escherichia coli* β-lactamases: what really matters. Front Microbiol. 2016;**7**:417. DOI: 10.3389/fmicb.2016.00417.

[69] Kumar A, Schweizer HP. Bacterial resistance to antibiotics: active efflux and reduced uptake. Adv Drug Deliv Rev. 2005;**57**:1486-1513.

[70] Poole K. Efflux pumps as antimicrobial resistance mechanisms. Ann Med. 2007;**39**:162-176. DOI: 10.1080/07853890701195262.

[71] Collu F, Cascella M. Multidrug resistance and efflux pumps: insights from molecular dynamics simulations. Curr Top Med Chem. 2013;**13**:3165-3183.

[72] Blair JM, Richmond GE, Piddock LJ. Multidrug efflux pumps in Gram-negative bacteria and their role in antibiotic resistance. Future Microbiol. 2014;**9**:1165-1177. DOI: 10.2217/fmb.14.66.

[73] Lubelski J, Konings WN, Driessen AJ. Distribution and physiology of ABC-type transporters contributing to multidrug resistance in bacteria. Microbiol Mol Biol Rev. 2007;**71**:463-476. DOI: 10.1128/MMBR.00001-07.

[74] Kuroda T, Tsuchiya T. Multidrug efflux transporters in the MATE family. Biochim Biophys Acta. 2009;**1794**:763-768. DOI: 10.1016/j.bbapap.2008.11.012.

[75] Swick MC, Morgan-Linnell SK, Carlson KM, Zechiedrich L. Expression of multidrug efflux pump genes *acrAB-tolC*, *mdfA*, and *norE* in *Escherichia coli* clinical isolates as a function of fluoroquinolone and multidrug resistance. Antimicrob Agents Chemother. 2011;**55**:921-924. DOI: 10.1128/AAC.00996-10.

[76] Kumar S, Mukherjee MM, Varela MF. Modulation of bacterial multidrug resistance efflux pumps of the major facilitator superfamily. Int J Bacteriol. 2013;**2013**. pii: 204141. DOI: 10.1155/2013/204141.

[77] Tuckman M, Petersen PJ, Howe, AY, Orlowski M, Mullen S, Chan K, et al. Occurrence of tetracycline resistance genes among *Escherichia coli* isolates from the phrase 3 clinical trials for tigecycline. Antimicrob Agents Chemother. 2007;**51**:3205-3211. DOI: 10.1128/AAC.00625-07.

[78] Bay DC, Rommens KL, Turner RJ. Small multidrug resistance proteins: a multidrug transporter family that continues to grow. Biochim Biophys Acta. 2008;**1778**:1814-1838. DOI: 10.1016/j.bbamem.2007.08.015.

[79] Piddock LJ. Clinically relevant chromosomally encoded multidrug resistance efflux pumps in bacteria. Clin Microbiol Rev. 2006;**19**:382-402. DOI: 10.1128/CMR.19.2.382-402.2006.

[80] Anes J, McCusker MP, Fanning S, Martins M. The ins and outs of RND efflux pumps in *Escherichia coli*. Front Microbiol. 2015;**6**:587. DOI: 10.3389/fmicb.2015.00587.

Chapter 6

Antibiotic Resistance among *Escherichia coli*: Isolates and Novel Approaches to the Control of *E. coli* Infections

Henrique C. Alves, Felipe de P. N. Cruz,
Pamela C. P. de Assis, José D. C. Pessoa,
Luis C. Trevelin, Angela M. de O. Leal and
Cristina P. de Sousa

Additional information is available at the end of the chapter

http://dx.doi.org/10.5772/67400

Abstract

Bacteria are the microorganisms that most frequently cause infectious diseases in humans. The synthesis of silver nanoparticles (AgNPs) has attracted interest due to the new and different physical and chemical characteristics with applications in new fields. AgNPs, alone or supported on ceramic, are used as antimicrobial fillers in textiles and polymers for food-packaging and biomedical applications, for antimicrobial paints, and potentially for drug delivery. The evaluation of mesoporous nanostructures or nanocomposites as FDU-12/lignin/silver was effective in inhibiting *Staphylococcus aureus, E. coli, Enterococcus faecalis*, and *Candida albicans*. The best results were achieved against the inhibition of *E. coli* and with the structures FDU-12/silver. In plates with FDU-12/lignin/silver, FDU-12, FDU-12/lignin, and the positive control, it was enumerated at 0, 6, 14, and 27 colonies, respectively. While the development of resistance to a new antibiotic is expected, the time course and degree of resistance are uncertain and depend on various factors. The application of AgNPs as nanocomposites can alter the expression of bacterial proteins and could be used for inactivation. This review explores such aspects and a number of factors arising like the use of nanostructures against *E. coli*, from the knowledge acquired.

Keywords: *Escherichia coli*, nanostructures, nanocomposites, FDU-12/lignin/silver, *E. coli* resistance

1. Introduction

Bacterial survival and persistence in an inappropriate substrate can be defined as the ability of bacteria to tolerate exposure to lethal concentrations of bactericidal antibiotics. This view was first noticed in 1944 regarding that treatment of cultures of *Staphylococcus aureus* with high concentrations of penicillin did not kill all the strains, and that a fraction of the order of 10^{-6} of these strains survived. Bacteria can cause frequently infections in humans, and the resistance to antibiotics is a primary cause of disease and sometimes death in the intensive-care units of hospitals worldwide [1] and the cause of numerous clinical problems [2]. The development and increase of resistance among pathogens causing nosocomial and community-acquired infections are known to be associated with the widespread utilization of antibiotics [3–5].

Antimicrobial is a general term for drugs, chemicals, and/or other substances that either kill or slow the microbial metabolism. Various antimicrobial agents that are in use today are antibiotic, antiviral, antifungal, and antiparisitic drugs. An antibiotic is a type of antimicrobial agent produced by a fungi or a bacterium that has a direct influence on other microbes, specifically bacteria. Many of antibiotic resistance genes are found on transposons, integrons, and/or plasmids that can be transferred to another bacteria belonging to the same or different species [6] and resistance elements can be transferred to the human commensal or pathogenic microbiome [7].

The genes conferring resistance to antibiotics have been widely distributed in the environment since before the introduction of antibiotic chemotherapies, but human activities are probably the major driven force of the resistant bacteria found in air and water, principally with *S. aureus* and *E. coli* isolates. The antibiotic presence in the environment can exert selective pressure on the organisms living closely, but the mechanisms of cross resistance to antibiotics are unknown [6].

Studies with animals [8] showed that the proximity with humans has the tendency to generate more antibiotic-resistant enteric bacteria as saw with African baboons. With birds, a study [9] showed that 8% of *E. coli* isolated from arctic region presented resistance. This can enhance the pressure of antibiotic resistance by an anthropogenic activity. In pristine environments, the determinants of an antibiotic resistance existed naturally and were probably subjected to horizontal gene transfer [10]. This predisposition for the genetic exchange of resistance elements has facilitated the antibiotic resistance in pathogenic bacteria.

Antibiotics kill or inhibit bacteria that are susceptible to that antibiotic. Bacteria that are intrinsically resistant or that can acquire resistance will survive and replace the drug-susceptible bacteria. The production of an antibiotic is associated with the presence of genes encoding one or more self-protection processes. Antibiotic biosynthesis gene clusters that encode resistance proteins specific to the compound made (modification of the compound or target) or multifunctional (efflux systems) are important systems. The resistance genes that are contiguous with the biosynthesis genes could be involved in regulation of the biosynthetic pathway.

There are consistent results [11] that showed that antibiotic resistance genes are found in natural sources. Another form of resistance in isolates not producing antibiotics is the mutation of the target gene product, which reduces or prevents inhibition by antibiotic binding. Spontaneous mutations causing resistance often lead to different bacterial phenotypes.

http://dx.doi.org/10.5772/67400

The presence of antibiotic resistance strains in environment may be understood as a response to the selective pressures. Thus, any antibiotic use will provide a selective pressure that perpetuates resistant bacteria. The introduction of antibiotics in the treatment of diseases that were prior incurable, enabled the effective treatment of these, promoting the increase in longevity. This kind of medicine is widely used in the treatment of people in the community and health services and is also used to treat animals in agricultural environments. Thus, the increasing levels of resistance are compromising the effectiveness of them. Therefore, it is essential that we assess the use of antibiotics carefully, regardless of setting, and use them only when necessary, to avoid promoting the development of resistance among bacteria [12].

Various infections are caused by important pathogens, such as *Staphylococcus aureus*, and up to 50% are resistant to stronger drugs, such as methicillin [13], and with *E. coli* [12, 14–16] the resistant trait is growing.

The food supply can be a source of antimicrobial-resistant and virulent *E. coli* strains that could be lethal to humans or, in a major scale, can cause intestinal as well as extra intestinal infections. *Escherichia coli* (**Figure 1**) is a ubiquitous and versatile microorganism, moving from commensal to opportunistic and specialized virulent bacteria, with potential to cause different diseases. To cause infection, harmless commensal *E. coli* can acquire a set of combination of mobile genetic elements to become a highly adapted pathogen capable of causing different diseases in different hosts, ranging from gastroenteritis to extra intestinal infections of the urinary tract, bloodstream, and central nervous system. Seven diarrheagenic and two extra intestinal *E. coli* pathovars can cause disease in various hosts.

Interestingly, one outbreak happens, caused by one not expected *E. coli* pathotype [18] in 2011. An uncommon high number of haemolytic uremic syndrome (HUS) cases were reported in

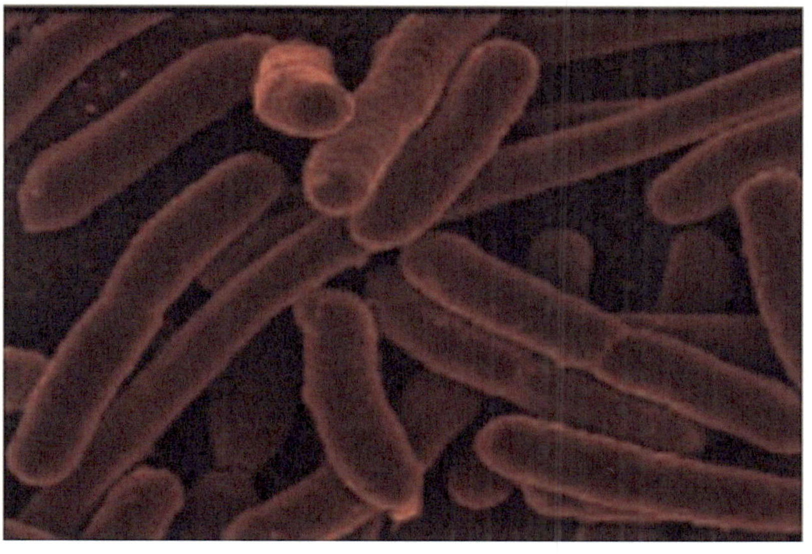

Figure 1. *E. coli* in scanning electronic microscopy [17].

Europe, most precisely in Germany. The implicated agent was an enterohemorrhagic *E. coli* (EHEC), which presented virulence traits of both, a verotoxigenic *E. coli* (VTEC) and enteroaggregative *E. coli* (EAEC).

A relevant study involving enterotoxigenic *E. coli* STb toxin was conducted in 2014 [19], regarding the STb toxigenicity. STb is a heat-resistant toxin responsible for diarrhea in farm animals and in humans as well. The toxic effect of STb in host cells is due to allowing the passage of electrolytes and water through the paracellular space. The authors [19] demonstrated that STb could promote the delocalization of transmembrane proteins such as claudin-1.

This event among others can prove how the versatility of this bacterium can reach a worldwide proportion, with a high concern for public health. These types of outbreaks are not solely a consequence of health conditions in developing countries. With the increase in international travel and trade globalization, diarrheagenic *E. coli* has become a worldwide public health threat [20].

On the other hand, antibiotic resistance rates in *E. coli* are rapidly rising, especially concerning to the use of fluoroquinolones and third- and fourth-generation cephalosporin. These strains are acquired predominantly in the community [12]. In these conditions, drug-resistant *E. coli* are readily acquired via the consumption of contaminated food and beverage. Some authors [14] studied 287 *E. coli* samples isolated from meats regarding their virulence factors. They observed that drug-resistant isolates had similar characteristics to those collected from the same types of meat.

This review shows the immune view of *E. coli*, and focus on the presence of these bacteria highlighting the acquisition of resistance and discussing various aspects of *E. coli* pathotypes. Because the antibiotic treatment is our primary method of threaten diseases, studies on this field are important to a better understanding of bacterial evasion, circumventing, and subverting mechanisms to acquire resistance characteristics.

2. Immune view

A good immune system is essential for the survival of any organism because of the protection against infectious beings. It is the principal infections evolution blocker that may cause elevated decease rate. This is a well-established fact for almost all known infective illness; the number of subjects in contact with the infectious agents is greater than those who really evolve diseases.

Contaminations occurred by no cell invasive bacteria are the most common. In these cases, the immune system of shield is mostly associated to the harborer's innate barriers, natural protection mechanisms, and antibody production. The importance of innate barriers (**Table 1**) in the combat against no cell invasive bacterial infections is well-known [21]. The integrity of skin and mucosa prevent adherence and penetration of bacteria; mucociliary movement eliminates bacteria from the respiratory tract; the stomach's acidic pH destroys some bacteria penetrating by the upper digestive tract; and in the saliva, eyes secretion, and prostatic secretion, lysozyme and other substances have antimicrobial activity.

http://dx.doi.org/10.5772/67400

I. Natural barriers against infection	II. Innate immunity	III. Acquired immunity
1. Integrity of skin and mucosa	1. Extracellular molecules (C reactive protein, complement)	1. Antibodies
2. Mucociliar movement	2. Natural killer cells, neutrophils, macrophages	2. Cytokines produced by T cells
3. pH variations	3. Chemokines, cytokines	–
4. Antimicrobial substances	–	–
Note: Ref. [21] with modifications.		

Table 1. Barriers against infectious microorganisms.

On the other hand, the main characteristic of intracellular bacteria is the ability to survive within the macrophages. In this context, some important pathogens are *L. monocytogenes, Mycobacterium tuberculosis* and, *M. leprae*. Invasion of the macrophage is also a parasite's getaway strategy. Though paradoxical, the last mechanism is benign to the harborer, while the lack of cell penetration by bacteria can induce a strong inflammatory effect and excessive injury to the host.

Adaptive immunity, principally by means of antibodies plays an important function versus bacteria outside of the cell. Antibodies may exert its inhibition in three steps: (i) opsonization, (ii) activation of the complementary system, and (iii) furthering the neutralization of bacteria or their metabolites.

Extracellular bacteria are prone to undoing when phagocytozed. So subverting this system, they developed substances such as evasive mechanism with an antiphagocytic system.

Antibodies directed against these substances not only avoid their action, also facilitate phagocytosis, while neutrophils and macrophages have receivers for the fc part of immunoglobulin (opsonization).

The antibodies also coassist in the destruction of complement by bacteria, and activate this system by the classical pathway. Through neutralization mechanism, IgA antibodies, in particular, can bind to bacteria and therefore prevent the latter from settling on the intestinal mucosa and the respiratory tract. Antibodies bind frequently to toxins produced from bacteria, such as tetanus (*Clostridium tetani*) and diphtheria toxin (*Corynebacterium diphtheriae*), and neutralize the action of these metabolites. The fine balance between health and disease is found in this scenario, in which deficiency is as much as excess may result in tissue damage.

3. *E. coli* antibiotic resistance

A mature human gut harbors a vast number of bacterial resident microbiota, accounting for more than 10^{14} individual bacteria. Notably, the composition of the microbiota is individual host specific and the type of species living in the gastrointestinal tract varies with the host age, diet, habits, health, and idiosyncratic status [22]. The intestinal mucosa is a first contact between the immune system and the external environment and plays a central role in a microbe and host cross talk [23]. The indigenous intestinal microbiota provides important protective, metabolic and trophic functions, principally offering resistance to colonization by exogenous microorganisms, and preventing invasion by incoming pathogens.

The intestinal epithelium can resist against microbial invasion, but through evolution mechanisms, potential pathogenic enteric microorganisms developed strategies to circumvent and subvert this strong barrier. As an initial step in the infection process, some pathogens target specific epithelial cell structures, as glycoprotein and glycolipid [24], which act as receptors for attachment, permitting the microorganisms to exploit the underlying signal transduction pathway.

Other strategies utilized by invasive pathogens such as *Salmonella enterica* serovar, *S. thyphimurium, Shigella* spp., and invasive *E. coli* orchestrated their entry into intestinal epithelial cells. This strategy uses the expression of a bacterial type III protein secretion system, to deliver various effectors proteins into the host cell [25]. This effectors protein subverts normal host cell processes by triggering a marked rearrangement of the host cytoskeleton. This procedure facilitates the pathogen to cross the epithelial barrier and induces an inflammatory host response [25].

The latter strategy can be done by direct cytotoxic injury, intracellular migration, disruption of the epithelial tight junctions, or indirectly by inducing neutrophil infiltration. Pathogenic *E. coli* have been shown to increase chloride ion secretion from intestinal epithelia by upregulating the expression of the receptor for the neuropeptide galanin-1 [26].

Enteric pathogens have the propriety to perturb the intestinal epithelial barrier and impact paracellular permeability, most often with an alteration in the arrangement of tight junctional component proteins by mechanisms that are unique for different pathogens. With respect to enteropathogenic *E. coli*, they disrupt the epithelial barrier by the phosphorylation of myosin light chains [27].

E. coli isolated from human and animal gut, and as well as from environmental sources presenting antibiotic resistance is a public health problem, especially in developing countries [28]. Work conducted in 2005 [29] showed that extended spectrum lactamase producing *E. coli* (ESBL) strains have spread as a hospital infection. The large plasmid genes coding this resistance also carry genes for resistance to other antibiotics [30]. The frequency of resistance to fluoroquinolone antibiotics (ciprofloxacin, levofloxacin, moxifloxacin, norfloxacin, and nalidixic acid) in *E. coli* has increased worldwide [31].

In one review about *E. coli* producing fimbrial or afimbrial adhesins [32], authors showed that some *E. coli* strains (ETEC STb positive) associated with diarrhea, presented an afimbrial adhesin, named AIDA-I (adhesion involved in diffuse adherence). This adhesin originally found in human *E. coli* isolates showed that the establishment of a persistent and chronic infection could also help the microorganism to resist antimicrobial agents and prevent effective treatment of diseased animals.

In 2010, some authors [33] detected high resistance rates among *E. coli* (up to 30%) to ampicillin, tetracycline, streptomycin, ciprofloxacin, enrofloxacin, and cotrimoxazol. These authors [33] also found lower resistance to gentamicin (6.5%) and chloramphenicol (3.2%).

Also in 2010, one study [34] reported that morbidity and mortality attributable to third -generation-cephalosporin-resistant *E. coli* are significant. They also believe that if prevailing resistance trends continue, high societal and economic costs can be expected and that better management of infections caused by resistant *E. coli* is becoming essential.

Work with neonates in a single center concluded that the use of minor antibiotic therapy with reducing preemptive treatment resulted in a moderate reduction of the antibiotic use and did not increase mortality [35].

Another study [36] was conducted to determine the antimicrobial susceptibility patterns among common pathogens in the intensive care unit of a university hospital in Iran between 2006 and 2009. Authors worked with 606 isolates from respiratory, urine, blood, and wound specimens of 456 patients. *E. coli* was present in 8.3% of isolates, and presented high antimicrobial resistance.

Scientists worked with 1163 clinical isolates in Taiwan [37]. The frequencies of Gram-positive and Gram-negative bacteria isolates were 30.4 and 56.2%, respectively. *Staphylococcus aureus* was the most common isolate among the Gram-positive organisms, while *Pseudomonas aeruginosa, E. coli,* and *Klebsiella pneumoniae* were the leading Gram-negative isolates.

The antimicrobial resistance in one intensive care unit in Canada was investigated. In 2008, it was found high antibiotic rates to *E. coli*: cefazolin, 20.1%; cefepime, 0.7%; ceftriaxone, 3.7%; gentamicin, 3.0%; fluoroquinolones, 21.1%; piperacillin-tazobactam, 1.9%; and trimethoprim-sulfamethoxazole, 24.8%. *E. coli* was the most prevalent Gram-negative bacterium [38].

According to a work conducted in 1975 [39], a hospital acquired urinary tract infection account for approximately 45% of nosocomial infection and 2–4% of the cases may develop septicemia. In this context, it was observed that 40% of the Gram-negative septicemia acquired in hospital originates in the urinary tract. This observation can enhance the *E. coli* importance for acquiring resistance. In 2009 was observed that, Gram-negative bacteria were the most frequent isolates, with *E. coli* being the most common followed by *Pseudomonas aeruginosa* and *Klebsiella* spp. *Candida albicans* accounted for almost 11% of the organisms, followed by *Acinetobacter baumanni* (**Table 2**) [39].

Bacteria and fungi	Total	Resistance to all	Sensibility
	N (%)	N (%)	N (%)
Escherichia coli	27 (49.1)	22 (81.5)	5 (18.5)
Pseudomonas aeruginosa	7 (12.7)	5 (71.4)	2 (28.6)
Klebsiella spp.	7 (12.7)	4 (57.1)	3 (42.9)
Candida albicans	6 (10.9)	–	–
Acinetobacter baumanni	3 (5.5)	3 (100)	0
Others	5 (9.1)	2 (40)	3 (60)
Total	55 (100)	36 (73.5)	13 (26.5)

Note: Ref. [39] with modifications.

Table 2. Profile resistance of main microorganisms isolated from hospitals

4. Mechanisms of antibiotic resistance in Gram-negative bacteria

Bacterial antimicrobial resistance in both the medical and agricultural fields has become a serious problem worldwide. Resistant bacteria isolated from agriculture, farm or hospital can transfer the resistance genes to human pathogens [40]. The selection pressure applied by the antibiotics that are used in clinical and agricultural settings has promoted the evolution and spread of genes that confer resistance, regardless of their origins. Several factors can be implicated with resistance, sensibility, and antibiotic resistance dissemination such as: (i) impermeable barriers [6]; in this case, some bacteria are intrinsically resistant to certain antibiotics because they have an impermeable membrane or lack the target of the antibiotic; (ii) multidrug resistance efflux pumps; these pumps protect the bacterial cell against toxic molecules. It is an active transport mechanism for outside the cell. Some transporters, such as those of the resistance-nodulation cell division family, can pump antibiotics directly outside the cell, whereas others, such as those of the major facilitator superfamily, secrete them into the bacterial periplasm; (iii) resistance mutations; these mutations can cause a modification in the target protein, for example, by disabling the antibiotic-binding without changing the protein functionality. Specific examples include mutations in the gyrase, which cause resistance to fluoroquinolones, in RNA polymerase subunit B, which cause resistance to rifampicin, and in the 30S ribosomal subunit protein S12 (encoded by *rpsL*), which cause resistance to streptomycin; and (iv) antibiotic inactivation; inactivation can occur by covalent modification of the antibiotic, such as that catalyzed by acetyltransferases acting on aminoglycoside antibiotics, or by degradation of the antibiotic, such as the hydrolytic degradation of the β-lactam ring on antibiotics by the β-lactamases. The emergence of drug resistance among diarrheagenic *E. coli* is important, and in infant, is a cause of morbidity and mortality principally in developing countries. Analyzing stools of infants in India was verified that about 90% of *E. coli* strains presented resistance to the most antibiotics tested [41]. All isolates were resistant to ampicillin, imipenem, cotrimoxazole, and sensitive to amikacin, and presented 29 different antibiotic profiles. Most of the isolated *E. coli* harbored plasmids (64%) and up to 76% could transfer their plasmids. The transconjugant strains were carrying plasmids and presented resistance to ampicillin, imipenem, and cotrimoxazole. The authors found an increase in the prevalence of drug resistance among *E. coli* isolates, and conjugation transfer of plasmids contributed to a rapid spread of an antibiotic resistance.

Cyclomodulins are a growing functional family of toxins, which hijack eukaryotic cell cycle. Four cyclomodulin types are actually known in *E. coli*: cytotoxic necrotizing factors (CNFs), cycle inhibiting factor (Cif), cytolethal distending toxins (CDTs), and the pks-encoded toxin.

One interesting work [42] isolated ceftriaxone-resistant *E. coli* from 1.5% of participants in Maryland and Michigan, United States. One *E. coli* isolate collected from an apparently healthy person, presented resistance to eight antibiotics, and the resistance genes were contained on an incompatibility plasmid. These plasmid types are common among *Enterobacteriaceae* and can carry multiple resistance genes, generating multidrug resistance [43]. In Krueger's work [42], the source of the extensively resistant *E. coli* is not known, but the isolated strain may have been acquired from food.

http://dx.doi.org/10.5772/67400

5. Diarrheagenic and extra intestinal *E. coli* pathotypes

Several distinct pathogenic categories (i.e., pathotypes or virotypes) of diarrheagenic *E. coli* strains are recognized. Each pathotype is defined by a characteristic set of virulence-associated determinants that act in a concert to determine the clinical, pathological, and epidemiological features of the disease they cause [44].

By definition, the virulence determinants of each *E. coli* pathotype are distinct. However, they can generally be categorized as either colonization factors (adhesins), which enable the bacteria to bind closely to the intestinal mucosa and resist removal by peristalsis, or secreted toxins, which interfere with the normal physiological processes of host cells. The key virulence determinants of the primary pathotypes of diarrheagenic *E. coli* are summarized in **Table 3**.

Pathotype	Common genotype	Most common presentation	Intestinal pathology	Susceptibile groups
EPEC	eae +, bfp +, EAF +	Non-specific gastroenteritis, noninflammatory diarrhea	Intimate adhesion, attaching–effacing lesions throughout the intestine, loss of brush border enterocyte	Children under 2 years of age in developing countries
ETEC	LT, ST, (STa, STb toxins)	Watery, cholera-like diarrhea, noninflammatory diarrhea	No notable change, adhesion to small intestinal mucosa	Children in developing countries; travelers
EHEC	eae +, stx +	Bloody diarrhea 'Hemorrhagic colitis';	attaching–effacing lesions confined to the large intestine; necrosis in severe cases; HUS, hemorrhagic colitis	Children and the elderly in industrialized countries
EIEC	Inv	Bacillary dysentery	Inflammation and disruption of the mucosa, mostly of the large intestine; necrosis and blood loss	All ages; more common in less-developed countries
EAEC	AA +, aaa −/aaa +	Persistent diarrhea Inflammation;	cytotoxic changes in enterocytes	Children in less-developed countries; travelers to those countries
A-EPEC	eae +, bfp (−/+), EAF −	Nonspecific gastroenteritis	Some lesions throughout the intestine; toxin production as EAST1	Children and adults; reservoir for human infection

Note: Ref. [44] with modifications.

Table 3. Key virulence determinants of diarrheagenic *E. coli*.

It can be seen in **Table 3**, that the number of virulence traits varies from each pathotype and have implications on intestinal pathology. Besides Enteropathogenic *E. coli* (EPEC) causing intimate adhesion, attaching-effacing lesions throughout the intestine and loss of brush enterocytes, Enterotoxigenic *E. coli* (ETEC) do not present notable change to intestinal mucosa. Enterohaemorragic *E. coli* (EHEC) provoke a similar intestinal pathology, with necrosis. Enteroinvasive *E. coli* (EIEC) cause inflammation and necrosis, but Enteroaggregative *E. coli* (EAEC) present enterocytes changes. Atypical *E. coli* (A-EPEC) and Diffusely adherent *E. coli* (DAEC) can cause lesions in the intestine.

Based on genetic variation within *E. coli*, it was found [45] that pathogenic strains have accelerated the rates of mutation and recombination and virulence is the driving force for more frequent recombination. These characteristics can impulse the bacterial population to acquire more resistance. Some studies [45–46] proposed a model where commensal *E. coli* maintains low frequencies of homologous recombination and acquisition of novel genes that result in virulence by horizontal genetic exchange. The pathogenic condition results in exposure to immune system barriers and antibiotic selection. These population presents higher mutation and recombination rates. Epidemic strains are exposed to stronger selection by pressures imposed by immune defenses and antibiotic use, resulting in highest levels of mutation, recombination, and infection.

In one study, conducted in Ontario, Canada, the authors [15] showed that the most common bacteria identified on urine culture over a 5 year period were *Escherichia coli* (71.6%), *Enterococcus* spp. (5.7%), and *Klebsiella* spp. (5.0%) and that these bacteria were frequently resistant to ampicillin (54.4%) and trimethoprim-sulfamethoxazole (TMP-SMX) (40.4%) [15].

Another study showed that resistance was more commonly seen in typical EPEC than in atypical pathotypes. The most prevalent resistances observed were to ampicillin, tetracycline, streptomycin, and the sulfonamides [16].

EPEC, an established etiological agent of human infantile diarrhea, is a pathogen that subverts intestinal epithelial cell function to produce distinctive "attaching and effacing" (A/E) lesions. These types of pathogens are typically found on the surface of the host epithelial cell. They can cause severe lesions on intestinal microvilli. Other pathogens can display similar characteristics, which includes *Hafnia alvei, Citrobacter rodentium*, and enterohemorrhagic *E. coli*.

The interactions between EPEC and host cells have been divided into three stages. Initial adherence to cultured epithelial cells is mediated by the formation of type IV fimbriae known as bundle forming pili (BFP) [47]. Initial adherence helps bring the bacteria in intimate contact with the host cell. BFPs mediate bacterial interactions in a human intestinal organ culture model [48].

The genetic answer for the formation of A/E lesions can be explained by the presence of the *locus* of enterocyte effacement (LEE) [49]. This cluster includes the genes of following bacterial proteins: *E. coli* attaching and effacing that encodes the protein intimin (*eae*); *E. coli* secretion (*escs*); *E. coli*-secreted protein (*esps*); secretion of *E. coli* proteins (*sep*), and translocated intimin receptor (Tir).

The second stage of EPEC pathogenesis involves the secretion of bacterial proteins, some into the host cell, including EspA, EspB, and EspD at the temperature of the body [50], and particularly the gastrointestinal tract, the expression of these proteins is maximal, which

http://dx.doi.org/10.5772/67400

implies that they may be involved in virulence. The translocation of these proteins is essential for activating a number of signal transduction pathways.

The third stage of EPEC interaction with the eukaryotic cells is characterized by the intimate attachment with the host cell. A 94-kDa outer membrane protein and intimin, encoded by the *eae* gene [51], binds to a 90-kDa tyrosine phosphorylated protein in the host membrane. This receptor is of bacterial origin and has been designated as the translocated intimin receptor (Tir). Tir is translocated from the bacterial cell into the host membrane, where it becomes phosphorylated on one or more tyrosine residues and functions as a receptor for its binding partner, intimin. The resultant tight association is accompanied by the formation of actin pedestals. The most remarkable change in the cellular structure of the eukaryotic cell is the formation of typical actin pedestals. Within 3 hours of infection by EPEC, host-cell actin, a-actinin, talin, erzin, and villin accumulate directly under the bacteria. EPEC presents a strong and intimate adhesion to the intestinal mucosa leading to dissolution of the brush border by inducing vesiculation of the microvilli. This is the attaching and effacement step, and in the jejunum and ileum results in a loss of brush border disaccharidase enzymes and a large area of absorptive surface.

Typical kinds of EPEC are EPECs that have lost the EAF plasmid. ETEC strains are a major cause of secretory diarrhea in both humans and animals. They produce heat-labile and/or heat-stable (STa and STb) toxins that also cause diarrhea. EHEC strains are implicated in foodborne diseases principally due to ingestion of uncooked minced meat and raw milk. These strains produce shiga-like toxin 1 (stx1), shiga-like toxin 2 (stx2), and variants thereof. These toxins can destroy colonic enterocytes and produce hemorrhagic colitis. EIEC can attach to enterocytes and penetrate by endocytosis and replicate therein. DAEC strains are diffusely adhering *E. coli* that are also implicated with episodes of diarrhea. EAEC damage and blunt colonic villi by hemorrhagic necrosis, although the precise pathogenic mechanisms are unclear. EAEC are a major cause of chronic diarrhea in children. ExPEC are the cause of a diverse spectrum of invasive human and animal infections, often leading to septicemia and sometimes to death.

Extraintestinal *E. coli* (ExPEC) strains have amazing behavior and possess virulence mechanisms to invade, colonize, and induce disease in sites outside of the gastrointestinal tract. Human diseases caused by the ExPEC include urinary tract infections, neonatal meningitis, sepsis, pneumonia, surgical site infections, as well as infections in other extraintestinal locations. ExPEC strains have been isolated from food products, in particular from raw meats, and poultry, indicating that these organisms potentially represent a new class of foodborne pathogens [52–53].

Extraintestinal *E. coli* infections are associated with specialized strains presenting antimicrobial resistance. The food supply may disseminate ExPEC and antimicrobial-resistant *E. coli*. Retail foods may be an important vehicle for community-wide dissemination of antimicrobial-resistant *E. coli* and ExPEC, which may represent a newly recognized group of medically significant foodborne pathogens.

E. coli contamination exhibited a prevalence gradient from miscellaneous foods (9%), through beef or pork (69%), to poultry (92%) [54]. Among *E. coli*-positive samples, similar prevalence gradients were detected for antimicrobial resistance (27, 85, and 94 of samples, respectively) and ExPEC contamination (4, 19, and 46%, respectively). Indirect evidence suggested on-farm selection of resistance.

Uropathogenic strains can invade bladder cells and at this local, form reservoirs, which is possibly the storage local of the bacterium. *E. coli* causing infant meningitis is resistant to host immune responses and has the ability to cross the blood-brain barrier and cause disease. ExPEC from human and avian hosts encounter similar challenges in establishing infection in extraintestinal locations.

Extended spectrum beta-lactamases (ESBLs) are the bacterial enzymes that make them resistant to advanced generation cephalosporins and might lead to the failure on therapy.

The importance of this resistance in one children population in India was studied. CTX-M-15 enzyme is increasingly being reported from this part of the world together with TEM-1 [55]. TEM-1 is the most commonly encountered beta-lactamase in Gram-negative bacteria. Up to 90% of ampicillin, resistance in *E. coli* is due to the production of TEM-1 and *E. coli* is the most common cause of neonatal sepsis. The authors found that 97 ESBL-producers were identified among 266 *E. coli* strains isolated from 238 neonates. The isolates were screened for blaCTX-M, blaTEM, armA, rmtA, and rmtB, the last three genes being responsible for aminoglycoside resistance. The authors [55] concluded that male neonates colonized or infected by ESBL-producing *E. coli* have longer stay in NICU compared to their female counterparts. This happened because of male neonates getting colonized and/or infected earlier than their female counterparts do. Plasmid-mediated-conjugal transfer was found to be the mechanism of transfer of blaCTX-M-15 resistance marker in the described setting [55].

Antimicrobial drug resistance is a large and growing problem among organisms that cause diarrheal disease. Although most diarrheal diseases are self-resolving and should not be treated with antimicrobial agents, invasive or protracted infections require chemotherapy and are typically managed empirically [56].

The more recently defined enteroaggregative *E. coli* are typically multidrug-resistant and are one of the most common causes of childhood diarrhea, particularly persistent infections [56]. Antimicrobial drug-resistant diarrheagenic *E. coli* pathotypes, including enteroaggregative *E. coli*, are also emerging as important diarrheal pathogens in AIDS patients [57].

According some data [18, 20] about *E. coli* outbreaks, new pathotypes can emerge and cause disease and death in different populations in both, developed [20] and in developing [53] countries. Other authors [58] observed that both EHEC O157 and non-O157 STEC infections can occur at the same time. These authors presented some interesting reasons to this, such as: (i) they are common and may be increasing in frequency; (ii) could be associated with high morbidity and mortality; (iii) utilizing ideal laboratory conditions these pathogens should be detected by both, culture procedures and using protocols to detect Shiga toxin; and (iv) these strains cannot be readily detected with certainty by selective targeting of patients age, time of year or presence of blood in the stool. These observations can be understood in a globalized world. Humans are embedded into the microbial world.

In healthy populations, saprophytic microorganisms constitute a rich source of genetic material which pathogens can readily acquire resistance. The study conducted by NIS in Nigeria showed

http://dx.doi.org/10.5772/67400

that resistance of commensal *E. coli* to almost all agents studied increased rapidly over time [59]. Additionally, urban residents in Nigeria, Ghana, and Zimbabwe were more likely to carry multidrug-resistant *E. coli* than were rural or provincial residents [60]. This finding has important consequences in light of the rapid rate of urbanization in these countries and other parts of the continent. Travel networks have become more efficient and are more extensively used.

Most antibiotic-producing strains carry genes encoding resistance to the antibiotics that they produce, and they are located in the same gene cluster as the antibiotic biosynthesis pathway genes. The sources by which antibiotic resistance genes can be found are presented in **Table 4**.

Resistance genes exist naturally in the environment owing to a range of selective pressures in nature. Humans have applied additional selective pressure for antibiotic resistance genes because of the large quantities produced, consumed, and applied in daily activities. Physical and biological forces also cause widespread dissemination of resistance throughout many natural environments.

In lifetime, humans are exposed to antibiotic resistance bacteria. The potential routes for human exposition with wild animals and its microbiota include [6]: (i) translocation of wildlife into suburban areas, habit destruction, pollution ,and changes to water storage, irrigation or climate changes; (ii) human contact with nature such as hunting and camping; (iii) consumption of exotic foods, bushmeat and game farms; (iv) acquisition of exotic pets and transport of live animals from long distances; (v) incorporation of animal's habitats in human life as zoos; and (vi) trapping of fur-bearing animals.

Some microorganisms and some environments harbor antibiotic resistance genes irrespective of the human use of antibiotics. The prevalence and diversity of resistance genes in the environment inspire hypotheses about the native roles of so-called resistance genes in natural microbial communities.

Selection for antibiotic resistance	Environment	Utilization
Nature	Medicine	Agriculture
Protection against endogenous antibiotics	Industrial antibiotic production	Utilization of antibiotics onto fields
Protection against naturally occurring antibiotics and heavy metals	Antibiotic consumption	Antibiotic consumption
Alternative cellular functions of the resistance protein	–	–
Spread of antibiotic resistance genes	–	–
Physical forces	Biological forces	–
Air currents	Human activities	–
Water	Animal presence	–

Note: Ref. [6] modified.

Table 4. Sources and movement of antibiotic resistance genes in the environment.

6. Antibiotic resistance requires a coordinated response

Antibiotic use in animals has led to the emergence of resistant bacteria, and sometimes these resistant bacteria can be transferred from animals to humans by direct contact or by handling and/or consuming contaminated food.

High levels of resistance were observed for tetracycline as well as intermediate resistance against tetracycline, amikacin, and gentamicin. Gentamicin was the most effective out of these antibiotics [61]. Some authors [62] have showed high rates of tetracycline resistance in strains of enteric *E. coli*. Preventing resistant infections provides the greatest opportunity to limit resistance. Strategies to prevent and control resistant bacteria vary by the pathogen and the setting in which the infection is acquired. Infections were diagnosed in 188 patients from a single healthcare institution [63]. The medical costs for antibiotic resistant infections were estimated between $13.35 and $18.75 million dollars. In United States, antibiotic resistance is also an economic burden on the healthcare system, in other words, resistant infections cost more to treat.

Unfortunately, infections caused by antibiotic resistant bacteria are an everyday occurrence in healthcare settings. In United States, an effort of the National Antimicrobial Resistance Monitoring System (NARMS) contributes to minimize the impact of resistance. NARMS consists in a lab-based system for surveillance. This system is presented in all 50 states and detects resistance in pathogens that are commonly transmitted from animals to humans or through food, such as *Salmonella, Campylobacter*, and *E. coli*. Outbreaks caused by resistant bacteria can occur in community settings where people are concentrated, such as athletic teams, childcare centers, and prisons, or in healthcare settings, including hospitals, long-term care facilities, and ambulatory care facilities. Because the impact of resistance is extensive, activities may be done. The action plan could focus on: (i) reducing inappropriate antimicrobial use; (ii) reducing the spread of antimicrobial resistant microorganisms in institutions, communities, and agriculture; (iii) encouraging the development of new antiinfective products, vaccines, and adjunct therapies; and (iv) supporting basic research on antimicrobial resistance.

Another interesting goal to the process used to inhibit pathogens is linked to ancient knowledge. Many plant products are known to be able to inhibit the growth of several pathogens [64]. These compounds are used by plants in defense mechanisms such as predation by herbivores, insects, and microbial infections.

On the other hand, some studies [65] have shown that microorganisms living in intimate interaction with the host plant without causing any apparent disease symptoms produce most of these compounds. These microorganisms are defined as endophytes [65].

Some studies [65] recently showed that the phytochemicals produced by endophytes have revolutionized the use of these microorganisms as a source of bioactive compounds in recent years [65]. Among the great diversity of the different biomes, many plants stand out for its medicinal properties.

Streptomyces tubercidicus can produce tubercidin. Scientists working with a strain isolated from the Brazilian tropical savannah tree (*Solanum lycocarpum* St. Hill), named this strain (RND-C) [66]. In this study, different fractions with strong antimicrobial activity against *E. coli* and

S. aureus were obtained. The fractions showed a diverse chemical structure and molecular weight, suggesting the presence of new bioactive compounds.

In another study [67], *Paenibacillus polymyxa* was isolated as an endophyte from *Prunus* spp. in the same environment (Brazilian tropical savannah) as *S. tubercidicus*. This study reported the isolation of potent bioactivity of small molecules (<403 Da), against *E. coli* and. *S. aureus*. The previous author with collaborators [68] conducted studies highlighting conditions for production and characterization of these bioactive substances isolated from *P. polymyxa* RNC-D. Recently, a new group [69, 70] showed as well that endophytes isolated from *Miconia albicans* had that potential to inhibit *E. coli* and other pathogens.

According to these data, the bioprospection of endophytes consists in a promising and unexplored reserve for phytochemical agents. Thus, there is a great opportunity to find new antimicrobial substances [64, 65].

7. Nanotechnology in health sciences

Nanotechnology is the technology that deals with materials and products at the nanoscale. It is able to provide more effective solutions to some of the biotechnology issues, such as the development of drugs, due to the reduction of the proportion between contact surfaces and volume of materials, optimizing their action and consequently reduces the consumption of substances and products.

Mesoporous nanostructures, as FDU-12 silica, have high specific surface area, mesoporous large volume, diameter, and adjustable pore surface properties that can be directed to the desired needs. They also have a great importance in catalysis processes, adsorption separation of large molecules, sensors, photonics, optical, drug release or drug, acoustic, nanoreactors, nanotechnology with advanced integrated systems, among others [71].

Lignin, besides being the second vegetal macromolecule found naturally in abundance, can functionalized mesoporous nanostructures, as it has in its structure phenolic and carboxylic groups. These groups are still capable of reducing metal to form nanoparticles and they also have the advantage coat of the silver nanoparticles.

8. Nanoparticles linked to silver

Metallic nanoparticles have different functions, like the following: (i) the marking of a particular stretch of DNA; (ii) the increase in resistance of metals and in the case of nanoparticles linked to silver; (iii) the antimicrobial action (both against Gram-negative bacteria, which have a thin layer of peptidoglycan and against Gram-positive, whose layer is thicker); and (iv) fungicide, which makes these particles a special nanostructured material to be incorporated into the control of such pathogens [72, 73].

However, there are no general consensuses about the mechanisms that can explain the action of silver nanoparticles in the inhibition of microbial growth. Some researchers claim that silver reacts with the thiol group of some vital enzymes to microorganisms and inactive them. Others claim dimerization of the pyrimidines of DNA, thus preventing the replication and thus their growth [74]. Another hypothesis is that the silver nanoparticle causes a change in the cell membrane, causing the output of reducing sugars of the membrane and thus causing cell death [75].

A study conducted by Xu et al. [76] concluded that reactive oxygen species (ROS) played a very important role in the mechanism of AgNPs antibacterial activity, because in anaerobic conditions the efficiency was significantly lower.

Recently [77], α-Ag_2WO_4 microcrystals were synthetized and tested for antimicrobial activity against *E. coli*. The successful of the inactivation was directly related to the presence of specific defects in crystal surfaces. This interaction crystal-bacteria leads to a production of OH* and O_2H^* radicals that interact with several components of bacteria such as peptidoglycan, DNA, cell wall, proteins, and other bacterial structures (**Figure 2**) [77].

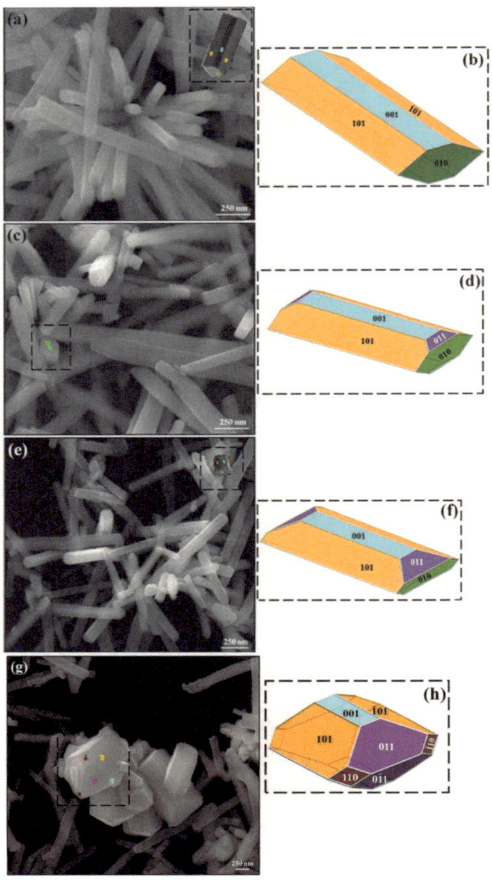

Figure 2. α-Ag_2WO_4 microcrystals in FE-SEM images (a, c, e, and g) and, respectively crystal shape (b, d, f, and h). The crystals were synthetized by MH method. The points highlighted in different colors corresponds each to its respective crystallographic planes [17].

It is known that silver is a toxic metal, for both humans at high concentrations, as for most microorganisms, it is the preferred substance for inhibition thereof, when compared to gold nanoparticles, zinc, and magnesium titanium [78].

The nanocomposites efficiency, containing silver, for the silver ion is much higher than the single metal species, as it has been proved in experiments [78]. It is not completely understood yet, but it is believed that connecting silver to other nanoparticles, such as silica and lignin, can inhibit the growth of microorganisms and these nanoparticles contribute to the destabilizing effect of the cell membrane.

9. Bioactivity of propolis nanoparticles against *E. coli*

Propolis is a natural resinous substance collected from the leaf buds of different tree species by honeybees and known for its biological properties (antibacterial, antifungal, and antioxidant) [79].

Some authors [80] evaluated the antimicrobial activity of propolis nanoparticles in comparison with ethanol-propolis extract against *E. coli*. Ethanol-propolis extract was obtained from green propolis resin, in absolute ethanol under agitation during 15 days. To obtain the propolis nanoparticles, ethanol-propolis extract at 13.75% (w/v) was mixed with polyvinyl-alcohol solution at 0.1% (w/v). The size of the nanoparticles was determined by dynamic light scattering (DLS), atomic force microscopy (AFM), and it was about 70 nm in average [80].

Antimicrobial activity of propolis nanoparticles and ethanol-propolis extract was tested against *E. coli*. Qualitative minimum inhibitory concentrations (MIC) of both solutions were evaluated by agar-well diffusion method, as shown in **Figure 3**. The result was 3.44% (w/v) for ethanol-propolis extract and 1.15% (w/v) for propolis nanoparticles.

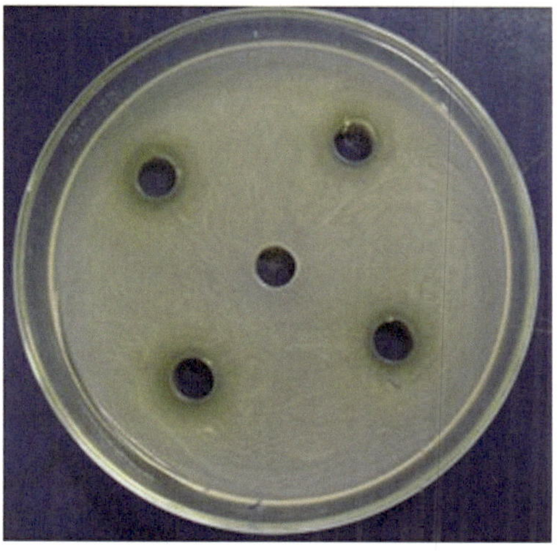

Figure 3. Determination of qualitative MIC of propolis nanoparticles against *E. coli* by agar-well diffusion method in plate dish [80].

The shown antimicrobial activity of propolis nanoparticles is of potential interest for direct applications or in film formulations, for example. Therefore, results obtained in this study, set the bases for future studies, using films as support for propolis nanoparticles, and for application in many products.

10. Conclusions

In the preantibiotic era [81], it was showed that from 30 lyophilized strains before 1950, four were multidrug resistant. The study of bacterial resistance can contribute to the discovery of the potential sources and novel alleles of antibiotic resistance genes. Considering that antibiotic treatment is our primary, and in many cases only, method of treating infectious diseases. We conclude that studies of environmental reservoirs of resistance are crucial to our future ability to fight infection. It is important to establish measures and politics to control the use of antibiotics, but an immediate modification of resistant profile in bacteria is not expected. Patients may follow procedures and use the antibiotics according prescription. The usual techniques of hand wash and use of barriers to prevent bacterial spread is important.

In the experiments, the FDU-12/silver nanoparticles showed the greatest inhibition in the growth of *E. coli*, as was observed fewer colonies or even their absence. Based on these results, we can infer that the best nanoparticle, among tested to inhibit the growth of *E. coli* is described above. The second nanocomposites with proven efficiency in inhibiting the growth of *E. coli* were nanoparticles containing only FDU-12, with an intermediate efficiency. The last nanoparticle studied, FDU-12/lignin/silver, showed the lowest efficiency in inhibiting the growth of *E. coli*, allowing a greater number of colonies to grow in the culture medium.

Author details

Henrique C. Alves[2,3,6], Felipe de P. N. Cruz[1,2,6], Pamela C. P. de Assis[1,2,6], José D. C. Pessoa[1,3], Luis C. Trevelin[1,4,6], Angela M. de O. Leal[1,5,6] and Cristina P. de Sousa[1,2,6]*

*Address all correspondence to: prokarya@ufscar.br

1 Biotechnology Post Graduation Program (PPGBiotec), São Carlos, Brazil

2 Microbiology and Biomolecules Laboratory (LaMiB), São Carlos, Brazil

3 Brazilian Agropecuary and Research Incorporation (Embrapa), São Carlos Brazil

4 Computer Department, São Carlos, Brazil

5 Medicine Department, São Carlos, Brazil

6 Federal University of São Carlos, Brazil

References

[1] Alekshun MN, Levy SB. Molecular mechanisms of antibacterial multidrug resistance. Cell. 2007;128:1037-1050.

[2] Gangoue-Pieboji J, Eze N, Djintchui AN, Ngamenis B, Tsabangl N, Pegnyemb DE, et al. The in-vitro antimicrobial activity of some traditionally used medicinal plants against β-lactam-resistant bacteria. J Infect Dev Ctries. 2009; 3(9):671-680.

[3] Pfaller MA, Jones RN, Marshall SA, Coffman SL, Hollis RJ, Edmond MB, et al. Inducible amp C beta-lactamase producing Gram-negative bacilli from blood stream infections: frequency, antimicrobial susceptibility, and molecular epidemiology in a national surveillance program (SCOPE). Diagn Microbiol Infect Dis. 1997; 28: 211-219.

[4] Jacoby TS, Kuchenbecker RS, Dos Santos RP, Magedanz L, Guzatto P, Moreira LB. Impact of hospital-wide infection rate, invasive procedures use and antimicrobial consumption on bacterial resistance inside an intensive care unit. J Hosp Infect. 2010; 75(1): 23-27.

[5] Kerwat K, Kerwat M, Graf J, Wulf H. Resistance to antibiotics and multiresistant pathogens. Anasthesiol Intensivmed Notfallmed Schmerzther. 2010; 45(4): 242-243.

[6] Allen HK, Donato J, Wang HH, Cloud-Hansen KA, Davies J, Handelsman J. Call of the wild: antibiotic resistance genes in natural environments. Nat Rev Microbiol. 2010; 8(4): 251-259.

[7] Aarestrup FM. Veterinary drug usage and antimicrobial resistance in bacteria of animal origin. Basic Clin Pharmacol Toxicol. 2005; 96: 271-281.

[8] Rwego IB, Isabirye-Basuta G, Gillespie TR, Goldberg TL. Gastrointestinal bacterial transmission among humans, mountain gorillas, and livestock in Bwindi Impenetrable National Park, Uganda. Conserv Biol. 2008; 22: 1600-1607.

[9] Sjolund M. et al. Dissemination of multidrug-resistant bacteria into the Arctic. Emerg Infect Dis. 2008; 14: 70-72.

[10] Hall BG, Barlow M. Evolution of the serine β-lactamases: past, present and future. Drug Resist. Updat. 2004; 7: 111-123.

[11] Frieden T. Antibiotic resistance and the threat to public health. Centers for Disease Control and Prevention. U.S. Department of Health and Human Services. CDC , Atlanta, US. 2010; 1-17.

[12] Laupland KB, Church DL, Vidakovich J, Mucenski M, Pitout JD. Community-onset extended-spectrum β-lactamase (ESBL)-producing *Escherichia coli*: importance of international travel. J Infect. 2008; 57: 441-448.

[13] Palumbi SR. Humans as the world's greatest evolutionary force. Science. 2001; 293: 1786-1790.

[14] Johnson JR, McCabe JS, White DG, Johnston B, Kuskowski MA, Mcdermott P. Molecular analysis of *Escherichia coli* from retail meats (2002-2004) from the United States National Antimicrobial Resistance Monitoring System. Clin Infect Dis. 2009; 49: 195-201.

[15] Kwan CW, Onyett H. Community-acquired urinary tract pathogens and their resistance patterns in hospitalized children in southeastern Ontario between 2002 and 2006. Paediatr Child Health. 2008; 13(9): 759-762.

[16] Scaletsky IC, Souza TB, Aranda KR, Okeke IN. Genetic elements associated with antimicrobial resistance in enteropathogenic *Escherichia coli* (EPEC) from Brazil. BMC Microbiol. 2010; 27: 10-25.

[17] Roca RA, Sczancoski JC, Nogueira IC, Fabbro MT, Alves HC, Gracia L, et al. Facet-dependent photocatalytic and antibacterial properties of α-Ag2WO4 crystals: combining experimental data and theoretical insights. Catal. Sci. Technol. 2015; 5: 4091-4107.

[18] Chattaway MA, Dallman T, Okeke IN, Wain J. Enteroaggregative *E. coli* O104 from an outbreak of HUS in Germany 2011, could it happen again?. J Infect Dev Ctries. 2011; 5(6): 425-436.

[19] Nassour H, Dubreuil JD. *Escherichia coli* STb enterotoxin dislodges claudin-1 from epithelial tight junctions. PLoS ONE. 2014; 9(11): e113273.

[20] Rubino S, Cappuccinelli P, Kelvin DJ. *Escherichia coli* (STEC) serotype O104 outbreak causing haemolytic syndrome (HUS) in Germany and France. J Infect Dev Ctries. 2011; 5(6): 437-440.

[21] Machado PRL, Araujo MIAS, Carvalho L, Carvalho EM. Mecanismos de resposta imune às infecções. Ann Bras Dermatol, Rio de Janeiro. 2004; 79(6): 647-664.

[22] Hooper LV, Midwedt T, Gordon JI. How host-microbial interactions shape the nutrient environment of the mammalian intestine. Ann Rev Nutr. 2002; 22: 283-307. DOI:10.1146/annurev.nutr.22.011602.092259.

[23] Srikanth CV, Mccormick BA. Interactions of the intestinal epithelium with the pathogen and the indigenous microbiota: a three-way crosstalk. Interdiscip Perspect Infect Dis. 2008; 2008: 626827. Epub 2008; 1-14.

[24] Schauer DB. Indigenous microflora: paving the way for pathogens?. Curr Biol. 1997; 7(2): R75–R77.

[25] Galan JE, Wolf-Watz H. Protein delivery into eukaryotic cells by type III secretion machines. Nature. 2006; 444(7119): 567-573.

[26] Benya RV, Marrero JA, Ostrovskiy DA, Koutsouris A, Hecht G. Human colonic epithelial cells express galanin-1 receptors, which when activated cause Cl^- secretion. Am J Physiol. 1999; 276(1): G64–G72.

[27] Yuha R, Koutsouris A, Savkovlc SD, Hecht G. Enteropathogenic *Escherichia coli*-induced myosin light chain phosphorylation alters intestinal epithelial permeability. Gastroenterology. 1997; 113(6): 1873-1882.

[28] Benz I, Schmidt MA. Cloning and expression of an adhesin (AIDA-I) involved in diffuse adhrence of enteropathogenic I. Infect Immunity. 1989; 57: 1506-1511.

[29] Pitout JDD, Nordmann P, Laupland KB, Poirel L. Emergence of *Enterobacteriaceae* producing extended-spectrum β-lactmases (ESBLs) in the community. J Antimicrob Chemother. 2005; 56: 52-59.

[30] Livermore DM, Woodford N. The ß-Lactamase Threat in *Enterobacteriaceae, Pseudomonas* and *Acinetobacter*. Trends Microbiol. 2006; 14: 413-420.

[31] Hopkins KL, Davies RH, Threlfall EJ. Mechanisms of quinolone resistance in *Escherichia coli* and Salmonella: recent developments. Int J Antimicrob Agents. 2005; 25: 358-373.

[32] Dubreuil JD. STb and AIDA-I: the missing link? Crit Rev Microbiol. 2010; 36(3): 212-220.

[33] Kmet V, Piatnicová E. Antibiotic resistance in commensal intestinal microflora. Folia Microbiol. 2010; 55(4): 332-335.

[34] De Kraker ME, Wolkewitz M, Davey PG, Koller W, Berger J, Nagler J, et al. Burden of antimicrobial resistance in European hospitals: excess mortality and length of hospital stay associated with bloodstream infections due to *Escherichia coli* resistant to third-generation cephalosporins. J Antimicrob Chemother. 2010; 66(2):398-407.

[35] Zingg W, Pfister R, Posfay-Barbe KM, Huttner B, Touveneau S, Pittet D. Secular trends in antibiotic use among neonates: 2001-2008. Pediatr Infect Dis J. 2011; 30(5):365-370.

[36] Mohammadtaheri Z, Pourpaki M, Mohammadi F, Namdar R, Masjedi MR. Surveillance of antimicrobial susceptibility among bacterial isolates from Intensive Care Unit patients of a Tertiary-Care University Hospital in Iran: 2006-2009. Chemotherapy. Nov 23, 2010; 56(6): 478-484.

[37] Lee CY, Chen PY, Huang FL, Lin CF. Microbiologic spectrum and susceptibility pattern of clinical isolates from the pediatric intensive care unit in a single medical center—6 years' experience. J Microbiol Immunol Infect. 2009; 42(2): 160-165.

[38] Zhanel GG, Decorby M, Laing N, Weshnoweski B, Vashisht R, Tailor F, et al. Canadian antimicrobial resistance alliance (CARA), Hoban DJ. Antimicrobial-resistant pathogens in intensive care units in Canada: results of the Canadian National Intensive Care Unit (CAN-ICU) study, 2005-2006. Antimicrob Agents Chemother. 2008 Apr; 52(4): 1430-1437.

[39] Kamat US, Fereirra A, Amonkar D, Motghare DD, Kulkarni MS. Epidemiology of hospital acquired urinary tract infections in a medical college hospital in Goa. Indian J. Urology. 2009; 25(1): 76-80.

[40] Rhodes G, et al. Distribution of oxytetracycline resistance plasmids between aeromonads in hospital and aquaculture environments: implication of Tn1721 in dissemination of the tetracycline resistance determinant Tet A. Appl. Environ. Microbiol. 2000; 66: 3883-3890.

[41] Uma B, Prabhakar K, Rajendran S, Kavitha K, Sarayu YL. Antibiotic sensitivity and plasmid profiles of *Escherichia coli* isolated from pediatric diarrhea. J Glob Infect Dis. July 2009; 1(2): 107-110.

[42] Krueger AL, Folster J, Medalla F, Joyce K, Perri MB, Johnson L, et al. Commensal *Escherichia coli* isolate resistant to eight classes of antimicrobial agents in the United States. Foodborne Pathog Dis. Feb 2011; 8(2): 329-332.

[43] Lindsey RL, Fedorka-Cray PJ, Frye JG, Meinersmann RJ. Inc A=C plasmids are prevalent in multidrug-resistant *Salmonella enterica* isolates. Appl Environ Microbiol. 2009; 75: 1908-1915.

[44] Robins-Browne RM, Hartland EL. *Escherichia coli* as a cause of diarrhea. J Gastroenterol Hepatol. 2002; 17: 467-475.

[45] Wirth T, Falush D, Lan R, Colles F, Mensa P, Wieler LH, et al. Sex and virulence *in E. coli*: an evolutionary perspective. Mol Microbiol. 2006; 60(5): 1136-1151.

[46] Hacker J, Kaper JB. Pathogenicity islands and the evolution of microbes. Ann Rev Microbiol. 2000; 54: 641-679.

[47] Giron JA, Ho AS, Schoolnik GK. An inducible bundleforming pilus of enteropathogenic *Escherichia coli*. Science. 1991; 254: 710-713.

[48] Hicks S, Frankel G, Kaper J, Dougan G, Philips AD. Role of intimin and bundle-forming pili in enteropathogenic *Escherichia coli* adhesion to pediatric intestinal tissue *in vivo*. Infect Immun. 1998; 66: 1570-1578.

[49] McDaniel TK, Kaper JB. A cloned pathogenicity island from enteropathogenic *Escherichia coli* confers the attaching and effacing phenotype on *E. coli* K-12. Mol Microbiol. 1997; 23: 399-407.

[50] Kenny B, Abe A, Stein M, Finlay BB. Enteropathogenic *Escherichia coli* protein secretion is induced in response to conditions similar to those in the gastrointestinal tract. Infect Immun. 1997; 65: 2606-2612.

[51] Jerse AE, Kaper JB. The *eae* gene of enteropathogenic *Escherichia coli* encodes a 94-kilodalton membrane protein, the expression of which is influenced by the EAF plasmid. Infect Immun. 1991; 59: 4302-4309.

[52] Smith JL, Fratamico PM, Gunther NW. Extraintestinal pathogenic *Escherichia coli*. Foodborne Pathog Dis. 2007;4(2): 134-163.

[53] Sousa CP. The versatile strategies of *Escherichia coli* pathotypes: a mini review. J Venom Animals Toxins Including Tropical Dis. 2006; 12: 363-373.

[54] Johnson JR, Kuskowski MA, Smith K, O'Bryan TT, Tatini S. Antimicrobial-resistant and extraintestinal pathogenic *Escherichia coli* in retail foods. J Infect Dis. April 1, 2005; 191(7): 1040-1049.

[55] Shakil S, Akram M, Ali SM, Khan AU. Acquisition of extended-spectrum β-lactamase producing *Escherichia coli* strains in male and female infants admitted to a neonatal intensive care unit: molecular epidemiology and analysis of risk factors. J Med Microbiol. 2010; 59: 948-954.

[56] Okeke IN, Nataro JP. Enteroaggregative *Escherichia coli*. Lancet Infect Dis. 2001; 1: 304-313.

[57] Gassama A, Sow PS, Fall F, Camara P, Gueye-N'diaye A, Seng R, et al. Ordinary and opportunistic enteropathogens associated with diarrhea in Senegalese adults in relation to a human immunodeficiency virus serostatus. Int J Infect Dis. 2001; 5: 192-198.

[58] Marcon MJ, Kiska DL, Riddell SW, Gilligan P. Should all stools be screened for shiga toxin-producing *Escherichia coli*?. J. Clin. Microbiol. Jul 2011; 49: 2390-2397.

[59] Okeke IN, Lamikanra A, Czeczulin J, Dubovsky F, Kaper JB, Nataro JP. Heterogeneous virulence of enteroaggregative *Escherichia coli* strains isolated from children in southwest Nigeria. J Infect Dis. 2000; 181: 252-260.

[60] Nys S, Okeke IN, Kariuki S, Dinant GJ, Driessen C, Stobberingh EE. Antibiotic resistance of fecal *Escherichia coli* from healthy volunteers from eight developing countries. J Antimicrob Chemother. 2004; 54: 952-955.

[61] Garcia PG, Silva VL, Diniz CG. Occurrence and antimicrobial drug susceptibility patterns of commensal and diarrheagenic *E. coli* in fecal microbiota from children with and without acute diarrhea. J Microbiol. 2011; 49(1): 46-52.

[62] Usein CR, Taty-Chitoiu D, Ciontea S, Condei M, Damian M. *Escherichia coli* pathotypes associated with diarrhea in Romanian children younger than 5 years of age. J. Infect. Dis. 2009; 62: 289-293.

[63] Roberts RR, Hota B, Ahmad I, Scott RD II, Foster SD, Abbasi F, et al. Hospital and societal costs of antimicrobial-resistant infections in a Chicago teaching hospital: implications for antibiotic stewardship. Clin. Infect. Dis. 2009; 49: 1175-84.

[64] Dubreuil JD. Antibacterial and antidiarrheal activities of plant products against enterotoxinogenic *Escherichia coli*. Toxins. 2013; 5: 2009-2041.

[65] Lacava PT, Sousa CP. Role of endophytic actinomycetes in crop protection: plant growth promotion and biological control. Plant Growth Promoting Actinobacteria. 1ed. Telangana, India: Springer Singapore. 2016; 1: 147-160.

[66] Ratti RP, Piza ACMT, Malpass AC, Hokka CO, Dubreuil JD, Sousa CP. Growing kinetics and antimicrobial activity of Streptomyces tubercidicus crude extracts. In: World Scientific Publishing Company Pte Ltd. (Org.). Microorganisms in Industry and Environment from scientific and industrial research to consumer products. Singapore: World Scientific Publishing Company Pte Ltd. 2010; 1: 589-592.

[67] Serrano NFG. Purificação e caracterização bioquímica de substâncias bioativas produzidas por endofítico isolado de *Prunus* spp. Dissertation, Federal University of São Carlos, Sao Carlos, Sao Paulo, Brazil. 2009.

[68] Serrano NFG, Rodrigues LRM, Hokka CO, Sousa CP, Teixeira JAC, Mussato SID. Optimal glucose and inoculum concentrations for production of bioactive molecules by *Paenibacillus polymyxa* RNC-D. Chem Papers (Online). 2012; 66: 1111-1117.

[69] Piza ACMT, Hokka CO, Sousa CP. Endophytic actinomycetes from *Miconia albicans* (Sw.) Triana (Melastomataceae) and evaluation of its antimicrobial activity. J Sci Res Reports. 2015; 4: 281-291.

[70] Piza ACMT, Lima LCPS, Hokka CO, Sousa CP. Endophytic *Nocardiopsis dassonvillei* and *Amycolatopsis orientalis* isolated from Brazilian tropical savannah presented antibiosis against pathogens. In: A. Méndez-Vilas. (Org.). Microbes in the spotlight: recent progress in the understanding of beneficial and harmful microorganisms. 1st ed. Boca Raton: BrownWalker Press. 2016; 1: 264-266.

[71] Lu J, et al. Ultrasensitive electrochemical immunosensor based on Au nanoparticles dotted carbon nanotube-graphene composite and functionalized mesoporous materials. Biosens Bioelectron. 2012; 33: 29-35.

[72] Klabunde KJ. Richards RM (Ed). Nanoscale materials in chemistry, Wiley. 2nd ed. 2009; 804 p.

[73] Morones JR, et al. The bactericidal effect of silver nanoparticles. Nanotechnology, Institute of Physics Publishing. 2005; 16: 2346-2353.

[74] Matsumura Y, et al. Mode of bactericidal action of silver zeolite and its comparison with that of silver nitrate. Appl Environ Microbiol Am Soc Microbiol. 2003; 69(7): 4278-4281.

[75] Li J, et al. Highly selective antibacterial activities of silver nanoparticles against *bacillus subtilis*. J Nanosci Nanotechnol. 2013; 13(10): 6806-6813.

[76] Xu H, Qu F, Xu H, Lai W, Andrew Wang Y, Aguilar ZP, et al. Role of reactive oxygen species in the antibacterial mechanism of silver nanoparticles on *Escherichia coli* O157:H7. Biometals. Feb 2012; 25(1): 45-53.

[77] Roca RA, Gouveia AF, Lemos PS, Gracia L, Andrés J, Longo E. Formation of ag nanoparticles on β-ag2wo4 through electron beam irradiation: a synergetic computational and experimental study. Inorg Chem. Aug 17, 2016; 55: 8661-8671.

[78] Rai M, Yadav A, Gade A. Silver nanoparticles as a new generation of antimicrobials. Biotechnol Adv. 2009; 27: 76-83.

[79] Koo H, Gomes BPFA, Rosalen PL, Ambrosano GMB, Park YK, Cury JA. *In vitro* antimicrobial activity of propolis and *Arnica montana* against oral pathogens. Arch Oral Biol. 2000; 45: 141-148.

[80] Alves HC, et al. Antimicrobial activity of propolis nanoparticles against some common meat contamination bacteria. Food Microbiology & Biotechnology, Portuguese Congress of Microbiology and Biotechnology. 2013; 44.

[81] Smith DH. R factor infection of *E. coli* lyophilized in 1946. J Bacteriol. 1967; 94: 2071-2072.

Section 2

Innovative Approaches to Detection and Application of E. coli in the Environment

E. coli as an Indicator of Contamination and Health Risk in Environmental Waters

Robert G. Price and Dirk Wildeboer

Additional information is available at the end of the chapter

http://dx.doi.org/10.5772/67330

Abstract

Good public health depends on regular monitoring of water quality as faecal contamination is a serious problem due to the potential for contracting disease. Bacterial contamination in water is measured using indicator organisms, notably *Escherichia coli and Enterococci* which are used as primary indicators of contamination in fresh and marine water quality, respectively, rather than the total coliforms present. Although most *E. coli and Enterococci* strains cause only mild infections, their presence is indicative of the potential presence of other more pathogenic organisms which are a danger to human health. The acceptable levels of indicator organisms are defined in legislation and are set for drinking, river, well and marine water. This chapter will consider current gold standard culture methods of analysis for *E. coli* and compare them with molecular DNA procedures. Established culture methods use β-D-glucuronidase to identify *E. coli* and β-D-galactosidase to detect coliforms. Emphasis will be placed on newer procedures that can be used onsite supported by laboratory procedures used for confirmation. Available rapid fluorimetric procedures which have been developed for use in the field, based on the assay of β-D-glucuronidase, will be discussed. The rapid advances in procedures using a molecular approach will be considered and compared with the more established methods for determining *E. coli* in water. It is essential that all these methods should be quantitative in order to comply with legal norms, and in this regard, the potential involvement of biosensor technology will be of great value in successfully transferring laboratory procedures to the field.

Keywords: water quality monitoring, *E. coli*, β-D-glucuronidase, faecal bacteria, rapid detection of contamination, biosensors

1. Introduction

Pathogen contamination of environmental waters is a major health risk and a threat to future supplies of water for living and recreational activities. Acceptable bacterial limits have been defined in legislation by among others WHO [1], US EPA [2] and the European Union [3]. Health risks can be assessed and monitored using a series of tests for specific indicators which are defined in regional legislation. Water-borne contamination and related diseases are discussed in detail elsewhere [4, 5]. A recent comprehensive review [6] considered recent reports on recreational water and infection comparing epidemiological studies and quantitative microbial risk assessment (QMRAs). While potential sources of contamination are considered in a review [7] which concentrates on the transport of pathogens in the agricultural setting and their health implications. In this chapter, we assess the methodology currently available for monitoring the presence of *Escherichia coli* in environmental waters. Although laboratory analyses will remain the reference procedures, the current trend is to develop onsite methodology which will yield more rapid results allowing more immediate action to be taken if contamination is found. This development also benefits, for example, developing countries where good laboratory procedures may not be easily accessible and accurate and reliable onsite technology will be the key to progress and improved public health.

E. coli are present in the intestine of men and animals and are released into the environment in faecal material. As faecal matter is the main source for disease-causing agents in water, faecal bacteria are widely used as indicators of contamination which can affect rivers, sea beaches, lakes, ground water, surface water, recreational water and the many and diverse activities associated with these [5]. Contamination can result from leakage of sewage, sewer overflow caused by storm events and accidental or deliberate release into receiving water bodies, as well as water draining from agricultural land or directly from livestock and birds [4, 8]. Sewage treatment plants can also be a source of pathogenic *E. coli* and these can spread in the river systems [9, 10]. Even low levels of contact with contaminated water in rivers [11] or beaches [12] are significant and can result in outbreak of gastroenteritis. However, the amount of water likely to be ingested is most important when determining the risk of certain activities (e.g. swimming, boating) [13]. Although coliforms do not usually cause serious illness they are used to indicate the presence of more pathogenic bacteria and viruses. The health risk to humans and animals can be assessed using a series of tests which are defined in regional legislation. Coliforms and in particular *E. coli* are the most valuable markers. *E. coli* is widely accepted as the better faecal indicator organism than total coliforms. Contamination of water supplies by pathogenic strains like *E. coli* O157:H7 is more serious but usually localised. A number of reports have shown that most *E. coli* (over 95%) express β-D-glucuronidase (GUD) activity [14] making this enzyme a sensitive and specific marker for *E. coli* detection and thus faecal pollution. The current acceptable upper limit for *E. coli* content in fresh surface water is 900 cfu/100 ml and 500 cfu/100 ml in marine water [3]. Although *E.coli* is the marker of choice a number of other markers are used in environmental monitoring. *Enterococci* for example are used as a maker for contamination particularly in marine waters [15]. Further details of other markers used in environmental monitoring are detailed in Price and Wildeboer [16].

The widespread use of antibiotics in agriculture and their release from sewage works has accelerated the development of antibiotic-resistant strains in environmental water bodies increasing the need for accurate and regular monitoring. A recent study [17] demonstrated the presence of bacteria resistant to a number of antibiotics, some of which were of faecal origin highlighting concerns about release and spread of antibiotic-resistant organisms in receiving waters. Another important aspect of faecal contamination of rivers and lakes is its effect on fish. This has both public health and economic impacts and is of critical importance in water bodies used for aquaculture [18–20]. The release of microorganisms into a lake or river and the use of antibiotics in fish farming can combine to create a perfect storm of an environment that is highly selective for the development of multi-drug resistant strains. Effective monitoring of water quality and rapid detection of contamination as well as more sustainable approaches and a reduction of drug use in aquaculture will need to go hand-in-hand to improve food safety and environmental health.

In this chapter, the different procedures currently available for monitoring *E. coli* will be critically assessed and particular emphasis will be on comparing recent and older methods for the detection *E. coli* (**Table 1**).

Culture-based methods	Sensitive, 1–2 days to obtain a result. Detects primary indicator organism and others present, relies on biochemical or immunological methods of identification, underestimates bacterial load as only viable organisms detected.
Chromogenic agars	Detects non-viable VBNC as well as viable bacteria, based on the assay of β-D-glucuronidase and β-D-glucuronidase.
API®ID Strip Range	Based on miniaturised laboratory techniques used as confirmatory tests.
Membrane filtration method	Reference method used for ISO standards. Culture on chromogenic media after filtration.
Most probable number	Depends on growth of target organism in liquid medium, more time consuming and labour intensive than MFM, not suitable for marine organisms.
Direct methods	Direct measurement of indicator enzyme activity in water, usually using fluorescent substrates for β-glucuronidase and β-galactosidase. Suitable for onsite monitoring.
Semi-automated methods	Commercial procedures, e.g. Colilert analysers, use selective media and fluorescent substrates, suitable for online monitoring, can give results within 24 h.
Nucleic acid-based procedures	Sensitive and rapid but when low numbers of bacteria are present and enrichment step is needed. Invaluable technique to identify individual pathogens, e.g. *E. coli* O157:H7.
Quantitative PCR	qPCR determines the number of genomes per volume of water for a bacterial species, can be coupled to fluorescence *in situ* hybridisation (FISH) or plate counting. FISH is used to identify different mixtures of bacteria in a sample, usually requires enrichment step.
qPCR and qPRT-PCR	A rapid sensitive method used in study of emerging as well as established pathogens. Needs further standardisation.
Biosensor techniques	Able to directly detect target bacteria and provide real-time results. Portable and easy to use for onsite testing. Avoids cultivation step and can measure viable and non-viable cells. Sensitive optical biosensors can detect 7 cfu/ml *E. coli* in water samples. Biosensors based on electrochemical immunosensors are also used while biosensors based on physicochemical methods, e.g. Raman spectroscopy are currently under development but probably would not be suitable for routine analysis.

Table 1. Established and developing methods used to monitor *E. coli* in environmental water.

2. Established analytical methods to detect *E. coli* in environmental waters

Methods involving culturing procedures are essentially laboratory based and, although they are sensitive, usually involve one or two days before the result is known. They can be used to detect the presence of a range of potential contaminating organisms in addition to the primary target organism. Culture procedures rely on either biochemical, immunological or molecular methods to identify the bacteria present. However, culture methods may underestimate the bacterial load or fail to grow relevant organisms as they measure only the viable organisms present in the samples that can be cultured. In environmental samples, a significant number of cells may not be detected despite being viable. Viable but non-culturable cells (VBNC) result from stress encountered in the environment or the condition and content of the samples [21]. Therefore, alternative new technologies that do not rely on growing the bacteria in culture are required; many of these involve nucleic acid based methods [6]. Chromogenic agar can detect non-growing cells by measuring the presence of an enzyme e.g. β-D-galactosidase for coliforms [22] and β-D-glucuronidase for *E. coli* [23]. A wide range of media is available for the characterisation of environmental microorganisms [24]. Detailed descriptions of standard laboratory procedures which are used in environmental studies including microscopic as well as biochemical characterisation are given in Alexander and Strete [25]. The rapid identification of known bacteria can be achieved using the API® ID Strip Range (BioMerieux, France) which consists of a series of miniaturised techniques based on established laboratory procedures.

The reference methods for detection and isolation of *E. coli* and coliforms in water are the membrane filtration method (ISO 9308-1:2014) and the multiple tube fermentation (Most Probable Number, MPN, ISO 9308-2:2012). ISO 9308-1:2014 is based on membrane filtration and subsequent culture on a chromogenic coliform-agar medium [26]. Due to the low selectivity of the differential agar medium, background growth can interfere with the reliable enumeration of *E. coli* and coliform bacteria, for example, in surface waters or shallow well waters. This method is not suitable for these types of water. As the MPN method (ISO 9308-2:2012) is based on the growth of the target organisms in liquid medium it is suitable for most waters but should not be used for enumeration of bacteria in marine samples as dilution of the sample is required. A recent study compared membrane filtration (MF) and multiple tube fermentation (MTF) procedures to analyse water obtained from a dockside and a beach in California [27]. The MF method gave more reliable and precise data than the MTF method. The later method was more time consuming, labour intensive and less precise. The MF procedure also has the advantage of being able to examine large volumes of water but it has limitations when dealing with turbid water samples. The *E. coli* and coliform content in water samples from five Environmental Protection Agency regions (EPA) in the USA were compared using the Colilert™ automated test and MTF procedure [28]. Similar results were obtained with both methods; however, the Colilert™ procedure was easier to perform and interpret.

Enumeration and characterisation of bacteria in environmental samples requires a tiered approach. The samples collected from, e.g., rivers are diluted or centrifuged to remove particulate matter followed by a filtration step; the bacteria retained on the membrane are incubated on a growth medium for up to 18 h. *E. coli* are selected on colony colour and identified using chromogenic agar, confirmation can be via API 20E strips or PCR. Some strains of *E. coli* which are β-D-glucuronidase negative, such as *E. coli* O157:H7, will not be detected as *E. coli* but, as they are β-D-galactosidase positive, they will appear as coliform bacteria on selected chromogenic agars [29]. A range of chromogenic agars are available for the detection of *E. coli* O157:H7 which have improved specificity when compared to cefixime-tellurite Sorbitol MacConkey (CT-SMAC) [30] when tested against eight environmental samples inoculated with *E. coli* [31].

Amirat *et al.* [32] used the membrane filtration procedure followed by culture on selective chromogenic media to monitor bacterial contamination of the river Thames. This procedure successfully identified *Salmonella, Enterococci, Klebsiella pneumoniae* and *E. coli*. Sixty percent of the samples were in excess of the EU standard for bathing water and the study demonstrated frequent sewage pollution of the Thames which was most noticeable after heavy rainfall. The relationship between sewage contamination of rivers and heavy rainfall has also been reported in other studies: Tryland *et al.* [33] used the Colifast early warning system while Kolarevic *et al.* [34] studied the river Tisa in India using the membrane filtration method. The MPN method was also used to demonstrate an increase in indicator organisms including *E. coli* 2 days after rainfall in the river Göta Älv in Sweden [35] and to measure faecal pollution and antibiotic resistance in the river Cauvery in India [36]. Faecal contamination of the river Danube was measured using the indicator organisms: coliforms and *Enterococci* [37]. A rapid onsite method for *E. coli*, ColiSense, is based on the direct fluorescent analysis of β-D-glucuronidase activity in recreational water samples [38]. Total time taken to complete the analysis was approximately 103 minutes of which 75 minutes were needed to complete the assay. The total time taken to obtain a result depends on the time to transport the sample from the test site to the laboratory and time for any pre-treatment steps. This method does offer greater rapidity and portability but there may be differences in the results obtained with this procedure than with standard culture procedures.

Monitoring of environmental water samples is usually carried out using culture-based faecal indicators of microbial contamination. However, these methods are expensive and time-consuming and recently efforts have been made to develop methods which give more rapid results at lower cost and greater specificity. Indirect detection of *E. coli* and total coliforms in water samples from Canadian fresh water beaches using a portable detection system has been described [39]. The detection procedure was based on the fluorescent detection of β-D-glucuronidase and β-D-glucuronidase using novel anthracene-based enzyme substrate. The method is able to detect single cells of either *E. coli* or total coliforms within 18 h and turbidity and colour and turbidity of the water samples does not affect the result. False-positive coliform results due to the presence of *Aeromonas spp.* could be eliminated by the inclusion of Cefsulodin in the growth medium.

A number of semi-automated systems are currently available which utilise selective growth media and fluorometric substrates. The Colifast Analyser system utilises 4-methylumbelliferone-β-D-glucuronide to detect *E. coli* and 4-nitrophenyl-β-D-galactoside to detect coliforms using defined substrate technology which is used for online monitoring. The endpoints are yellow for total coliforms and fluorescent for *E. coli*. There is also a micro hand held version available. Results can be obtained using this procedure within 2–12 h. An alternative system, Colilert® 3000 (Seres, France) utilises fluorescent or chromogenic substrates and can deliver results within 24 h. These methods correlate well with standard laboratory methods although the results were two to three orders of magnitude higher than MTF and MPN methods probably due to the presence of *Aeromonas spp.* and *Vibrio spp.* (natural inhabitants of the surface water) known to interfere with the Colilert test [40]. A comprehensive study by Schang [41] compared four methods to analyse riverine, estuarine and marine environments near Melbourne, Australia. They compared the industry-standard IDEXX (Colilert®) culture-based method with three alternative approaches: the TECTA™ automated system uses fluorometric assays [42] and while still under development they found a good correlation between the IDEXX and TECTA™ procedures while the later had the advantage of a faster turnaround time. Good correlation was found between the IDEXX method and the US EPA Method 1611 for qPCR detection of *Enterococci*. Good correlation was found between next-generation-sequencing (NGS) and the culture-based procedures; however, the cost of NGS is too high at present, but future developments might make the use of this procedure suitable for routine screening.

The use of indicator organisms is well established and will probably continue as the gold standard of microbial contamination until reliable alternative procedures are developed. There are however several promising areas of development which are considered in the sections below which provide valuable supplementary information and have the potential to evolve in specific easy to use onsite procedures. Culture procedures take a minimum of 24 h to complete and the availability of more rapid techniques will allow earlier appropriate management decisions to be made.

3. Molecular techniques for bacterial identification in environmental waters

Molecular techniques for the specific detection and quantification of bacteria are highly sensitive, rapid and specific, they can be readily automated and standardised so have some advantages over the standard culture-based techniques. Detection does not rely on the target organisms being viable and multiply under culture conditions or on the expression and activity of enzymes or other biochemical markers. However, where low numbers of bacteria are present, an enrichment step is often required limiting the aforementioned advantages. Quantitative PCR methods provide accurate numbers of genomes present and multiplex approaches can simultaneously identify the target organism and test for genes associated with pathogenicity or antibiotic resistance [43, 44] and host-specific detection thus linking the contamination to a source [45–47]. Both sample clean-up and PCR protocols have recently been developed to be fast and simplified and requiring a limited set of laboratory resources thus making molecular analysis a more attractive option for routine monitoring and even field testing. The development of automated DNA extraction and PCR methods have been utilised to develop an autonomous system for the *in situ* detection of faecal indicator bacteria [48] showing the future potential for bringing molecular analysis out of the laboratory and constructing robotic analysers.

Recent advances in sequencing technology and the decrease in costs for whole genome sequencing have made this technology the forefront of investigations into outbreaks of infectious diseases and food or water contamination [49–51]. Rapid identification can be achieved and the outbreak quickly be traced to its source allowing for more effective treatment and containment. This provides an entirely new and effective tool that allows tracing a faecal contamination of water to its source. Measures can then be put in place to contain the current release, prevent future events and if the cause is found to be a careless or deliberate release, legal proceeding can be initiated. However, for routine monitoring of water quality this technology is not a viable alternative as it is more expensive, requires specialist equipment and trained analysts and does not provide rapid or onsite results.

The coupling of microarray technology with PCR enhances detection and identification of bacterial contaminants in water samples. Several commercial kits are now available for the assay of *shiga* toxin producing *E. coli* O157:H7 in environmental samples. More recently, detection techniques using biosensors have shown potential for onsite monitoring. These combine a rapid biochemical reaction with a physicochemical signal that is proportional to the concentration of the target molecule and thus the number of bacteria present in a sample. The biomarkers targeted are most commonly the enzymes established in laboratory-based assays. We have shown that a direct assay of 1 ml river water sample for β-D-glucuronidase activity analysed with a portable fluorimeter can achieve detection limits of 7 cfu/ml within 30 min [52], the ColiSense system described by Heery [38] combines incubation and fluorescent detection in a portable device achieving below 100 cfu/ml in 75 min and a recent study by Hesari [53] describes a biosensor, sensitive enough for the detection of *E. coli* in drinking water with a significant fluorescent signal generated in under 2 h and no sample processing. Wutor [54] describes a biosensor targeting β-D-galactosidase that can detect 1 cfu/100 ml in 15 min using voltammetry to detect the enzyme activity. A system that combines concentration of *E. coli* with a colorimetric detection of enzyme activity and is easy to use, portable and not requiring any instrumentation was recently developed and commercialised [55]. Several immunosensors have also been developed, mostly in order to detect specific bacterial antigens correlated with virulence. A detection limit of 100 cfu/ml is achieved by a specific immunosensor for *E. coli* O157:H7 [56], and with a gold-nanoparticle sensor described more recently, *E. coli* O157:H7 were detected as low as 10 cfu/ml in 1 h [57]. An electrochemical biosensor capable of specifically detecting ESBL *E. coli* strains was developed and achieved a detection limit of 5000 cfu/ml [58]. A third type of biosensors targets nucleic acids and Paniel [59] has shown that both optical and electrochemical detection methods can achieve detection limits below 20 cfu/ml *E. coli* in seawater. Capacitors can be utilised to detect whole cells and a recent paper describes a biosensor that can specifically detect *E. coli* to a limit of 70 cfu/ml in river water by combining a capacitive biosensor with microcontact imprinting [60]. A number of different biosensor systems for the detection of bacteria in water and studies evaluating these are reviewed by Lopez-Roldan [61].

Proteomics methods have been developed and extensive databases created allowing the identification of microorganisms directly in complex samples. Several studies have shown how MALDI-TOF-MS (Matrix-Assisted Laser Desorption Ionisation Time-of-flight Mass Spectrometry) can be employed to identify organisms at species level, and detect virulence and resistance markers in environmental waters [62, 63]. A study by Loff [64] compares proteomics analysis with molecular and biochemical methods for the detection of microorganisms commonly associated with water safety. It can be expected that future developments of this technology will widen its application in many diagnostic and analytical applications.

It has to be noted that the identification of organisms and detection of virulence or resistance by both molecular and proteomics approaches relies on the comparison of results with existing databases. This limits to the identification of known strains and characterised genes and proteins and is thus unlikely to achieve detection of uncultivable microorganisms. However, a combination of recent advances in bioinformatics and novel methods like the one described by Kaeberlein [65] have increased our knowledge about the microbial world and extended our database resources. Molecular and proteomics methods have shown great potential in the identification in temporal and special distribution of microorganisms in the aquatic environment and to combine species identification with detection of virulence and drug resistance. Future developments are likely to combine the best of both worlds to achieve robust assessment of water quality by quantifying indicator organisms to detect contamination and identify virulence and resistance markers to assess public health risks and inform stakeholders on the need and nature of required interventions.

4. Disadvantages in relying solely on *E. coli* to monitor water contamination

Although historically total coliforms, faecal coliforms, *Enterococci* and *E. coli* have all been used as indicator organism for faecal water pollution and currently employed methods continue to largely rely on these, it is clear that alternative indicators need to be developed to address limitations in identifying other water contaminants of considerable public health concerns. Water-borne diseases including diarrhoea and gastrointestinal illness can be caused by bacteria, viruses and protozoa [4]. Approximately 3.4 million people, mainly children, die from water-borne diseases [66] and solely relying on *E. coli* can result in misleading information [67]. Major etiological agents including *Giardia, Cryptosporidium, Vibrio cholerae* and *Salmonella* would be missed by current testing procedures. Often outbreaks are due to local flood or storm events or releases of untreated sewage which result in significant contamination of environmental water. Worldwide morbidity and mortality caused by contaminated drinking water is of considerable magnitude. The WHO ranks diarrhoeal diseases sixths highest in the list of causes of environmental deaths with an estimate of 846,000 deaths annually [68]. This highlights the need for a concentrated effort to make both recreational and drinking water safe in both developing and developed countries [4]. The development of methods detecting a wide range of significant pathogens is most likely to be achieved by extraction and antibody based detection, as described for pathogenic protozoa [69] or molecular techniques such as PCR, shown for *Cryptosporidium parvum* and *Giardia lamblia* [70], and with further developments of NGS and MALDI. However, the advantage of the currently used *E. coli*–based procedures is their simplicity, low cost and functionality for rapid onsite detection. Additional more broad ranging tests would need to be rigorously assessed in a wide variety of environmental situations before they could be adapted as international standards. There is, therefore, a clear need to re-examine the precision and reproducibility of both culture and molecular-based methods in the assessment of environmental samples to take into account local variations and design new methods to be applicable for a wide range of scenarios in order to make a significant contribution to improving water safety globally.

5. Conclusions

Sensitive and frequent monitoring of environmental waters is essential to minimise adverse effect on human health. The current approach to monitoring for contamination in environmental waters is shown in **Figure 1**.

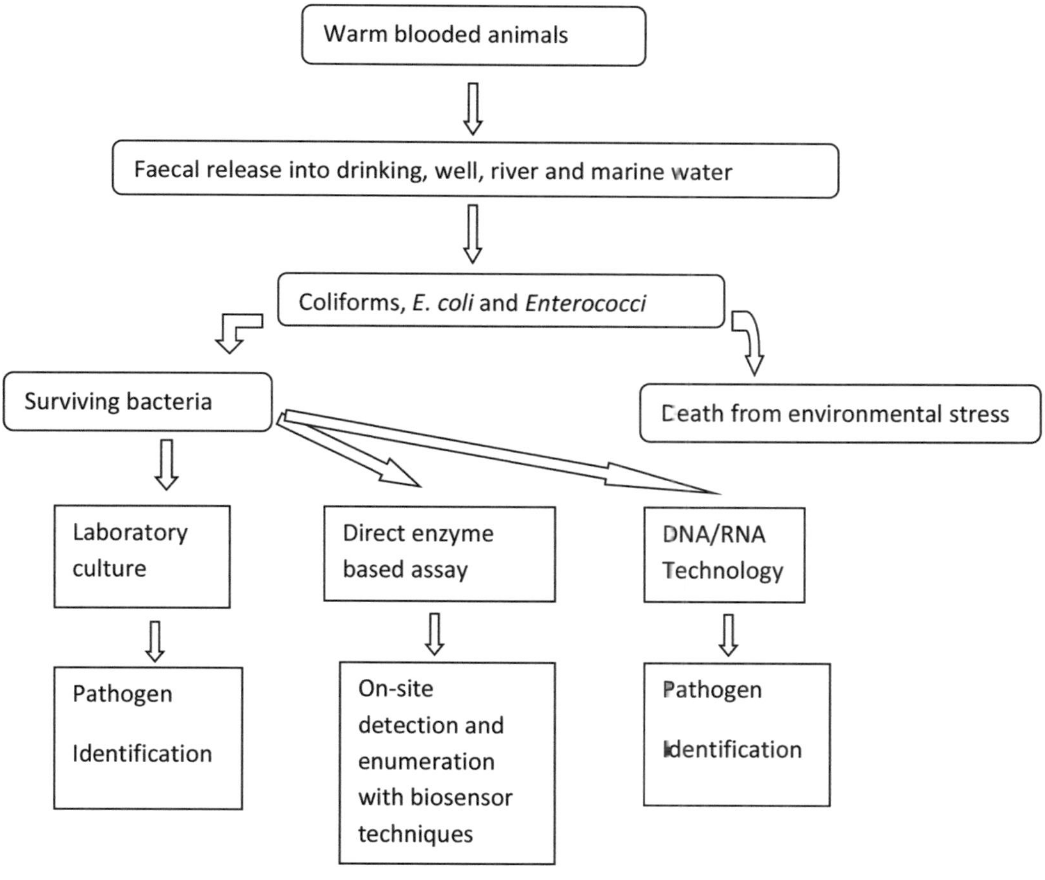

Figure 1. Current approach to monitoring and identifying bacteria in environmental water.

A wide range of techniques are now available for monitoring but culture-based techniques are used to define the legally accepted limits of environmental water contamination. The quantification of the indicator organisms *E. coli* and *Enterococci* are used to detect faecal pollution. Routine analysis is still largely based on the enumeration of these two intestinal organisms by culture coupled with the detection of β-D-galactosidase and β-D-glucuronidase activity. A secondary objective of environmental monitoring is the identification and quantification of bacteria present in water samples and this is best achieved by molecular methods. Whereas culture methods have the limitation of only providing information the day after collection of the sample, all the other methods currently available have some limitations as well when used for environmental samples. In the case of molecular methods this is the need to concentrate the sample or amplify the DNA, further the highly specific target sequences that are used could result in an underestimation of the actual level of indicator organism. The most promising area is the development of a wide range of biosensor systems which show promising simplicity for direct and *in situ* analysis.

Author details

Robert G. Price[1*] and Dirk Wildeboer[2]

*Address all correspondence to: robert.price@kcl.ac.uk

1 Faculty of Life Sciences and Medicine, Diabetes and Nutritional Sciences Division King's College London, London, UK

2 Faculty of Science and Technology, Natural Sciences Department, Middlesex University, The Burroughs, London, UK

References

[1] WHO Chapter 4: Faecal pollution and water quality. In: Guidelines for safe recreational water environments. World Health Organisation, 2003. Available from: http://www.who.int/water_sanitiation_health/bathing/srwe1/en.

[2] US EPA Recreational water quality criteria. Office of Water. 2012; 820-F-12-058.

[3] EU Directive 2006/7/EC (2006) of the European Parliament and of the Council of 15 February 2006 concerning the management of bathing water quality. The European Parliament and the Council of the European Union: Official Journal of the European Union. 2006; L64/37.

[4] Pandey PK, Kass PH, Supir ML, Biswas S, Singh VP. Contamination of water resources by pathogenic bacteria. AMB Express 2014;**4**:51.

[5] Ishi S, Sadowsky MJ. *Escherichia coli* in the environment: Implications for water quality and human health. Microbes Environ. 2008;**23**:101-108.

[6] Fewtrell L, Kay D. Recreational water and infection: a review of recent findings. Curr Environ Health. 2015; **Rpt 2**:85-94.

[7] Bradford SA, Morales VL, Zhang W, Harvey RW, Packman AI, Mohanram A, Welty C. Transport and fate of microbial pathogens in agricultural settings. Crit. Rev. Environ. Sci. Technol. 2012; **43**:775-893.

[8] Cornejova T, Venglovsky J, Gregova G, Kmetova M, Kmet V. Extended spectrum beta-lactamases in *Escherichia coli* from municipal wastewater. Ann. Agric. Environ. Med. 2015;**22**(3),447-450.

[9] Anastasi EM, Matthews B, Stratton HM, Katouli M. Pathogenic Escherichia coli found in sewage treatment plants and environmental waters. Appl. Environ. Microbiol. 2012;**78**(16), 5536-5541.

[10] Eichmiller JJ, Hicks R, Sadowsky MJ. Distribution of genetic markers of fecal pollution on a freshwater sandy shoreline in proximity to wastewater effluent. Environ. Sci. Technol. 2013;**47**(7), 3395-3402.

[11] Madoux-Humery A-S, Dorner S, Sauve S, Aboulfadl K, Galarneau M, Servais P, Prevost M. The effects of combined sewer overflow on riverine sources of drinking water. Water Res 2016;**92**:218-227.

[12] Boehm A, Sassoubre LM. *Enterococci* as indicators of environmental contamination. In: Commensals to leading to causes of drug resistant infections. Gilmore MS, Clewell DB, Ike Y. (editors), Boston, Mass: Eye and Ear Infirmary, 2014.

[13] Dorevitch S, Pratap P, Wroblewski M, Hryhorczuk DO, Li H, Liu LC, Scheff PA. Health risks of limited-contact water recreation. Environ Health Perspect. 2012;**120**:192-197.

[14] Manafi M, Kneifel W, Bascombe S. Fluorogenic and chromogenic substrates used in bacterial diagnosis. Microbiol. Rev. 1991;**55**:2011-234.

[15] Ferguson DM, Moore DF, Getrich MA, Zhowandai MH. Enumeration and Speciation of *Enterococci* in marine and intertidal sediments and coastal waters in Southern California. J. Appl. Microbiol. 2005;**99**:598-608.

[16] Price RG, Wildeboer D. methods of analysis of bacterial contamination in environmental waters. In: Coliforms: occurrence, detection methods and environmental impact. Editor G McCoy. New York, USA: Nova Sci. Publ. 2015;pp. 27-52.

[17] Mulamattathil SG, Bezuidenhout C, Mbewe M, Collins NA. Isolation of environmental bacteria from surface and drinking water in Mafikeng, South Africa, and characterisation using their antibiotic resistance profiles. J Pathog 2014;Article ID 371208, 11 pages. http://dx.doi.org/10.1155/2014/371208.

[18] Ibrahim AB, Mohd Khan A, Norrakiah AS. Microbiological risk assessment of fresh water aquaculture fish: From farm to table. Adv. Environ.. Biol. 2014; **8**(14),105-111.

[19] Kapetanovic D, Dragun Z, Smrzlic IV, Valic D, Teskeredžic E. The microbial marine water quality associated with capture-based bluefin tuna aquaculture: a case study in Adratic sea (CROATIA). Fresen. Environ. Bull. 2013;**22**(8),2214-2220.

[20] Mahmood MA, Abdelsalam M, Mahdy OA, El Miniawy HMF, Ahmed ZAM, Osman AH, Mohamed HMH, Khattab AM, Zaki Ewiss MA. Infectious bacterial pathogens, parasites and pathological correlations of sewage pollution as an important threat to farmed fishes in Egypt. Environ. Pollut. 2016; **219:** 939-948.

[21] McPeters GA, Cameron SC, Le Chevallier MW. Influence of diluents, media and membrane filters on detection of injured waterborne coliform bacteria. Appl. Environ. Microbiol. 1982;**43:**97-103.

[22] Browne NK, Huang Z, Dockrell M, Hashmi P, Price RG. Evaluation of new chromogenic substrates for the detection of coliforms. J. Appl. Microbiol. 2010;**108**:1823-1838.

[23] Cassar R, Cuschieri P. Comparison of Salmonella chromogenic medium with DCLS Agar for the isolation of *Salmonella* species from Stool Specimens. J. Clin. Microbiol. 2003;**41**:3229-3232.

[24] Atlas RM. Handbook of microbiological media, 4th Ed., Boca Raton, USA: CRC Press, 2010.

[25] Alexander SK, Strete D. Microbiology. A photographic atlas for the laboratory. New Jersey, USA: Pearson, 2000.

[26] ISO (2015) International Standards Organisation: ISO/TC 147/SC 4–Microbiological methods. Available at: http://www.iso.org/iso/home/store/catalogue_tc/catalogue_tc_browse.htm?commid=52944&published=on

[27] Nadaozie PC. Comparative study of two conventional methods used for coliform enumeration from Port Harcourt waters. OALib J.. 2016;**3**. http://dx.doi.org/10.4236/oalib.1102500.

[28] Edberg SC, Allen MJ, Smith DB and the Natl. Collaborative Study. National field evaluation of a defined substrate method for the simultaneous enumeration of total coliforms and *Escherichia coli* from drinking water: comparison with the standard Multiple Tube Fermentation Method. Appl. Environ. Microbiol. 1988;**54**:1595-1601.

[29] Heijnen L, Medena G. Quantitative detection of *E. coli, E. coli* O157 and other shiga toxin producing *E. coli* in water samples using a culture method with real-time PCR. J. Water Health. 2006; **4**(4):487-498.

[30] Chapman PA. Methods available for the detection of *Escherichia coli* O157 in clinical, food and environmental samples. World J. Microbial. Biotechnol. 2000;**16**:733-740.

[31] Ngwa GA, Schop R, Weir S, Leon-Velarde CG, Odumeru JA. Detection and enumeration of *E. coli* O157:H7 in water samples by culture and molecular methods. J Microbiol. Methods. 2013;**15**:164-72.

[32] Amirat L, Wildeboer D, Abuknesha RA, Price RG. *Esherichia coli* contamination of the river Thames in different seasons and weather conditions. Water Environ. J. 2012;**26**:482-489.

[33] Tryland I, Surman S, Berg JD. Monitoring faecal contamination of the Thames estuary using semi-automated early warning system. Water Sci. Technol. 2002;**46**:25-31.

[34] Kolarevic S, Knezevic-Vukcevic J, Paunovic M, Gaeic Z, Vukovic-Gacie B. Assessment of the microbiological quality of the river Tisa in Serbia. Water Res. Manage. 2011;**1**:57-61.

[35] Tornevi A, Bergstedt O, Forsberg B. Precipitation effects on microbial pollution in a river: lag structures and seasonal effect modifications. PLoS One 2014; e 9:e98546.

[36] Skariyachan S, Mahajananakatti AB, Grandhi NJ, Prasanna A, Sen B, Sharma N, Vasist KS, Narayanappa S. Environmental monitoring of bacterial contamination and antibiotic resistance patterns of the faecal coliforms isolated from Cauvery River, a major drinking water source in Karnataka, India. Environ. Monit. Assess. 2015;**187**:279.

[37] Pall E, Niculaen M, Kiss T, Sandru CD, Spinu M. Human impact on the microbiological water quality of the rivers. J. Med. Microbiol. 2013;**62**:1630-1640.

[38] Heery B, Briciu-Burghina C, Zhang D, Duffy G, Brabazon D, O'Connor N, Regan F. ColiSense, today's sample today: a rapid on-site detection of β-D-glucuronidase activity in surface water as a surrogate for *E. coli*. Talanta 2016;**148**:75-83.

[39] Hewage N, Saleh M. Evaluation of the pathogen detect system and anthracene-based enzyme substrates for the detection and differentiation of *E. coli* and coliforms in water samples. J Water Resour Protect. 2015;**7**:689-701.

[40] Zuckerman U, Hart I, Armon R. Field evaluation of ground raw and treated water and comparison with standard membrane filtration methods. Water Air Soil Pollut. 2008;**188**:3-8.

[41] Schang C, Henry R, Kolotelo PA, Prosser T, Crosbie N, Grant T, Cottam D, O'Brien PO, Coutts S, Deletic A, McCarthy T. Evaluation of techniques for measuring microbial hazards in bathing waters: a comparative study. PLoS One 2016; DOI:10.1371/journal. one.01558481-19.

[42] Bramburger AJ, Brown RS, Haley J, Ridal JJ. A new, automated rapid fluorimetric method for the detection of *Escherichia coli* in recreational waters. J. Great Lakes Res. 2015; **41**:298-302.

[43] Aw TG, Rose JB. Detection of pathogens in water: from phylochips to qPCR to pyrosequencing. Curr. Opin. Biotechnol. 2012;**23**(3),422-430.

[44] Carlos C, Alexandrino F, Stoppe NC, Sato MI, Ottoboni LM. Use of *Escherichia coli* BOX-PCR fingerprints to identify sources of fecal contamination of water bodies in the State of Sao Paulo, Brazil. J. Environ. Manage. 2012;**93**(1),38-43.

[45] Drozd M, Merrick NN, Sanad YM, Dick LK, Dick WA, Rajashekara G. Evaluating the occurrence of host-specific, general fecal indicators, and bacterial pathogens in a mixed-use watershed. J. Environ. Qual. 2013;**42**(3),713-725.

[46] Ervin JS, Russell TL, Layton BA, Yamahara KM, Wang D, Sassoubre LM, Cao Y, Kelty CA, Sivaganesan M, Boehm AB, Holden PA, Weisberg SB, Shanks OC. Characterization of fecal concentrations in human and other animal sources by physical, culture-based, and quantitative real-time PCR methods. Water Res. 2013;**47**(18):6873-6882.

[47] Harwood VJ, Staley C, Badgley BD, Borges K, Korajkic A. Microbial Source Tracking Markers for Detection of Fecal Contamination in Environmental Waters: Relationships to Pathogens and Human Health Outcomes. FEMS Microbiol. Rev. 2014;**38**(1):1-40.

[48] Yamahara KM, Demir-Hilton E, Preston CM, Marin R 3rd, Pargett D, Roman B, Jensen S, Birch JM, Boehm AB, Scholin CA. Simultaneous monitoring of faecal indicators and harmful algae using an *in-situ* autonomous sensor. Lett. Appl. Microbiol. 2015;**61**(2):130-138.

[49] Allard MW, Strain E, Melka D, Bunning K, Musser SM, Brown EW, Timme R. Practical value of food pathogen traceability through building a whole-genome sequencing network and database. J. Clin. Microbiol. 2016;**54**(8):1975-1983.

[50] Bentley SD, Parkhill J. Genomic perspectives on the evolution and spread of bacterial pathogens. Proc. Roy. Soc. B: Biol. Sci. 2015;**282**(1821). doi: 10.1098/rspb.2015.0488.

[51] Parsons BD, Zelyas N, Berenger BM, Chui L. Detection, characterization, and typing of shiga toxin-producing *Escherichia coli*. Front. Microbiol. 2016;**7**(APR), art. no. 478.

[52] Wildeboer D, Amirat L, Price RG and Abuknesha RA. Rapid detection of Escherichia coli in water using a hand-held fluorescence detector. Water Res. 2010;**44**(8): 2621-2628.

[53] Hesari N, Alum A, Elzein, M, Abbaszadegan M. A biosensor platform for rapid detection of E. coli in drinking water. Enzyme Microb. Technol. 2016;**83**:22-28.

[54] Wutor VC, Togo CA, Limson JL, Pletschke BI. A novel biosensor for the detection and monitoring of β-D-galactosidase of faecal origin in water. Enzyme Microb. Technol. 2007;**40**:1512-1517.

[55] Gunda NSK, Chavali R, Mitra SK. A hydrogel based rapid test method for detection of *Escherichia coli (E. coli)* in contaminated water samples. Analyst 2016;**141**(10):2920-2929.

[56] Chowdhury AD, De A, Chaudhuri CR, Bandyopadhyay K, Sen P. Label free polyaniline based impedimetric biosensor for detection of *E. coli* O157:H7 Bacteria. Sens. Actuat. B: Chem. 2012; **171-172**: 916-923.

[57] Wang, Y, Alocilja EC. Gold nanoparticle-labeled biosensor for rapid and sensitive detection of bacterial pathogens. J. Biol. Eng. 2015; **9**(1). doi: 10.1186/s13036-015-0014-z.

[58] Rochelet M, Solanas S, Betelli L, Neuwirth C, Vienney F, Hartmann A. Amperometric detection of extended-spectrum small beta-lactamase activity: application to the characterization of resistant *E. coli* strains. Analyst. 2015;**140**(10):3551-3556.

[59] Paniel N, Baudart J, Hayat A, Barthelmebs L. Aptasensor and genosensor methods for the detection of microbes in real world samples. Methods 2013;**64**:224-229.

[60] Idil N, Hedström M, Denizli A, Mattiasson B. Whole cell based microcontact imprinted capacitive biosensor for the detection of *Escherichia coli*. Biosens. Bioelectron. 2017;**87**:807-815.

[61] Lopez-Roldan R, Tusell P, Cortina J.L, Courtois S, Cortina JL. On-line bacteriological detection in water. TrAC—Trends Anal. Chem. 2013;**44**:46-57.

[62] Gemmell ME, Schmidt S. Is the microbiological quality of the Msunduzi River (KwaZulu-Natal, South Africa) suitable for domestic, recreational, and agricultural purposes? Environ. Sci. Pollut. Res. 2013;**20**(9):6551-6562.

[63] Thevenon F, Regier N, Benagli C, Tonolla M, Adatte T, Wildi W, Poté J. Characterization of fecal indicator bacteria in sediments cores from the largest freshwater lake of Western Europe (Lake Geneva, Switzerland). Ecotoxicol. Environ. Saf. 2012; **78**:50-56.

[64] Loff M, Mare L, De Kwaadsteniet M, Khan W. 3M™ Molecular Detection system versus MALDI-TOF mass spectrometry and molecular techniques for the identification of *Escherichia coli* 0157: H7, *Salmonella spp.* and *Listeria* spp. J. Microbiol. Methods. 2014;**101**(1):33-43.

[65] Kaeberlein T, Lewis K, Epstein SS. Isolating "uncultivatable" microorganisms in pure culture in a simulated natural environment. Science 2002;**296**(5570):1127-1129.

[66] Chlorination Chemistry Council. Drinking water chlorination—a review of disinfection practices and issues. Available from: http://www.waterandhealth.org/drinkingwater/wp.html

[67] Gordon DM. Geographical structure and host specificity in bacteria and the implications for tracing the source of coliform contamination. Microbiology. 2001; **147**:1079-1085.

[68] Prüss-Ustün A, Wolf J, Corvlan C, Bos M, Neira M. Preventing disease through healthy environments. A global assessment of the burden of disease from environmental risks. Geneva: Word Health Organisation, 2016. Available from: http://apps.who.int/iris/bitstream/10665/204585/1/9789241565196_eng.pdf?ua=1

[69] Lora-Suarez F, Rivera R, Triviño-Valencia J, Gomez-Marin JE. Detection of protozoa in water samples by formalin/ether concentration method. Water Res. 2016;**100**:377-381.

[70] Kumar T, Majid MAA, Onichandran S, Jaturas N, Andiappan H, Salibay CC, Tabo HAL, Tabo N, Dungca JZ, Tangpong J, Phiriyasamith S, Yuttayong B, Polseela R, Do BN, Sawangjaroen N, Tan T, Lim YAL, Nissapatorn V. Presence of Cryptosporidium parvum and Giardia lamblia in water samples from Southeast Asia: towards an integrated water detection system. Infect. Dis. Poverty 2016;**5**(1):3.

Chapter 8

Detection Methods for Lipopolysaccharides: Past and Present

Loreen R. Stromberg, Heather M. Mendez and Harshini Mukundan

Additional information is available at the end of the chapter

http://dx.doi.org/10.5772/intechopen.68311

Abstract

Lipopolysaccharide (LPS) is the primary component of the outer membrane of Gram-negative bacteria. LPS aids in protecting bacterial cells, and also defines the unique serogroups used to classify bacteria. Additionally, LPS is an endotoxin and the primary stimulator of innate immune cells in mammals, making it an ideal candidate for early detection of pathogens. However, the majority of methods for detection of LPS focus on detection of the endotoxic component of the molecule, lipid A. Since lipid A is largely conserved among bacterial species and serogroups, these detection approaches are highly nonspecific. Thus, the importance of identifying the O-polysaccharide antigenic portion of LPS, which confers serogroup specificity, has received a great deal of attention in recent years. However, methods that are highly selective to the O-antigens are typically less sensitive than those that target the endotoxin. Here we present a history and comparison of the sensitivity of these methods and their value for detecting bacteria in a variety of different sample types.

Keywords: lipopolysaccharide, endotoxin, O-antigen, Serogroup, biodetection

1. Introduction

The increasing occurrence of infectious disease is a global issue. Emerging pathogens with increasing levels of drug resistance are a continuing danger to both public health and agriculture. Accurate and rapid detection of pathogens is critical to implement preventative measures to mitigate this problem. Despite this urgent need, conventional methods for bacterial detection require cell culture and serology, which can take several weeks. As new pathogens emerge, it is even more important that our detection technologies evolve to keep pace with the need to discriminate pathogen from host flora. This requires an understanding of pathogen biology, the types of samples they occur in, and their mechanism of immune interaction within the hosts [1].

The innate immune system is able to discriminate pathogens from nonpathogens, and rapidly sense pathogen biomarkers in the complex milieu of the host. Exploiting this recognition via measurement of pathogen signatures, can provide an optimal strategy for discriminatory biodetection. A primary category of such biomarkers is virulence signatures termed pathogen-associated molecular patterns (PAMPs) [2]. PAMPs are evolutionarily conserved molecules that bind pattern-recognition receptors in the host, and activate the innate immune response [2, 3], providing a means for both early and specific pathogen detection. Biochemically, PAMPs are a diverse array of proteins, lipopeptides, lipoglycans, peptidoglycans, teichoic acids, and nucleic acids [4]. However, many detection methods have largely focused on proteins and nucleic acids [1, 5], ignoring other categories of PAMPs [2, 6–8]. Also, their small size, biochemistry, and low concentration in hosts make them difficult to target in detection assays [8, 9].

Classified as a lipogylcan, lipopolysaccharides (LPS) are small amphiphilic molecules that are associated with Gram-negative bacteria [7, 10]. LPS is an indicator of active infection, is serogroup-specific [11–13], more stable than its protein counterparts, and is released early in infection, making it an ideal candidate for detection and diagnostics. LPS serves as a biomarker that aids in serological discrimination of Gram-negative bacteria; this allows for identification and characterization of pathotypes that are essential for timely mitigation and treatment of infections. Since LPS is a pathogen-specific biomarker, it is an indicator of acute infection, which is an advantage over serological assays. In addition to medical diagnostics, LPS detection provides a method for detecting *Escherichia coli* in the food-industry, which is often associated with food-borne illnesses. Finally, LPS is also a virulence factor whose structure and function determines *E. coli* serogroup, a factor which has ramifications on vaccine design and therapeutic interventions. While many methods for LPS detection exist, most of them are not optimized for amphiphilic detection in physiological samples. An ideal measurement for LPS should be sensitive enough to detect low concentrations of the amphiphile in aqueous physiological milieu (e.g., blood), and use antibodies or ligands that provide serogroup selectivity [14]. Coupling sensitive detection platforms with surfaces designed to maximize the binding of amphiphilic PAMPs is a potential solution to achieve such an ideal.

2. Sources of lipopolysaccharides

Bacteria are classified into Gram-negative and Gram-positive [15], which release amphiphilic virulence factors such as LPS, lipoarabinomannan (LAM), and lipoteichoic acid (LTA) in the host. Species of pathogenic Gram-negative bacteria of concern to human health, include *Acinetobacter* [16], *Burkholderia* [17], *Bordetella* [18], *Campylobacter* [19–21], *Chlamydia* [22, 23], *E. coli* [20, 24], *Helicobacter* [25, 26], *Hemophilius* [27], *Klebsiella* [28], *Legionella* [20, 29], *Moraxella* [30], *Neisseria* [31], *Pseudomonas* [32], *Proteus* [33], *Salmonella* [20, 34], *Shigella* [35], *Yersinia* [36], and others, grouped into the Enterobacteriaceae family. These pathogens are contaminants in food, water, and soil, used as agents of bioterrorism, and can cause nosocomial infections [5]. Detection of these organisms, particularly *E. coli*, is an important aspect for epidemiology, disease control, and treatment.

Herein, we present a comprehensive description of the structural and biochemical properties of LPS, current methods for its detection, and potential approaches to overcome the current limitations for direct detection of the molecule in physiological matrices.

3. Lipopolysaccharide structures and conformations

Lipopolysaccharides have been the subject of intense study for over half a century [37–39]. LPS is the prototypical lipoglycan with an overall net negative charge [40–42], and is the primary component of the outer membrane of nearly all Gram-negative bacteria [11]. The bacterial membrane of each *E. coli* cell is composed of approximately 10^6 lipid A moieties and 10^7 glycerophospholipid molecules, comprising approximately three-quarters of the outer membrane [43–45]. Thus, there are approximately 62 pg of LPS per cell (for *E. coli* in log phase growth) [46]. LPS has an amphipathic tripartite structure (**Figure 1**). Lipid A is the most conserved portion of the LPS molecule, and consists of six, sometimes seven, fatty acid tails (*E. coli* and *Salmonella*, respectively), which gives the molecule its hydrophobic properties [10, 43, 45]. Lipid A is also called endotoxin [43], and is responsible for the biological effects of LPS

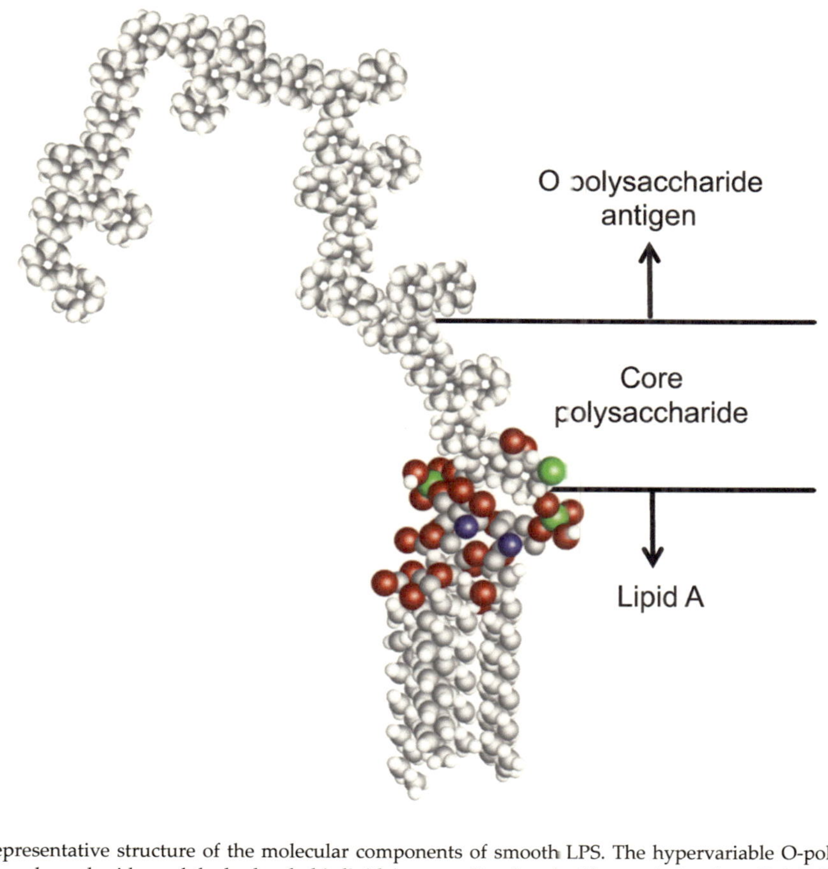

Figure 1. Representative structure of the molecular components of smooth LPS. The hypervariable O-polysaccharide antigen, core polysaccharide, and the hydrophobic lipid A group. Reprinted with permission from Ref. [74].

caused by its binding to the mammalian innate immune receptor, toll-like receptor 4 (TLR4) [11, 44, 47, 48]. Structurally, lipid A is covalently bound to the core polysaccharide, which is further divided into the inner and outer core polysaccharides, with the outer core being less conserved in both sugar moieties and location of glycosidic linkages [45, 49, 50].

There are two main forms of LPS—smooth (S-form) and rough (R-form) [42, 45, 46]. The distal end of LPS extends to a long chain O-polysaccharide antigen (O-ag(s)) in organisms possessing S-form, which is an indicator of virulence [51, 52]. R-form LPS is devoid of the O-ag [45], but can still induce an immunogenic response [53]. The O-ag is hyper-variable, and made up of repeating subunits, each composed of 1–7 glycosyl residues [45, 54]. As many as 40 size variations in subunit repeats of the O-ag have been reported just for *E. coli* O111:B4 [55], and 180 O-ag have been identified overall for *E. coli* species [47, 54]. The sugars (colitose, paratose, tyvelose, and abequose) that make the O-ag unique are seldom found elsewhere [54]. Other variations to the polysaccharide are implemented through addition of noncarbohydrate entities, such as acetyl or methyl groups [54]. These variations make discriminative detection of enteric bacteria feasible [56], but complicate antigen characterization. Therefore, LPS serves as an ideal target for early detection and identification of Gram-negative pathogens.

In aqueous solutions, amphiphiles like LPS can present in a micellar conformation [48, 55, 57–59]. This occurs at a concentration specific to the amphiphile [55], and is known as the critical micelle concentration (CMC). At or above the CMC, there is an equilibrium state between monomers, micelles or supramolecular aggregates, depending on environmental conditions [48, 55–57, 60–63]. This amphiphilic biochemistry and structural variability complicates determination of the exact molecular weight of S-form LPS. As such, LPS concentrations are reported in weight per volume, or in endotoxin units (EU), a measure of activity. As degree of endotoxicity can vary according to bacterial origin, a rough estimate of 100 pg = 1 EU is used in many cases to facilitate unit conversion [64, 65].

The large oligosaccharide region on S-form LPS makes the molecule amphipathic [54], which influences the shape of micelles in solution. Lipid A is largely responsible for shaping the LPS micelle [10, 45, 46, 56, 66–68], although other factors can also contribute. Lipid A is conserved within species in the number of fatty acid chains and the degree of saturation [44, 66] within those chains [22, 47, 69]. Shapes for LPS micelles include cubic, lamellar, and hexagonal inverted structures [56, 67, 70, 71]. Whether aggregate or monomeric forms (or both) of LPS is required for innate immune activation is debatable [56, 72, 73]. Since this process occurs in aqueous blood, it is unlikely that the molecule is presented as a monomer, unless associated with serum binding proteins.

Variation in LPS micelles [55] modifies presentation of O-ag-specific epitopes to antibodies, making detection challenging [74, 75]. This is specifically true when the heterogeneous presentation of linear [76] and conformational epitopes [49, 77] present on LPS molecules are considered. The primary structure of LPS varies in the core polysaccharide, within and between species [47, 55]. Core polysaccharides are primarily made up of common sugars such as heptose and 2-deoxy-D-*manno*octulosonic acid (a.k.a. KDO), which can be functionalized with phosphate or ethanolamine groups [45, 50, 78]. This feature contributes to varying charge distributions and differential size ratio of the hydrophobic to hydrophilic regions which influences micelle assembly [10, 59, 79, 80]. Other factors that contribute to micelle shape [10, 79] are pH [61], ion concentration [81–86], and temperature [62]. These biochemical properties drive host-pathogen interactions and should be considered in the design of detection strategies.

4. Detection methods for lipopolysaccharides and similar amphiphiles

There have been many efforts to establish rapid and reliable detection methods for LPS in clinical samples [10, 46] and for testing pharmacological products such as infusion fluids, sterile injectables, medical device implants, and others [87]. These methods can be broadly divided into six overlapping categories: *in vivo* and *in vitro* tests, immunoassays and their derivatives; biological, chemical, and cell-based sensors. These methods span a broad range of sensitivity, but many lack the ability to differentiate between LPS serogroups.

4.1. Limulus amoebocyte lysate assay and the rabbit pyrogen test

The first method approved by the US Food and Drug Administration for LPS detection was called the rabbit pyrogen test [88–90], which simply measures the ability of an endotoxin to induce fever in an animal. Any febrile response was attributed to the presence of endotoxin [89–91]. The test, clearly, is activity-based, and nonspecific. In the case of Hepatitis B vaccine manufacturing, the rabbit pyrogen test is still the standard method for determining endotoxin contamination [91], but the test is cost prohibitive and is minimally utilized today, except in some parenteral devices [10].

In 1956, Bang discovered that amoebocytes from *Limulus polyphemus* (a.k.a. horseshoe crab) agglutinate upon addition of endotoxin [46], as a result of a protease cascade [10]. Bang and Levin [46, 92] subsequently used this concept to devise a method for endotoxin detection. Since the lysates of amoebocytes were required, it was called the limulus amoebocyte lysate (LAL) assay, and is the gold standard for the detection of lipid A. The LAL assay is prone to variability and can be inhibited through several mechanisms. The United States Pharmacopeia and the Code of Federal Regulations have consequently published guidances for the manufacturing and testing of assays for use on human products [93, 94]. Despite some challenges, the LAL assay is more rapid, cost effective, and reportedly 300 times more sensitive [46] than the rabbit pyrogen test [46].

Variants of the LAL assay use turbidimetric [95], chromogenic [46], or viscosity [10] measurements to determine results [10, 46]. A turbidimetric gel clot has more coagulen, and measures the change in turbidity over time, but does not form a solid clot [46, 95]. The viscosity assay, however, measures the degree of clotting via the change in viscosity. The chromogenic assay can be endpoint or kinetic, and utilizes a *p*-nitroaniline substrate, which is cleaved by an LAL proenzyme, providing a colorimetric readout [46]. The sensitivity of LAL assays is dependent on the sample type, processing method and time, as well as the dilution factor [46]. Additionally, the source of the LAL reagent plays a factor, as it is apparent when comparing the different limits of detection (LoD) reported for endotoxin standards. A survey of the relative sensitivities of the LAL assay is shown in **Table 1**.

Description	**Sample**	**Detection method**	**Species**	**Sensitivity (ng/mL)***	**Specific**	**Source**
Rabbit pyrogen	Purified endotoxin	Febrile response	–	–	No	[89]
LAL	Plasma	Gelation	Multiple species	0.5–5.0	No	[96]
LAL	Blood, plasma	Gelation	*E. coli*	0.5–5.0	No	[92]
LAL	Serum plasma	Optical density	*E. coli*	0.025–0.5	No	[100]
LAL	Urine	Gelation	*E. coli*	0.5	No	[204]
LAL	Urine	Optical density	Multiple species	2.0	No	[98]
LAL	Spinal fluid/ plasma	Optical density	*E. coli, Haemophilus influenzae B*	0.1	No	[101]
LAL	Ascites	Gelation	*E. coli*	0.5	No	[104]
LAL	Cerebral/synovial	–	*E. coli*	1.0	No	[103]
LAL	Seawater	Optical density	*E. coli*	2.3	No	[41]
LAL	Purified endotoxin	Gelation	*E. coli*	1.0	No	[95]
LAL	Purified endotoxin	Gelation	*Salmonella minnesota*	10^{-11}	No	[111]
LAL	Ground beef	Gelation	*Enterobacter aerogenes*	–	No	[205]
LAL	Ground beef	Gelation	Multiple species	51.0 ng/g	No	[108]
LAL	Milk	Chromogenic	*Pseudomonas putida*	0.01	No	[107]
LAL	Purified endotoxin	Gelation	*E. coli* O114	100	No	[206]
LAL-magnetoelastic sensor	Purified LPS	resonant frequency	*E. coli* O111:B4	0.0105 EU/ mL	No	[207]
ENDOLisa® (LAL)	Purified endotoxin	Fluorescence	*E. coli* spp., *Salmonella* spp.	0.05–500 EU/ mL	No	[129]
ELISA	Milk	Abs at 405 nm	*E. coli*	100–200		[165]
LPS pull down-sandwich ELISA	Pure cultures	Abs at 450 nm	*E. coli* O157	–		[125]
LPS pull down-sandwich ELISA	Purified LPS	Abs at 450 nm	*Salmonella* spp. (31 total)	1.0	Yes	[126]
Premier EIA *E. coli* O157	Stool extract	Spectro-photometric	*E. coli* O157	–	Yes	[122]
LPS pull down	Purified endotoxin	RIA	*E. coli* O114	300	No	[206]
LPS pull down-ion (NTA-Cu)	Purified LPS	EIS	*E. coli* O55:B5	0.0001–0.1	No	[161]
Diaphorase functionalized surface	Purified LPS	Chemical	*E. coli* O127:B8	50	Maybe	[87]

Description	Sample	Detection method	Species	Sensitivity (ng/mL)*	Specific	Source
LPS pull down-SAMs with synthetic peptide	Purified LPS	Electro-chemistry	*E. coli* ATCC 35218	21.8 pg/mL	No	[189]
LPS pull down-SAMs with aptamer	Purified LPS	EIS	*E. coli* O55:B5	0.1–1.0	Maybe	[159]
LPS pull down-gold electrode w/ aptamer	Purified LPS	EIS and cyclic voltammetry	*E. coli* O55:B5	0.001–1.0	No	[160]
LPS aptamer sandwich	Purified LPS	Electro-chemistry	–	10 fg/mL	Maybe	[188]
LPS pull down-gold electrodes w/ PmB	Purified LPS	EIS	*E. coli* O111:B4	0.2	No	[162]
Polydiacetylene liposomes	Purified LPS (5 groups)	Change in Abs	*E. coli* spp, *Salmonella* spp	2.22 mg/mL	Yes	[191]
Impedance enthothelial biosensor	Purified LPS in culture medium+	Resistivity of cell monolayer	–	500	No	[169]
Macrophage microarrays on gold electrodes	Purified LPS in culture medium	FTIR	*E. coli* O111:B4	0.1 μg/mL	No	[200]
Primary culture HDME cells	Purified LPS	Fluorescence	*E. coli* O111:B4	1.0 μg/mL	No	[171]
Engineered cells secrete alkaline phosphatase	Purified LPS in culture medium+	Electro-chemistry	–	0.1	No	[170]
LPS pull down-PmB	Purified LPS	Evanescent sensing	*E. coli* O128:B12	25	No	[75]
LPS pull down-TLR4/MD2 on gold electrodes	Purified LPS	Electro-chemistry	*E. coli* O55:B5	0.0005 EU/mL	No	[180]
LPS pull down-membrane insertion	Purified LPS (3 groups)	Evanescent sensing	*E. coli*	420	Yes	[74]
LPS pull down-antibody	Pure cultures in ground beef	Evanescent sensing	*E. coli* O157	–	Yes	[166]
LPS pull down-proanthocyanidin	FITC-labeled LPS	Fluorescence	*E. coli* O55:B5	–	No	[192]
Copolythiophene interacts with LPS	Purified LPS	Fluorescence	*E. coli* O55:B5	$2.5E^{-5}$–2.0 μM	No	[164]
Polydiacetylene liposomes	–	Fluorescence	–	0.1 μM	No	[190]
Peptide-based fluorescence	Purified LPS	FRET-increase	*E. coli* O111:B4	0.15–2.0 μM	No	[194]
Pyrenyl-derived long-chain quaternary ammonium probe	Purified LPS	Fluorescence	*E. coli* O55:B5	100 nM	No	[193]

Description	Sample	Detection method	Species	Sensitivity (ng/mL)*	Specific	Source
LPS pull down-peptide on Graphene Oxide	Purified LPS (4 groups)	Fluorescence	Several species	130 pM	No	[195]
LPS pull down-PmB capture	Purified LPS spiked in blood	Acoustic sensing	*E. coli* O55:B5	1.0	No	[196]
LPS pull down-CD14 capture	Biotin-LPS	Luminescence	–	10.0	No	[176]
LPS pull down Polyaniline + ConA lectin	Purified LPS and LTA	EIS	*E. coli*, *S. aureus*	50.0	No	[208]
Aptamer sandwich on beads	Purified LPS	Fluorescence	*E. coli* O55:B5	0.01	Maybe	[163]
LPS pull down endotoxin neutralizing protein	Purified LPS	Capacitance	*E. coli*	10^{-13} M	No	[181]
LPS pull down CramoLL lectin	Purified LPS (4 types)	EIS	*E. coli* *Salmonella* *Klebsiella* *Serratia*	25.0 μg/mL	No	[185]

*Unless otherwise indicated.

Table 1. Overview of sensitivities and specificities for LPS detection methods.

In 1970, Levin discovered that samples tested in whole blood would not render a positive result [92], but if plasma was extracted in chloroform and diluted 1–10%, then endotoxin activity could be detected in the 0.5–5 ng/mL range [92, 96]. Levin correctly assumed that components of whole blood were bound to endotoxin, thereby inhibiting the reaction with the LAL reagent [46, 92, 97], or changing the reaction kinetics [46]. This is evident when the amphiphilic nature of LPS and the aqueous nature of blood are considered. In addition to blood and plasma [46, 92, 96], the LAL assay has been used in urine [46, 98], cerebral spinal fluid, synovial fluid, ascites fluid, vaginal and cervical fluids, broncho-alveolar lavage samples, seawater [46], bovine milk [99], and beef tissue [100, 101]. Virtually all of these have reported ng/mL LoDs, for endotoxin, but none are serogroup-specific. Researchers have used heat [46, 102], chemical treatment with chloroform [103], acids [104, 105], alkali [106, 107], or ether [108] to improve sensitivity with some success when using heat or chemical extraction of the endotoxin [46, 109]. However, the results show poor reproducibility between researchers (**Table 1**). Yin and Galanos [106] reported a sensitivity of 10^{-11} ng/mL for *Salmonella* spp., while Cooper et al. [89] reported 1.0 ng/mL for *E. coli* endotoxin. This disparity leaves a lot of questions and draws attention to the fact that small changes in preparation, heat or chemical treatments, usage of plastics instead of silanized glass, or addition of surfactants can result in altered assay sensitivity. This variation can also be explained by the variable biosynthesis of lipid A, as shown with *Salmonella* [47, 110]. Additionally, LAL can yield false positives upon reacting with other polysaccharides or β-(1,3)-glucans [10, 46] and depends on the source of bacteria, as LPS/endotoxin can vary in toxicity [10, 56, 79, 68], in regards to immune stimulation [41, 46, 111].

Thus, the LAL assay and rabbit pyrogen test, both based on the native immune responses of the horseshoe crab or rabbit, exhibit significant variability in outcomes. Despite these, the LAL is still very useful for quickly detecting contamination. For example, in 1981, Jay [101] used the LAL test to determine both microbial counts and endotoxin load in 153 samples of store bought ground beef with a mean sensitivity of 7.9 μg/mL (endotoxin/beef sample) in 1 h. In 1985, Nachum and Shanbrom [46] used a chromogenic LAL system to detect between 2 and 175 ng/mL of endotoxin in 324 patient urine samples, with the assay taking between 2 and 4 h. Timely detection is valuable to both patient care and product viability. Despite being an ideal test for the presence of endotoxin, determining identity of pathogens still requires culture or enrichment.

4.2. Immunoassays for LPS detection and antibody selection

Developed in 1971 [112, 113], the enzyme-linked immunosorbent assays (ELISAs) are based on the immune reaction between antigen and antibody, with each assay being tailored for the unique antigen being tested. ELISAs were evaluated for *Salmonella* O-ags very early in development [114]. However, ELISAs for lipoglycans such as LPS suffer from low sensitivity and reproducibility [115–117]. One of the primary reasons for sensitivity issues is the amphipathic biochemistry of these molecules, leading to inconsistent binding on ELISA plates [118], and variable conformations of epitope binding sites [12, 119].

There exist two primary types of LPS-ELISAs, which detect either the LPS antigen, or LPS antibody titers. With the former, the plate surface is typically coated with a primary capture antibody specific to LPS, or with the sample to be tested [118]. After antigen capture, an epitope-specific antibody is used to detect LPS. The detection antibody can be directly labeled with an enzyme [113] or secondary antibody for colorimetric detection [120, 121]. In 1998, Mackenzie et al. [122] reported on the effectiveness of a commercial assay to screen stool samples for *E. coli* O157 antigens, and found that re-testing samples provided inconsistent results. It was speculated that this was due to inefficient washing of the microwells, yet the amphiphilic antigen preparation and its presentation to antibodies could have contributed to assay inconsistencies. It was also not considered that LPS is notorious for nonspecific and inconsistent binding on microplates [10, 116, 118]. In clinical samples, the association of LPS with host carrier molecules may affect its ability to adhere to capture surfaces [123, 124], as proteins will preferentially bind to the plate. Some groups have also reported cross reactivity or false positives with LPS sandwich ELISAs [125, 126]. Choi et al. [126] developed a sensitive capture ELISA with 24 species of *Salmonella*, but cross reactivity was observed. To mitigate cross reactivity, attempts have been made to substitute antibodies with other ligands. Grallert et al. [127, 128] coated microplates with proteins isolated from bacteriophages, which are specific to core polysaccharides in order to capture LPS, followed by detection with Factor C (a component of the LAL assay). This sandwich ENDOLisa®, a microplate assay for direct detection of endotoxin, reports sensitivity between 0.05 and 500 EU/mL. This technology is sold as the Endotoxin Sample Preparation (ESP™) kit, and is one of the few kits available for direct detection of endotoxin in blood or serum [129]. However, the assay is unable to differentiate between serogroups.

The second type of ELISA measures LPS antibody titers to screen for Gram-negative bacterial infections. Here, the surface of the plate is functionalized with the antigen to pull down antibodies (Immunglobulins A, G, and M (IgG, IgA, IgM)) from serum. Since this method is based on adaptive immunity, there is a lag between initial exposure to the pathogen, and increased antibody titers [130], making early detection difficult. This assay is not specific for active infection, but has been used to monitor population health and track epidemiology of infections. Screening has been used to detect exposure of military personnel to *Shigella* [131], obstetric patients with *Chlamydia* spp. [132], patients with *Salmonella* [133], and other pathogens [114, 134–137]. Suthienkul et al. [136] used an indirect ELISA to passively adsorb LPS onto polystyrene plates, and measure associated IgG/IgM titers in cholera patients. The results indicated discrepancies between the titers of IgG and IgM in young versus older patients, which could either be due to the inconsistency of LPS coating or associated with cross reactivity [138]. Suthienkul also acknowledged that antibody levels in infants screened could be inherited from the mother [136, 139].

Functionalizing ELISA plates with amphiphilic LPS is a technical challenge [12], since the surfaces are optimized for protein binding. In the late 1970s, it was discovered that polymyxin B (an antibiotic, PmB) interacted with LPS monomers in a 1:1 ratio [86, 140], and can be used to functionalize surfaces for Gram-negative detection [119]. However, PmB recognizes the conserved lipid A group of LPS, and does not allow for discriminative detection. Takahashi et al. [118] showed that precoating the plate with high molecular weight poly-L-lysine increases surface adsorption and allows for detection of 1 μg/mL LPS, with no cross reactivity. Others have studied the effects of ions such as calcium and magnesium [141], trichloroacetic acid [142], mixing the antigen in chloroform/ethanol, and drying on the plate surface [135], or complexing LPS with a protein such as bovine serum albumin [143] to improve performance and reproducibility. Functionalization of ELISA plates with proteins known to bind LPS, such as high- or low-density lipoproteins (HDL, LDL), chylomicrons, and LPS-binding protein (LBP) have also been evaluated [123, 124] and offers promise for the reliable detection of LPS antigen in complex samples.

Other limitations for LPS detection include the fact that many LPS antigens have not been isolated [144] and thus are not available for the development of screening assays, limiting accessibility of specific antibodies as well [145–150]. However, there is also a need to refine methods for selection of tailored antibodies. While there are variations [10], ELISA plates are typically functionalized with whole dead bacteria to screen monoclonal antibody cultures [145, 146, 148], giving rise to potentially cross reactive clones [10, 144] that are then screened against a multitude of bacterial strains [146, 149, 150]. It is noted that it is impossible to screen clones against all epitopes of LPS, even amongst the many *E. coli* serotypes. In 2000, Jauho et al. [12] addressed this issue by covalently linking purified LPS O-ags to polystyrene ELISA plates using anthraquinone and UV irradiation. This technique could prove useful in developing serogroup-specific antibodies against LPS, as conserved antigens like lipid A and core polysaccharide are absent. Alternative methods for antibody screening have utilized immunoblotting [144, 149, 151–153] and flow cytometry [154–156]. In addition, ELISAs can suffer from high background due to nonspecific interactions limiting their sensitivity [10, 122, 135, 157]. Particularly,

http://dx.doi.org/10.5772/intechopen.68311

endogenous endotoxin present in reagents, on glassware, or plastics [158], may contribute to false positive results. Factors identified above have to be carefully considered in the development of ELISAs targeting LPS.

4.3. Biological and chemical-based LPS sensing

Many advanced methods such as electrochemical impedance spectroscopy (EIS) [159–161], antimicrobials [75, 162], aptamers [163], synthetic polymers [164], optical immunoassays [122, 125, 165], waveguide technology [75, 166, 167], lipid bilayers [9, 74, 168], and *in vitro* [169–171] assays have been applied for LPS detection. These technologies involve functionalizing biosensors with proteins or molecules to pull down LPS from a sample.

LBP [10], a relatively small protein (~60 kDa) that transports LPS in blood, shuttles the antigen to the cluster of differentiation 14 (CD14) protein in the extracellular matrix, or to the membrane of immune cells, such as macrophages [10]. After LPS binds CD14, it is passed to the hydrophobic binding pocket of myeloid differentiation factor 2 (MD-2) [7, 10], a necessary cofactor for the activation of TLR4. Also, the serum carrier lipoproteins (HDL and LDL), are carriers for LPS in blood. In addition to these, LPS has been demonstrated to bind aptamers [159, 160], various peptides [87, 109, 162, 172], and metal/cation complexes [84, 86, 161, 173–175]. Such carrier moieties are exploited in the development of novel detection methods for LPS, as outlined below.

For electrochemical (EC) sensing of LPS, a recognition ligand (similar to ELISA) and a transducer are required to measure the variation in signal [161]. For fluorescence-based sensing, a receptor captures LPS, while another molecule emits a fluorescent signal when bound to the antigen. Burkhardt et al. [176] used solubilized LBP to transfer LPS to a CD14 functionalized surface, with a LoD of 10 ng/mL using an electro-chemiluminescent assay. This method enforces the role of LBP as a lipid transfer protein, as demonstrated by Wurfel et al. [177, 178] and shows that CD14 can bind monomeric LPS in the absence of TLR4 [179]. Highly sensitive (LoD = 0.0005 EU) EC sensors have also been developed using a recombinant TLR4 + MD-2 complex for recognition of LPS [180]. Yet, these assays are unable to discriminate between LPS serogroups. Priano et al. [10] developed a competitive EC assay using recombinant endotoxin-neutralizing protein (ENP) on a dextran matrix, with a detection range of 1–100 ng/mL. ENP has also been used in a capacitive biosensor with an extremely low LoD (1.0×10^{-13} M) [181]. The sensitivity differences may be due to variations in surface functionalization. Priano et al. [10] used the dextran matrix, and Limbut et al. [181] used self-assembled monolayers, which provide low background interference [182–184]. Inoue and Takano [10] used a recombinant factor C in an EC hybrid LAL biosensor, with a sensitivity range of 5×10^{-4}–1.0 EU/mL [10]. Kato [87] and Iijima [10] labeled PmB with ferrocene-bound LPS in solution, and captured it on a nanocarbon-film electrode with a detection range of 2–50 ng/mL in 5 minutes [10]. Ding et al. [162] functionalized an electrode with PmB and performed EIS with a detection range of 0.2–0.8 ng/mL which is more sensitive, but has a smaller range. A broader detection range was demonstrated by Rahman et al. [172] who functionalized interdigitated electrodes with PmB and tested 0.1–1000 μg/mL of LPS O111:B4 in food samples, using impedance spectroscopy. Sugar binding proteins, such as lectins and polyaniline coated electrodes, have been used for detecting LPS [10], as with an EIS sensor functionalized with the lectin, cramoLL, with a detection range of 25–200 μg/mL [185].

Several assays have been developed using aptamers as the detection ligand. Su et al. [160, 186, 187] used aptamers attached to gold nanoparticles to detect LPS using EIS, with an impressive detection limit of 0.1 pg/mL [10]. Aptamers have also been used in a magnetic aptasensor to detect LPS in medias containing BSA, sucrose, glucose, or RNA [163], and provide a detection range of 0.01–1.0 × 10^6 ng/mL (LPS O55:B5) by flow cytometry within 1 minute. Bai et al. [188] developed an EC sensor where aptamers that bind LPS were hybridized with capture probes, which were hybridized to complementary DNA sequences on gold nanoparticles with a very sensitive range (10 fg/mL up to 50 ng/mL). However, multiple aptamer libraries against O-ag would be essential before this method could be implemented for serogroup discrimination. Modifications to improve sensitivity include use of SAMs to functionalize sensors with peptides [189], PmB [162], antibodies [10], and aptamers [159]. Despite optimal surface capture methods, some of these assays suffer from poor detection limits or range of performance [10, 159].

Investigators have utilized the interaction of LPS with synthetic systems such as copolythiophene copolymers [164] and polydiacetylene liposomes [190, 191]. Johnson et al. [192] demonstrated an endotoxin capture technique by functionalizing a bead matrix with proanthocyanidins and binding with fluorescein isothiocyanate-labeled LPS [192]. Pyrenyl-derived quaternary ammonium probes, developed by Zeng et al. [193] exhibited fluorescence when bound to LPS and detected nanomolar concentrations, while fluorescently labeled CD14 synthetic peptides demonstrated an increase in Förster resonance energy transfer when bound to LPS, but were only able to detect μM concentrations [194]. Lim et al. [195] used a functionalized graphene oxide to develop a fluorescence quench-recovery method for LPS, targeting the lipid A component. Thompson et al. [196] designed a tandem system to both detect (LoD = 1.0 ng/mL) and filter LPS from blood using piezoelectric quartz discs functionalized with PmB.

Other methods have taken advantage of the amphipathic nature of LPS. Harmon et al. [197] demonstrated that disrupting the hydrophobic association of LPS with liposomes increases the sensitivity of the LAL assay. Stromberg et al. [74, 198] were able to detect 4.20 μg/mL of amphiphilic LPS O157 in beef lysates on a waveguide biosensor using a technique called membrane insertion, which has previously been applied to other amphiphiles such as LAM and phenolic glycolipids [8, 9, 199]. Membrane insertion uses the natural association of amphiphiles with a lipid bilayer to facilitate detection and fluorescent detection of a labeled antibody is performed within an evanescent field [168, 199]. Many biosensors report exquisite sensitivity, even down to the picogram [164] and femtomolar [9, 168, 199] range, but very few are capable of physiological presentation of amphiphiles to facilitate discriminative detection of O-ag groups [74, 167, 198].

4.4. Cell-based LPS detection systems

Cell systems are ideal for recognizing endotoxin, although interpreting the signal response can be challenging. Bouafsoun et al. [169] functionalized the surface of an impedance biosensor with endothelial cells, and measured the decrease in impedance with LPS binding, with a sensitivity of 500 ng/mL. Veiseh et al. [200] patterned macrophage cells onto gold electrodes to detect LPS concentrations of 0.1–10 μg/mL. However, cells were concurrently stained with necrosis and apoptosis markers in parallel studies, and no staining effect could be seen in cells using concentrations less than 10 μg/mL. This is an interesting effect, as in many *in vitro* studies, cytokine response is induced at much lower concentrations of endotoxin [97, 201, 202]. It can be deduced that Veiseh used serum supplemented media in the experiments, and the lipoproteins and LBP in serum could have a protective effect on cells [46, 202, 203], and attenuated assay sensitivity. The most sensitive cell-based assay was developed by Inoue et al. [170] with a LoD of 0.1–1.0 ng/mL. Here, cells were engineered to secrete alkaline phosphatase in the presence of LPS, and patterned on the surface of an amperometric biosensor to measure voltage change upon LPS binding. Cell-based *in vitro* assays are prone to errors and contamination, so developing a robust and fieldable assay based on this technology is not plausible. However, by studying LPS in cell-based systems, knowledge about interactions with receptors and cell membranes can be gained, which can facilitate better detection methods.

5. Conclusions

Many novel approaches have been used for the detection of amphiphilic LPS, not all of which are functional in physiological matrices or have the required sensitivity or ease of use. One major reason for this is the failure to incorporate the amphiphilic properties of the antigen into assay design. The presentation, conformation, and host-interactions of the antigens should be considered for the development of effective assays. While both LAL and EC assays are the most sensitive for testing endotoxicity, identifying O-ag with a high degree of selectivity remains elusive, and limited to methods that use specific recognition ligands, such as membrane insertion and ELISAs. By far, the greatest limitation has been the lack of sensitive and selective ligands for the serogroup-specific detection of the antigen. Thus, as repositories of these necessary recognition molecules expand to include more serogroups, so too will our ability to selectively detect LPS.

Acknowledgements

This work was supported by the Agriculture and Food Research Initiative Competitive Grant no. 2012-68003-30155 from the United States Department of Agriculture's National Institute of Food and Agriculture.

Author details

Loreen R. Stromberg[1,2,3], Heather M. Mendez[1,2,3] and Harshini Mukundan[1,2,3]*

*Address all correspondence to: harshini@lanl.gov

1 Center for Biomedical Engineering, University of New Mexico, Albuquerque, USA

2 Physical Chemistry and Applied Spectroscopy, Los Alamos National Laboratory, Los Alamos, USA

3 New Mexico Consortium, Los Alamos, USA

References

[1] Love TE, Jones B. Introduction to pathogenic bacteria. Principles of Bacterial Detection: Biosensors, Recognition Receptors and Microsystems. New York, NY: Springer New York; 2008. pp. 3-13

[2] Kumagai Y, Takeuchi O, Akira S. Pathogen recognition by innate receptors. The Journal of Infectious Diseases. 2008;**14**:86-92

[3] Broz P, Monack DM. Newly described pattern recognition receptors team up against intracellular pathogens. Nature Reviews Immunology. 2013;**13**:551-565

[4] Miyake K. Innate recognition of lipopolysaccharide by Toll-like receptor 4-MD-2. Trends in Microbiology. 2004;**12**:186-192

[5] Deisingh AK, Thompson M. Biosensors for the detection of bacteria. Canadian Journal of Microbiology. 2004;**50**:69-77

[6] Kawai T, Akira S. TLR signaling. Seminars in Immunology. 2007;**19**:24-32

[7] Kumar H, Kawai T, Akira S. Pathogen recognition by the innate immune system. International Reviews of Immunology. 2011;**30**:16-34

[8] Sakamuri RM, Price DN, Lee M, Cho SN, Barry CE, Via LE, et al. Association of lipoarabinomannan with high density lipoprotein in blood: Implications for diagnostics. Tuberculosis. 2013;**93**:301-307

[9] Sakamuri RM, Capek P, Dickerson TJ, Barry CE, Mukundan H, Swanson BI. Detection of stealthy small amphiphilic biomarkers. Journal of Microbiological Methods. 2014;**103**: 112-117

[10] Su W, Ding X. Methods of endotoxin detection. Journal of Laboratory Automation. 2015;**20**: 354-364

[11] Alexander C, Rietschel ET. Bacterial lipopolysaccharides and innate immunity. Journal of Endotoxin Research. 2001;**7**:167-202

[12] Jauho ES, Boas U, Wiuff C, Wredstrøm K, Pedersen B, Andresen LO, et al. New technology for regiospecific covalent coupling of polysaccharide antigens in ELISA for serological detection. Journal of Immunological Methods. 2000;**242**:133-143

[13] Munford RS. Sensing Gram-Negative bacterial lipopolysaccharides: A human disease determinant? Infection and Immunity. 2008;**76**:454-465

[14] Schreiber A, Humbert M, Benz A, Dietrich U. 3D-Epitope-Explorer (3DEX): Localization of conformational epitopes within three-dimensional structures of proteins. Journal of Computational Chemistry. 2005;**26**:879-887

[15] Beveridge TJ. Structures of Gram-negative cell walls and their derived membrane vesicles. Journal of Bacteriology. 1999;**181**:4725-4733

[16] Joly-Guillou M-L. Clinical impact and pathogenicity of *Acinetobacter*. Clinical Microbiology and Infection, European Journal of Clinical Microbiology & Infectious Diseases. 2005;**11**:868-873

[17] Wiersinga WJ, van der Poll T, White NJ, Day NP, Peacock SJ. Melioidosis: Insights into the pathogenicity of *Burkholderia pseudomallei*. Nature Reviews Microbiology. 2006;**4**:272-282

[18] Mattoo S, Foreman-Wykert AK, Cotter PA. Mechanisms of *Bordetella* pathogenesis. Frontiers in Bioscience. 2001;**6**:E168–E186

[19] Brooks BW, Devenish J, Lutze-Wallace CL, Milnes D, Robertson, RH, Berlie-Surujballi G. Evaluation of a monoclonal antibody-based enzyme-linked immunosorbent assay for detection of *Campylobacter fetus* in bovine preputial washing and vaginal mucus samples. Veterinary Microbiology. 2004;**103**:77-84

[20] Lazcka O, Del Campo FJ, Muñoz FX. Pathogen detection: A perspective of traditional methods and biosensors. Biosensors & Bioelectronics. 2007;**22**:1205-1217

[21] Ketley JM. Pathogenesis of enteric infection by *Campylobacter*. Microbiology. 1997;**143**:5-21

[22] Lüderitz O, Freudenberg MA, Galanos C, Lehmann V, Rietschel ET, Shaw DH. Lipopolysaccharides of Gram-Negative Bacteria. Current Topics in Membranes and Transport. Elsevier; 1982. pp. 79-151

[23] Belland RJ, Ouellette SP, Gieffers J, Byrne GI. *Chlamydia pneumoniae* and atherosclerosis. Cell Microbiology. 2004;**6**:117-127

[24] Leimbach A, Hacker J, Dobrindt U. *E. coli* as an All-Rounder: The Thin Line Between Commensalism and Pathogenicity. Berlin, Heidelberg: Springer; microbiology and immunology. 2013;**358**:3-32

[25] Moran AP, Lindner B, Walsh EJ. Structural characterization of the lipid A component of *Helicobacter pylori* rough- and smooth-form lipopolysaccharides. Journal of Bacteriology. 1997;**179**:6453-6463

[26] Yamaoka Y, Graham DY. *Helicobacter pylori* virulence and cancer pathogenesis. Future Oncology. 2014;**10**:1487-1500

[27] Livorsi DJ, Macneil JR, Cohn AC, Bareta J, Zansky S, Petit S, et al. Invasive *Haemophilus influenzae* in the United States, 1999-2008: Epidemiology and outcomes. Journal of Infection. Elsevier Ltd. 2012;**65**:496-504

[28] Meatherall BL, Gregson D, Ross T, Pitout JDD, Laupland KB. Incidence, risk factors, and outcomes of *Klebsiella pneumoniae* bacteremia. American Journal of Medicine. 2009;**122**:866-873

[29] Newton HJ, Ang DKY, van Driel IR, Hartland EL. Molecular pathogenesis of infections caused by *Legionella pneumophila*. Clinical Microbiology Reviews. 2010;**23**:274-298

[30] Laura Perez Vidakovics M, Riesbeck K. Virulence mechanisms of *Moraxella* in the pathogenesis of infection. Current Opinion in Infectious Diseases. 2009;**22**:279-285

[31] Stephens DS. Biology and pathogenesis of the evolutionarily successful, obligate human bacterium *Neisseria meningitidis.* Vaccine. 2009;**27**:B71–B77

[32] Mahajan-Miklos S, Tan MW, Rahme LG, Ausubel FM. Molecular mechanisms of bacterial virulence elucidated using a *Pseudomonas aeruginosa-Caenorhabditis elegans* pathogenesis model. Cell. 1999;**96**:47-56

[33] Mobley HL, Belas R. Swarming and pathogenicity of *Proteus mirabilis* in the urinary tract. Trends Microbiology. 1995;**3**:280-284

[34] Mather AE, Reid S, Maskell DJ, Parkhill J, Fookes MC, Harris S, et al. Distinguishable epidemics within different hosts of the multidrug resistant zoonotic pathogen *Salmonella Typhimurium* DT104. Science. 2013;**341**(6153):1514

[35] Caboni M, Pédron T, Rossi O, Goulding D, Pickard D, Citiulo F, et al. An O antigen capsule modulates bacterial pathogenesis in *Shigella sonnei*. Koehler TM, editor. PLoS Pathogens. 2015;**11**:e1004749

[36] Fábrega A, Vila J. *Yersinia enterocolitica*: Pathogenesis, virulence and antimicrobial resistance. Medicina Clinica. SEGO. 2012;**30**:24-32

[37] Bennett IL, Cluff LE. Bacterial pyrogens. Pharmacological Reviews. 1957;**9**:427-475

[38] Westphal O, Westphal U. The history of pyrogen research. Microbiology. 1977;**1977**: 221-238

[39] Beutler B, Rietschel ET. Innate immune sensing and its roots: The story of endotoxin. Nature Reviews Immunology. 2003;**3**:169-176

[40] Olins AL, Warner RC. Physicochemical studies on a lipopolysaccharide from the cell wall of *Azotobacter vinelandii*. Journal of Biological Chemistry. 1967;**242**(21):4994-5001

[41] Schromm AB, Bradenburg K, Loppnow H, Zähringer U, Rietschel ET, Carroll SF, et al. The charge of endotoxin molecules influences their conformation and IL-6-inducing capacity. Journal of Immunology. 1998;**161**:5464-5471

[42] Bishop RE. Fundamentals of endotoxin structure and function. In: Herwald RW, editor. Contributions to Microbiology. Basel: Karger; 2005. pp. 1-27

[43] Meredith TC, Aggarwal P, Mamat U, Lindner B, Woodard RW. Redefining the requisite lipopolysaccharide structure in *Escherichia coli*. ACS Chemical Biology. 2006;**1**:33-42

[44] Raetz CRH, Guan Z, Ingram BO, Six DA, Song F, Wang X, et al. Discovery of new biosynthetic pathways: The lipid A story. Journal of Lipid Research. 2009;**50**(Suppl):S103-S108

[45] Raetz CRH, Whitfield C. Lipopolysaccharide endotoxins. Annual Review of Biochemistry. 2002;**71**:635-700

[46] Hurley JC. Endotoxemia: Methods of detection and clinical correlates. Clinical Microbiology Reviews. 1995;**8**:268-292

[47] Erridge C, Bennett-Guerrero E, Poxton IR. Structure and function of lipopolysaccharides. Microbes and Infection. 2002;**4**:837-851

[48] Aurell CA, Wistrom AO. Critical aggregation concentrations of Gram-negative bacterial lipopolysaccharides (LPS). Biochemical and Biophysical Research Communications. 1998;**253**:119-123

[49] Plested JS, Makepeace K, Jennings MP, Gidney MA, Lacelle S, Brisson J, et al. Conservation and accessibility of an inner core lipopolysaccharide epitope of *Neisseria meningitidis*. Infection and Immunity. 1999;**67**:5417-5426

[50] Silipo A, Molinaro A. The diversity of the core oligosaccharide in lipopolysaccharides. Subcellular Biochemistry. Dordrecht: Springer Netherlands. 2010;**53**:69-99

[51] Nevola JJ, Stocker BA, Laux DC, Cohen PS. Colonization of the mouse intestine by an avirulent *Salmonella typhimurium* strain and its lipopolysaccharide-defective mutants. Infection and Immunity. 1985;**50**:152-159

[52] Murray GL, Attridge SR, Morona R. Regulation of *Salmonella typhimurium* lipopolysaccharide O antigen chain length is required for virulence; identification of FepE as a second Wzz. Molecular Microbiology. 2003;**47**:1395-1406

[53] De Bagüés M, Elzer PH, Jones SM. Vaccination with *Brucella abortus* rough mutant RB51 protects BALB/c mice against virulent strains of *Brucella abortus, Brucella melitensis*, and *Brucella ovis*. Infection and Immunity. 1994;**62**(11):4990-4996

[54] Stenutz R, Weintraub A, Widmalm G. The structures of *Escherichia coli* O-polysaccharide antigens. FEMS Microbiology Reviews. 2006;**30**:382-403

[55] Goldman RC, Leive L. Heterogeneity of antigenic-side-chain length in lipopolysaccharide from *Escherichia coli* 0111 and *Salmonella typhimurium* LT2. European Journal of Biochemistry. 1980;**107**:145-153

[56] Bradenburg K, Schromm AB, Gutsmann T. Endotoxins: Relationship between structure, function, and activity. Structure. Dordrecht: Springer Netherlands. 2004;**53**:53-67

[57] Bergstrand A, Svanberg C, Langton M, Nydén M. Aggregation behavior and size of lipopolysaccharide from *Escherichia coli* O55:B5. Colloids and Surfaces B: Biointerfaces. 2006;**53**:9-14

[58] Santos NC, Silva AC, Castanho MARB, Martins Silva J, Saldanha C. Evaluation of lipopolysaccharide aggregation by light scattering spectroscopy. ChemBioChem. 2003; **4**:96-100

[59] Israelachvili J. Intermolecular and Surface Forces. 2nd ed. London: Academic Press; 1991

[60] Ruckenstein E, Nagarajan R. Critical micelle concentration. Transition point for micellar size distribution. Journal of Physical Chemistry (American Chemical Society). 1975;**79**: 2622-2626

[61] Din ZZ, Mukerjee P, Kastowsky M, Takayama K. Effect of pH on solubility and ionic state of lipopolysaccharide obtained from the deep rough mutant of Escherichia coli. Biochemistry. 1993;**32**:4579-4586

[62] Sasaki H, White SH. Aggregation behavior of an Ultra-Pure lipopolysaccharide that stimulates TLR-4 receptors. Biophysical Journal. 2008;**95**:986-993

[63] Moroi Y. CMC range due to polydispersity of micelles. Journal of Colloid and Interface Science. 1991;**141**:581-583

[64] Krüger D. Assessing the quality of medicinal products containing ingredients obtained by gene technology. Drugs Made in Germany. 1989;**32**(2):64-67

[65] Hirayama C, Sakata M. Chromatographic removal of endotoxin from protein solutions by polymer particles. Journal of Chromatography B Analytical Technologies Biomedical and Life Sciences. 2002;**781**:419-432

[66] Netea MG, van Deuren M, Kullberg BJ, Cavaillon J-M, Van der Meer JWM. Does the shape of lipid A determine the interaction of LPS with Toll-like receptors? Trends in Immunology. 2002;**23**:135-139

[67] Seydel U, Schromm AB, Blunck R, Bradenburg K. Chemical structure, molecular conformation, and bioactivity of endotoxins. Chemical Immunology. 2000;**74**:5-24

[68] Nagarajan R. Molecular packing parameter and surfactant Self-Assembly: The neglected role of the surfactant tail †. Langmuir. 2002;**18**:31-38

[69] Rietschel ET, Brade H, Brade L, Kaca W, Kawahara K, Lindner B, et al. Newer aspects of the chemical structure and biological activity of bacterial endotoxins. Progress in Clinical and Biological Research. 1985;**189**:31-51

[70] Jucker BA, Harms H, Zehnder A. Polymer interactions between five gram-negative bacteria and glass investigated using LPS micelles and vesicles as model systems. Colloids and Surfaces B: Biointerfaces. 1998;**11**:33-45

[71] Petsch D, Anspach FB. Endotoxin removal from protein solutions. Journal of Biotechnology. 2000;**76**:97-119

[72] Mueller M, Lindner B, Kusumoto S, Fukase K, Schromm AB, Seydel U. Aggregates are the biologically active units of endotoxin. Journal of Biological Chemistry. 2004;**279**: 26307-26313

[73] Vasselon T, Hailman E, Thieringer R, Detmers PA. Internalization of monomeric lipopolysaccharide occurs after transfer out of cell surface CD14. Journal of Experimental Medicine. 1999;**190**:509-521

[74] Stromberg LR, Hengartner NW, Swingle KL, Moxley RA, Graves SW, Montaño GA, et al. Membrane insertion for the detection of lipopolysaccharides: Exploring the dynamics of Amphiphile-in-Lipid Assays. Gasset M, editor. PLoS ONE. 2016;**11**:e0156295

[75] James EA, Schmeltzer K, Ligler FS. Detection of endotoxin using an evanescent wave fiber-optic biosensor. Applied Biochemistry and Biotechnology. 1996;**60**:189-202

[76] Kannenberg EL, Perotto S, Bianciotto V, Rathbun EA, Brewin NJ. Lipopolysaccharide epitope expression of Rhizobium bacteroids as revealed by *in situ* immunolabelling of pea root nodule sections. Journal of Bacteriology. 1994;**176**:2021-2032

[77] Haselhorst T, Espinosa J-F, Jiménez-Barbero J, Sokolowski T, Kosma P, Brade H, et al. NMR experiments reveal distinct Antibody-Bound conformations of a synthetic disaccharide representing a general structural element of bacterial lipopolysaccharide epitopes. Biochemistry. 1999;**38**:6449-6459

[78] Hershberger C, Binkley SB. Chemistry and Metabolism of 3-Deoxy-d-mannooctulosonic acid I. Sterochemical determination. Journal of Biological Chemistry. 1968;**243**(7): 1578-1584

[79] Brandenburg K, Andrä J, Müller M, Koch MHJ, Garidel P. Physicochemical properties of bacterial glycopolymers in relation to bioactivity. Carbohydrate Research. 2003;**338**:2477-2489

[80] Aurell CA, Hawley ME, Wistrom AO. Direct visualization of Gram-negative bacterial lipopolysaccharide self-assembly. Molecular Cell Biology Research Communications. 1999;**2**:42-46

[81] Adams PG, Lamoureux L, Swingle KL, Mukundan H, Montaño GA. Lipopolysaccharide-induced dynamic lipid membrane reorganization: Tubules, perforations, and stacks. Biophysical Journal. 2014;**106**:2395-2407

[82] van Alphen L, Verkleij A, Burnell E, Lugtenberg B. 31P nuclear magnetic resonance and freeze-fracture electron microscopy studies on *Escherichia coli*. II. Lipopolysaccharide and lipopolysaccharide-phospholipid complexes. Biochimica et Biophysica Acta (BBA) - Biomembranes. 1980;**597**:502-517

[83] Coughlin RT, Haug A, McGroarty EJ. Physical properties of defined lipopolysaccharide salts. Biochemistry. 1983;**22**:2007-2013

[84] Coughlin RT, Tonsager S, McGroarty EJ. Quantitation of metal cations bound to membranes and extracted lipopolysaccharide of *Escherichia coli*. Biochemistry. 1983;**22**: 2002-2007

[85] Naumann D, Schultz C, Sabisch A, Kastowsky M, Labischinski H. New insights into the phase behaviour of a complex anionic amphiphile: Architecture and dynamics of bacterial deep rough lipopolysaccharide membranes as seen by FTIR, X-ray, and molecular modelling techniques. Journal of Molecular Structure. 1989;**214**:213-246

[86] Schindler M, Osborn MJ. Interaction of divalent cations and polymyxin B with lipopolysaccharide. Biochemistry. 1979;**18**:4425-4430

[87] Kato D, Iijima S, Kurita R, Sato Y, Jia J, Yabuki S, et al. Electrochemically amplified detection for lipopolysaccharide using ferrocenylboronic acid. Biosensors & Bioelectronics. 2007;**22**:1527-1531

[88] McClosky WT, Price CW, Van Winkle W, Welch H, Calvery HO. Results of first U. S. P. Collaborative study of pyrogens. Journal of the American Pharmaceutical Association (Scientific edition). 1943;**32**:69-73

[89] Cooper JF, Levin J, Wagner HN. Quantitative comparison of *in vitro* and *in vivo* methods for the detection of endotoxin. Journal of Laboratory and Clinical Medicine. 1971;**78**:138-148

[90] Roberts KJ. Endotoxins: Pyrogens, LAL testing and depyrogenation. Williams KL, editor. CRC Press, Taylor & Fancis Group LLC; 2007. pp. 261-284

[91] Park C-Y, Jung S-H, Bak J-P, Lee S-S, Rhee D-K. Comparison of the rabbit pyrogen test and Limulus amoebocyte lysate (LAL) assay for endotoxin in hepatitis B vaccines and the effect of aluminum hydroxide. Biologicals. 2005;**33**:145-151

[92] Levin J, Tomasulo PA, Oser RS. Detection of endotoxin in human blood and demonstration of an inhibitor. Journal of Laboratory and Clinical Medicine. 1970;**75**:903-911

[93] Pharmacopeial Convention US. 85> Bacterial Endotoxins Test. 2011. The United States Pharmacopeial Convention (P)\\usp-netapp2\share\SHARE\USPNF\PRINTQ\pager\xmlIn\AO_20111014080832_M98830.xml

[94] U.S. Department of Health and Human Services, U.S. Food and Drug Administration. Guidance for Industry. 21 CFR; Dec 8, 1987 pp. 1-54.

[95] Novitsky TJ, Roslansky PF. Quantification of endotoxin inhibition in serum and plasma using a turbidimetric LAL assay. Progress in Clinical and Biological Research. 1985;**189**:181-196

[96] Levin J, Poore TE, Zauber NP, Zauber NP, Oser RS. Detection of endotoxin in the blood of patients with sepsis due to Gram-negative bacteria. The New England Journal of Medicine. 1970;**283**:1313-1316

[97] Cavaillon JM, Fitting C, Haeffner-Cavaillon N, Kirsch SJ, Warren HS. Cytokine response by monocytes and macrophages to free and lipoprotein-bound lipopolysaccharide. Infection and Immunity. 1990;**58**:2375-2382

[98] Nachum R, Shanbrom E. Rapid detection of Gram-negative bacteriuria by limulus amoebocyte lysate assay. Journal of Clinical Microbiology. 1981;**13**:158-162

[99] Svensson A, Hahn-Hägerdal B. Comparison of a gelation and a chromogenic Limulus (LAL) assay for the detection of Gram-negative bacteria, and the application of the latter assay to milk. Journal of Dairy Research. 1987;**54**:267-273

[100] Jay JM, Margitic S, Shereda AL, Covington HV. Determining endotoxin content of ground beef by the Limulus amoebocyte lysate test as a rapid indicator of microbial quality. Applied and Environmental Microbiology. 1979;**38**:885-890

[101] Jay JM. Rapid estimation of microbial numbers in fresh ground beef by use of the Limulus test. Journal of Food Protection. 1981;**44**:275-278

[102] Goto H, Nakamura S. Dry up method as a revised Limulus test with a new technique for gelatin inhibitor removing. The Japanese Journal of Experimental Medicine. 1979;**49**:19-25

http://dx.doi.org/10.5772/intechopen.68311

[103] Hartman I, Ziv G, Saran A. Application of the Limulus amoebocyte lysate test to the detection of Gram-negative bacterial endotoxins in normal and mastitic milk. Research in Veterinary Science. 1976;**20**:342-343

[104] Reinhold RB, Fine J. A technique for quantitative measurement of endotoxin in human plasma. Proceedings of the Society for Experimental Biology and Medicine. 1971. 334-340

[105] Maxie MG, Valli VE. Studies with radioactive endotoxin. III. Localization of 3H-labelled endotoxin in the formed elements of the blood and detection of endotoxin in calf blood with the Limulus amebocyte lysate. Canadian Journal of Comparative Medicine-Revue Canadienne De Medecine Comparee. 1974;**38**:383-390

[106] Yin ET, Galanos C, Kinsky S, Bradshaw RA, Wessler S, Lüderitz O, et al. Picogram-sensitive assay for endotoxin: Gelation of Limulus polyphemus blood cell lysate induced by purified lipopolysaccharides and lipid A from Gram-negative bacteria. Biochimica et Biophysica Acta. 1972;**261**:284-289

[107] Takagi K, Moriya A, Tamura H, Nakahara C. Quantitative measurement of endotoxin in human blood using synthetic chromogenic substrate for horseshoe crab clotting enzyme: A comparison of methods of blood. Thrombosis Research. 1981;**23**:51-57

[108] Niwa M, Hiramatsu T, Waguri O. Proceedings: Quantitative aspects of the gelation reaction of horseshoe crab amoebocyte and bacterial endotoxin. Symp. Toxins. jpn j of medical sci biology. 1974;**28**:98-100

[109] Tsuji K, Martin PA, Gaunnac GL. Recovery of endotoxin from human plasma by acid oxidative treatmtnets as monitored by an automated microtiter plate-chromogenic substrate limulus amebocyte lysate (LAL) assay method. Progress in Clinical and Biological Research. 1986;**231**: 443-457

[110] Karibian D, Deprun C, Caroff M. Comparison of lipids A of several *Salmonella* and *Escherichia* strains by 252Cf plasma desorption mass spectrometry. Journal of Bacteriology. 1993;**175**: 2988-2993

[111] Schletter J, Heine H, Ulmer AJ, Rietschel ET. Molecular mechanisms of endotoxin activity. Archives of Microbiology. 1995;**164**:383-389

[112] Engvall E, Perlmann P. Enzyme-linked immunosorbent assay, ELISA III: Quantitation of specific antibodies by enzyme-labeled anti-immunoglobulin in antigen-coated tubes. Journal of Immunology. 1972;**109**:129-135

[113] Van Weemen BK, Schuurs AHWM. Immunoassay using antigen-enzyme conjugates. FEBS Letters. 1971;**15**:232-236

[114] Carlsson HE, Lindberg AA, Hammarström S. Titration of antibodies to *Salmonella* O antigens by enzyme-linked immunosorbent assay. Infection and Immunity. 1972;**6**:703-708

[115] Nielsen B, Baggesen D, Bager F, Haugegaard J, Lind P. The serological response to *Salmonella* serovars typhimurium and infantis in experimentally infected pigs. The time course followed with an indirect anti-LPS ELISA and bacteriological examinations. Veterinary Microbiology. 1995;**47**: 205-218

[116] Nalepka JL, Greenfield EM. Detection of bacterial endotoxin in human tissues. Biotech niques. 2004;**37**:413-417

[117] Reither K, Saathoff E, Jung J, Minja LT, Kroidl I, Saad E, et al. Low sensitivity of a urine LAM-ELISA in the diagnosis of pulmonary tuberculosis. BMC Infectious Diseases. 2009;**9**:141

[118] Takahashi K, Fukada M, Kawai M, Yokochi T. Detection of lipopolysaccharide (LPS) and identification of its serotype by an enzyme-linked immunosorbent assay (ELISA) using poly-l-lysine. Journal of Immunological Methods. 1992;**153**:67-71

[119] Scott BB, Barclay GR. Endotoxin-polymyxin complexes in an improved enzyme-linked immunosorbent assay for IgG antibodies in blood donor sera to Gram-Negative endotoxin core glycolipids. Vox Sanguinis. 1987;**52**:272-280

[120] Sternberger LA. The unlabeled antibody (PAP) method. Journal of Histochemistry & Cytochemistry. 1979;**27**:1657-1657

[121] Hsu SM, Raine L, Fanger H. The use of antiavidin antibody and avidin-biotin-peroxidase complex in immunoperoxidase technics. American Journal of Clinical Pathology. 1981;**75**:816-821

[122] Mackenzie A, Lebel P, Orrbine E, Rowe PC, Hyde L, Chan F, et al. Sensitivities and Specificities of premier *E. coli* O157 and premier EHEC enzyme immunoassays for diagnosis of infection with verotoxin (Shiga-Like Toxin)-producing *Escherichia coli*. Journal of Clinical Microbiology. 1998;**36**:1608-1611

[123] Vreugdenhil AC, Snoek AM, van 't Veer C, Greve JW, Buurman WA. LPS-binding protein circulates in association with apoB-containing lipoproteins and enhances endotoxin-LDL/VLDL interaction. Journal of Clinical Investigation. 2001;**107**:225-234

[124] Vreugdenhil A, Rousseau CH. Lipopolysaccharide (LPS)-binding protein mediates LPS detoxification by chylomicrons. Journal of Immunology. 2003;**170**:1399-1405

[125] Kerr P, Chart H, Finlay D, Pollock DA, MacKie DP, Ball HJ. Development of a monoclonal sandwich ELISA for the detection of animal and human *Escherichia coli* O157 strains. Journal of Applied Microbiology. 2001;**90**:543-549

[126] Choi D, Tsang RS, Ng MH. Sandwich capture ELISA by a murine monoclonal antibody against a genus-specific LPS epitope for the detection of different common serotypes of salmonellas. Journal of Applied Bacteriology. 1992;**72**:134-138

[127] Schütz M, Meyer R, Grallert H, Miller S. Method for Detecting and for Removing Endotoxin [Internet]. 2010. US Patent Office; US20090017445 A1

[128] Schütz M, Meyer R, Grallert H, Miller S. Method for identifying and for extracting endotoxin. 2009. US Patent Office; 7,585,620

[129] Grallert H, Leopoldseder S, Schuett M, Kurze P, Buchberger B. EndoLISA®: A novel and reliable method for endotoxin detection. Nature Reviews Immunology. Nature Publishing Group. 2011:**8**:iii-v

[130] Alberts B. Molecular Biology of the Cell. 5th ed. Garland Science; 2008. pp. 1539-1557

[131] Hyams KC, Malone JD, Bourgeois AL, Hawkins R, Hale TL, Murphy JR. Serum antibody to lipopolysaccharide antigens of *Shigella* species among U.S. military personnel deployed to Saudi Arabia and Kuwait during Operations Desert Shield and Desert Storm. Clinical and Diagnostic Laboratory Immunology. 1995;**2**:700-703

[132] Blatz R, Aseffa A, Gedefaw M, Rühle HJ, Forberg J, Christian AR. Prevalence of Chlamydia specific antibodies among obstetric and gynecological outpatients in Gondar, North-west Ethiopia. Ethiopia Medical Journal. 2001;**39**:293-303

[133] House D, Wain J, Ho VA, Diep TS, Chinh NT, Bay PV, et al. Serology of typhoid fever in an area of endemicity and its relevance to diagnosis. Journal of Clinical Microbiology. 2001;**39**:1002-1007

[134] Chaicumpa W, Ngren-ngarmlert W, Kalambaheti T, Ruangkunaporn Y, Chongsa-Nguan M, Tapchaisri P, et al. Monoclonal antibody-based dot-blot ELISA for the detection of *Salmonella* in foods. Asian Pacific Journal of Allergy and Immunology. 1995;**13**:159-166

[135] Freudenberg MA, Fomsgaard A, Mitov I, Galanos C. ELISA for antibodies to lipid A, lipopolysaccharides and other hydrophobic antigens. Infection. 1989;**17**:322-328

[136] Suthienkul O, Poomchart A, Kositanont U, Siripanichgon K, Vathanophas K. ELISA for seroepidemiological study of exposure to *Vibrio cholerae* of population in Krabi Province, Thailand. Asian Pacific Journal of Allergy and Immunology. 1992;**10**:55-60

[137] Chaicumpa W, Ruangkunaporn Y, Burr D, Chongsa-Nguan M, Echeverria P. Diagnosis of typhoid fever by detection of *S typhi* antigen in urine Journal of Clinical Microbiology. 1992;**30**:2513-2515

[138] Covinsky M, Laterza O, Pfeifer JD, Farkas-Szallasi T, Scott MG. An IgM lambda antibody to *Escherichia coli* produces false-positive results in multiple immunometric assays. Clinical Chemistry. 2000;**46**:1157-1161

[139] Ben-Hur H, Gurevich P, Elhayany A, Avinoach I, Schneider D, Zusman I. Transport of maternal immunoglobulins through the human placental barrier in normal pregnancy and during inflammation. International Journal of Molecular Medicine. 2005;**16**:401-407

[140] Morrison DC, Jacobs DM. Binding of polymyxin B to the lipid A portion of bacterial lipopolysaccharides. Immunochemistry. 1976;**13**:813-818

[141] Mattsby-Baltzer I, Jakobsson A, Sörbo J. Endotoxin is angiogenic. International Journal of Experimental Pathology. 1994;**75**:191-196

[142] Hardy E, Ohlin M, Llano M. Enhanced ELISA sensitivity using TCA for efficient coating of biologically active lipopolysaccharides or lipid A to the solid phase. Journal of Immunological Methods. 1994;**176**:111-116

[143] Weintraub A, Widmalm G, Jansson PE, Jansson M. Vibrio cholerae O139 Bengal possesses a capsular polysaccharide which may confer increased virulence. Microbial Pathogenesis. 1994;**16**:235-241

[144] Stromberg LR, Stromberg ZR, Banisadr A, Graves SW, Moxley RA, Mukundan H. Purification and characterization of lipopolysaccharides from six strains of non-O157 Shiga toxin-producing *Escherichia coli*. Journal of Microbiological Methods. 2015;**116**:1-7

[145] Brooks BW, Lutze-wallace CL, Blais B, Gauthier M, Deschênes M. Monoclonal antibodies to lipopolysaccharide O antigens of enterohemorrhagic *Escherichia coli* strains in serogroups O26, O45, O103, O111, O121, and O145. Journal of Food Protection. 2015;**78**: 1252-1258

[146] Westerman RB, He Y, Keen JE, Littledike ET, Kwang J. Production and characterization of monoclonal antibodies specific for the lipopolysaccharide of *Escherichia coli* O157. Journal of Clinical Microbiology. 1997;**35**:679-684

[147] Coughlin RT, Bogard WC. Immunoprotective murine monoclonal antibodies specific for the outer-core polysaccharide and for the O-antigen of *Escherichia coli* 0111: B4 lipopolysaccharide (LPS). Journal of Immunology. 1987;**139**(2):557-561

[148] Rivera-Betancourt M, Keen JE. Murine monoclonal antibodies against *Escherichia coli* O4 lipopolysaccharide and H5 flagellin. Journal of Clinical Microbiology. 2001;**39**:3409-3413

[149] Mutharia LM, Crockford G, Bogard WC, Hancock RE. Monoclonal antibodies specific for *Escherichia coli* J5 lipopolysaccharide: Cross-reaction with other Gram-negative bacterial species. Infection and Immunity. 1984;**45**:631-636

[150] Bogard WCW, Dunn DLD, Abernethy KK, Kilgarriff CC, Kung PCP. Isolation and characterization of murine monoclonal antibodies specific for gram-negative bacterial lipopolysaccharide: Association of cross-genus reactivity with lipid A specificity. Infection and Immunity. 1987;**55**:899-908

[151] de Jongh-Leuvenink J, Vreede RW, Marcelis JH, de Vos M, Verhoef J. Detection of antibodies against lipopolysaccharides of *Escherichia coli* and *Salmonella* R and S strains by immunoblotting. Infection and Immunity. 1985;**50**:716-720

[152] Gibb AP, Barclay GR, Poxton IR, di Padova F. Frequencies of lipopolysaccharide core types among clinical isolates of *Escherichia coli* defined with monoclonal antibodies. Journal of Infectious Diseases. 1992;**166**:1051-1057

[153] Porat YB, Zan-Bar I, Ravid A. Quantitative dot-blot assay for low titer anti-lipopolysaccharide antibodies in human plasma. Journal of Immunological Methods. 1995;**180**:213-218

[154] Evans ME, Pollack M, Hardegen NJ, Koles NL, Guelde G, Chia JK. Fluorescence-activated cell sorter analysis of binding by lipopolysaccharide-specific monoclonal antibodies to Gram-negative bacteria. Journal of Infectious Diseases. 1990;**162**:148-155

[155] Evans ME, Pollack M, Koles NL, Hardegen NJ, Panopoulos D. Lipopolysaccharide heterogeneity in *Escherichia coli* J5 variants: Analysis by flow cytometry. Journal of Infectious Diseases. 1992;**166**:803-811

[156] Nelson D. Flow cytometry in bacteriology. Reviews in Medical Microbiology. 1993;**4**: 215-221

[157] Péterfi Z, Kocsis B. Comparison of blocking agents for an elisa for Lps. Journal of Immunoassay. 2000;**21**:341-354

[158] Gorbet MB, Sefton MV. Endotoxin: The uninvited guest Biomaterials. 2005;**26**:6811-6817

[159] Kim S-E, Su W, Cho M, Lee Y, Choe W-S. Harnessing aptamers for electrochemical detection of endotoxin. Analytical Biochemistry. Elsevier Inc. 2012;**424**:12-20

[160] Su W, Lin M, Lee H, Cho M, Choe W-S, Lee Y. Determination of endotoxin through an aptamer-based impedance biosensor. Biosensors & Bioelectronics. Elsevier B.V. 2012;**32**:32-36

[161] Cho M, Chun L, Lin M, Choe W, Nam J, Lee Y. Sensitive electrochemical sensor for detection of lipopolysaccharide on metal complex immobilized gold electrode. Sensors and Actuators B: Chemical. Elsevier B.V. 2012;**174**:490-494

[162] Ding SJ, Chang BW, Wu CC, Chen CJ. A new method for detection of endotoxin on polymyxin B-immobilized gold electrodes. Electrochemistry Communications. 2007;**9**: 1206-1211

[163] Zuo M-Y, Chen L-J, Jiang H, Tan L, Luo Z-F, Wang Y-M. Detecting endotoxin with a flow cytometry-based magnetic aptasensor. Analytical Biochemistry. 2014;**466**:38-43

[164] Lan M, Wu J, Liu W, Zhang W, Ge J, Zhang H, et al. Copolythiophene-derived colorimetric and fluorometric sensor for visually supersensitive determination of lipopolysaccharide. Journal of the American Chemical Society. 2012;**134**:6685-6694

[165] Mohammed AH, McCallus DE, Norcross NL. Development and evaluation of an enzyme-linked immunosorbent assay for endotoxin in milk. Veterinary Microbiology. 1988;**18**:27-39

[166] DeMarco DR, Lim DV. Detection of *Escherichia coli* O157: H7 in 10-and 25-gram ground beef samples with an evanescent-wave biosensor with silica and polystyrene waveguides. Journal of Food Protection. 2002;**65**:596-602

[167] Lamoureux L, Adams P, Banisadr A. An optical biosensor for detection of pathogen biomarkers from Shiga toxin-producing *Escherichia coli* in ground beef samples. Proceedings of SPIE. 2015; 931004

[168] Mukundan H, Price DN, Goertz M, Parthasarathi R, Montaño GA, Kumar S, et al. Understanding the interaction of Lipoarabinomannan with membrane mimetic architectures. Tuberculosis. Elsevier Ltd; 2012;**92**:38-47

[169] Bouafsoun A, Othmane A, Jaffrezic-Renault N. Impedance endothelial cell biosensor for lipopolysaccharide detection. Materials Science and Engineering: C. 2008;**28**:653-661

[170] Inoue KY, Yasukawa T, Shiku H, Matsue T. Cell-based electrochemical assay for endotoxin using a secreted alkaline phosphatase reporter system. Electrochemistry. 2008;**76**:525-528

[171] Unger RE, Peters K, Sartoris A, Freese C, Kirkpatrick CJ. Human endothelial cell-based assay for endotoxin as sensitive as the conventional Limulus Amebocyte Lysate assay. Biomaterials. 2014;**35**:3180-3187

[172] Rahman MSA, Mukhopadhyay SC, Yu P-L, Goicoechea J, Matias IR, Gooneratne CP, et al. Detection of bacterial endotoxin in food: New planar interdigital sensors based approach. Journal of Food Engineering. Elsevier Ltd. 2013;**114**:346-360

[173] Ganesh V, Bodewits K, Bartholdson SJ, Natale D, Campopiano DJ, Mareque-Rivas JC. Effective binding and sensing of lipopolysaccharide: Combining complementary pattern recognition receptors. Angewandte Chemie International Edition. 2009;**48**:356-360

[174] Beveridge TJ, Koval SF. Binding of metals to cell envelopes of *Escherichia coli* K-12. Applied and Environmental Microbiology. 1981;**42**(2):325-335

[175] Langley S, Beveridge TJ. Effect of O-side-chain-lipopolysaccharide chemistry on metal binding. Applied and Environmental Microbiology. 1999;**65**:489-498

[176] Burkhardt M, LopezAcosta A, Reiter K, Lopez V, Lees A. Purification of soluble CD14 fusion proteins and use in an electrochemiluminescent assay for lipopolysaccharide binding. Protein Expression and Purification. 2007;**51**:96-101

[177] Wurfel MM, Wright SD. Lipopolysaccharide-binding protein and soluble CD14 transfer lipopolysaccharide to phospholipid bilayers: Preferential interaction with particular classes of lipid. Journal of Immunology. 1997;**158**:3925-3934

[178] Fitzgerald KA, Rowe DC, Golenbock DT. Endotoxin recognition and signal transduction by the TLR4/MD2-complex. Microbes and Infection. 2004;**6**:1361-1367

[179] Yu B, Hailman E, Wright SD. Lipopolysaccharide binding protein and soluble CD14 catalyze exchange of phospholipids. Journal of Clinical Investigation. 1997;**99**:315-324

[180] Yeo TY, Choi JS, Lee BK, Kim BS, Yoon HI, Lee HY, et al. Electrochemical endotoxin sensors based on TLR4/MD-2 complexes immobilized on gold electrodes. Biosensors & Bioelectronics. Elsevier B.V. 2011;**28**:139-145

[181] Limbut W, Hedström M, Thavarungkul P, Kanatharana P, Mattiasson B. Capacitive biosensor for detection of endotoxin. Analytical and Bioanalytical Chemistry. 2007;**389**: 517-525

[182] Anderson AS, Dattelbaum AM, Montaño GA, Price DN, Schmidt JG, Martinez JS, et al. Functional PEG-modified thin films for biological detection. Langmuir. 2008;**24**: 2240-2247

[183] Kwon SJ, Kim E, Yang H, Kwak J. An electrochemical immunosensor using ferrocenyl-tethered dendrimer. Analyst. 2006;**131**:402-406

[184] Senaratne W, Andruzzi L, Ober CK. Self-Assembled monolayers and polymer brushes in biotechnology: Current applications and future perspectives. Biomacromolecules. 2005;**6**:2427-2448

[185] Oliveira MDL, Andrade CAS, Correia MTS, Coelho LCBE, Singh PR, Zeng X. Impedimetric biosensor based on self-assembled hybrid cystein-gold nanoparticles and CramoLL lectin for bacterial lipopolysaccharide recognition. Journal of Colloid and Interface Science. 2011;**362**:194-201

[186] Su W, Kim SE, Cho M, Nam JD, Choe WS, Lee Y. Selective detection of endotoxin using an impedance aptasensor with electrochemically deposited gold nanoparticles. Innate Immunity. 2013;**19**:388-397

[187] Su W, Cho M, Nam J-D, Choe W-S, Lee Y. Aptamer-Assisted gold Nanoparticles/PEDOT platform for ultrasensitive detection of LPS. Electroanalysis. 2013;**25**:380-386

[188] Bai L, Chai Y, Pu X, Yuan R. A signal-on electrochemical aptasensor for ultrasensitive detection of endotoxin using three-way DNA junction-aided enzymatic recycling and graphene nanohybrid for amplification. Nanoscale. 2014;**6**:2902-2908

[189] Zuzuarregui A, Souto D, Pérez-Lorenzo E, Arizti F, Sánchez-Gómez S, Martínez de Tejada G, et al. Novel integrated and portable endotoxin detection system based on an electrochemical biosensor. Analyst. 2015;**140**:654-660

[190] Wu J, Zawistowski A, Ehrmann M, Yi T, Schmuck C. Peptide functionalized polydiacetylene liposomes act as a fluorescent Turn-On sensor for bacterial lipopolysaccharide. Journal of the American Chemical Society. 2011;**133**:9720-9723

[191] Rangin M, Basu A. Lipopolysaccharide identification with functionalized polydiacetylene liposome sensors. Journal of the American Chemical Society. 2004;**126**:5038-5039

[192] Johnson BJ, Delehanty JB, Lin B, Ligler FS. Immobilized proanthocyanidins for the capture of bacterial lipopolysaccharides. Analytical Chemistry. 2008;**80**:2113-2117

[193] Zeng L, Wu J, Dai Q, Liu W, Wang P, Lee C-S. Sensing of bacterial endotoxin in aqueous solution by supramolecular assembly of pyrene derivative. Organic Letters. 2010;**12**:4014-4017

[194] Voss S, Fischer R, Jung G, Wiesmüller K-H, Brock R. A fluorescence-based synthetic LPS sensor. Journal of the American Chemical Society. 2007;**129**:554-561

[195] Lim SK, Chen P, Lee FL, Moochhala S, Liedberg B. Peptide-assembled graphene oxide as a fluorescent turn-on sensor for lipopolysaccharide (endotoxin) detection. Analytical Chemistry. 2015;**87**:9408-9412

[196] Thompson M, Blaszykowski C, Sheikh S, Romaschin A. A true theranostic approach to medicine: Towards tandem sensor detection and removal of endotoxin in blood. Biosensors & Bioelectronics. 2015;**67**:3-10

[197] Harmon P, Cabral-Lilly D, Reed RA, Maurio FP, Franklin JC, Janoff A. The release and detection of endotoxin from liposomes. Analytical Biochemistry. 1997;**250**:139-146

[198] Stromberg LR. Differential interactions of lipopolysaccharides with lipid bilayers: Applications for pathogen detection. [Doctoral Dissertation]. 2016. 1-296

[199] Sakamuri RM, Wolfenden MS, Anderson AS, Swanson BI, Schmidt JS, Mukundan H. Novel optical strategies for biodetection. Proceedings of SPIE. 2013. 881209

[200] Veiseh M, Veiseh O, Martin MC, Bertozzi C, Zhang M. Single-cell-based sensors and synchrotron FTIR spectroscopy: A hybrid system towards bacterial detection. Biosensors & Bioelectronics. 2007;**23**:253-260

[201] Shanmugam A, Rajoria S, George AL, Mittelman A, Suriano R, Tiwari RK. Synthetic Toll like receptor-4 (TLR-4) agonist peptides as a novel class of adjuvants. PLoS ONE. 2012;**7**:e30839

[202] Lamping N, Dettmer R, Schröder NW, Pfeil D, Hallatschek W, Burger R, et al. LPS-binding protein protects mice from septic shock caused by LPS or Gram-negative bacteria. Journal of Clinical Investigation. 1998;**101**:2065-2071

[203] Chien JY, Jerng JS, Yu CJ, Yang PC. Low serum level of high-density lipoprotein cholesterol is a poor prognostic factor for severe sepsis. Critical Care Medicine. 2005;**33**:1688-1693

[204] Cooperstock MS, Tucker RP, Baublis JV. Possible pathogenic role of endotoxin in Reye's syndrome. The Lancet. 1975;**1**:1272-1274

[205] Jay JM. Limulus lysate endotoxin assay as a test of microbial quality of ground Beef. Journal of Applied Bacteriology. 1977;**43**:99-109

[206] Kimura H. Measurement of endotoxin. II. Comparison of reactivities measured by radioimmunoassay and with the Limulus test. Acta Medica Okayama. 1976;**30**:257-270

[207] Ong KG, Leland JM, Zeng K, Barrett G, Zourob M, Grimes CA. A rapid highly-sensitive endotoxin detection system. Biosensors & Bioelectronics. 2006;**21**:2270-2274

[208] da Silva JSL, Oliveira MDL, de Melo CP, Andrade CAS. Impedimetric sensor of bacterial toxins based on mixed (Concanavalin A)/polyaniline films. Colloids and Surfaces B: Biointerfaces. 2014;**117**:549-554

Chapter 9

Effect of Environmental Conditions on *Escherichia coli* Survival in Seawater

Slaven Jozić and Mladen Šolić

Additional information is available at the end of the chapter

http://dx.doi.org/10.5772/67912

Abstract

We investigated separate and simultaneous effect of temperature, salinity and solar radiation, as well as bacterial strain and origin on *Escherichia coli* (*E. coli*) survival in seawater in experimental conditions. The experiments were carried out by placing the bottles filled with seawater of different salinity (15.0, 30.0 and 36.5 psu) and contaminated by bacterial cultures in three light-protected air incubators set to different temperatures (6, 12, 18 and 24°C), or by placing the bottles in plastic containers filled with water of controlled temperature and exposing them to direct solar light. In experiments in the dark, two typed and two wild *E. coli* strains were tested. The mean T_{90} values were 33.55 h for *E. coli* ATCC 8739, 42.50 h for *E. coli* ATCC 35218, 72.8 h for *E. coli* originating from seagull feces and 278.6 h for *E. coli* originating from sewage, indicating differences between survival abilities among strains. The effect of temperature on T_{90} was significant only in seagull *E. coli* at 36.5 psu and sewage *E. coli* at 30.0 psu and was positive. The effect of salinity was significant only in seagull strain and also was positive. No interactive effect of temperature and salinity was recorded. Experiments in the presence of solar radiation, carried out with two ATCC *E. coli* strains, demonstrated its dominate harmful effect on bacterial cells, reducing T_{90} of both strains to 0.30–0.82 h for *E. coli* ATCC 35218 and 0.31–5.93 h for *E. coli* ATCC 8739. Within the ultraviolet A (UVA) and photosynthetically active radiation (PAR) spectrum of solar radiation, the wavelengths of 320–360 nm were found as most bactericidal. By comparing survival of cultivated *E. coli* cells to those in natural seawater samples, significantly higher survival *E. coli* cells in natural seawater samples was found.

Keywords: *Escherichia coli*, bacterial strain, survival, temperature, salinity, solar radiation

1. Introduction

Fecal pollution of seawater can present a serious problem due to potentially introducing of intestinal pathogens—bacterial, viral, and parasitic. Because of a wide variety of pathogenic microorganisms that can enter the sea, time-consuming and complex procedures of their determination, the assessment of microbiological quality of seawater has traditionally been based on the determination of indicator microorganisms, bacteria that suggest the presence of pathogens [1]. In the last decade, European Union member states have accepted *Escherichia coli* as the indicator for assessment of microbiological quality of bathing and shellfish waters [2, 3]. Apart from its human and warm-blooded animal feces origin, selection of *E. coli* as indicator organisms is based on scientific understanding and reliable research of one of the most important criteria which good indicator have to meet: resistance to environmental conditions.

When released into the sea, *E. coli* cells are exposed to the impact of a very hostile environment. That impact is reflected in the negative effect of the complex array of biotic and abiotic factors of the marine environment. Among abiotic factors, the effect of temperature, salinity, and particularly solar radiation is most pronounced [4–7]. The distribution and abundance of indicator bacteria in seawater depend mostly on their input, but also on the intensity of aforementioned environmental factors [8] and bacterial cell adaptation capacity. Due to their minor adaptation capacity to marine conditions, *E. coli* cells suffer a sublethal injury and enter a dormant, viable but nonculturable state, in which they can still maintain some metabolic activity [9–11], infective capacity and potential for pathogenicity [12, 13]. The "viable but non-culturable" state concept was introduced to describe cells that remain metabolically active but are unable to divide in or on nutritional media that normally support their growth. The capacity to form colonies on a solid medium is the first ability that enteric bacteria lose in seawater [14]. That means that they cannot be detected during standard routine monitoring by culturing method unless resuscitation methods on liquid media were used. With the prolonged exposure, particularly in the presence of solar radiation, *E. coli* cells are irreversibly inactivated and they die [15]. For how long they will maintain culturability on standard media depends on many factors, such as the intensity of environmental factors and the characteristics of the bacterial cell, where besides the origin and previous growth history, the bacterial strain plays an important role [7, 16, 17]. Although there are many studies in which the effects of the aforementioned factors have been addressed, their simultaneous effects have been poorly investigated. In this chapter, the separate and combined effect of temperature, salinity and solar radiation, as well as the growth history, strain and origin of *E. coli* cells on their survival in seawater were presented. Since microbial pollution of bathing waters is routinely monitored by culturing methods on standard solid media, and viable but nonculturable cells usually cannot be detected, for the purposes of this chapter, the term "survive" means to maintain culturability.

2. Materials and methods

2.1. Experiments with pure bacterial cultures

Bacterial cultures used in experiments were always freshly prepared by incubation of pure culture on mineral-modified glutamate broth (MMGB). Bacterial suspensions were taken in the exponential phase of growth and serially diluted in phosphate buffer solution. After

http://dx.doi.org/10.5772/67912

determination of the concentration of *E. coli* cells by epifluorescence microscopy method, appropriate dilution, cca 10^3 CFU/mL, was kept at 4°C until the beginning of the experiments (cca 20 h).

Experiments in the dark were performed in two sets. In the first set, experiments were carried out at six different experimental conditions corresponding to Adriatic sea natural range of temperatures (12°C—mean winter temperature, 18°C—mean spring and autumn temperature and 24°C—mean summer temperature) and salinities (30.0 psu—lower salinity corresponding to areas near the mouth of rivers or sewage outfalls and 36.5 psu—typical salinity in coastal seawater). Two different *E. coli* strains were used: *E. coli* ATCC 35218 originating from canine feces and *E. coli* ATCC 8739, originating from human feces. Bacterial suspension was added to 500 mL borosilicate glass bottles containing autoclaved seawater of appropriate salinity (30.0 and 36.5 psu). Bacterial concentration in bottles was targeted to 10^3 CFU *E. coli*/100 mL. The bottles were then stirred and placed in a temperature controlled air incubators at three different temperatures (12, 18 and 24°C).

In the second set, additional experiments were performed at lower temperature (6°C) and lower salinity (15 psu). Two new bacterial strains were also introduced—wild *E. coli* strain isolated from sewage and wild *E. coli* strain isolated from seagull feces.

Experiments in the presence of solar radiation were performed with two ATCC *E. coli* strains, also combining the same temperatures (12, 18 and 24°C) and salinities (30.0 and 36.5 psu). Bacterial suspension was added to 500 mL ultraviolet B (UVB)—blocking borosilicate glass bottles containing autoclaved seawater of appropriate salinity. Bacterial concentration in bottles was also targeted to 10^3 CFU *E. coli*/100 mL. The bottles were then stirred and left in dark for 15 min to homogenize. Bacterial cells in bottles were then exposed to different intensities of the natural range and spectrum of solar radiation. The exposure to solar light was carried out in two ways: by placing the bottles in 50 L (60 × 30 × 30 cm) transparent plastic containers, filled with water of appropriate and controlled temperature, and placed on the open space in front of the laboratory;—by hanging the bottles from research vessel, vertically on rope to different depths (0.2, 5, 15 and 30 m) of the water column, to expose them to different intensities of solar light (for *E. coli* ATCC 8739 only). In both cases, the irradiance, Ed ($\mu Wcm^{-2}nm^{-1}$), of ultraviolet A (UVA) and photosynthetically active radiation (PAR) was measured by optical radiometer PRR800 (Biospherical Inc.).

All experiments were performed in triplicates. The initial concentrations of culturable *E. coli* cells in all experiments were determined by taking 10 mL subsamples 15 min after adding bacterial suspension. After exposing the bottles to desired conditions, the concentrations of *E. coli* were monitored by taking 10 mL subsamples every 24 h in experiments performed in the dark and every 10 or 20 min in experiments performed in solar light.

2.2. Experiments with natural samples

Natural samples of moderately polluted seawater were collected near sewage outfalls and were stored at 4°C. Sampling was performed in the morning (9 o'clock AM) and at noon. The number of culturable *E. coli* was determined after sampling and every 24 h until their reduction to zero. After isolation and counting on selective agar plates, one colony of *E. coli* cells that survived T_{90} (the time required to reduce culturability by 90%) or longest was randomly selected from each plate of samples collected in the morning. Cultures were incubated on MMGB and processed in the same way as pure cultures of ATCC strains. A bacterial suspension was added to 500 mL borosilicate bottles, containing autoclaved, 36.5 psu seawater, and stored in dark at 4°C. The number of culturable *E. coli* was determined every 24 h until their reduction to zero.

2.3. *E. coli* determination

The concentration of *E. coli* in suspensions was determined by the direct method of epifluorescence microscopy [18]. The number of culturable *E. coli* cells in suspension and seawater was determined by the modified ISO/TS 16649-1 method [19] using membrane filtration technique and expressed as CFU *E. coli*/100 mL.

2.4. Statistical analysis

Data were processed using statistical package Statistica 8.0 (StatSoft Inc., 2007). High and significant ($R^2 > 0.9$, $p < 0.01$) fittings of raw die-off data of *E. coli* to exponential function, which can be expressed by Eq. (1), were found in the dark as well as in the presence of solar radiation. Consequently, T_{90} was derived from Eq. (1) and was calculated by Eq. (2),

$$N_t = N_0 e^{kt} \tag{1}$$

$$T_{90} = \frac{-\ln(0.1)}{k} \tag{2}$$

where N_0 and N_t are the number of culturable *E. coli* at the beginning of the experiment and at the time of subsampling (t).

The inactivation energy S_{90} (the insolation required to reduce culturability by 90%) was calculated by Eq. (3),

$$S_{90}(\mathrm{Whm^{-2}}) = \sum_{n=0}^{T_{90}} E_n T_n \tag{3}$$

where E_n ($\mathrm{Wm^{-2}}$) = the intensity of solar radiation.

3. Results and discussion

3.1. Experiments in the absence of solar radiation

In the natural range of temperature and salinity, the T_{90} values in this study were 31.9–51.7 h (mean 42.5 h) for *E. coli* ATCC 35218 and 29.4–37.9 h (mean 33.55 h) for *E. coli* ATCC 8739 (**Figure 1**). The results were mostly consistent with the results of previous studies. The T_{90} values of *E. coli* reported in earlier studies were from 26 h, which was found in estuarine water at 20°C [20], to 115 h, which was found for fecal coliforms in seawater at 8–10°C [5].

The results of two-way ANOVA revealed that there were no statistically significant ($p > 0.05$) separate and/or interactive effects of the variations in temperature and salinity in their natural range, on changes in T_{90} values of ATCC *E. coli* strains. Unlike the T_{90} values, these results were not consistent with those of previous studies. In general, most studies showed enhanced stability of indicator bacteria at lower temperatures [4, 5], although Anderson et al. [21] found a lower stability and negative effect. The increased inactivation of indicator microorganisms at higher temperatures was mostly attributed to increased metabolic activities in terms of reduced nutrient concentration [22], increasing predation, grazing and the deleterious effect of solar radiation [23]. One of the possible explanations for the absence of clear effect of temperature in our experiments might be the absence of grazing and predation, since seawater was sterilized by autoclaving. Anderson et al. [21] attributed a positive effect of temperature in their study mostly to sublethal stress that was induced by laboratory manipulation and related to the pre-exposure history of the used isolates. In our additional experiments with *E. coli* ATCC 8739 at 6°C, significantly higher T_{90} values were recorded (**Figure 1**), indicating more significant negative effect of temperature in its natural range than at lower values. A positive effect of temperature in whole measured range was observed in seagull *E. coli* at 36.5 psu and sewage *E. coli* at 30.0 psu (**Figure 2**).

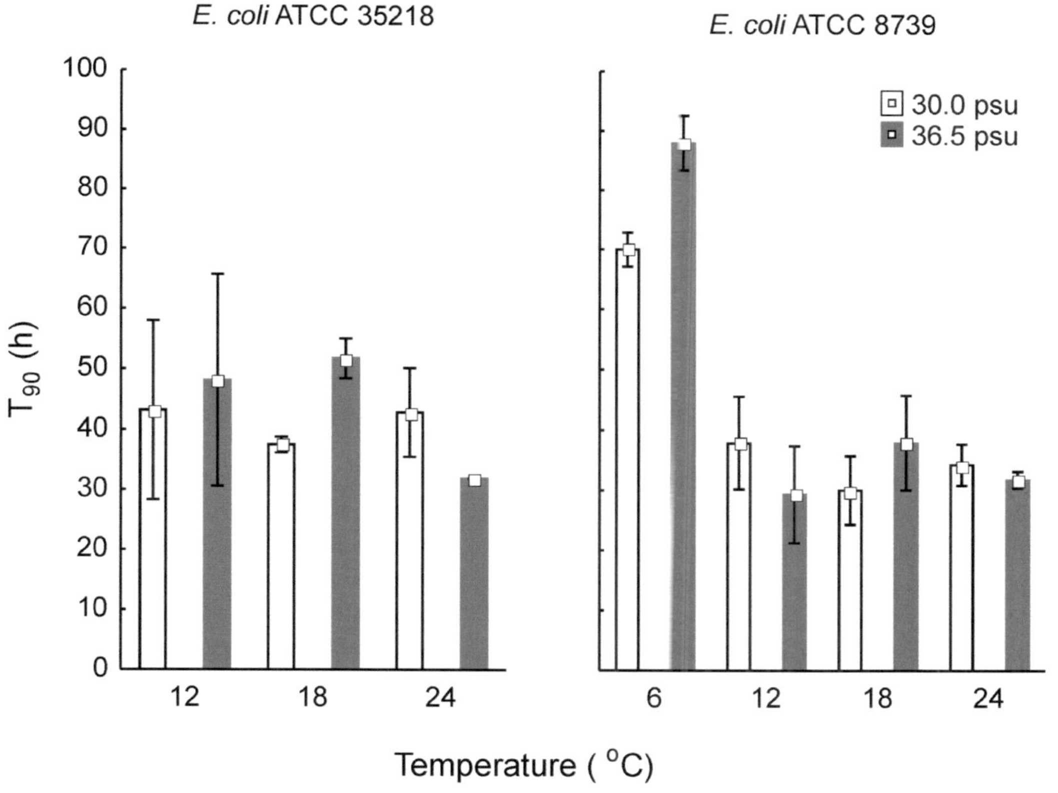

Figure 1. Effect of temperature and salinity on the survival of ATCC 8739 and ATCC 35218 *E. coli* strains in the absence of solar radiation (mean values ± SD).

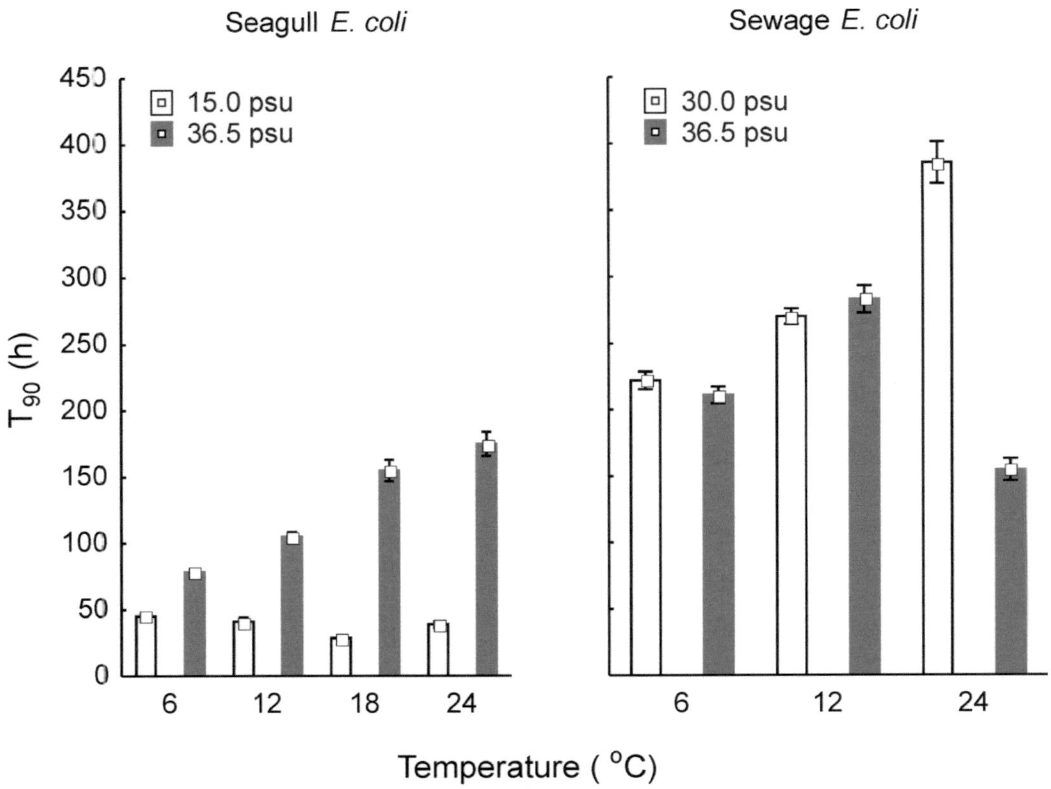

Figure 2. Effect of temperature and salinity on the survival of *E. coli* strains originating from seagull feces and sewage in the absence of solar radiation (mean values ± SD).

Most studies showed a negative correlation between survival time of indicator bacteria, including *E. coli*, and salinity [3, 7, 24, 25]. Troussellier et al. [26] found negative effect of salinity only in the presence of solar light. An unclear correlation between T_{90} and salinity in our study was partly attributed to a narrow salinity range. In order to extend the range of salinity and to clarify its effect on T_{90}, we performed additional experiments with *E. coli* ATCC 8739 at 15 psu. At higher temperatures (18 and 24°C), negative effect of lower salinity was less pronounced than the effect of salinity in its natural range, while at 6°C, lower salinity significantly lowered T_{90}, making the effect of salinity additionally unclear (**Figure 3**). A negative effect of salinity is attributed to specific characteristics of sea water, such as osmotic pressure [27] and the toxicity of inorganic salts [6]. Survival largely depends on the osmoregulatory ability of each strain or group of bacteria [28]. In order to equalize osmotic pressure and avoid drastic loss of water from the cytoplasm, bacterial cells can accumulate or synthesize specific osmoprotectant molecules [29] which increase cell resistance to seawater. This depends, among other things, on preadaptation media. Since *E. coli* in experiments was incubated on MMGB media, accumulation of glutamate, which is recognized as osmoprotectant [30], probably caused an unclear effect of salinity on *E. coli* survival.

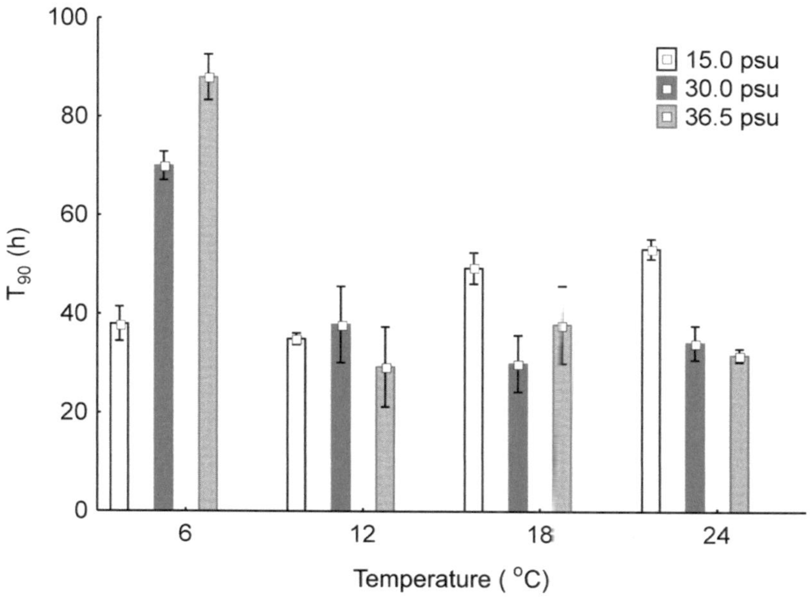

Figure 3. Effect of temperature and salinity in its wider range (15.0, 30.0 and 36.5 psu) on the survival of ATCC 8739 *E. coli* strain in the absence of solar radiation (mean values ± SD).

Although not statistically significant, *E. coli* ATCC 35218 survived longer than *E. coli* ATCC 8739 in almost all tested conditions. A significantly higher T_{90} was found in pure culture of *E. coli* isolated from seagull feces, 28.5–173 h (mean 72.8 h) and particularly in *E. coli* isolated from sewage outfall, 150–390 h (mean 278.6) (**Figure 3**). This suggested the importance of cell strain and origin to their survival in sea water and partially contributed to better understanding of the variations in results of previous studies. Since all tested *E. coli* strains were exposed to the same environmental conditions, the obtained results probably illustrated the extensive genetic and phenotypic diversity exhibited within *E. coli* strains, which could explain the different survival abilities in this study and aquatic environments generally [31]. On the basis of genomic information, *E. coli* species have been divided into eight phylogenetic groups, A, B1, B2, C, D, E, F, and clade I [32]. Strains belonging to phylogroups A and B1 are highly adapted to humans and vertebrate animals, the A phylogroup strains being predominant in humans and the B1 strains in animals [33, 34]. Significant differences in survival in water environment were found among strains belonging to different phylogroups. Recent studies showed that *E. coli* B1 strains can persist longer in water than strains of the other phylogroups [31] and supported the hypothesis that persistent genotypes have an adaptive advantage in the secondary habitat outside the host [35]. Consequently, once released into water, *E. coli* strains could be selected on the basis of their survival ability, and the resulting population differed from the original one in terms of phenotypic traits. *E. coli* strain isolated from sewage outfall and used in this study was in the seawater for an unknown period and probably passed selection that explains its superiority in survival over other tested strains.

Anderson et al. [7] found significant differences in the survival of indicator bacteria, *E. coli* and enterococci, depending on their origin. Among three investigated sources of bacteria; soil, sewage and dog feces, bacteria that originated from soil showed the highest resistance to environmental factors. These results are very important, particularly because apart human feces, there are many potential sources of enteric bacteria that enter the sea, such as untreated piggery effluents [36], and the feces of wild birds [37] and other warm-blooded animals.

In seagull *E. coli*, a positive effect of salinity was recorded in whole range of temperature, and at 36.5 psu higher temperature enhanced bacteria survival (**Figure 2**). Some *E. coli* cells may adapt to a range of concentrations of sodium chloride, possibly by means of osmoregulatory mechanism induced by salts or some structural modification in the outer membrane of bacteria [27]. Seagulls are marine birds and sea environment is their natural habitat. They feed mainly marine animals that contain high content of sodium chloride and drink both, fresh and seawater. Before being processed and excreted through salt gland in order to maintain osmotic balance, sodium chloride is present in intestinal tract content in a relative high concentration [38]. Consequently, seagull intestinal microflora, including *E. coli*, is highly adapted to saline environment. Such cells probably survive longer in seawater than other cells. Seagulls present a big problem to shellfish farms because they usually gather on buoys and other farm constructions, and huge quantities of feces enter the sea and contaminate it. Since up to 10^7 CFU *E. coli* g^{-1} was found in seagull feces in this study, and the results suggested better survival of *E. coli* originating from seagull feces, there is higher probability of their accumulation in filter feeding bivalves than *E. coli* that survive shorter.

3.2. Experiments in the presence of solar radiation

The intensity of solar radiation in this study was in the range 258–693 Wm^{-2}, with a mean contribution of the UVA spectrum of 9.3–11.1%. In the experiments carried out in the laboratory, a strong ($R^2 > 0.82$) and statistically significant ($p < 0.01$) negative correlation between the T_{90} of *E. coli* and the intensity of the UVA spectrum of solar radiation was found (**Figure 4**). The T_{90} of *E. coli* ATCC 35218 was in the range 0.30–0.82 h, whereas the T_{90} of *E. coli* ATCC 8739 ranged from 0.31 to 5.93 h. A significant, 15- to 70-fold reduction in T_{90}, compared with that recorded in the absence of solar radiation indicated the dominant effect of solar radiation on the survival of *E. coli* in seawater. Multiple linear regressions were used to investigate the combined effect of temperature, salinity, and the intensity of solar radiation on changes in the T_{90} of *E. coli* (**Table 1**). High and statistically significant ($p < 0.01$) coefficients of multiple determination (R^2) were found, which revealed that most of the variance in T_{90} can be explained by independent variables. However, only variations in solar radiation had a significant effect on T_{90}.

Because of inadequate weather conditions (a relative cloudy sky), in situ experiments were carried out at lower intensities of solar radiation. We also found a strong vertical decline in the intensity of solar radiation (UVA and PAR) and a significant decrease in the contribution of the UVA spectrum in the water column (**Figures 5** and **6**). Therefore, only a few data from surface layer could be used in our calculations. Unlike the experiments carried out in the laboratory, T_{90} of *E. coli* fitted exponential function (**Figure 7**) which can be expressed by Eq. (4).

http://dx.doi.org/10.5772/67912

$$T_{90}(h) = 31.305\, e^{-0.17 E_{UVA}} \tag{4}$$

According to the function, when $E_{UVA} = 0\ Wm^{-2}$, T_{90} value of *E. coli* ATCC 8739 amounted to 31.305, which corresponds to its value in the previous experiments in the absence of sunlight (**Figure 1**), which confirms the validity of function.

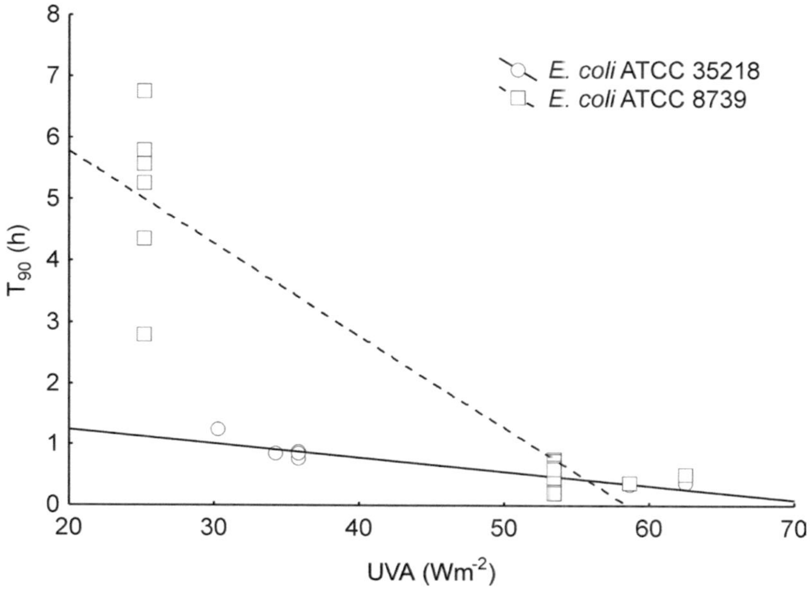

Figure 4. Effect of the UVA part of the solar radiation spectrum on the survival of ATCC 8739 and ATCC 35218 *E. coli* strains.

Variable	r_p	Beta	a	b	R^2
E. coli ATCC 35218					
T	−0.116	−0.208	1.183	−0.011	0.8797*
S	0.380	0.143		0.011	
UVA	−0.830*	−0.955		−0.024	
PAR	0.211	0.323		0.001	
***E. coli* ATCC 8739**					
T	−0.463	−1.043	7.882	−0.488	0.911*
S	0.319	0.107		0.711	
UVA	−0.8465*	−0.816		−0.131	
PAR	0.438	0.924		0.017	

*p < 0.01.

Table 1. Simultaneous effect of temperature (T), salinity (S), and solar radiation (UVA and PAR) on the T_{90} of *E. coli* (r_p—coefficient of partial correlation; beta-regression coefficients; a—intercept; b—coefficient of multiple linear regression; R^2—coefficient of multiple determination).

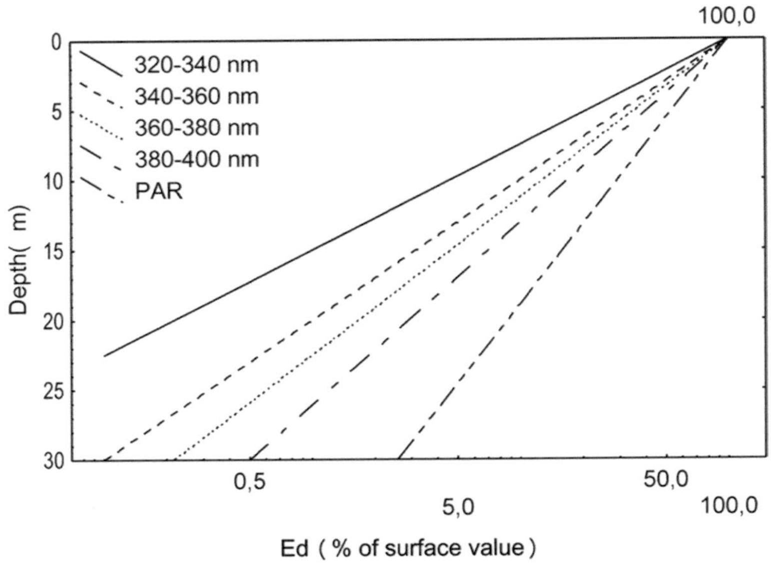

Figure 5. Attenuation of irradiance (% of surface value) as a function of sea depth.

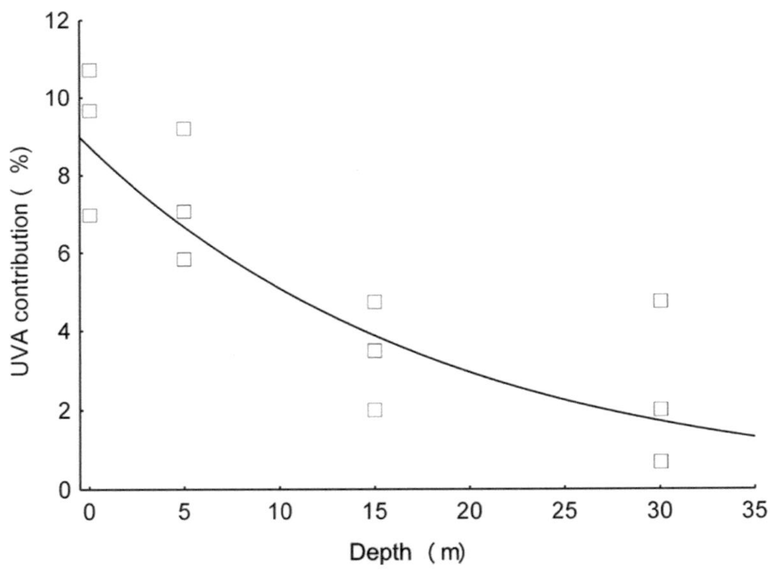

Figure 6. The reduction in the contribution of the UVA component of solar radiation as a function of sea depth.

The negative effect of sunlight exposure was also confirmed in the study with wild cultures of *E. coli* kept at 4°C. A significantly lower survival (T_{90} = 98 ± 22 h, n = 18) was found in *E. coli* sampled at noon than in those sampled in the morning (T_{90} = 153 ± 35 h, n = 18). This might be attributed to prolonged exposure to solar radiation and its higher intensity.

http://dx.doi.org/10.5772/67912

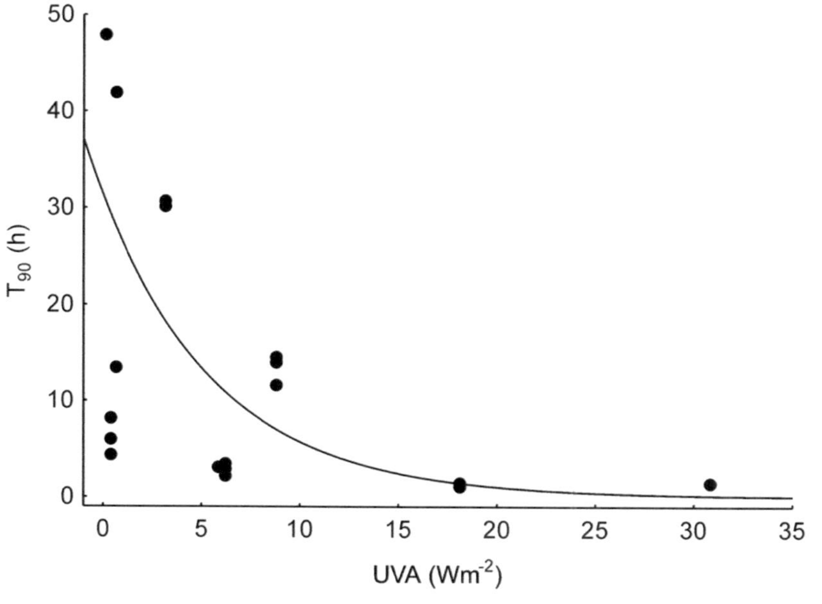

Figure 7. Effect of the lower intensity of UVA part of the solar radiation spectrum on the survival of ATCC 8739 *E. coli* strain.

Solar light is considered to be the most important factor to bacterial reduction in the sea, although its effects are restricted to shallow depths [5], also observed in this study. The negative effects of solar radiation to bacterial cells operate via two different mechanisms: firstly, direct photobiological mechanisms break DNA bonds in bacterial cells [39, 40], while secondly, indirect photochemical mechanisms damage bacterial cells by photosensitized reactions initiated by some of endogenous and/or exogenous sensitizers [41]. Photochemical mechanisms become more important at higher wavelengths, and it is more injurious in the presence of oxygen [5]. Both effects cause a rapid decrease in colony forming ability [25, 26]. Dominant toxic effect of sunlight was also observed in previous studies. Šolić and Krstulović [4] found that within the investigated range of intensity of solar radiation (510–830 Wm^{-2}), the T_{90} of fecal coliforms exponentially decreased by about 40% when the intensity of solar radiation increased by 100 Wm^{-2}. Large differences (30- to 40-fold) in survival with or without exposure to sunlight were observed by Fujioka et al. [25], who noted a T_{90} of fecal coliforms exposed to solar radiation in the range of 0.5–1.5 h. The reduction in survival time in the presence of solar radiation was also recorded by Chandran and Hatha [20], where the T_{90} of *E. coli* was reduced from 26 h in the dark to 4 h in the presence of solar radiation.

According to Davies-Colley et al. [42], T_{90} is a better indicator for expressing inactivation in the absence of solar radiation and also inactivation caused by solar radiation of an equable and higher irradiance, whereas the S_{90} better expresses the inactivation caused by solar radiation of variable intensity, as exists in nature. The energy of solar radiation absorbed by bacterial cells and which is responsible for cell injury is a product of the intensity of solar radiation and exposure time.

The mean values of S_{90} recorded in this study were 250 Whm^{-2} for *E. coli* ATCC 35218, and 610 Whm^{-2} for *E. coli* ATCC 8739. We found a medium-strong ($R^2 = 0.457$) and strong ($R^2 = 0.8282$) statistically significant ($p < 0.01$) negative linear correlation between the intensity of the UVA spectrum of solar radiation and S_{90} values for both *E. coli* strains (**Figure 8**).

A high and significant correlation between the intensity of the UVA spectrum of solar radiation with T_{90} and S_{90} in this study suggests that within the studied spectrum of solar radiation, this part of the measured spectrum was most responsible for the inactivation of microorganisms. The linear regression-slope coefficients suggested the wavelengths 320–360 nm to be the most bactericidal within the UVA spectrum (**Table 2**).

Acra et al. [43] found that up to 70% of the solar inactivation of bacteria can be attributed to the effect of the UVA part of the solar radiation spectrum, whereas Sinton et al. [5] found that 50% of the inactivation of indicator microorganisms could be attributed to solar radiation wavelengths up to 360 nm, with a wavelength of about 330 nm being most bactericidal. Calkins and Barcelo [44] find the UVB (280–330 nm) portion of the solar spectrum the most bactericidal, causing direct photobiological DNA damage. Although bactericidal effect of solar radiation is mainly associated with shorten wavelengths, the synergistic effect of UVB, UVA, and PAR explained most variations found in culturability of *E. coli* [45].

The values of S_{90} observed in this study were significantly lower than those in similar studies. S_{90} of fecal coliforms found by Gameson [22] was 1.290 Whm^{-2}, whereas Sinton et al. [5] found a significantly higher value, 1.660 Whm^{-2} (6.0 MJm^{-2}). Significant differences could be

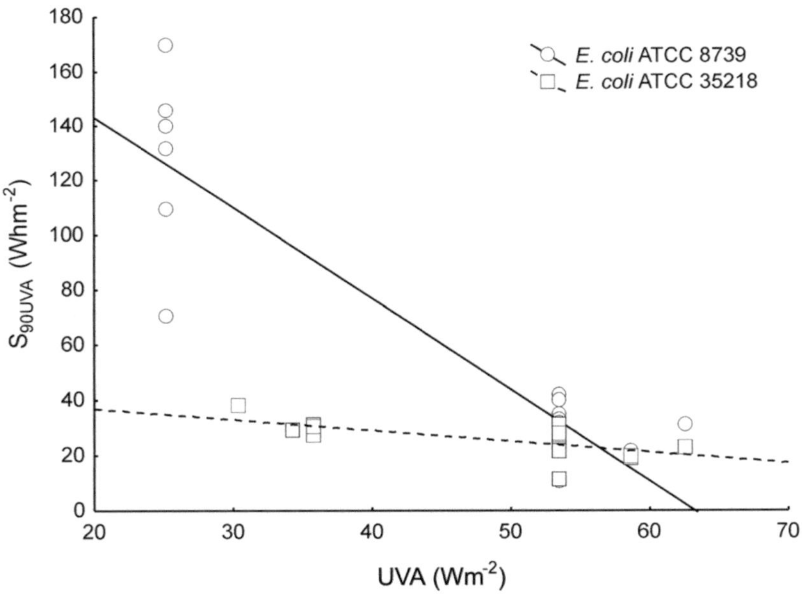

Figure 8. The S_{90} of ATCC 8739 and ATCC 35218 *E. coli* strains as a function of the intensity of the UVA part of the solar radiation spectrum.

	Wavelength (nm)				
	320–340	340–360	360–380	380–400	400–700 (PAR)
E. coli ATCC 35218					
b	−0.147	−0.124	−0.072	−0.052	−0.001
R^2	0.442	0.663	0.848	0.348	0.192
p	<0.01	<0.01	<0.01	<0.01	>0.05
E. coli ATCC 8739					
b	−1.095	−0.812	−0.488	−0.364	−0.014
R^2	0.741	0.834	0.851	0.864	0.635
p	<0.01	<0.01	<0.01	<0.01	<0.01

Table 2. Contribution of different wavelengths of measured solar radiation to T_{90} of *E. coli* expressed through slopes of linear regression (b—coefficient of multiple linear regression; R^2—coefficient of multiple determination; *p*—level of significance).

attributed to the different intensity of solar radiation and to variations in intensity, but also to different groups of microorganisms tested.

Lower T_{90} and S_{90} values in this study might partly be explained by the previous growth history of cell cultures until exposure to the environment, different origin and strain of bacterial cells, as well as by the different intensity of solar radiation and other environmental factors. There are many ways in which bacterial cells can enter the sea. In some cases, they are discharged directly from boats or bathers, and in others, they remain for different periods in wastewater reservoirs and/or are carried out in the sea through natural rivers or artificial conduits [14]. The change from a nutrient-rich environment to nutrient-poor one, places *E. coli* cells under starvation stress, which is less pronounced in bacteria from the stationary-phase because they have already experienced a starvation adaptation period. As a response to starvation stress, bacterial cells can induce protective mechanisms against UVA stress [46]. Furthermore, starved cultures taken in the stationary-phase of growth also showed higher osmotic [47] and temperature [48] resistance than those taken in a logarithmic-phase. This is due to specific protein synthesis during stationary-phase starvation [43]. In this study, *E. coli* cells were taken during the logarithmic-phase and were directly transferred to phosphate buffer without washing of nutrients. Since these cells did not experience starvation during the growth phase or during culture transfer, this probably made them less resistant to the negative effects of seawater and oxidative processes of solar radiation than cells that had experienced starvation [47, 49, 50]. Consequently, wild bacterial cells that have not experienced growth in a rich medium and are taken from the stationary phase of growth should show a higher resistance than cultivated cells, as was confirmed in this study. We found a statistically significant, at least threefold lower T_{90} (50.6 ± 6 h, n = 18) in cultivated wild *E. coli* cells than in their mother cells that were isolated from seawater (153.3 ± 35 h, n = 18), although the latter were pre-exposed to solar light and hostile environment for unknown period before seawater samples collected.

As mentioned previously, *E. coli* ATCC 35218 survived longer than *E. coli* ATCC 8739 in almost all experimental conditions in the dark, but if exposed to solar radiation, *E. coli* ATCC 35218 survived significantly shorter than *E. coli* ATCC 8739. This suggests that these microorganisms probably do not have equally developed mechanisms of protection against various abiotic environmental factors and that the protection rate also depends on which mechanism is more effective under the same conditions.

4. Conclusions

This study showed that in the absence of solar radiation, there were no statistically significant effects of temperature and salinity in their natural range (12, 18 and 24°C; 30.0 and 36.5 psu) on the survival of two ATCC strains. The survival of *E. coli* ATCC 8739 was enhanced only at 6°C, suggesting a negative effect of temperature at temperatures lower than natural range. At 15.0 psu, significantly lower T_{90} values of *E. coli* ATCC 8739 were observed at lower temperatures (6 and 12°C) than at higher ones (18 and 24°C). In the natural range of temperature and salinity, mean T_{90} values varied significantly, but only as a function of bacterial strain and origin. The importance of bacterial strain and origin for the survival of *E. coli* was demonstrated by significantly longer survival of *E. coli* cells isolated from seagull feces and sewage outfall. In the same conditions, their survival surpassed the survival of ATCC strains up to 10-fold. A dominate effect of solar light on *E. coli* survival was confirmed by recording a more rapid *E. coli* died-off in cells exposed to a natural range of solar radiation. The T_{90} was 15- to 70-fold shorter than in the absence of solar radiation. Within the investigated range of solar radiation (320–700 nm), only the effect of UVA spectrum was found to be statistically significant. The wavelengths 320–360 were the most bactericidal. The bacterial strain that had a shorter T_{90} in the absence of solar radiation showed a significantly higher T_{90} and S_{90} when exposed to solar light, suggesting different mechanisms of adaptation to studied abiotic environmental factors and a different efficiency of mechanisms under the same conditions. Cultivated bacteria showed threefold shorter T_{90} than their mother cells isolated from seawater. This suggested the importance of previous growth history of bacterial cells prior to exposure to the environment, for their adaptation capacity. The observed superiority of wild bacterial cultures over cultivated ones was probably a result of starvation experience during the stationary-phase, and/or due to a lack of nutrients.

Author details

Slaven Jozić* and Mladen Šolić

*Address all correspondence to: sjozic@izor.hr

Institute of Oceanography and Fisheries, Split, Croatia

References

[1] Berg G, editor. The indicator system. Indicators of Viruses in Water and Food. Ann Arbor: Ann Arbor Science Publishers; 1978. pp. 1-13. doi:10.1002/jobm.19800200609

[2] The European Parliament and the Council of the European Union. Regulation (EC) No 854/2004 of the European Parliament and of the Council of 29 April 2004 laying down specific rules for the organisation of official controls on products of animal origin intended for human consumption. Official Journal of the European Union. 2004;L226:83-127.

[3] The European Parliament and the Council of the European Union. Directive 2006/7/EC of 15 February 2006 concerning the management of bathing water quality and repealing directive 76/160/EEC. Official Journal of the European Union. 2006;L64:37-51.

[4] Šolić M, Krstulović N. Separate and combined effects of solar radiation, temperature, salinity and pH on the survival of faecal coliforms in seawater. Marine Pollution Bulletin. 1992;24(8):411-416. doi:10.1016/0025-326X(92)90503-X

[5] Sinton LW, Davies-Coley RJ, Bell RG. Inactivation of enterococci and fecal coliforms from sewage and meatworks effluents in seawater chambers. Applied and Environmental Microbiology. 1994;60(6):2040-2048.

[6] Carlucci AF, Pramer D. An evaluation of factors affecting the survival of Escherichia coli in sea water. II. Salinity, pH and nutrients. Applied Microbiology. 1960;8(4):247-250.

[7] Anderson KL, Whitlock JE, Harwood DJ. Persistence and differential survival of fecal indicator bacteria in subtropical waters and sediments. Applied and Environmental Microbiology. 2005;71(6):3041-3048. doi:10.1128/AEM.71.6.3041-3048.2005

[8] Sivri N, Balci M, Durmus T, Seker DZ, Balkis N. Analysis of enteric bacteria distribution in the Gulf of Gemlik (Marmara Sea) by means of GIS. Fresenius Environmental Bulletin. 2012;21(11):3224-3232.

[9] Anderson IC, Rhodes M, Kator HI. Sublethal stress in *Escherichia coli*: a function of salinity. Applied and Environmental Microbiology. 1979;38(6):1147-1152.

[10] Kapuscinski RB, Mitchell R. Solar radiation induces sublethal injury in *Escherichia coli* in seawater. Applied and Environmental Microbiology. 1981;41(3):670-674.

[11] Barcina I, González JM, Iriberri J, Egea L. Survival strategy of *Escherichia coli* and *Enterococcus faecalis* in illuminated fresh and marine systems. Journal of Applied Bacteriology. 1990;68(2):189-98. doi:10.1111/j.1365-2672.1990.tb02565.x

[12] Grimes DJ, Atwell RW, Brayton PR, Palmer LM. Rollins, DM, Roszak DB, Singleton FL, Tamplin ML, Colwell RR. The fate of enteric pathogenic bacteria in estuarine and marine environments. Microbiological Sciences. 1986;3(11):324-329.

[13] Singh A, R Yeager, McFeters GA. Assessment of in vivo revival, growth, and pathogenicity of *Escherichia coli* strains after copper- and chlorine-induced injury. Applied and Environmental Microbiology. 1986;52(4):832-837.

[14] Rozen Y, Belkin S. Survival of enteric bacteria in seawater. FEMS Microbiology Reviews. 2001;25(5):513-529. doi:10.1111/j.1574-6976.2001.tb00589.x

[15] Fujioka RS, Narikawa OT. Effect of sunlight on enumeration of indicator bacteria under field conditions. Applied and Environmental Microbiology. 1982;44(2):395-401.

[16] Whittam TS. Clonal dynamics of *Escherichia coli* in its natural habitat. Antonie van Leeuwenhoek. 1989;55(1):23-32.

[17] Topp E, Welsh M, Tien YC, Dang A, Lazarovits G, Conn K, Zhu H. Strain-dependent variability in growth and survival of *Escherichia coli* in agricultural soil. FEMS Microbiology Ecology. 2003;44(3):303-308. doi:10.1016/S0168-6496(03)00055-2

[18] Porter KG, Feig YS. The use of DAPI for identifying and counting aquatic microflora. Limnology and Oceanography. 1980;25(5):943-948. doi:10.4319/lo.1980.25.5.0943

[19] ISO 16649-1. Microbiology of food and animal feeding stuff—Horizontal method for the enumeration of β-glucuronidase-positive *Escherichia coli*—Part 1: Colony-count technique at 44°C using membranes and 5-bromo-4-chloro-3-indolyl-β-D-glucuronide. International Organization for Standardization; 2001. 9 p.

[20] Chandran A, Hatha AAM. Survival of *Escherichia coli* in a tropical estuary. The South Pacific Journal of Natural Science. 2003;21(1):41-46. doi:10.1071/SP03008

[21] Anderson IC, Rhodes MW, Kator HI. Seasonal variation in survival of Escherichia coli exposed in situ in membrane diffusion chambers containing filtered and nonfiltered estuarine water. Applied and Environmental Microbiology. 1983;45(6):1877-1883. doi: 0099-2240/83/061877-07$02.00/0

[22] Gameson ALH. Bacterial mortality. Part 3. In: Investigations of sewage discharges to some British coastal waters. Water Research centre Technical Report TR 201. Medmenham, United Kingdom: Water Research Centre Environment; 1986. pp. 1-74.

[23] Sinton LW. Biotic and abiotic effects. In: Belkin S, Colwell RR, editors. Oceans and Health: Pathogens in the Marine Environment. New York: Springer; 2005. pp. 69-92. doi:10.1007/b102184

[24] Evison LM. Comparative studies on the survival of indicator organisms and pathogens in fresh and sea water. Water Science and Technology. 1988;20(11-12):309-315.

[25] Fujioka RS, Hashimoto HH, Siwak EB, Reginald HF. Effect of sunlight on survival of indicator bacteria in seawater. Applied and Environmental Microbiology. 1981;41(3):690-696.

[26] Troussellier M, Bonnefont JL, Courties C, et al. Responses of enteric bacteria to environmental stresses in seawater. Oceanologica Acta. 1998;21(6):965-981. doi:10.1016/S0399-1784(99)80019-X

[27] Gauthier MJ, Munro PM, Mohajer S. Influence of salts and sodium chloride on the recovery of *Escherichia coli* from seawater. Current Microbiology. 1987;15(1):5-10. doi:10.1007/BF01577205

[28] Oren A, Vlodavsky L. Survival of *Escherichia coli* and *Vibrio harveyi* in Dead Sea water. FEMS Microbiology Letters. 1985;31(6):365-371. doi:10.1111/j.1574-6968.1985.tb01173.x

[29] Csonka LN, Epstein W. Osmoregulation. In: Neidhardt FC, Curtiss R, Ingraham JL, Lin ECC, Low KB, Magasanik B, Rezniko, WS, Riley M, Schaechter M, Umbarger HE, editors. *Escherichia coli* and *Salmonella*: Cellular and Molecular Biology, Vol. 1. Washington, DC: ASM Press; 1996. pp. 1210-1223.

[30] Gauthier MJ, Flatau GN, Le Rudulier D, Clement RL, Combarro MP. Intracellular accumulation of potassium and glutamate specifically enhances survival of *Escherichia coli* in seawater. Applied and Environmental Microbiology. 1991;57(1):272-276.

[31] Berthe T, Ratajczak M, Clermont O, Denamur E, Petit F. Evidence for coexistence of distinct *Escherichia coli* populations invarious aquatic environments and their survival in estuary water. Applied and Environmental Microbiology. 2013;79(15):4684-4693. doi:10.1128/AEM.00698-13

[32] Clermont O, Christenson JK, Denamur E, Gordon DM. The Clermont *Escherichia coli* phylotyping method revisited: improvement of specificity and detection of new phylo-groups. Environmental Microbiology Reports. 2013;5(1):58-65. doi:10.1111/1758-2229.12019

[33] Duriez P, Clermont O, Bonacorsi S, Bingen E, Chaventre A, Elion J, Picard B, Denamur E. Commensal *Escherichia coli* isolates are phylogenetically distributed among geographically distinct human populations. Microbiology. 2001;147(6):1671-1676. doi:10.1099/00221287-147-6-1671

[34] Gordon DM, Cowling A. The distribution and genetic structure of *Escherichia coli* in Australian vertebrates: host and geographic effects. Microbiology. 2003;149(12):3575-3586. doi:10.1099/mic.0.26486-0

[35] Walk ST, Alm EW, Calhoun LM, Mladonicky JM, Whittam TS. Genetic diversity and population structure of *Escherichia coli* isolated from freshwater beaches. Environmental Microbiology. 2007;9(9):2274-2288. doi:10.1111/j.1462-2920.2007.01341.x

[36] Chinivasagam HN, Thomas RJ, Casey K, McGaham E, Gardner EA, Rafiee M, Blackall PJ. Microbiological status of piggery effluent from 13 piggeries in the south east Queensland region of Australia. Journal of Applied Microbiology. 2004;97(5):883-891. doi:10.1111/j.1365-2672.2004.02382.x

[37] Gülhan T, Boynukara B, Durmus A, Kiziroglu I, Sancak YC. Enteric bacteria and some pathogenic properties of *Enterococcus faecalis, Enterococcus faecium* and *Escherichia coli* strains isolated from wild ducks and gulls. Fresenius Environmental Bulletin. 2012;21(7a):1961-1966.

[38] Robinson Hughes M. Cloacal and salt-gland ion excretion in the seagull, Larus glaucescens, acclimated to increasing concentrations of sea water. Comparative Biochemistry and Physiology. 1970;32(2):315-325. doi:10.1016/0010-406X(70)90944-8

[39] Jagger J. Solar-UV Actions on Living Cells, 1st ed. New York: Praeger; 1985. 202 p.

[40] Eisenstark A. Bacterial genes involved in response to near-ultraviolet radiation. Advances in Genetics. 1989;26:99-147. doi:10.1016/S0065-2660(08)60224-2

[41] Curtis TP, Mara DD, Silva SA. Influence of pH, oxygen, and humic substances on ability of sunlight to damage fecal coliforms in waste stabilization pond water. Applied and Environmental Microbiology. 1992;58(4):1335-1343.

[42] Davies-Colley RJ, Bell RG, Donnison AM. Sunlight inactivation of enterococci and fecal coliforms in sewage effluent diluted in seawater. Applied and Environmental Microbiology. 1994;60(6):2049-2058.

[43] Acra A, Raffoul Z, Karahagopian Y. Solar Disinfection of Drinking Water and Oral Rehydration Solutions: Guidelines for Household Application in Developing Countries. Beirut: UNICEF; 1984. 66 p.

[44] Calkins S, Barcelo JA. Action spectra. In: Calkins J, editor. The Role of Solar Ultraviolet Radiation in Marine Ecosystems. New York and London: Plenum Press; 1982. pp. 143-150. doi 10.1007/978-1-4684-8133-4

[45] Muela A, García-Bringas I, Barcina I. The effect of simulated solar radiation on *Escherichia coli*: the relative roles of UV-B, UV-A, and photosynthetically active radiation. Microbial Ecology. 2000:39(1):65-71. doi:10.1007/s002489900181

[46] Berney M, Weilenmann HU, Ihssen J, Bassin C, Egli T. Specific growth rate determines the sensitivity of *Escherichia coli* to thermal, UVA, and solar disinfection. Applied and Environmental Microbiology. 2006;72(4):2586-2593. doi:10.1128/AEM.72.4. 2586-2593.2006

[47] Jenkins DE, Chaisson SA, Matin A. Starvation-induced cross protection against osmotic challenge in *Escherichia coli*. Journal of Bacteriology. 1990;172(5):2779-2781. doi: 10.1128/jb.170.9.3910-3914.1988

[48] Jenkins DE, Schultz JE, Matin A. Starvation-induced cross protection against heat or H_2O_2 challenge in *Escherichia coli*. Journal of Bacteriology. 1988;170(9):3910-3914. doi: 10.1128/jb.170.9.3910-3914.1988

[49] Kjelleberg S, Hermanosson M. Starvation-induced effects on bacterial surface characteristics. Applied and Environmental Microbiology. 1984;48(3):497-503.

[50] Siegele DA, Kolter S. Life after log. Journal of Bacteriology. 1992;174(2):345-348. doi: 10.1128/jb.174.2.345-348.1992

Chapter 10

Isolation and Characterization of *Escherichia coli* from Animals, Humans, and Environment

Athumani Msalale Lupindu

Additional information is available at the end of the chapter

http://dx.doi.org/10.5772/67390

Abstract

Working on a diverse species of bacteria that have hundreds of pathotypes representing hundreds of strains and many closely related family members is a challenge. Appropriate research design is required not only to achieve valid desired outcome but also to minimize the use of resources, including time to outcome and intervention. This chapter outlines basics of *Escherichia coli* isolation and characterization strategies that can assist in research designing that matches the set objectives. Types of samples to be collected, collection and storage strategies, and processing of samples are described. Different approaches to isolation, confirmation and concentration of various *E. coli* strains are summarized in this chapter. Characterization and typing of *E. coli* isolates by biochemical, serological, and molecular methods have been explained so that an appropriate choice is made to suite a specific *E. coli* strain/pathotype. Some clues on sample and isolate preservation for future use are outlined, and general precautions regarding *E. coli* handling are also presented to the researcher to avoid improper planning and execution of *E. coli*-related research. Given different options, the best *E. coli* research design, however, should try as much as possible to shorten the length of time to outcomes.

Keywords: *E. coli*, β-glucuronidase, Enterobacteriaceae, cryoprotectant, IMViC

1. Introduction

Escherichia coli is Gram-negative, facultative anaerobic, and rod-shaped bacterium of the genus *Escherichia*. This is a large diverse group of bacteria commonly found in the lower intestine of warm-blooded organisms. Most of them are commensals inhabiting the lower gastrointestinal tract (GIT) of mammals. The other strains that are pathogenic are categorized into two groups, according to the site of infection. *E. coli* that infect and cause disease syndromes in the gastrointestinal tract are intestinal pathogenic *E. coli* (IPEC). Those that cause disease syndromes in systems other than gastrointestinal tract are called extra-intestinal *E. coli* (EXPEC). The commensal group form part of gut microbiota and is used as indicator bacteria for fecal contamination.

Pathogenic *E. coli* group consist of many strains, which for simplicity, can be grouped according to the virulence factors they possess or pathological effects they cause. The intestinal pathogenic *E. coli* include enterotoxigenic *E. coli* (ETEC), enteroaggregative *E. coli* (EAEC), enteropathogenic *E. coli* (EPEC), enteroinvasive *E. coli* (EIEC), diffusely adherent *E. coli* (DAEC), and verocytotoxigenic *E. coli* (VTEC) according to O'Sullivan et al. [24]. Extra-intestinal pathogenic *E. coli* includes uropathogenic *E. coli* (UPEC), neonatal meningitis-associated *E. coli* (NMEC), and sepsis-causing *E. coli* (SEPEC) [1].

Most pathogenic *E. coli* are transmitted by fecal-oral route from food materials, water, animals, and environment. Depending on the pathotype and the system, *E. coli* infection may cause a range of syndromes including watery, mucoid, or bloody diarrhea; abdominal cramps; urinary tract infection syndromes; and meningitis. Complications to pathogenic *E. coli* infection may lead to hemorrhagic uremic syndrome (HUS). These syndromes have been reported as food poisoning outbreak, travel-related illness, or animal or contaminated environment contact-related diseases. Global *E. coli*-related morbidities and mortalities are high. The estimates for the year 2010 show that there were 321,969,086 cases of *E. coli* food-borne illness which is 16.1% of global food-borne diseases. Also there were 196,617 deaths attributable to *E. coli*-related food-borne poisoning which is 0.02% of global mortalities due to food poisoning [2]. This situation calls for regular and continuous investigations to diagnose, treat, and prevent *E. coli*-related diseases.

Inappropriate planning of research due to lack of knowledge may lead to undesired outcomes. For instance, if one aims at assessing the magnitude of shading of diarrheagenic *E. coli* in cattle feces, he or she may end up with underestimated results if he or she chooses to use sorbitol MacConkey agar as a screening media because not all diarrheagenic *E. coli* are sorbitol fermenters. Likewise, if one is looking for *E. coli* O157:H7 in a sample, the use of media that discriminate bacteria according to the presence of β-glucuronidase activities may lead to missing the desired outcome since *E. coli* O157:H7 do not possess such an enzyme. This chapter, therefore, outlines approaches to isolate and characterize *E. coli* from animals, humans, and the environment so that planning and implementation of *E. coli*-related research can match the set objectives and desired outcome.

2. Collection and storage of sample for *E. coli* isolation

2.1. Sample collection

E. coli predominantly inhabit the gastrointestinal tract of mammals and are shed to the environment through feces. The feces from mammals can be collected for the purpose of *E. coli* isolation. In this case, fresh fecal material from individual humans or animals can be used.

http://dx.doi.org/10.5772/67390

Dry or sunburnt fecal samples may lead to false negative results. Shading of *E. coli* in feces makes this microorganism abundantly available in the environment. As a result, *E. coli* can be recovered from water, soil, contaminated food material, and surfaces.

Sampling of the soil for isolation of *E. coli* requires taking the sample 2–5 cm beneath the surface. Top soils may contain dead bacteria. Water samples can be collected for *E. coli* detection. *E. coli* can also be isolated from contaminated surfaces of both animate and inanimate materials. Animate surfaces include human or animal body surface. Food surfaces or working structures such as table, knives, and clothes can be a good source of *E. coli*. Food surfaces such as meat, eggs, or fish can be used to isolate *E. coli*, depending on the objective of the study. Animal fecal sample can be taken from the rectum (large animals) or fresh droppings can be collected by fingers of a gloved hand. Human stool can be put in a container with a stopper. Water samples can be collected by different methods according to nature of the water body. Still surface can be collected by hand deep method, whereas flowing water sample collection requires depth-and-width-integrating methods. In this type of water body, for example, a stream, 5–10, or more samples are collected across the vertical depth and width [3]. Samples from surfaces such as hide, table, knife, and the likes can be obtained by sweeping a buffered peptone water with premoistened swabs or sponge on the sampling surface in a Z-pattern [4]. The sponge or swabs that covers approximately 400–1000 cm^2 are then put in 100 ml of tryptic soya broth for further processing.

2.2. Sample storage

Samples for *E. coli* isolation are best processed right after collection, normally within 24 h. This includes inoculation into enrichment or inoculation onto solid culture media. When situation does not allow, a sample can be stored at low temperatures that restrict further cell division, but at the same time, allows survival of the bacteria. Surface water samples for *E. coli* isolation stored at below 10°C, but not freezing, can give comparably good results for up to 48 h after collection [5].

Sometimes analysis of fecal samples immediately after collection is impractical due to temporal and spatial challenges or assessment of old samples can be a requirement. In this case, fecal/stool samples should be stored for later laboratory isolation or old samples that were appropriately stored are recalled. Fecal samples will maintain *E. coli* population density, clonal characteristics, and diversity as fresh samples when stored in glycerol broth at lower temperatures than −70°C for 30 days up to 1 year. The fecal sample may form 10% of final concentration in 10% glycerol broth. However, storage of this sample at −20°C for the same time period will lead to a decrease in bacteria population density but increased diversity [6, 7]. Moreover, samples stored in glycerol broth will have more similar *E. coli* isolates to isolates from the fresh original sample than those from samples stored without mixing with glycerol, and if samples are repeatedly thawed, then addition of glycerol broth is recommended. Pure samples stored for a long time without glycerol lead to decrease in *E. coli* number [6]. Therefore, longer storage of fecal samples without appropriate processing may lead to inaccurate results.

3. Isolation of *E. coli* and quality control

3.1. Isolation of *E. coli*

Different options are available for the isolation of *E. coli*. The choice depends on target strain and objective of isolation. The ability to ferment lactose gives an option to use MacConkey agar to discriminate *E. coli* from other nonlactose fermenting coliforms from fecal, stool, food, water, and soil samples. Sample suspension (for solid samples) is made at any concentration, for example, 5% in normal saline or phosphate buffer solution and inoculated onto MacConkey agar followed by 18–24 h incubation at 37°C. Pink, round medium-sized colonies are picked as *E. coli* suspect colonies. All *E. coli* strains can be captured on MacConkey agar, and this approach gives a wide spectrum of strains to work on. Incubation of inoculated culture media at 45°C selects for thermophilic *E. coli* strains.

The concentration of sample suspension may be set at different levels such as 1 g of solid sample in 19 ml of normal saline or phosphate buffer solution (5%), 1 g in 9 ml (10%) or 1 g in 4 ml of diluent (20%). However, the concentration of sample suspension will affect the number of colonies on the culture plate. This is well evidenced in bacteria count procedures whereby higher dilution, like 10^5, will give lower number of bacteria than low dilutions, for example, 10^1. This is because the bacteria growth rate depends on initial cell density in the sample [8].

Sample suspension can be enriched by 24 h incubation at 37°C in nondifferential broth such as Muller-Hinton or nutrient broth. This procedure will allow multiplication of *E. coli* and hence increase the chance of *E. coli* isolation especially when infrequent strains, such as pathogens, are the target. The generation (doubling) time for *E. coli* at 37°C incubation is 17–18 min [8], therefore, in 18–24 h incubation there will be 60–80 *E. coli* cell generations. However, clonal variability will decrease when samples are enriched because same bacteria increase in number. Therefore, this procedure is suitable when the research aims at a mere presence of a single specific strain and not its variants.

The weight of the sample and the volume of diluent used in making the sample suspension may affect the probability of bacteria recovery. Large sample weight normally increases the sensitivity of the isolation procedure. For example, in *E. coli* studies to isolate nonsorbitol-fermenting Shiga toxin-producing *E. coli* (NSF STEC) whereby *E. coli* broth was used to enrich fecal samples, different prevalence measure was obtained. When 10 g of sample was suspended in 90 ml of *E. coli* broth, the prevalence of Shiga toxin-producing *E. coli* (STEC) obtained was 1.3% [9], while the suspension of 20 g in 180 ml of same diluent resulted into a prevalence 11.1% NSF STEC [10].

Purification of *E. coli* colonies can be done in nondifferential media such as blood or nutrient agars. Depending on the degree of colony density, a series of inoculations can be desired until pure, single, or solitary colonies are obtained.

3.2. Quality control

These are procedures undertaken to validate the accuracy of the bacteria isolates. Among the measures of quality control in isolation of *E. coli* include incubation of uninoculated media

http://dx.doi.org/10.5772/67390

plates at 37°C overnight. The media plates should have no microbial growth after incubation. This will ensure that the isolates obtained after inoculation come from the samples and not due to contamination. Moreover, uninoculated media plate should be incubated simultaneously with inoculated media plates. Use of reference positive controls strains, e.g. *E. coli* ATCC 25922, will also help to ensure the isolates are the targeted bacteria.

For water samples, quality control measures may involve the use of blank and sample replicates. The true samples and the blanks are simultaneously incubated. The blank sample will tell that the sampling equipment has not been contaminated The replicate results will assess the presence of variation for which explanations should be sorted out.

4. Confirmation of *E. coli* isolates

Confirmation of *E. coli* isolates can be done by biochemical, enzymatic, or molecular methods. The choice of the method depends on many factors including availability of resources. The confirmation methods include biochemical methods, such as IMViC and Analytical Profile Index 20E (API 20E) systems, enzymatic methods, for example, use of brilliance *E. coli* agar or Petrifilm Select *E. coli* count plate, and molecular techniques such as MALD-TOF.

4.1. IMViC tests

E. coli isolates can be confirmed biochemically by the use of a traditional method called IMViC tests. This is a set of four tests that are used to differentiate members of the family Enterobacteriaceae. IMViC is an abbreviation that stands for the Indole, Methyl red, Voges-Proskauer, and Citrate utilization tests. In Indole test, the bacteria are tested for their ability to produce indole from tryptophan (amino acid) using the enzyme tryptophanase.

The indole reacts with the aldehyde in the Kovac's reagent to give a red or a pink ring at the top of the tube. Peptone water in a tube, which contains tryptophan, is inoculated with bacteria isolate to be tested. The mixture is incubated overnight at 37°C. Then, a few drops of Kovac's reagent are added to the mixture and formation of a red or a pink colored ring at the top is a positive reaction. *E. coli* are indole-positive bacteria

Methyl red test detects the ability of a bacterium to produce acid from glucose fermentation. Methyl red, a pH indicator, remains red in color at a pH less or equal to 4.4. The bacterium to be tested is inoculated into glucose phosphate (MRVP) broth, which contains glucose and a phosphate buffer and incubated at 37°C for 48 h. Three to five drops of MR reagent are added to the tube. Red color development is a positive reaction that occurs when the bacteria have produced enough acid to neutralize the phosphate buffer. Yellow discoloration occurs to MR-negative bacteria. *E. coli* are MR-positive bacteria.

Voges-Proskauer test is used to detect the presence of acetoin in the bacteria-containing media. Acetoin is oxidized to diacetyl in the presence of air and sodium hydroxide. Diacetyl, in the presence of alpha-naphthol, reacts with guanidine to produce red color. In order to perform VP test, the test bacterium is inoculated into glucose phosphate (MRVP) broth in a tube and incubated for 72 h.

Addition of 15 drops of alpha-naphthol to the test broth is followed by shaking. Then add five drops of 40% potassium hydroxide (KOH) to the broth and shake well. Allow the tube to stand for 15 min to see a positive red discoloration, after 1 h of no color change the isolate is categorized as VP negative. *E. coli* is VP negative.

Citrate utilization test detects the ability of the bacteria to use citrate as its sole source of carbon and energy. Citrate agar media contains a pH indicator called bromthymol blue. The agar media changes from green to blue at an alkaline pH. Streak a loopful of bacteria onto a citrate agar slant without stabbing the butt and incubate at 37°C for 24 h with a loose cap. Citrate in the media breaks down to oxaloacetate and acetate due to action of an enzyme citritase. Oxaloacetate is further broken down to pyruvate and CO_2. Production of Na_2CO_3 from sodium citrate changes the media into alkaline pH, and hence color change from green to blue. Blue color formation is a positive reaction, whereas the slant remaining green colored is a feature for negative test. *E. coli* is citrate negative.

This conventional IMViC test method gives results (**Table 1**) that are similar to an agar plate IMViC method [11]. *E. coli* and *Proteus vulgaris* show the same IMViC pattern, but *Proteus* spp. are lactose-negative, motile, and show swarming behavior.

4.2. The API 20E system

Analytical Profile Index 20E is a set of biochemical tests specific for differentiating between members of the Gram-negative bacterial family Enterobacteriaceae. It is used for rapid identification of already known bacteria. API 20E system is made up of 20 small reaction tubes that contain dehydrated substrates for detection of the enzymatic fermentation of sugars by the test isolates. This fermentation occurs during incubation, and the resulting pH change is detected by an indicator. It is important to confirm that the test culture is of an Enterobacteriaceae first, by doing a quick oxidase test. Enterobacteriaceae are oxidase negative.

Inoculate the suspension of a pure culture into each of the 20 reaction tubes and Incubate the tray at 37°C for 18–24 h. You can read the color change in some compartments right after

Bacterium	Indole	MR	VP	Citrate
Escherichia coli	+	+	–	–
Klebsiella pneumoniae	–	–	+	+
Enterobacter aerogenes	–	–	+	+
Salmonella species	–	+	–	+
Shigella species	–	+	–	–
Proteus vulgaris	+	+	–	–
Proteus mirabilis	–	+	–	+
Citrobacter freundii	–	+	–	+

Table 1. MViC test results of some members of family Enterobacteriaceae (Adapted from Powers and Latt [11]).

http://dx.doi.org/10.5772/67390

incubation, but some may require additional reagents. Mark each test as positive or negative on the lid of the tray and score them. Add up the scores, the maximum score being seven, to get a 7-digit code that is used to identify the bacteria by using the online database.

4.3. Enzymatic activities

Strict selective media that check for specific enzymatic activities in *E. coli* can be used to confirm *E. coli* isolates. For instance, brilliance *E. coli* agar or Petrifilm Select *E. coli* count plate can be used to check for presence and activity of β-glucuronidase enzyme. Beta-glucuronidase enzyme, which is specific to *E. coli*, cleaves glucuronide substrate resulting in purple and blue-green colonies in Brilliance *E. coli* agar and Petrifilm *E. coli* Select count plates, respectively. Non-*E. coli* coliforms have ß-galactosidase only, which enable them to break down lactose, whereas most of *E. coli* have both β-galactosidase and β-glucuronidase. However, *E. coli* O157 are glucuronidase negative; therefore, these media are not appropriate for initial screening of *E. coli* population but can be used to differentiate *E. coli* O157 from confirmed *E. coli* population.

4.4. MALD-TOF mass spectrometry

Matrix-Assisted Laser Desorption/Ionization Time-of-Flight (MALD-TOF) mass spectrometry is a rapid and accurate method for microorganism identification. Principally, the biomolecules are allowed to gain or lose electrons (ionization) and then sorted based on their mass to charge ratio, when subjected to electric or magnetic field. The spectrum generated is analyzed and compared to stored profiles using software. These spectra, which are species-specific, can be used to confirm microorganism, for example, *E. coli* or discriminating closely related species such as *E. coli* and Shigella.

5. Convergence of *E. coli* isolates

E. coli form a large diverse species of bacteria that is difficult to handle when targeting a specific strain. Working on any *E. coli*-suspect colony from less discriminatory procedures prolong the time interval to isolate confirmation and utilizes more resources. The use of selective media helps to achieve this goal, but only when target *E. coli* strain is well defined. Otherwise, other approaches should be employed. Selection of *E. coli* isolates with some common features may be used to narrow down the population size. Converging similar *E. coli* isolates can be done by employing different procedures that utilize antimicrobial resistance, enzymatic, and immunogenic reactions and genetic characteristics of specific *E. coli* to mention a few. The choice of the method of converging *E. coli* isolates depends on different factors including study objectives, bacteria characteristics, skill, and resource availability.

Resistance to a single antimicrobial agent or combined resistance to more than one antimicrobial agent can be used to get *E. coli* isolates with common features. Resistance to common antimicrobial agents used in an area can be used to screen *E. coli* isolates before further analyses. For example, in a study to assess genetic similarities between *E. coli* isolates from humans, cattle, and the environment, Lupindu and his colleagues [12] chose to isolate *E. coli* with resistance to tetracycline and ampicillin to concentrate *E. coli* from the general population. *E. coli* isolated from MacConkey agar was subjected to ampicillin-tetracycline solution using Petrifilm Select *E. coli* count (SEC) plate. Out of 1046 *E. coli* isolated from MacConkey agar, 118 isolates were resistant to ampicillin-tetracycline drug combination. Antimicrobial stock solution and bacteria inoculation were executed as previously described in Ref. [13]. One milliliter of antimicrobial stock solution containing 0.32 mg ampicillin and 0.64 mg was placed on the bottom lid. After 2 h of absorption of the antimicrobial solution, 2 μl of standardized sample suspension was spot-inoculated onto the antimicrobial embedded lower lid of Petrifilm SEC plate. The upper lid was closed after 10 min, and the plate incubated at 42°C for 24 h. Round, medium-sized *E. coli* colonies appear dark-green due to the presence of β-glucuronidase activity on glucuronide substrate in indicator embedded medium. This procedure was also used to confirm the *E. coli* isolates that were further analyzed by PFGE for their genetic relatedness.

Ability of some *E. coli* strains to ferment different sugars can be used to concentrate strains of interest. All *E. coli* are lactose fermenters, but only some can ferment sorbitol. Sorbitol (instead of lactose) is mixed with MacConkey agar to form sorbitol MacConkey agar. This media can be used to discriminate sorbitol fermenting *E. coli* from nonsorbitol fermenters (NSF) and hence narrow down the *E. coli* population to a group of interest. The most common pathogenic *E. coli* that can be targeted by this procedure is *E. coli* O157:H7. Majority of *E. coli* O157:H7 and a few other diarrheagenic *E. coli* strains do not ferment sorbitol. Many studies to isolate *E. coli* O157:H7 have used sorbitol MacConkey agar. For example, Lupindu and friends [14], instead of focusing on every brown-colored, medium-sized round colony grown on MacConkey agar, they went for nonsorbitol fermenters in search for O157:H7. Sorbitol MacConkey agar was supplemented with antimicrobials cefexime and tellurite to inhibit growth of other bacteria such as *Aeromonas* and *Proteus* species and thus improving the recognition of nonsorbitol fermenting *E. coli*. The plates were inoculated with sample suspension and incubated at 37°C for 24 h. Nonsorbitol fermenting bacteria appeared colorless. NSF *E. coli* were confirmed by biochemical method. In this procedure, where one isolate was selected from each sample, the authors managed to recover 143 NSF *E. coli* isolates from the total of 1046 samples analyzed. The NSF *E. coli* isolates were further analyzed by molecular techniques, for example, PCR and DNA hybridization and serology to determine their virulence genes and pathotypes. Of 95 NSF *E. coli* isolates from cattle, 4 (4.2%) were *E. coli* O157:H7, carrying *vtx2c* genes.

Concentration of *E. coli* isolates can be achieved by molecular techniques where a specific part of the DNA is compared for different isolates. PFGE is one of the commonly used methods to bring together *E. coli* isolates with similar attribute prior to further analyses. Specific base pair sites of the DNA are cut by special enzymes, amplified, and electrophoresed by applying electric voltage in three directions periodically. It is suitable even for comparison of large DNA fragments up to 20 kb. PFGE can be reliably used as final analyses in the outbreak investigation in Ref. [12], but sequencing is becoming an adjunct to PFGE whereby isolates with identical PFGE bands are further subtyped by sequencing to give a more detailed discrimination in Ref. [15]. In outbreak situations, isolates are fingerprinted by PFGE, but detailed discrimination among isolates especially from different outbreak in different locations is obtained by

http://dx.doi.org/10.5772/67390

sequencing. For example, Turabelidze and colleagues [16] sequenced pathogenic *E. coli* that was congregated by PFGE. It was reported that these isolates had identical PFGE band, but their differences were revealed by sequencing. Likewise, Trees et al. [17] sequenced 240 isolates related to outbreaks from different sources by PFGE fingerprinting. As a result, whole genome sequencing of 228 isolates showed that they were Shiga toxin-producing *E. coli*, whereas other 12 isolates were non-Shiga toxin-producing diarrheagenic *E. coli*.

Moreover, *E. coli* isolates can be brought together by making use of common antigenic features they possess. Antibodies specific to the bacteria antigen are used to trap the bacteria in enrichment broth. Magnetic beads are coated with specific antibodies for specific bacteria antigen. When beads are applied to the culture broth, antigen will attract antibody resulting in bacteria-bead complex. The complexes are brought together by a magnetic field and concentrate at the bottom of the tube. After decantation, concentrated bacteria-bead complexes are inoculated on a solid media and incubated at 37°C for 24 h. The culture is then analyzed by other methods such as PCR or sequencing. Immunomagnetic separation (IMS) can be used to isolate different bacterial and fungal species. Different strains of Shiga toxin-producing *E. coli* can be isolated by this procedure. These include all Shiga toxin-producing *E. coli* with somatic antigen O157, O26, O45, O103, O111, O113, O121, and O145 [18].

Chromogenic media can also be used to concentrate bacteria possessing some enzymes whose action on sugars brings changes that are detected and depicted by indicating color change. *E. coli* are distinguished from other coliforms by the presence of β-glucuronidase activity on glucuronide. Examples of chromogenic media for coliform discrimination are Brilliance *E. coli* agar and Petrifilm Select *E. coli* count plate. Apart from differentiating the coliforms, these media can be used to sort out between β-glucuronidase positive and negative *E. coli* since there are a few *E. coli* strains that are β-glucuronidase negative, for example, *E. coli* O157:H7 [19]. Beta-glucuronidase positive isolates will appear purple on Brilliance *E. coli* agar or dark-green on Petrifilm Select *E. coli* count plate. The use of chromogenic media is usually followed by analyses by other techniques, for example, PCR, PFGE, or sequencing [20].

6. Storage of *E. coli* isolates

Preservation of bacteria aims at slowing the rate of harmful reactions in bacteria cultures so as to maintain viability and genetic attributes for future use. When imminent analyses require intact live cell, the storage method becomes very important. Different methods can be used to store pure *E. coli* and other bacteria isolates for future analyses [21]. Removal of water from the bacteria culture (drying) can be one option in preserving bacteria cells, while low temperature storage can also reduce the rate of chemical reaction in the cell culture and hence prolong bacteria viability. Drying of the bacteria cells may involve freeze and vacuum drying. In freeze drying, also called lyophilization or cryodesiccation, bacteria are suspended in a medium which maintain their viability through freezing, water removal, and storage. Principally, the bacteria in 15% glycerol suspension are frozen on dry ice or liquid nitrogen and subjected to high vacuum line that allows bacteria to dry through water sublimation. In vacuum drying, the bacteria are dried over calcium chloride in vacuum. Both freeze and vacuum-dried bacteria cultures are stored at 4°C for long time. Low temperature storage of bacteria involves keeping bacteria at low temperatures, ranging from 4 to −80°C. Freezing usually requires addition of glycerol or sugars as cryoprotectants. Deep freezing is the most common preservation method, which maintains both survival and similarity of bacteria population compared with other methods. The choice of the method of preservation depends on several factors, including the nature of bacteria, desired length of time of storage, analysis strategy, and study objectives.

Short period preservation, for example, for days or a week, bacteria can be stored under refrigeration temperatures. Pure bacteria culture is grown on agar slants or plates of nondifferential media and stored at 4°C. Screw-capped tubes are recommended when agar slants are used in bacteria preservation. Cultures on Petri dishes should be protected from contamination and rapid drying by sealing the plates with parafilm and stored inverted. Screw-capped tubes with hot sterile media are inclined at an angle to allow the media to solidify into a slant. A loopful of pure bacteria culture is inoculated onto the slant surface and incubated at 37°C for 24 h. The slant is then refrigerated for future use of bacteria.

Freezing is another method used to store bacteria whereby, the degree of coldness corresponds to length of storage period. The colder the storage temperature, the longer the culture will retain viable cells. Freezing temperatures of −20 to −40°C, which is achieved by most laboratory freezers, can be used to preserve bacteria for up to 1 year. Low temperature of −80°C can preserve bacteria for longer than 3 years, whereas cryofreezing at temperatures below −130°C, usually in liquid nitrogen, can preserve bacteria for more than 10 years.

Freezing may damage or kill bacteria cells due to resultant physical and chemical processes taking place. During freezing, water in the bacteria cell is converted to ice and solutes accumulate in the residual free water. Ice crystals formed can damage the cell membrane and the negative solute concentration can denature cell biomolecules. Cryoprotectants such as glycerol lower the freezing point of the bacteria suspension and thus prevent extracellular ice crystal formation and build-up of negative salt concentration. Besides, the lethal intracellular freezing is usually avoided by slow cooling or progressive freezing that allows sufficient water to leave the cell during freezing of extracellular fluid. A slow progressive freezing at a cooling rate of 1°C/min can be achieved by using a rate controlled freezer. Alternatively, similar results can be obtained by "snap freezing." Bacteria cells are snap-frozen by immersing the well-labeled 15% glycerol cell suspension containing cryotubes in dry ice or liquid nitrogen before storing them in freezer (−20 to −80°C) or in liquid nitrogen tank (−196°C) [22].

Bacteria cultures for freeze preservation can be prepared by inoculating a loopful of bacteria culture into nondifferential sterile broth such as nutrient broth followed by 37°C incubation for 24 h. This broth with pure bacteria culture is mixed with glycerol to make it 15–20% glycerol. Pure glycerol is a thick viscous liquid that needs dilution for practical handling. One-to-one dilution of pure glycerol with sterile normal saline is usually required, for example, 100 ml of glycerol is mixed with 100 ml of normal saline. As a result, for any required amount of pure glycerol, the diluted volume should be doubled. For example, if you want to store bacteria in 20% glycerol broth in a cryovial of 2 ml capacity, you need to put 600 μl of culture broth into a cryovial and add 400 μl of diluted glycerol. This 1 ml culture broth of 20% glycerol can be stored at −20, −80, or −196°C.

All *E. coli* strains can be revived by inoculation on blood agar, nutrient agar, or any nonselective media. A loopful of culture is inoculated onto the agar and incubated at 37°C for 18–24 h. Do not allow to thaw whenever frozen cultures intended for further storage are in use.

7. Characterization of *E. coli* isolates

Characterization includes detection of bacteria isolates from different sources and typing of bacteria isolates of same species. *E. coli* can be characterized by different methods, depending on what attribute is targeted. The methods are categorized as serology, molecular techniques, or cytopathic assays. Molecular characterization includes numerous techniques such as PCR, DNA hybridization, PFGE, restricted fragment length polymorphism (RFLP) and multilocus variable-number tandem repeat analysis (MLVA) to mention a few. These variable methods of bacteria typing have previously been summarized and compared in Ref. [19]. A combination of different methods can be used to complement each other especially when accurate diagnosis is required in a public health threat. A good example of combination of different characterization methods is the work reported by Sabat et al. [23], whereby isolates confirmed to possess somatic antigen O157 by agglutination test were further characterized by PCR subtyping of verotoxigenic (vtx) genes, O:H serotyping, Vero cell assay, sorbitol fermentation, β-glucuronidase activity, dot blot hybridization, and PFGE.

7.1. Serotyping

Presence of antigenic components that characterize a specific *E. coli* strain can be detected by using specific antibodies, for instance, presence of somatic antigen O, capsular antigen K, and flagella antigen H can be detected by agglutination tests and using specific antisera. The somatic and flagella antigens are tested against each specific antiserum, or they are tested against pools of antisera first and then tested against each of the specific antisera from the positive pools. The number of positive antisera is used in O and H antigen nomenclature, for example, *E. coli* O113:H21, O142:H34, and O157:H7. There are more than 180 O somatic antigens and more than 50 H-flagella antigens that are known and used as reference in *E. coli* serotyping. [24]. *E. coli* antigen serotyping has been described in detail by Ørskov and Ørskov [25].

7.2. Polymerase chain reaction (PCR)

Polymerase chain reaction is performed to characterize *E. coli* strains by targeting different virulence genes coding for different virulence factors. Common virulence factors for IPEC include verocytotoxin1, verocytotoxin 2, intimin, heat-stable enterotoxin, human variant, heat-stable enterotoxin, porcine variant, heat labile enterotoxin, and invasive plasmid antigen (**Table 2**). These virulence genes can be detected using multiplex DEC PCR kit as previously described in Ref. [26].

EXPEC commonly carry virulence factor causing urinary tract or nervous tissue infection characterized by syndromes such as urosepsis, pyelonephritis, prostatitis, cystitis, and meningitis. More than 30 virulence factors carried by EXPEC have been reported in Refs. [27, 28].

Virulence factor	Gene target	Primer sequence (5′-)	Amplicon size (bp)
Verocytotoxin 1	*vtx1*	GTTTGCAGTTGATGTCAGAGGGA	260
		CAACGAATGGCGATTTATCTGC	
Verocytotoxin 2	*vtx2*	GCCTGTCGCCAGTTATCTGACA	420
		GGAATGCAAATCAGTCGTCACTC	
Intimin	*Eae*	GGYCAGCGTTTTTTCCTTCCTG	377
		TCGTCACCARAGGAATCGGAG	
Heat-stable enterotoxin-human	*estA*-human	TTTCGCTCAGGATGCTAAACCAG	151
		CAGGATTACAACACAATTCACAGCAGTA	
Heat-stable enterotoxin-porcine	*estA*-porcine	CTTTCCCCTCTTTTAGTCAGTCAACTG	160
		CAGGATTACAACAAAGTTCACAGCAG	
Heat-labile enterotoxin	*eltA*	AAACCGGCTTTGTCAGATATGATGA	479
		TGTGCTCAGATTCTGGGTCTCCT	
Invasive plasmid antigen	*ipaH*	TTGACCGCCTTTCCGATACC	647
		ATCCGCATCACCGCTCAGAC	

Table 2. Gene target, primer sequence, and amplicon size for common intestinal pathogenic *E. coli* virulence factors (Adapted from Persson et al. [26]).

These include *papA*, *papC*, *papEF*, *papG*, *papG* II (±III), *papG* III (±II), *papG* II + III, *sfa*, *focDE*, *sfaS*, *focG*, *afa/draBC*, *iha*, *bmaE*, *gafD*, *fimH*, *hlyD*, *cnf1*, *cdtB*, *fyuA*, *iutA*, *iroN*, *ireA*, *kpsM* II, K1 *kpsM*, K2 *kpsM*, *kpsMT* III, *rfc*, *cvaC*, *traT*, *iss*, *ibeA*, *ompT*, H7 *fliC*, *malX*, and *ibeA*. Commercial multiplex PCR kits are available for detection different virulence genes for EXPEC.

Verocytotoxin (*vtx*) genes form the most variable group of IPEC virulence factors that can further be characterized by PCR into *vtx1* and *vtx2*. Within *vtx1* and *vtx2* groups further subtyping can be done as previously described in Ref. [29]. As a result, 10 subtypes have been identified, three for *vtx1* (*vtx1a*, *vtx1c* and *vtx1d*) and seven for *vtx2* (*vtx2a*, *vtx2b*, *vtx2c*, *vtx2d*, *vtx2e*, *vtx2f* and *vtx2g*). This subtyping is important because the subtype differ in virulence and disease syndrome they cause. Moreover, these details are needed when comparison of isolates from different cases/outbreaks is desired.

Detection of virulence factors and genetic relatedness of *E. coli* isolates can also be assessed by DNA hybridization. This a phenomenon whereby a single strand of DNA anneals to a complementary single-stranded DNA fragment (probe) to form a hybrid. Since the probe is labeled, formation of a hybrid molecule is detected and hence showing presence of its complementary (target) nucleic acid strand. Apart from detection of conventional virulence genes, DNA hybridization can be used as a complementary to PCR to check for additional virulence factors [14, 30]. Analyses of additional virulence factors by hybridization can assist in differentiation of closely related isolates. For instance, EPEC pathotypes possess *eae* gene, and they can be differentiate into classical EPEC and A/EEC through DNA hybridization. Classical EPEC possesses *bfp* that codes for bundle-forming pili (BFP) [14, 31]. Different DNA probes can be used in hybridization such as *vtx1*, *vtx2*, *eae*, enterohaemolysin (*ehxA*), EPEC adherence factor (*EAF*), bundle-forming pilus (*bfpA*), *saa*, *astA*, *and vtx2f*. The protocols for DNA hybridization have previously explained in Refs. [30, 32, 33].

7.3. DNA sequencing

This is the determination of precise order of bases in the nucleotides that make a specific segment of a DNA. Apart from characterization of genetic material for the purpose of identification of *E. coli* strain, DNA sequencing assist in comparison of genetic makeup from different sources, for example, in assessment of the association of different disease outbreak. Generally, sequencing use electrophoresis to separate pieces of DNA into bands. DNA molecules move through the gel when an electric current is applied and molecules are separated according to size, small molecules move faster. During sequencing, bases are tagged with fluorescence dyes, each base type producing a different color, for example, thymine = blue, cytosine = green, adenine = red, and guanine = yellow. Artificial modified bases are added to the DNA mixture. DNA molecules will undergo copying many times. When one of the modified bases is incorporated into the DNA molecule, elongation of the chain stops and all DNA pieces in that batch will have an ending with that particular modified base. The next batch of DNA copy will have a different artificial base at the end and so on. As a result, different DNA batches will end with different base T, A, G, and C, each with a specific color. So the base sequence in the assembled DNA material will be determined by a color pattern of the last (modified) base. The information is stored in computer memory and used for interpretation. This is a traditional Sanger sequencing. Besides, the fast advancing technology is taking the investigative life science from a few DNA fragments analysis into another level of whole genome sequencing. Next Generation Sequencing analyses the entire genome in a short time of single sequencing run. As a result, analysis and comparison of whole genome of isolates lead to correct diagnostic inference. Principally, next generation sequencing is similar to conventional Sanger method, but the former, through sequencing by synthesis, allows detection of single bases as they are incorporated into a growing DNA strand until the whole genome is read. Moreover, millions of reactions take place in parallel and many samples can be analyzed at once.

Sequencing is superior to other methods in characterization of genetic material. For example, whole genome sequencing can detect false positive and false negative clonal relationship of isolates from PFGE fingerprinting [34]. Regardless of the approach to the genome as a whole, the actual process of DNA sequencing is the same. Guidelines and protocols for sequencing are described in detail by a number of researchers in Refs. [35, 36], such that it is possible for many laboratories to manage the procedure.

7.4. Phenotypic characterization of *E. coli*

The genetic expression of *E. coli*, especially pathogenic *E. coli*, can be evaluated by applying the toxin extract from the bacteria to the monolayer Vero cell culture. Cytopathic effects to the cells will indicate virulence activities of the genes. Details of cytotoxic effect assay on Vero cell have been documented in Ref. [37]. Mouse inoculation can also be done to assess virulence of genes.

8. Common *E. coli* pathotypes

Intestinal pathogenic *E. coli* form a large proportion of pathogenic *E. coli*. They include VTEC, EPEC, ETEC, EAEC, DAEC, and EIEC.

Verocytotoxigenic *E. coli* (VTEC) produces verocytotoxins also known as Shiga toxins. The most common VTEC is O157:H7 strain. VTEC are characterized by possession of genes encoding for *vtx1* and *vtx2*, although they carry other virulence genes such as *eae* and *ehxA*. Animals are principal reservoirs of VTEC, and the main route of transmission is fecal-oral. In humans, especially children and elderly, VTEC cause abdominal cramps associated with diarrhea or dysentery. Complicated cases of VTEC infection may lead to HUS. VTEC can be isolated from different sources by different approaches, but the choice will depend on the objectives. Reliance on sugar fermentation ability, for example, sorbitol or presence of specific enzymes, for example, beta-glucuronidase, may lead to focus on specific fraction of the pathogen. On the other hand, targeting verocytotoxin-producing genes will give the overall burden of VTEC from a target source. In this scenario, the use of IMS technique may be recommended [28]. Characterization of isolates for VTEC detection may include immunological methods by using specific antibodies against target VTEC strain or PCR by targeting specific genes. VTEC isolates typing can be done by serology, using specific antisera, PFGE, DNA hybridization, and sequencing.

Enteropathogenic *E. coli* (EPEC) possess *eae* just as do some VTEC strains. As a result they cause attaching and effacing lesion and hence diarrhea. Classical EPEC differs from atypical EPEC (A/EEC) by possession of *bfpA* gene. However, atypical EPEC is a more prevalent cause of diarrhea [38]. Human EPEC infection follows fecal-oral route and isolation can be done from different sources such as water, food, animal, and environment. However, characterization emphasize should be put on distinguishing EPEC from VTEC by presence of *eae* gene and absence of vtx genes. Also, classical EPEC and atypical EPEC should be differentiated by assessing the presence of *bfpA* gene that encode for bundle-forming pili. These features can be determined by characterization procedures such as PCR and DNA hybridization [14]. PFGE typing can be applied to compare strains during outbreaks.

Enterotoxigenic *E. coli* (ETEC) are responsible for watery diarrhea in humans due to impaired sodium absorption and enhanced chloride secretion caused by enterotoxins. Fecal-oral contamination is responsible for transmission through food and water, and the syndrome is common to travellers and children. A simple procedure for detection of ETEC from stool has been described earlier in Ref. [38]. Heat-stable and heat-labile enterotoxins encoded by heat-stable enterotoxin (*estA*) and heat-labile enterotoxin (*eltA*) genes, respectively, are responsible. These genes can be easily detected by serological assays [39] and multiplex DEC PCR.

Enteroaggregative *E. coli* (EAEC) causes acute and persistent diarrhea in humans. This group has diverse strains differing in many aspects but have a common feature of forming a "stacked brick" pattern of adhesion to the human epithelial cell line HEp-2. This feature is used in HeLa cell adherence method to detect EAEC strains [40]. They often produce heat-stable toxin EAST1, Shigella enterotoxin (ShET1), and Haemolysin E, which cause host cell damage and induce inflammation leading to diarrhea especially in travellers, children, and immunocompromised patients. The EAEC strains are found in mixed infections whereby isolation by MacConkey ager, detection by conventional biochemical methods, and PCR and typing by PFGE are possible [41].

Diffusely adherent *E. coli* (DAEC) are responsible for acute diarrhea in humans. DAEC are characterized by the ability to adhere to Hep-2 cells in a diffuse fashion as confirmed by HeLa cells assays. Isolation is done conventionally and detection by PCR can be done by targeting Afa/Dr genes [42].

Enteroinvasive *E. coli* (EIEC) cause profuse diarrhea or dysentery in human through mechanical damage of host epithelial cell by using adhesin protein for binding and invading/entering intestinal cells. They do not produce toxin. EIEC resembles Shigella species biochemically and genetically. Most of them do not ferment lactose. Following conventional isolation methods, EIEC are detected by invasion plasmid antigens (*ipaH*) gene-targeted PCR [43]. The invasiveness of EIEC can be assessed by plaque formation on HeLa cell or guinea pig conjunctivitis assays.

Extra-intestinal pathogenic *E. coli* (EXPEC) cause a wide range of bacteraemia-associated disease syndromes. EXPEC have been isolated in patients with cystitis, pyelonephritis, or prostatitis [28]. Other syndromes associated with EXPEC include septic arthritis or pyomyositis, nontraumatic meningitis, or hematogenous osteomyelitis and pneumonia [44]. This group is comprised of UPEC, NMEC, and SEPEC [1]. Infection normally follows fecal-oral route.

Samples to collect will depend on infected system; urine samples can be collected for urinary tract infection-related syndromes, such as cystitis, Pyelonephritis, or Prostatitis [28], whereas blood, joint fluid, psoas fluid, or sputum are target samples when nonurinary syndromes are concerned [44]. Isolation of *E. coli* for EXPEC detection can follow methods that have been mentioned previously for other pathotypes. Detection of EXPEC can be done by multiplex PCR targeting different genes some of which have been previously described and dot blot hybridization [1, 20, 27, 28]. Typing of isolates from different sources can be done by different procedures including PFGE [20].

9. The viable but nonculturable (VBNC) state

E. coli viability has been reported to decrease when the cells are exposed to direct sunlight because they enter a viable but nonculturable (VBNC) state, while retaining pathogenic ability [45]. Some factors that are directly or indirectly linked to sample collection, storage, or processing may contribute toward *E. coli* entering VBNC state. These include nutrient starvation, elevated or lowered osmotic concentration, oxygen concentration, exposure to heavy metals or food preservatives, direct sunlight, and incubation outside normal temperature range [46]. These factors may lead to false-negative outcomes because *E. coli* does not grow on standard laboratory media when they are under VBNC state. When some of VBNC inducing factors are difficult to avoid, then *E. coli* detection methods that do not rely on viable or live cells, for example, DNA-dependent methods such as PCR, can be a perfect option.

10. Conclusion

Dealing with a diverse group of bacteria like *E. coli* may present a challenge. Knowledge on basics of *E. coli* in terms of isolation and characterization may help in planning, setting objectives, and execution of *E. coli*-related research. One should bear in mind that choice of one isolation or characterization approach may lead to a different output compared to another approach.

The current procedures for *E. coli* isolation and characterization take at least 72 h and sometimes even more time. The need to work on viable bacteria cells may be contributing much to this lengthy procedure. Working on the genetic material right from the sample could help to shorten the time spent from isolation of *E. coli* from sample to outcome. This should be the direction of future research.

Author details

Athumani Msalale Lupindu

Address all correspondence to: amsalale@yahoo.com

Department of Veterinary Medicine and Public Health, College of Veterinary and Medical Sciences, Sokoine University of Agriculture, Morogoro, Tanzania

References

[1] Köhler CD, Dobrindt U. What defines extraintestinal pathogenic *Escherichia coli*? International Journal of Medical Microbiology. 2011;**301**:642-647. DOI: 10.1016/j.ijmm.2011.09.006

[2] Kirk MD, Pires SM, Black RE, Caipo M, Crump JA, Devleesschauwer, B, et al. World Health Organization estimates of the global and regional disease burden of 22 foodborne bacterial, protozoal, and viral diseases, 2010: a data synthesis. PLoS Medicine. 2015;**12**(12):e1001921. DOI: 10.1371/journal.pmed.1001921

[3] US Geological Survey. USGS Water-Quality Information [Internet]. 2007 [Updated: May, 2014]. Available from: http://water.usgs.gov/owq/FieldManual/Chapter7/index.html [Accessed: 7 August, 2016]

[4] Arthur TM, Nou X, Kalchayanand N, Bosilevac JM, Wheeler T, Koohmaraie M. Survival of *Escherichia coli* O157:H7 on cattle hides. Applied and Environmental Microbiology. 2011;**77**(9):3002-3008. DOI: 10.1128/AEM.02238-10

[5] Pope M, Bussen M, Feige M, Shadix L, Gonder S, Rodgers C, et al. Assessment of the effects of holding time and temperature on *Escherichia coli* densities in surface water samples. Applied Environmental Microbiology. 2003;**69**(10):6201-6207. DOI: 10.1128/AEM.69.10.6201-6207.2003

[6] Achá SJ, Kühn I, Mbazima G, Colque-Navarro P, Möllby R. Changes of viability and composition of the *Escherichia coli* flora in faecal samples during long time storage. Journal of Microbiological Methods. 2005;**63**:229-238. DOI: 10.1016/j.mimet.2005.04.024

[7] Masters N, Christie M, Stratton H, Katouli M. Viability and stability of *E. coli* and enterococci populations in fecal samples upon freezing. Canadian Journal of Microbiology. 2015;**61**(7):495-501. DOI: 10.1139/cjm-2015-0020

[8] Irwin PL, Nguyen LHT, Paoli GC, Chen CY. Evidence for a bimodal distribution of *Escherichia coli* doubling times below a threshold initial cell concentration. BMC Microbiology. 2010;**10**(1):207. DOI: 10.1186/1471-2180-10-207

[9] Sargeant JM, Gillespie JR, Oberst RD, Phebus RK, Hyatt DR, Bohra LK, et al. Results of a longitudinal study of the prevalence of *Escherichia coli* O157: H7 on cow-calf farms. American Journal of Veterinary Research. 2000;**61**(11):1375-1379. DOI: 10.2460/ajvr.2000.61.1375

[10] Heuvelink AE, Van Den Biggelaar FLAM, De Boer E, Herbes RG, Melchers WJG, Huis JHJ, et al. Isolation and characterization of verocytotoxin-producing *Escherichia coli* O157 strains from Dutch cattle and sheep. Journal of Clinical Microbiology. 1998;**36**(4):878-882.

[11] Powers EM, Latt TG. Simplified 48-hour IMVic test: an agar plate method. Applied and Environmental Microbiology. 1977;**34**(3):274-279.

[12] Lupindu AM, Dalsgaard A, Msoffe PLM, Ngowi HA, Mtambo MM, Olsen JE. Transmission of antibiotic-resistant *Escherichia coli* between cattle, humans and the environment in

peri-urban livestock keeping communities in Morogoro, Tanzania. Preventive Veterinary Medicine. 2015;**118**(4):477-482. DOI: 10.1016/j.prevetmed.2014.12.005

[13] Wu S, Chouliara E, Jensen LB, Dalsgaard A. Evaluation of petrifilm™ select *E. coli* count plate medium to discriminate antimicrobial resistant *Escherichia coli*. Acta Veterinaria Scandinavica. 2008;**50**(1):38. DOI: 10.1186/1751-0147-50-38

[14] Lupindu AM, Olsen JE, Ngowi HA, Msoffe PLM, Mtambo MM, Scheutz F, et al. Occurrence and characterization of shiga toxin-producing *Escherichia coli* O157:H7 and other non-sorbitol-fermenting *E. coli* in cattle and humans in urban areas of Morogoro, Tanzania. Vector-Borne and Zoonotic Diseases. 2014;**14**(7):503-510. DOI: 10.1089/vbz.2013.1502

[15] Miller JM. Whole-genome mapping: a new paradigm in strain-typing technology. Journal of Clinical Microbiology. 2013;**51**(4):1066-1070. DOI: 10.1128/JCM.00093-13

[16] Turabelidze G, Lawrence SJ, Gao H, Sodergren E, Weinstock GM, Abubucker S, et al. Precise dissection of an *Escherichia coli* O157:H7 outbreak by single nucleotide polymorphism analysis. Journal of Clinical Microbiology. 2013;**51**(12):3950-3954. DOI: 10.1128/JCM.01930-13

[17] Trees E, Strockbine N, Changayil S, Ranganathan S, Zhao K, Weil R, et al. Genome sequences of 228 shiga toxin-producing *Escherichia coli* isolates and 12 isolates representing other diarrheagenic *E. coli* pathotypes. Genome Announcements. 2014;**2**(4):e00718–e00714. DOI: 10.1128/genomeA.00718-14

[18] DebRoy C, Roberts E, Valadez AM, Dudley EG, Cutter CN. Detection of shiga toxin-producing *Escherichia coli* O26, O45, O103, O111, O113, O121, O145, and O157 serogroups by multiplex polymerase chain reaction of the wzx gene of the O-antigen gene cluster. Foodborne Pathogens and Disease. 2011;**8**(5):651-652. DOI: 10.1089/fpd.2010.0769

[19] Soborg B, Lassen SG, Muller L, Jensen T, Ethelberg S, Molbak K, et al. A verocytotoxin producing *E. coli* outbreak with a surprisingly high risk of haemolytic uraemic syndrome, Denmark, September–October 2012. Euro Surveillance. 2013;**18**(2):20350

[20] Mohamed M, Owens K, Gajewski A, Clabots C, Johnston B, Thuras P, et al. Extraintestinal Pathogenic and Antimicrobial-Resistant *Escherichia coli* Contamination of 56 Public Restrooms in the Greater Minneapolis-St. Paul Metropolitan Area. Applied and Environmental Microbiology. 2015;**81**(13):4498-4506. DOI: 10.1128/AEM.00638-15

[21] Jahn M, Seifert J, Hübschmann T, von Bergen M, Harms H, Müller S. Comparison of preservation methods for bacterial cells in cytomics and proteomics. Journal of Integrated Omics. 2013;**3**(1):25-33. DOI: 10.5584/jiomics.v3i1.115

[22] Bonavia A, Thompson M, Schryver B, Ehrhardt R. Bacteria cryopreservation protocol. Protocol Exchange. 2012. DOI: 10.1038/protex.2012.006

[23] Sabat AJ, Budimir A, Nashev D, Sá-Leão R, van Dijl JM, Laurent F, et al. Overview of molecular typing methods for outbreak detection and epidemiological surveillance. Euro Surveillance. 2013;**18**(4):pii: 20380.

[24] O'Sullivan J, Bolton DJ, Duffy G, Baylis C, Tozzoli R, Wasteson Y, et al., editors. Methods for Detection and Molecular Characterisation of Pathogenic *Escherichia coli*. Dublin: Pathogenic *Escherichia coli* Network (PEN); 2007. 34 p.

[25] Ørskov F, Ørskov I. Serotyping of *Escherichia coli*. In: Bergan T., editor. Methods in Microbiology. 1st ed. London: Academic Press; 1984. p. 43-112. DOI: 10.1016/S0580-9517(08)70447-1

[26] Persson S, Olsen KEP, Scheutz A, Krogfelt KA, Gerner-Smidt P. A method for fast and simple detection of major diarrhoeagenic *Escherichia coli* in the routine diagnostic laboratory. Clinical Microbiology and Infection. 2007;**13**:516-524. DOI: 10.1111/j.1469-0691.2007.01692.x

[27] Johnson JR, Stell AL. Extended virulence genotypes of *Escherichia coli* strains from patients with urosepsis in relation to phylogeny and host compromise. Journal of Infectious Diseases. 2000;**181**(1):261-272. DOI: 10.1086/315217

[28] Johnson JR, Kuskowski MA, Gajewski A, Soto S, Horcajada JP, de Anta MTJ, et al. Extended virulence genotypes and phylogenetic background of *Escherichia coli* isolates from patients with cystitis, pyelonephritis, or prostatitis. Journal of Infectious Diseases. 2005;**191**(1):46-50. DOI: 10.1086/426450

[29] Scheutz F, Teel LD, Beutin L, Piérard D, Buvens G, Karch H, et al. Multicenter evaluation of a sequence-based protocol for subtyping Shiga toxins and standardizing Stx nomenclature. Journal of Clinical Microbiology. 2012;**50**(9):2951-2963. DOI: 10.1128/JCM.00860-12

[30] Gerrish RS, Lee JE, Reed J, Williams J, Farrell LD, Spiegel KM, et al. PCR versus hybridization for detecting virulence genes of enterohemorrhagic *Escherichia coli*. Emerging Infectious Diseases. 2007;**13**(8):1253-1255. DOI: 10.3201/eid1308.060428

[31] Jensen C, Ethelberg S, Olesen B, Schiellerup P, Olsen KEP, Scheutz F, et al. Attaching and effacing *Escherichia coli* isolates from Danish children: clinical significance and microbiological characteristics. Clinical Microbiology and Infection. 2007;**13**(9):863-872. DOI: 10.1111/j.1469-0691.2007.01773.x

[32] Scaletsky ICA, Fabbricotti SH, Aranda KR, Morais MB, Fagundes-Neto U. Comparison of DNA hybridization and PCR assays for detection of putative pathogenic enteroadherent *Escherichia coli*. Journal of Clinical Microbiology. 2002;**40**(4):1254-1258. DOI: 10.1128/JCM.40.4.1254-1258.2002

[33] Anjum MF, Lucchini S, Thompson A, Hinton JC, Woodward MJ. Comparative genomic indexing reveals the phylogenomics of *Escherichia coli* pathogens. Infection and Immunity. 2003;**71**(8):4674-4683. DOI: 10.1128/IAI.71.8.4674-4683.2003

[34] Salipante SJ, SenGupta DJ, Cummings LA, Land TA, Hoogestraat Dr, Cookson BT. Application of whole-genome sequencing for bacterial strain typing in molecular epidemiology. Journal of Clinical Microbiology. 2015;**53**(4):1072-1079. DOI: 10.1128/JCM.03385-14

[35] Metzker ML. Sequencing technologies—the next generation. Nature Reviews Genetics. 2010;**11**(1):31-46. DOI: 10.1038/nrg2626

[36] Kwong JC, McCallum N, Sintchenko V, Howden BP. Whole genome sequencing in clinical and public health microbiology. Pathology—Journal of the RCPA . 2015;**47**(3):199-210. DOI: 10.1097/PAT.0000000000000235

[37] El-Housseiny GS, Aboulwafa MM, Hassouna NA. Cytotoxic activities of some *Escherichia coli* isolates: possible mechanisms and approaches for inhibition. Journal of American Science. 2010;**6**(10):269-283.

[38] Ochoa TJ, Contreras CA. Enteropathogenic *E. coli* (EPEC) infection in children. Current Opinion in Infectious Diseases. 2011;**24**(5):478-483. DOI: 10.1097/QCO.0b013e32834a8b8b

[39] Işeri L, Apan TZ, Aksoy A, Koç F, Göçmen JS, Nuristani D. The prevalence of enterotoxigenic *E. coli* isolated from the stools of children aged 0-10 years with diarrhea in mid-Anatolia region, Turkey. Brazilian Journal of Microbiology. 2011;**42**(1):243-247. DOI: 10.1590/S1517-83822011000100030

[40] Aslani MM, Alikhani MY, Zavari A, Yousefi R, Zamani AR. Characterization of enteroaggregative *Escherichia coli* (EAEC) clinical isolates and their antibiotic resistance pattern. International Journal of Infectious Diseases. 2011;**15**(2):e136-e139. DOI: 10.1016/j.ijid.2010.10.002

[41] Sarantuya J, Nishi J, Wakimoto N, Erdene S, Nataro JP, Sheikh J, et al. Typical enteroaggregative *Escherichia coli* is the most prevalent pathotype among *E. coli* strains causing diarrhea in Mongolian children. Journal of Clinical Microbiology. 2004;**42**(1):133-139. DOI: 10.1128/JCM.42.1.133-139.2004

[42] Mansan-Almeida R, Pereira AL, Giugliano LG. Diffusely adherent *Escherichia coli* strains isolated from children and adults constitute two different populations. BMC Microbiology. 2013;**13**(22):1. DOI: 10.1186/1471-2180-13-22

[43] van den Beld M, Reubsaet FAG. Differentiation between Shigella, enteroinvasive *Escherichia coli* (EIEC) and noninvasive *Escherichia coli*. European Journal of Clinical Microbiology and Infectious Diseases. 2012;**31**(6):899-904. DOI: 10.1007/s10096-011-1395-7

[44] Johnson JR, Gajewski A, Lesse AJ, Russo TA. Extraintestinal pathogenic *Escherichia coli* as a cause of invasive nonurinary infections. Journal of Clinical Microbiology. 2003;**41**(12):5798-5802. DOI: 10.1128/JCM.41.12.5798-5802.2003

[45] Pommepuy M, Butin M, Derrien A, Gourmelon M, Colwell, RR, Cormier M. Retention of enteropathogenicity by viable but nonculturable *Escherichia coli* exposed to seawater and sunlight. Applied and Environmental Microbiology. 1996;**62**(12):4621-4626.

[46] Oliver JD. Recent findings on the viable but nonculturable state in pathogenic bacteria. FEMS Microbiology Reviews. 2010;**34**(4):415-425. DOI: 10.1111/j.1574-6976.2009.00200.x

Chapter 11

Escherichia coli Inactivation Using Pressurized Carbon Dioxide as an Innovative Method for Water Disinfection

Tsuyoshi Imai and Thanh-Loc Thi Dang

Additional information is available at the end of the chapter

http://dx.doi.org/10.5772/intechopen.68310

Abstract

Advanced water disinfection technologies that do not produce harmful by-products would be highly desirable. This study presents results for the use of pressurized carbon dioxide (CO_2) and a liquid-film-forming apparatus for disinfection of seawater. The sensitivity of *Escherichia coli* to the pressurized CO_2 was examined for various conditions of pressure, temperature, working volume ratios (WVRs), flow rates, and pressure cycling. Morphology of *E. coli* was observed by using scanning electron microscopy (SEM). A strong correlation between the *E. coli* inactivation efficiency and pressure cycling was detected ($p < 0.001$). The frequency and magnitude of pressure cycling were the key factors responsible for high rates of *E. coli* inactivation during the pressurized CO_2 treatment. The results from linear regression analyses suggest that the model can explain about 91% of the *E. coli* inactivation efficiency ($p < 0.001$). The pressurized CO_2 treatment (at 0.7 MPa, 20°C, 50% WVR) in the process involving pressure cycling ($\Delta P = 0.12$ MPa, 15 cycles) resulted in complete inactivation (5.2 log reduction) of *E. coli* within 3 min. These findings suggest that pressurized CO_2 could be a potentially useful disinfection method for water treatment.

Keywords: bactericidal performance, *Escherichia coli*, inactivation effect, pressurized carbon dioxide, water disinfection

1. Introduction

For more than a century, chlorination has been the most common method used worldwide for drinking water disinfection. Chlorine and chlorine-based compounds are widely used for the control of waterborne pathogens because of their high oxidizing potential, low cost, and residual disinfectant properties that prevent microbial recontamination. Unfortunately, the chemical reaction between chlorine and organic compounds in water generates carcinogenic agents such as trihalomethanes and halogenic acetic acids [1, 2]. Furthermore, some resistant microorganisms may only be inactivated with very high chlorine doses, which can exacerbate the formation of disinfection by-products (DBPs) [3]. Presently, growing concerns about the potential hazards associated with DBPs have boosted efforts to develop chlorination alternatives. Ozonation is effective at inhibiting a variety of pathogens; however, its disadvantages include the high cost and the potential formation of DBPs such as bromate in seawater [4, 5]. Other water treatment methods such as ultraviolet (UV) radiation, ultrasound, cavitation, or heat application can be used for the inactivation of organisms. Although these methods do not produce DBPs or other problematic chemical residues, they require substantial energy consumption and have high operational costs [5]. Besides, the efficiency of UV disinfection is greatly dependent on water quality because the activity of UV light is substantially decreased by turbidity or organic matter present in water [5].

Sterilization by using pressurized CO_2 has been an active research field for decades [6, 7]. CO_2 has been used extensively to sterilize dried food and liquid products via a nonthermal sterilization method [8] because of its effectiveness in inactivating microbes, nontoxicity, and low cost [9]. Prior research on high-pressure CO_2 treatments has investigated the effects of several factors such as pressure, temperature, type of microorganisms, agitation speed, decompression rate, and pressure cycling on the inactivation capacity of this method [6, 8, 10–15]. Most studies have reported that high-pressure operating conditions (4–50 MPa) are required to inactivate significant numbers of pathogens [7, 9]. Subsequently, certain concerns involving high-pressure operations (i.e., the need for heavy-duty pressure equipment, high initial investment costs, energy consumption concerns, and pressure control and management issues) have hampered the implementation of high pressurized CO_2 preservation technology at a large scale within the food industry.

In recent years, pressurized CO_2 has shown great potential as a sustainable disinfection technology in water and wastewater treatment applications [16–22] largely because this method does not generate DBPs [9, 22]. Kobayashi et al. [16, 17] employed CO_2 microbubbles in the treatment of drinking water and succeeded in inhibiting *Escherichia coli* within 13.3 min. However, the pressure (10 MPa) and temperature (35–55°C) requirements for effective inactivation [16, 17] are still high from a practical standpoint. Our research group has developed a novel method that uses low-pressure CO_2 treatments (0.2–1.0 MPa) based on technology that produces high amounts of dissolved gas in water to inactive bacteria and bacteriophages in freshwater [19–21] and seawater [23, 24]. Cheng et al. [19] suggested that the sudden discharge and resulting reduction of pressure could cause cells to rupture via a mechanical mechanism, and further, that this would be lethal to cells at high levels of dissolved CO_2 at 0.3–0.6 MPa and room temperature. Vo et al. [20, 21] demonstrated that acidified water and cellular lipid extraction caused by pressurized CO_2 at 0.7 MPa and room temperature were major factors for efficient disinfection within a treatment time of 25 min.

Previous research has shown that pressure cycling is a potential means to improve bacterial inactivation during pressurized CO_2 treatments [8–10, 13, 15]; nevertheless, the inactivation mechanism is still unknown for this process. Pressure cycling is defined as a repetitive procedure that involves the decompression and compression of CO_2 [9, 10]. Evidence so far suggests that the decompression process may lead to mechanically induced explosive cell ruptures [14], while the compression process may intensify the mass transfer of CO_2 across cell membranes [11–13]. In previous works, the pressure cycling procedure has been conducted with high-pressure operations (8–550 MPa) and with CO_2 discharges between each cycle of decompression and compression [8, 10, 13, 15]. Despite the good bactericidal performance of pressurized CO_2 technology enhanced by pressure cycling [11–13, 15], the high pressure and CO_2 release requirements are drawbacks owing to the costly and complex operating procedures. Presently, it is not clear whether pressure cycling with low-pressure CO_2 treatments (<1.0 MPa) will enhance the bactericidal activity. Therefore, in this study, we examined the effect of pressure cycling on the bactericidal performance of CO_2 at low pressures and with no release of CO_2 between each cycle of raised/lowered pressure.

This study investigated the use of pressurized CO_2 at less than 1.0 MPa for seawater disinfection applications such as ballast water treatment. Comparisons of *E. coli* inactivation caused by pressurized CO_2 and pressurized air were evaluated in both natural seawater and artificial seawater. The inactivation performance of pressurized CO_2 against *E. coli* was examined for various conditions of pressure, temperature, flow rates, and working volume ratios (WVRs). In particular, the influence of pressure cycling on *E. coli* inactivation was evaluated. Changes in cell morphology after pressurized CO_2 treatment were assessed by scanning electron microscopy (SEM). The research objective was to evaluate the bactericidal effectiveness of pressurized CO_2 for disinfecting water, with the goal of addressing the abovementioned emerging problems associated with water disinfection technology.

2. Novel idea: apparatus for forming highly dissolved gas in water

For pressurized CO_2 methods in the field of food preservation, the interaction efficiency between CO_2 and pathogens in the foodstuffs is probably limited at low pressures and ambient temperatures, and consequently, high-pressure (4–50 MPa) or ultra-high-pressure (200–700 MPa) conditions are vital for sufficient inactivation. However, to be more attractive in terms of its economic feasibility, pressurized CO_2 technology needs to be implemented at lower pressures. In this study, we employed the use of a liquid-film-forming apparatus, which enabled improvements in the interaction efficiency but with lower pressures (<1 MPa) for the water disinfection purposes.

The experimental apparatus for disinfection was a stainless steel chamber with an internal volume of 10 L and pressure tolerance up to 1.0 MPa. The device was designed with a solid stream nozzle and shield to enable vigorous agitation of the influent in such a way that produced liquid films along with fine bubbles (**Figures 1–3**). The device was supplemented with CO_2 pressure prior to the treatments. Sample water was then pumped into the device at high speed through a small nozzle and directed onto the shield. The highly pressurized fluid stream thus collided with the bubble-generating shield. Subsequently, numerous gas bubbles,

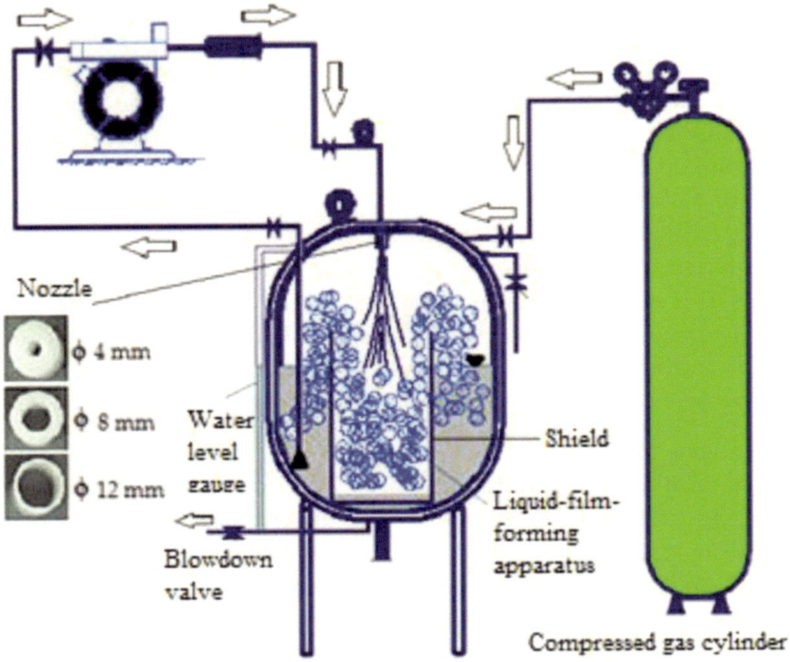

Figure 1. Apparatus for forming highly dissolved gas in water.

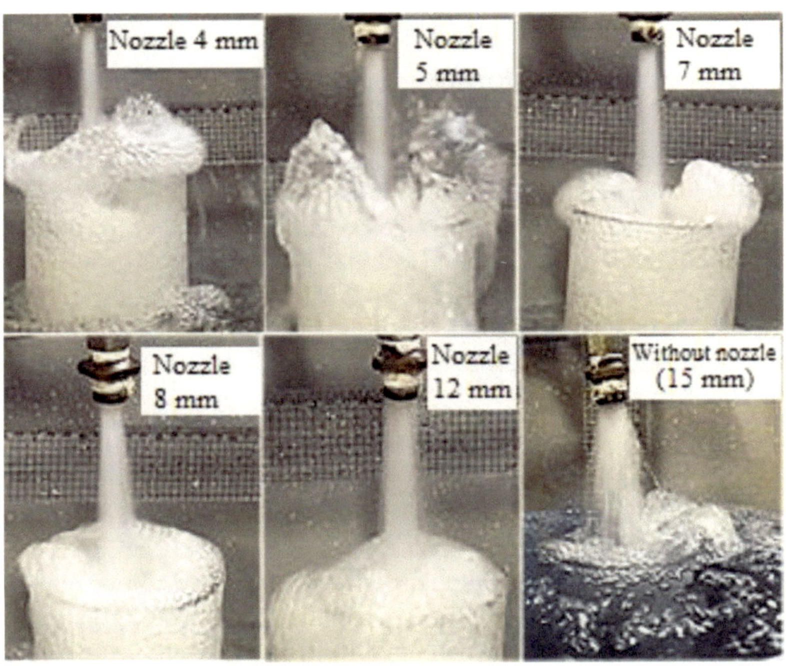

Figure 2. Representative pictures of liquid film formation with various nozzle diameters at a normal pressure in the pipeline.

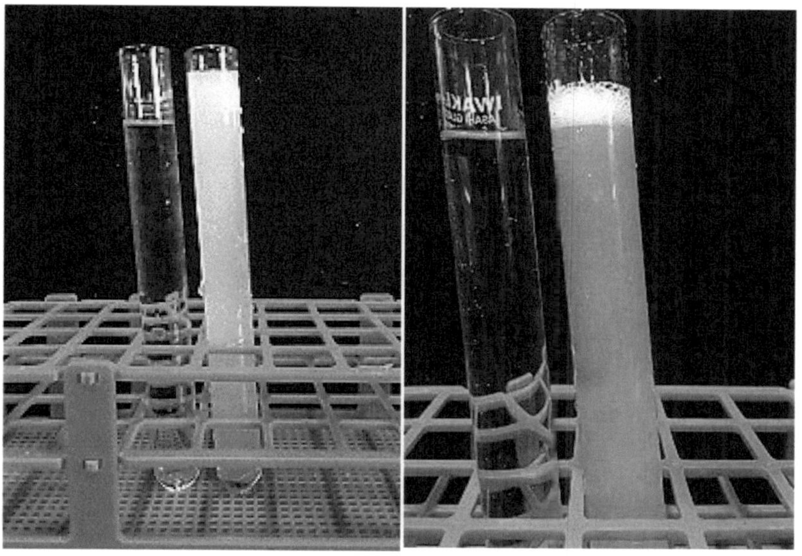

Figure 3. Pictures of an untreated sample and a CO_2-treated sample (the latter contains many small bubbles).

which were generated from inside the shield, were entrained by the ascending bubbles and overcame the shield; these bubbles then floated into the main chamber (outside the shield). Hence, CO_2 transfers took place both within the interior and exterior sides of the thin liquid films. The presence of numerous small bubbles also enhanced the contact area between gas and water and facilitated CO_2 dissolution into water. We hypothesized that the available interfacial contact area between CO_2 and the cell suspension was greatly multiplied in this setup and that the CO_2 transfer efficiency was high. Despite the lower pressures used, the high contact efficiency promoted by this apparatus enabled ample penetration of CO_2 into the cell membranes of *E. coli*.

3. Materials and methods

3.1. Microorganism preparation and enumeration

Stock cultures of *E. coli* (ATCC 11303) were propagated in Luria-Bertani (LB) broth (Wako Chemical Co., Ltd., Osaka, Japan) containing 30 g L^{-1} sodium chloride and incubated for 24 h at 37°C by using a reciprocal shaker set to rotate at 150 rpm. The initial enumeration was approximately 10^9–10^{10} CFU mL^{-1}. The permanent stock was maintained in 20% glycerol at −80°C.

The *E. coli* inoculum for each disinfection experiment was prepared by inoculating 100 μL of bacterial glycerol stock into 100 mL of LB broth containing 30 g L^{-1} sodium chloride. The culture was then incubated for 20 h at 37°C with continuous shaking at 150 rpm. Cells were harvested and washed three times with a 0.9% (w/v) saline solution followed by centrifugation (10 min at 8000 g at room temperature) in a CF15D2 centrifuge (Hitachi, Japan). The pellet was re-suspended in 100 mL saline solution.

E. coli were enumerated by using the plate count technique. Briefly, the samples were diluted into a series of 10-fold dilutions by using autoclaved artificial seawater at 3.4% salinity, and 100 μL of either a diluted or an undiluted sample was plated on LB agar (Wako). For samples with a low number of viable cells, 1 mL of the undiluted sample was poured into agar maintained at 45°C. Colonies growing on each plate were counted after incubating the plates overnight at 37°C. Each sample was analyzed in triplicate.

3.2. Seawater sample preparation

The artificial seawater was prepared by adding artificial sea salt (GEX Inc., Osaka, Japan) to distilled water to obtain a final salinity of 3.4%, as measured with a salinity meter (YK-31SA, Lutron Electronic Enterprice Co., Ltd., Taiwan). As for the preparation of filtered natural seawater, natural seawater (pH = 8.3, salinity 3.3%) was first filtered through a glass fiber filter (GA-100, Advantec, Toyo); then, the seawater was filtered through a membrane filter with a pore size of 0.45 μm (Millipore, Ireland). For all experiments, prepared *E. coli* cultures were added into the artificial/filtered seawater to obtain a bacterial concentration of 5–6 $\log_{10}$ CFU mL^{-1}. The solution was stirred for 30 min to acclimatize the bacteria before starting the experiments. For each batch mode operation, 12 L of samples were prepared, of which 4–5 L were used to restart the system. The pH and temperature of samples were measured with a pH meter (Horiba D-51, Japan).

3.3. Experimental setup

Disinfection experiments were conducted in batch mode (**Figure 4**). Sample water, as the influent, was pumped in one shot into the device. Following the first influx of water, pressurized CO_2 was also injected into the main chamber. System pressure was adjusted by a gas pressure regulator and gas exhaust valve. The fluid was then circulated by pumping inside the system for 25 min. A pump was used to apply a higher pressure than that inside the main chamber to accelerate gas solubilization in water. During the treatment period, the outer wall of the device was kept in contact with cool water by using a water jacket to maintain the initial temperature of the sample at ±1.0°C. The treated water was then collected from a bottom valve of the device.

3.4. Procedure for disinfection experiments

3.4.1. Experimental procedure for investigating the effects of pressure and temperature

To investigate the effects of pressure and temperature, 7 L of sample were pumped into the main chamber by using a 0.2 kW pump (Iwaya-WPT-202), and the fluid was circulated inside the system at a flow rate of 14 L min^{-1} (hydraulic retention time, HRT = 0.5 min). The pump was used to apply 0.12 MPa higher pressure than that inside the main chamber. The sensitivity of bacteria to pressurized CO_2 treatments under different conditions was determined by varying the CO_2 pressure (0.2–0.9 MPa) and seawater temperature (11–28°C) for a 25-min treatment period [23]. Each experiment was conducted in triplicate.

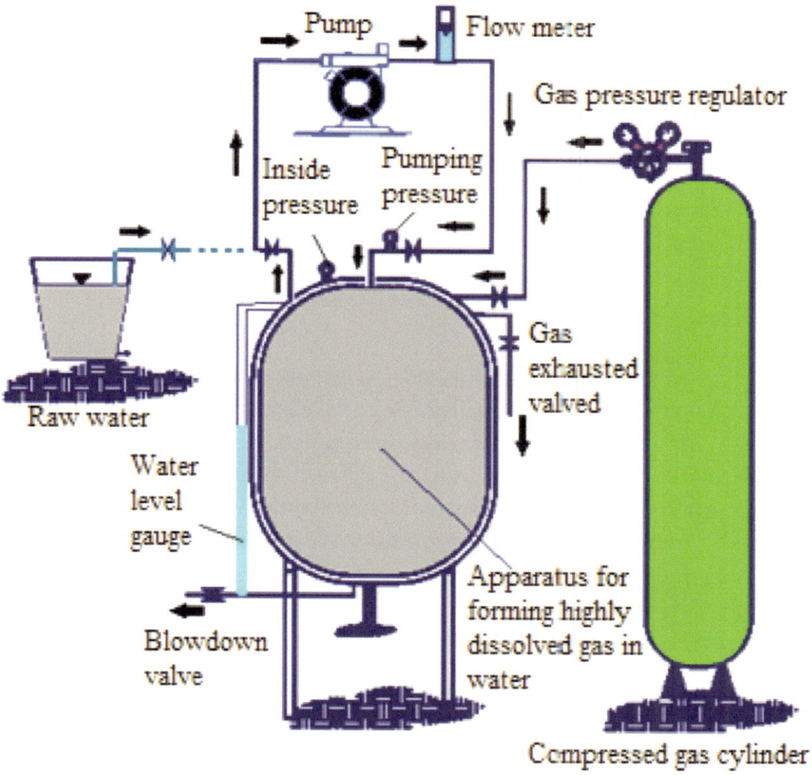

Figure 4. Setup of the water treatment apparatus.

3.4.2. Experimental procedure for investigating the effect of pressure cycling

In previous works, the pressure cycling procedure was conducted with high-pressure operations (8–550 MPa) and with CO_2 discharges between each cycle of decompression and compression [8, 10, 13, 15]. However, such high pressure and CO_2 release are undesirable from an economic standpoint. In order to overcome the above disadvantages, in the present study, we employed a process involving pressure cycling for *E. coli* inactivation but used lower pressures (<1 MPa) and no discharge of CO_2 between each cycle of raised and lowered pressure.

To investigate the effect of pressure cycling, two pumps (0.20 kW, Iwaya-WPT-202, Japan; 0.75 kW, 32 mm × 32 mm SUP-324 M, Toshiba, Japan) and nozzles with various sizes (15 mm height × 4–8 mm diameter) were used to change the flow rate and pressure power of the input (a treatment without a nozzle was also used, whereby the diameter of the pipeline inlet was 15 mm). Pumping pressure and system pressure were measured by pressure gages. The pressure difference ΔP = pumping pressure (MPa) − pressure inside the main chamber (MPa). The water flow rate was measured by a flow meter (GPI, Nippon Flow Cell Co., Ltd., Japan). The recycle number was calculated in relation to the treatment time and HRT, wherein HRT = sample volume/flow rate.

3.4.3. Experimental procedure for investigating the effect of the working volume ratio

The WVR is defined as the ratio between the sample volume and apparatus volume. To examine the effect of WVR, different sample volumes (5, 6, 7, and 8 L) were used to vary the sample volume ratios (50, 60, 70, and 80%). The experiment was conducted with the following two flow rate levels: 14 and 25 L min^{-1}. The water level was measured by using a gauge to evaluate the effect of WVR on the bubble-generating shield inside the main chamber. The HRT and recycle number were calculated as described in Section 3.4.2.

3.5. Scanning electron microscopy

Changes in cell morphology after pressurized CO_2 treatment were assessed by using SEM. The pellets of *E. coli* were immobilized with 2.5% glutaraldehyde in phosphate buffered saline (PBS) for 3 h at 4°C and then rinsed with PBS three times. Next, the samples were soaked in 1.0% osmium tetroxide in cacodylate buffer for 90 min and then washed three times with cacodylate buffer for removal of the fixative. After fixation, the cells were dehydrated by consecutive soaking in increasing concentrations of ethanol solutions (50, 70, 80, 90, 95, and 100%), and this was followed by an ethanol/t-butyl alcohol (v/v = 1:1) treatment for 30 min. The prepared cells were then soaked in t-butyl alcohol two times for 1 h, freeze-dried for 2 h, and sputter coated with gold-palladium. Finally, the cells were examined by using a scanning electron microscope (QuantaTM 3D, FEI Co., USA) at 20 kV [23].

3.6. Statistical analysis

The statistical analysis was done by using the statistical computer program R (version 3.2.2, available at http://cran.R-project.org). Multicollinearity regression was performed to evaluate statistically significant variables of the system with a significance level of 0.05. Predicted values of inactivation efficacy were based on the following first-order regression model:

$$y_i = \beta_0 + \sum \beta_i x_i \quad (1)$$

where y_i represents the predicted responses, x_i is a parameter, β_0 is the model intercept, and β_i is the linear coefficient.

4. Results and discussion

4.1. Bactericidal performance of pressurized CO_2 and pressurized air against *E. coli* in seawater

Bactericidal effects of pressurized CO_2 in comparison with pressurized air against ***E. coli*** in seawater were investigated at three pressure conditions (0.3, 0.7, and 0.9 MPa) and at 20 ± 1°C (**Figure 5**). In general, the disinfection efficiency of the pressurized CO_2 treatment was not different between filtered seawater and artificial seawater. At every operating pressure, the *E. coli* inactivation efficiency of pressurized CO_2 was always higher than that of pressurized air.

http://dx.doi.org/10.5772/intechopen.68310

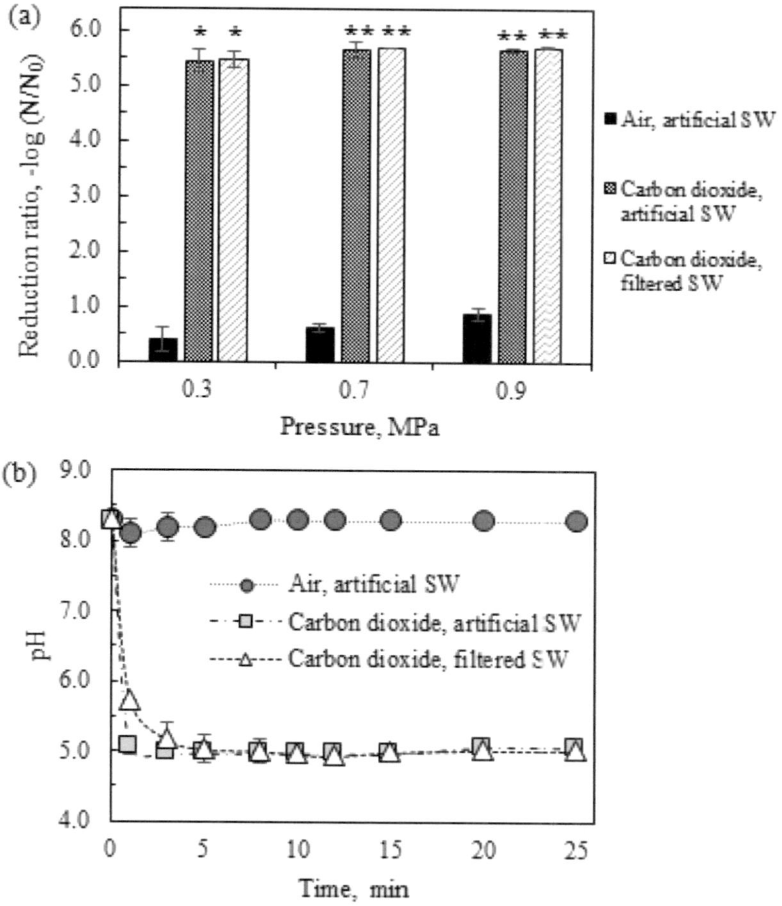

Figure 5. Effect of pressurized CO_2 and pressurized air on (a) *E. coli* inactivation and (b) the pH of seawater (SW). Operating conditions: 0.3–0.9 MPa, 20 ± 1°C, and a working volume ratio (WVR) of 70%. Asterisks (*) and (**) indicate that the *E. coli* load was completely inactivated after 25 and 10 min, respectively.

Approximately 5.4–5.7 log reductions of the *E. coli* load were achieved within 10–25 min by the pressurized CO_2 treatment (this involved complete inactivation of bacterial cells), whereas only 0.4–0.9 log reductions were achieved after 25 min by the pressurized air treatment; these tests involved pressures of 0.3–0.9 MPa (**Figure 5a**).

Pressurized CO_2 reduced the pH of both filtered seawater and artificial seawater to around 5.0 after the first few minutes of exposure time, whereas the pH of pressurized air-treated seawater remained around 8.3 during the treatment period (**Figure 5b**). It has been hypothesized that the decrease in pH caused by pressurized CO_2 is probably a major factor driving the bacterial inactivation process [12, 20, 21, 25]. However, Dang et al. [24] demonstrated that the low pH alone is not the main cause of the bactericidal activity. Perhaps with the concomitant presence of pressure and dissolved CO_2, the low pH prompted the *E. coli* cells to become more permeable, thereby stimulating the process of CO_2 penetration into the cells [24].

4.2. Effects of pressure and temperature

E. coli was disinfected in various pressure conditions (0.2–0.9 MPa) at 20°C (**Figure 6**). In general, *E. coli* inactivation significantly increased with increasing pressure, and higher pressures required shorter exposure times to achieve the same log reduction. For example, a treatment application period of 25 min was required to reduce the *E. coli* load by approximately 5.0 log with pressure applications of 0.2–0.4 MPa, whereas pressure applications of 0.5 and 0.6 MPa resulted in a reduction of the treatment period to 20 and 15 min, respectively. The treatment period was further reduced to 10 min with pressure applications of 0.7–0.9 MPa. However, the increased pressure application from 0.7 to 0.9 MPa did not result in significant increase in the rate of bacterial inactivation. These data indicated that the optimal CO_2 pressure for inactivating *E. coli* was in the range of 0.7–0.9 MPa, and hence, 0.7 MPa was chosen as the optimal pressure condition for effective bactericidal activity [23].

The disinfection efficiency of pressurized CO_2 substantially increased with increasing temperatures (11–28°C) at 0.7 MPa (**Figure 7**). The *E. coli* load was reduced by more than 5.0 log within 25 min of treatment at 11°C, whereas only 20, 12, and 10 min of pressurized CO_2 treatment at 15, 18, and 20–28°C, respectively, were required to reduce the *E. coli* load to a similar extent [23]. Taken together, these findings suggest that *E. coli* inactivation by pressurized CO_2 could be efficiently conducted at low-pressure (0.7 MPa) and ambient temperature

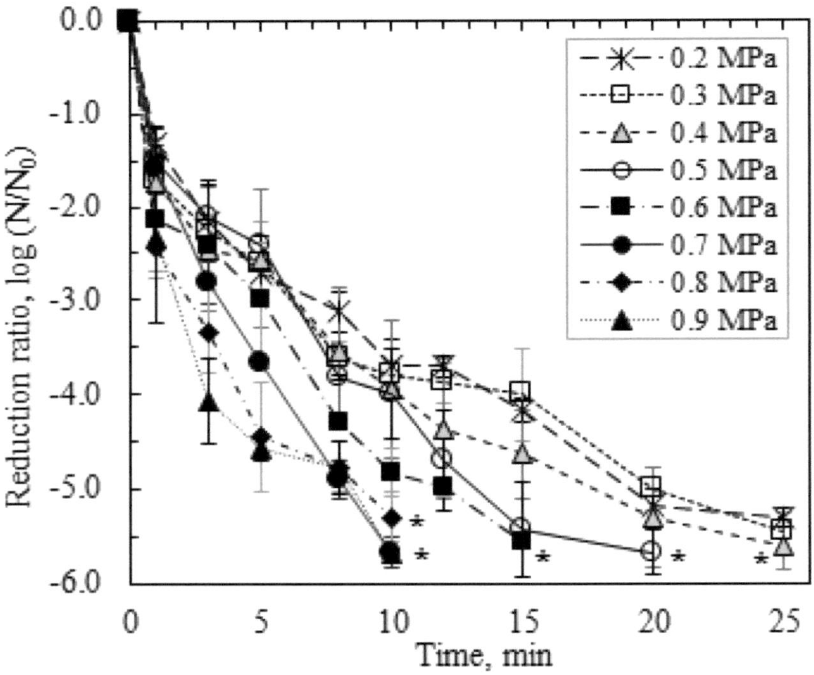

Figure 6. Effect of pressure on *E. coli* inactivation during the pressurized CO_2 treatment at 20 ± 1.0°C and a working volume ratio (WVR) of 70% [23]. Asterisks (*) indicate that no colonies were detected.

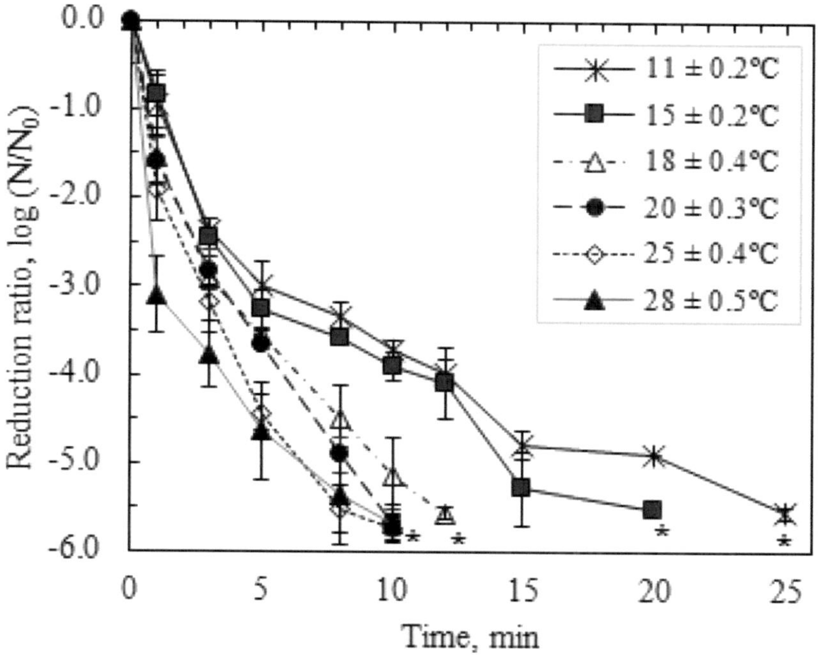

Figure 7. Inactivation of *E. coli* in seawater at various temperatures by using the pressurized CO_2 treatment at 0.7 MPa and a working volume ratio (WVR) of 70% [23]. Asterisks (*) indicate that no colonies were detected.

conditions. On the other hand, after disinfection and decompression, the pressurized CO_2-treated samples were placed at normal conditions to assess the viability of the remaining bacteria. After the 5-d holding period, the number of *E. coli* in the treated samples had not increased, i.e., no regrowth of bacteria was observed.

CO_2 is lipo-hydrophilic in nature, and it can easily penetrate into the phospholipid bilayer of cell membranes [26]. Thus, the increase in CO_2 pressure and temperature may stimulate the diffusion of CO_2 into cells and may increase the fluidity of cell membranes [11, 27]. In the present study, the solubility of CO_2 into seawater was considerably improved by using the liquid-film-forming apparatus. Hence, we speculate that simultaneous effects of pressure, temperature, and high efficiency of contact with this apparatus may have stimulated the process of CO_2 penetration into *E. coli* cells, thereby accelerating the efficiency of the pressurized CO_2 treatment [23].

4.3. Effect of pressure cycling

4.3.1. *Effect of pressure cycling at various pump powers and nozzle diameters*

The effect of pressure cycling on *E. coli* inactivation was investigated by using various nozzle diameters (4–8 mm) (a treatment without a nozzle was also tested, where the diameter of the pipeline inlet was 15 mm) and two pump powers (0.20 and 0.75 kW) to change both the flow rate and ΔP of the input. The disinfection experiments were conducted under 0.7 MPa of pressurized CO_2 at 20 ± 1°C with a WVR of 70% for a duration of 25 min (**Figure 8**). In general, larger nozzle diameters led to higher flow rates (**Figure 8c**) and faster fluid recycling in the treatment system (**Figure 8d**). In contrast, increases in the nozzle diameter reduced the pressure difference ΔP (**Figure 8c**). Furthermore, at the same nozzle diameter, stronger pumping powers improved not only the flow rate but also the pressure difference ΔP of the input (**Figure 8c**). At every nozzle diameter, operation of the pump with 0.75 kW of power (**Figure 8b**) yielded greater inactivation efficiencies than those with 0.20 kW of power (**Figure 8a**).

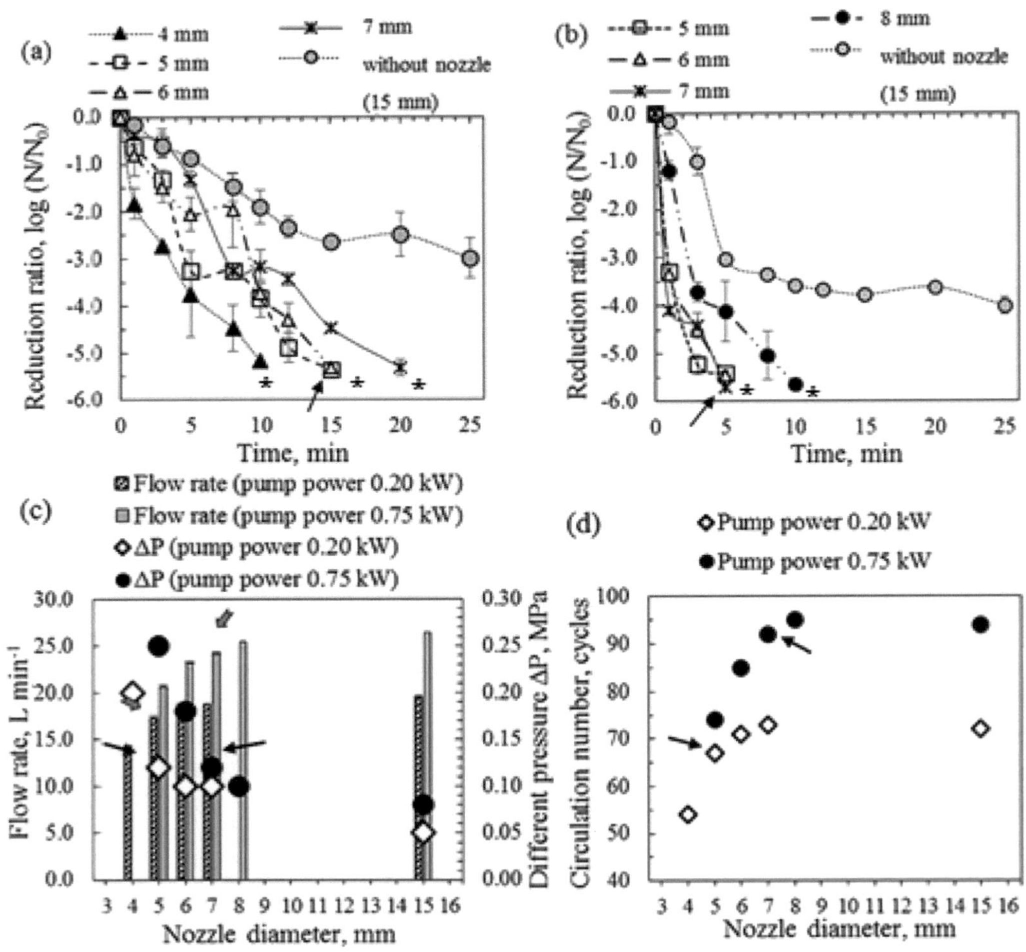

Figure 8. Effect of pressure cycling on the inactivation of *E. coli* in seawater. Effect of (a) 0.20 kW pump power and (b) 0.75 kW pump power along with various nozzle diameters on the inactivation with pressurized CO_2. Influence of different pump powers and nozzle diameters on the (c) flow rate and pressure difference ΔP, and (d) the circulation number. Operating conditions: 0.7 MPa, 20 ± 1°C, and a working volume ratio (WVR) of 70% within a duration of 25 min. Asterisks (*) indicate that no colonies were detected.

http://dx.doi.org/10.5772/intechopen.68310

It is hypothesized that pressure cycling enhances the inactivation efficiency by facilitating the mass transfer of CO_2 into bacterial cell membranes [9, 10]. Thus, an increase in water flow rate can be expected to improve the *E. coli* inactivation. However, our results show that the *E. coli* inactivation efficiency did not increase with higher flow rates or faster recirculation. When 0.20 kW of pumping power was used (**Figure 8a**), the length of treatment periods required for complete inactivation of the *E. coli* load by more than 5.0 log increased with the greater nozzle sizes (i.e., 10 min with the 4-mm nozzle, 15 min with the 5–6-mm nozzles, and 20 min with the 7-mm nozzle, which corresponded to flow rates of 14, 17–19, and 19 L min^{-1}, respectively). Furthermore, the reduction in *E. coli* load was only 3.0 log after 25 min when the device was operated without a nozzle (flow rate = 20 L min^{-1}). A similar finding was found when the pump was operated at 0.75 kW of power (**Figure 8b**); at the higher power, more than a 5.0 log reduction was achieved within 5 min with the 5-mm nozzle (flow rate = 21 L min^{-1}), whereas only a 4.0 log reduction was obtained after 25 min in the treatment lacking a nozzle (flow rate = 26 L min^{-1}). These results indicate that the bactericidal performance of pressurized CO_2 associated with pressure cycling can probably not be attributed to the flow rate alone.

On the other hand, the disinfection efficiency substantially increased with the higher ΔP (**Figure 8**). A 5.4 log reduction in *E. coli* load was achieved within 5 min by the treatment with a ΔP of 0.25 MPa, whereas only a 3.0 log reduction was attained after 25 min by the treatment with a ΔP of 0.05 MPa. When operating the device with the same pump power, as noted above, a larger nozzle diameter resulted in higher water flow rates but weaker ΔP values. Hence, the reduction of ΔP may be considered as a key reason for the phenomenon of low inactivation efficiency at high flow rates. This suggests that the disinfection effect of pressure cycling might be influenced by not only by the frequency of circulation but also by the ΔP.

Noticeably, at the same ΔP value, a faster frequency of circulation substantially augmented the *E. coli* inactivation efficiency (**Figure 8**). For instance, at the same ΔP of 0.12 MPa (generated by a 5-mm nozzle and 0.20 kW pump, and a 7-mm nozzle and 0.75 kW pump), the periods required for complete inactivation of *E. coli* were reduced from 15 to 5 min when the frequency of pressure cycling was raised from 67 cycles/25 min to 92 cycles/25 min, respectively. A similar association between the disinfection efficiency and frequency of pressure cycling was found at ΔP = 0.10 MPa (generated by a 6-mm nozzle and 0.20 kW pump and a 8-mm nozzle and 0.75 kW pump); the associated treatment periods were 15 and 10 min for the recycle numbers corresponding to 71 cycles/25 min and 95 cycles/25 min, respectively. These results affirm the effect of pressure cycling on *E. coli* inactivation during pressurized CO_2 treatment.

Table 1 summarizes the coefficients of correlation for the inactivation efficiency and parameters associated with pressure cycling, including the nozzle diameter (x_1), pressure difference ΔP (x_2), flow rate (x_3), and recycle number (x_4). Based on the Pearson matrix correlation results, *E. coli* inactivation efficiencies were correlated with ΔP values ($r = 0.63$, $p < 0.0001$) and recycle numbers ($r = 0.66$, $p < 0.0001$). The flow rate showed a weak correlation with the inactivation efficiency ($r = 0.09$, $p = 0.3$). Meanwhile, an inverse correlation ($r = -0.35$, $p = 0.0004$) was found between the nozzle diameter and disinfection efficiency. These data indicate that operations with a high flow rate, high ΔP value, large recycle number, and small nozzle diameter will yield greater inactivation efficiencies.

Factor	Symbol code	Unit	*r*	*t*-statistic	*p*-value
Nozzle diameter	x_1	mm	–0.35	–3.64	0.0004*
Pressure difference ΔP	x_2	Pa	0.63	8.08	1.69e-12*
Flow rate	x_3	L min^{-1}	0.09	1.05	0.30
Recycle number	x_4	cycles	0.66	8.73	6.928e-14*

*$p < 0.05$ (significant at the 95% confidence level); df = 98.

Table 1. Correlation coefficients among various operating parameters associated with pressure cycling and the *E. coli* inactivation efficiency.

Regression coefficients, *t*-values, and *p*-values were analyzed for the four factors as shown in **Table 2**. The outcome of the multicollinearity regression model analysis ($R^2 = 0.77$, $p < 0.001$) suggests that the model can explain 77% of the inactivation efficiency of *E. coli*. With bootstrap analysis, the results of multivariate regression analyses were validated. The variables of x_1, x_2, x_3, and x_4 that were found to be associated with pressure cycling in the original analyses were significantly associated with pressure cycling in approximately 8, 28, 3, and 37%, respectively, of the 1000 iterations of the multivariate analyses. Taken together, these findings suggest that the frequency of recirculation (x_4) and the ΔP magnitude of the input (x_2) were key factors that drove the effectiveness pressure cycling.

Although the use of small nozzle diameters was associated with effective inactivation, operating conditions at high ΔP values and low flow rates may be more complex and of lesser economical interest. The highest inactivation efficiency was observed when 5–7 mm nozzle diameters and the 0.75 kW pump were used (**Figure 8b**). Since a large processing capacity is of great commercial interest, the 7 mm nozzle and 0.75 kW pump were used for subsequent experiments.

4.3.2. *Effect of pressure cycling at various WVRs*

The effect of WVR was investigated at four ratios (50, 60, 70, and 80%) by applying a pressure of 0.7 MPa at a temperature of 20 ± 1°C and two flow rates (14 and 25 L min^{-1}) for 25 min (**Figure 9**). As shown in **Figure 9c**, decreasing WVR from 80 to 50% resulted in a decrease in

Source	Coefficient	*t*-statistic	*p*-value
Intercept	–0.63	–0.99	0.33
x_1	–0.13	–3.59	0.0005*
x_2	0.01	7.32	7.8e-11*
x_3	0.10	3.40	0.001*
x_4	0.05	11.29	<2e-16*

*Significant at the 95% confidence level; multiple $R^2 = 0.77$; adjusted $R^2 = 0.76$.
F-statistic = 78.77 with 4 and 95 degrees of freedom, $p < 2.2e\text{-}16$.

Table 2. Regression results showing the influence of operating parameters associated with pressure cycling on the inactivation efficiency (at 20 ± 1°C, system pressure = 0.7 MPa, and working volume ratio (WVR) = 70%).

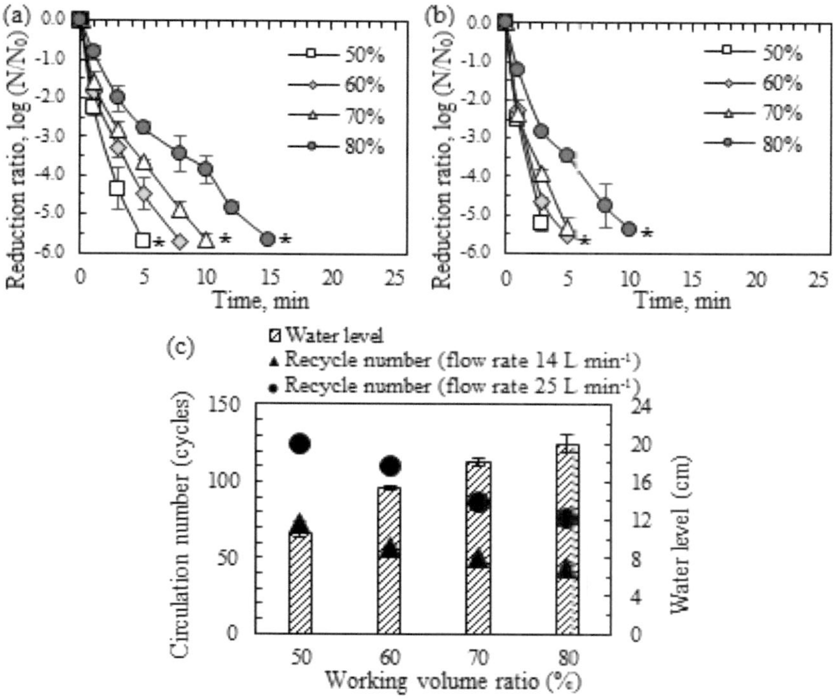

Figure 9. Effect of the working volume ratio (WVR) on the inactivation of *E. coli* in seawater by pressurized CO_2 at 0.7 MPa and 20 ± 1°C with (a) a flow rate of 14 L min^{-1} [23] and (b) a flow rate of 25 L min^{-1}. (c) Influence of the WVR on the circulation number and water level in the main chamber. Asterisks (*) indicate that no colonies were detected.

the water level (22–11 cm) and a faster frequency of pressure cycling. In regard to pressure cycling, the circulation number increased from 44 to 72 cycles with the flow rate of 14 L min^{-1}, and from 78 to 125 cycles with the flow rate of 25 L min^{-1}.

E. coli inactivation efficacy of pressurized CO_2 significantly increased with decreases in the WVR (**Figure 9**). Besides, at every WVR, operations with a high flow rate greatly enhanced the disinfection efficiency. When operating the device with a flow rate of 14 L min^{-1}, an approximate 5.7 log reduction of *E. coli* was achieved within 15 min at 80% WVR, whereas only 5 min was required at 50% WVR to reduce the *E. coli* load to a similar extent (**Figure 9a**; [23]). A similar tendency was found in the case of the 25 L min^{-1} flow rate (**Figure 9b**). The durations required for complete inactivation of *E. coli* were 10 min at 80%, 5 min at 60–70%, and 3 min at 50%.

Pressure cycling boosts the inactivation efficiency by providing a driving force for CO_2 transfer efficiency [9–13]. Recall that at the same flow rate and ΔP, a decrease in WVR increased the frequency of pressure cycling. Hence, it is hypothesized that a smaller WVR may have stimulated the CO_2 transfer across cell membranes and thus improved the bactericidal performance of pressurized CO_2 [11, 28, 29]. In this study, the low inactivation efficiency with a large WVR (i.e., 80%) may be related to the high water level (20–22 cm; **Figure 9c**), which led to submergence of the shield inside the device; this may have in turn decreased bubble formation via shield interactions [23, 24]. In contrast, the operations with smaller WVRs helped not only to promote a greater efficiency for CO_2 bubble generation but also increased the speed of the pressure cycling. Consequently, CO_2 supported by the high pressure and high efficiency of interactions in the apparatus easily penetrated into the cell membranes, thereby accelerating the *E. coli* inactivation efficiency.

Regarding the effect of WVR in pressure cycling treatments, Pearson regression tests showed that *E. coli* inactivation efficiency was strongly correlated with the recycle number ($r = 0.95$, $p < 0.001$). The regression coefficient, *t*-value, and *p*-value were analyzed with regard to the recycle number at various WVRs and flow rates (**Table 3**). According to the regression analysis, the experimental results fit the linear model shown in the following equation:

$$Y = 0.736 + 0.285 \times x_4 \quad (2)$$

Here, x_4 is the recycle number (cycles), and Y is reduction ratio ($-\log N/N_0$) of *E. coli* caused by pressurized CO_2.

As shown in **Table 3**, the *t* values of the regression model were positive and significant ($p < 0.05$), thus indicating that the model result was significant. The outcome of the linear regression model analysis ($R^2 = 0.91$, $p < 0.001$) suggests that 91% of the variation in the *E. coli* inactivation efficiency was explained by the frequency of pressure cycling ($\Delta P = 0.12$ MPa, flow rate = 14–25 L min^{-1}). Predicted values of *E. coli* reduction ratios were calculated based on Eq. (2), and the data are summarized in **Table 4** along with the experimental results. The predicted values were fairly similar to the experimental results, thus suggesting that the model could adequately describe the strong relationship between pressure cycling and bactericidal activity ($p < 0.05$). Taken together, these findings affirm that at the same ΔP, faster pressure cycling can achieve a greater *E. coli* inactivation efficiency.

Dillow et al. [13] reported that an increase of pressure cycling from 3 to 6 cycles using supercritical CO_2 (at 20.5 MPa and 34°C) within 0.6 h increased the inactivation from 3 to 9 log reductions. Silva et al. [10] found that an 8.0 log reduction could be achieved with pressure cycling (5 cycles/140 min) and supercritical CO_2 at 8 MPa, whereas a 5.0 log reduction was observed with 1 cycle/28 min and 8 MPa. However, high pressure and CO_2 discharge are not interesting from both economic and practical viewpoints. As demonstrated in the present study where CO_2 discharge was eliminated during the treatment process, pressure cycling at a low pressure (0.7 MPa) is a promising method to enhance the bactericidal activity of pressurized CO_2.

Coefficients	Estimate	Standard error	*t*-statistic	*p*-value	R^2
Intercept	0.736	0.195	3.77	0.0009*	
x_4	0.285	0.019	15.30	7.2e-14*	0.91

*95% confidence level.

Table 3. Regression results showing the influence of pressure cycling on the inactivation efficiency (at 20 ± 1°C, system pressure = 0.7 MPa, $\Delta P = 0.12$ MPa, flow rate = 14 to 25 L min^{-1}, and initial bacterial concentration = 5–6 $\log_{10}$ CFU mL^{-1}).

Flow rate, L min^{-1}	HRT, min	Variables		Responses Y: Reduction ratio, $-\log(N_t/N_0)$	
		WVR, %	x_4, cycles	Experimental	Predicted
25[a]	0.20	50	15[c]	5.2 ± 0.2	5.0*
25[a]	0.24	60	21[d]	5.5 ± 0.0	6.4*
25[a]	0.28	70	18[d]	5.3 ± 0.2	5.8*
14[b]	0.36	50	14[d]	5.7 ± 0.1	4.7*
14[b]	0.43	60	19[e]	5.7 ± 0.0	6.1*
14[b]	0.50	70	20[f]	5.7 ± 0.2	6.5*

HRT, hydraulic retention time

*Predicted values calculated based on Eq. (2).

[a, b]Generated by a 7-mm nozzle and 0.75 kW pump, and a 5-mm nozzle and 0.20 kW pump, respectively.

[c, d, e, f]Exposure times were 3, 5, 8, and 10 min, respectively, when bacteria were completely inactivated.

Table 4. Validation of model regression for the inactivation efficiency responses to pressure cycling as a function of various working volume ratios (WVRs) and flow rates (at 20 ± 1°C, system pressure = 0.7 MPa, ΔP = 0.12 MPa, and initial bacterial concentration = 5–6 $\log_{10}$ CFU mL^{-1}).

4.4. SEM analyses

Comparative SEM images of untreated samples and samples treated with pressurized CO_2 (0.7 MPa and 20°C for a duration of 25 min) revealed changes in the morphology of *E. coli* cells (**Figure 10**). The *E. coli* cells treated with pressurized CO_2 presented several small vesicles on the cell surface, and some treated cells appeared to be lysed (**Figure 10b**); in contrast, the untreated *E. coli* cells did not have such structures on the surface (**Figure 10a**) [23]. These results suggest that the pressurized CO_2-treated *E. coli* cells may have been disrupted [19, 20, 23], and that intracellular substance may have leaked out, possibly because of the alterations in cell permeability [20, 23, 30]. The findings also affirm the excellent bactericidal performance of the pressurized CO_2 treatment.

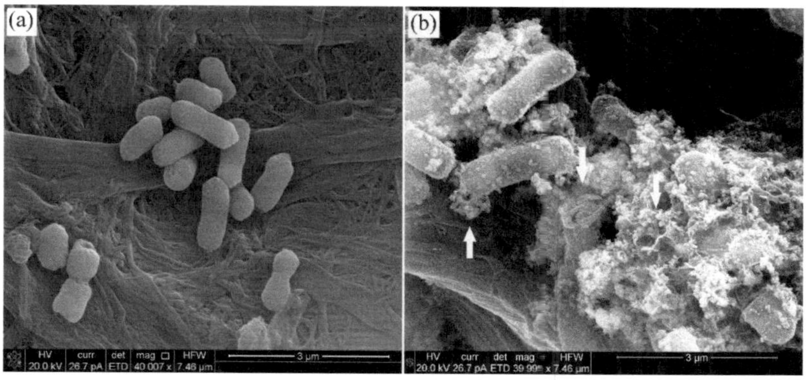

Figure 10. Representative scanning electron microscopy (SEM) images of *E. coli* cells that were (a) untreated and (b) treated by pressurized CO_2 at 0.7 MPa and 20°C for a duration of 25 min [23].

5. Summary

Pressurized CO_2 treatments can be used to eliminate *E. coli* from seawater. In this study, the inactivation efficiency was substantially enhanced by pressure cycling, which was conducted at a low pressure (0.7 MPa) and without CO_2 release during the treatment period. Bactericidal performance of pressure cycling was concomitantly influenced by two key factors involving the frequency of recirculation and ΔP ($p < 0.001$). At the same ΔP, an increase in the frequency of pressure cycling significantly improved the *E. coli* inactivation efficiency ($p < 0.001$). Additionally, the sensitivity of *E. coli* to pressurized CO_2 treatments substantially increased with increased pressures (0.2–0.9 MPa) and temperatures (11–28°C). Under identical treatment conditions (0.7 MPa, 20°C, 25 L min^{-1}, and 50% WVR), more than 5.0 log reductions in the load of *E. coli* were achieved after treatments for 3 min by using pressure cycling ($\Delta P = 0.12$ MPa, 15 cycles). Overall, these findings suggest that pressurized CO_2 technology would be feasible for water disinfection applications such as those used in ballast water treatment.

Acknowledgements

This study was supported by the Ministry of Education and Training of Vietnam under the Ph.D. Program No. 911, Yamaguchi University (Japan), and the Takahashi Industrial and Economic Research Foundation.

Author details

Tsuyoshi Imai[1]* and Thanh-Loc Thi Dang[2,3]

*Address all correspondence to: imai@yamaguchi-u.ac.jp

1 Division of Construction and Environmental Engineering, Graduate School of Sciences and Technology for Innovation, Yamaguchi University, Ube, Yamaguchi, Japan

2 Division of Environmental Science and Engineering, Graduate School of Science and Engineering, Yamaguchi University, Ube, Yamaguchi, Japan

3 Department of Environmental Science, College of Sciences, Hue University, Hue, Vietnam

References

[1] Boorman GA, Dellarco V, Dunnick JK, Chapin RE, Hunter S, Hauchman F. Drinking water disinfection byproducts: Review and approach to toxicity evaluation. Environmental Health Perspectives. 1999;**107**(Suppl 1)217-217

[2] Fabbricino M, Korshin GV. Formation of disinfection by-products and applicability of differential absorbance spectroscopy to monitor halogenation in chlorinated coastal and deep ocean seawater. Desalination. 2005;**176**69-69. DOI: 10.1016/j.desal.2004.10.026

[3] LeChevallier MW, Au K, editors. Water Treatment and Pathogen Control: Process Efficiency in Achieving Safe Drinking-water. WHO Drinking-water Quality Series. World Health Organization: IWA Publishing; 2004. p. 112. DOI: 10.2166/9781780405858

[4] Von Gunten U. Ozonation of drinking water: Part II. Disinfection and by-product formation in presence of bromide, iodide or chlorine. Water Research. 2003;**37**1487-1487. DOI: 10.1016/S0043-1354(02)00458-X

[5] Werschkun B, Sommer Y, Banerji S. Disinfection by-products in ballast water treatment: An evaluation of regulatory data. Water Research. 2012;**46**4901-4901. DOI: 10.1016/j.watres.2012.05.034

[6] Haas GJ, Prescott HE, Dudley E, Dik R, Hintlian C, Keane L. Inactivation of microorganisms by carbon dioxide under pressure. Journal of Food Safety. 1989;**9**265-265. DOI: 10.1111/j.1745-4565.1989.tb00525.x

[7] Garcia-Gonzalez L, Geeraerd AH, Spilimbergo S, Elst K, Van Ginneken L, Debevere J, Van Impe J, Devlieghere F. High pressure carbon dioxide inactivation of microorganisms in foods: The past, the present and the future. International Journal of Food Microbiology. 2007;**117**28-28. DOI: 10.1016/j.ijfoodmicro.2007.02.018

[8] Spilimbergo S, Elvassore N, Bertucco A. Microbial inactivation by high-pressure. The Journal of Supercritical Fluids. 2002;**22**63-63. DOI: 10.1016/S0896-8446(01)00106-1

[9] Zhang J, Davis TA, Matthews MA, Drews MJ, LaBerge M, An YH. Sterilization using high-pressure carbon dioxide. The Journal of Supercritical Fluids. 2006;**38**372-372. DOI: 10.1016/j.supflu.2005.05.005

[10] Silva JM, Rigo AA, Dalmolin IA, Debien I, Cansian RL, Oliveira JV, Mazutti MA. Effect of pressure, depressurization rate and pressure cycling on the inactivation of *Escherichia coli* by supercritical carbon dioxide. Food Control. 2013;**29**81-81. DOI: 10.1016/j.foodcont.2012.05.068

[11] Hong SI, Park WS, Pyun YR. Inactivation of *Lactobacillus* sp. from kimchi by high pressure carbon dioxide. LWT-Food Science and Technology. 1997;**30**685-685. DOI: 10.1006/fstl.1997.0250

[12] Hong SI, Pyun YR. Inactivation kinetics of *Lactobacillus plantarum* by high pressure carbon dioxide. Journal Food Science. 1999;**64**733-733. DOI: 10.1111/j.1365-2621.1999.tb15120.x

[13] Dillow AK, Dehghani F, Hrkach JS, Foster NR, Langer R. Bacterial inactivation by using near and supercritical carbon dioxide. Proceedings of the National Academic of Sciences of the United States of America. 1999;**96**10348-10348. DOI: 10.1073/pnas.96.18.10344

[14] Fraser D. Bursting bacteria by release of gas pressure. Nature. 1951;**167**34-34. DOI: 10.1038/167033b0

[15] Ferreira EHdR, Rosenthal A, Calado V, Saraiva J, Mendo S. *Byssochlamys nivea* inactivation in pineapple juice and nectar using high pressure cycles. Journal of Food Engineering. 2009;**95**669-669. DOI:10.1016/j.jfoodeng.2009.06.053

[16] Kobayashi F, Hayata Y, Kohara K, Muto N, Osajima Y. Application of supercritical CO_2 bubbling to inactivate *E. coli* and coliform bacteria in drinking water. Food Science and Technology Research. 2007;**13**22-22. DOI: 10.3136/fstr.13.20

[17] Kobayashi F, Yamaza F, Ikeura H, Hayata Y, Muto N, Osajima Y. Inactivation of microorganisms in untreated water by a continuous flow system with supercritical CO_2 bubbling. Journal of Water and Environment Technology. 2009a;**7**250-250. DOI: 10.2965/jwet.2009.241

[18] Kobayashi F, Hayata Y, Ikeura H, Tamaki M, Muto N, Osajima Y. Inactivation of *Escherichia coli* by CO_2 microbubbles at a lower pressure and near room temperature. Transactions of the ASABE. 2009b;**52**1626-1626. DOI: 10.13031/2013.29113

[19] Cheng X, Imai T, Teeka J, Yamaguchi J, Hirose M, Higuchi T, Sekine M. Inactivation of *Escherichia coli* and bacteriophage T4 by high levels of dissolved CO_2. Applied Microbiology and Biotechnology. 2011;**90**1500-1500. DOI: 10.1007/s00253-011-3163-0

[20] Vo HT, Imai T, Teeka J, Sekine M, Kanno A, Le TV, Higuchi T, Phummala K, Yamamoto K. Comparison of disinfection effect of pressurized gases of CO_2, N_2O, and N_2 on *Escherichia coli*. Water Research. 2013a;**47**4293-4293. DOI: 10.1016/j.watres.2013.04.053

[21] Vo HT, Imai T, Yamamoto H, Le TV, Higuchi T, Kanno A, Yamamoto K, Sekine M. Disinfection using pressurized carbon dioxide microbubbles to inactivate *Escherichia coli*, bacteriophage MS2 and T4. Journal of Water Environment Technology. 2013b;**11**505-505. DOI: 10.2965/jwet.2013.497

[22] Vo HT, Imai T, Ho TT, Dang TTL, Hoang SA. Potential application of high pressure carbon dioxide in treated wastewater and water disinfection: Recent overview and further trends. Journal Environmental Science. 2015;**36**47-47. DOI: 10.1016/j.jes.2015.04.006

[23] Dang TTL, Imai T, Le TV, Vo HT, Higuchi T, Yamamoto K, Kanno A, Sekine M. Disinfection effect of pressurized carbon dioxide on *Escherichia coli* and *Enterococcus* sp. in seawater. Water Science and Technology: Water Supply. 2016a;16(6)1735-1744. DOI: 10.2166/ws.2016.086

[24] Dang TTL, Imai T, Le TV, Nishihara S, Higuchi T, Nguyen KDM, Kanno A, Yamamoto K, Sekine M. Effect of pressure and pressure cycling on disinfection of *Enterococcus* sp. in seawater using pressurized carbon dioxide with different content rates. Journal of Environmental Science and Health, Part A. 2016b;51(11)930-937. DOI: 10.1080/10934529.2016.1191309

[25] Hutkins RW, Nannen NL. pH homeostasis in lactic-acid bacteria. Journal of Dairy Science. 1993;**76**2365-2365. DOI: 10.3168/jds.S0022-0302(93)77573-6

[26] Isenschmid A, Marison IW, von Stockar U. The influence of pressure and temperature of compressed CO_2 on the survival of yeast cells. Journal of Biotechnology. 1995;**39**237-237. DOI: 10.1016/0168-1656(95)00018-L

[27] Oulé MK, Tano K, Bernier AM, Arul J. *Escherichia coli* inactivation mechanism by pressurized CO_2. Canadian Journal of Microbiology. 2006;**52**1217-1217. DOI: 10.1139/w06-078

[28] Lin HM, Yang Z, Chen LF. Inactivation of *Leuconostoc dextranicum* with carbon dioxide under pressure. The Chemical Engineering Journal. 1993;**52**:B29-B34. DOI: 10.1016/0300-9467(93)80047-R

[29] Garcia-Gonzalez L, Geeraerd AH, Elst K, Van Ginneken L, Van Impe JF, Devlieghere F. Inactivation of naturally occurring microorganisms in liquid whole egg using high pressure carbon dioxide processing as an alternative to heat pasteurization. The Journal of Supercritical Fluids. 2009;**51**82-82. DOI: 10.1016/j.supflu.2009.06.020

[30] Kim SR, Rhee MS, Kim BC, Lee H, Kim KH. Modeling of the inactivation of *Salmonella typhimurium* by supercritical carbon dioxide in physiological saline and phosphate-buffered saline. Journal Microbiology Methods. 2007;**70**141-141. DOI: 10.1016/j.mimet.2007.04.003

Chapter 12

Evaluating Meta-Analysis Research of *Escherichia coli*

Noel Pabalan, Eloisa Singian, Lani Tabangay and Hamdi Jarjanazi

Additional information is available at the end of the chapter

http://dx.doi.org/10.5772/67337

Abstract

This chapter summarizes the progress in *Escherichia coli* research that used the meta-analysis approach. Using systematic searches for *E. coli* literature, we tracked meta-analysis publications and analyzed them based on a number of parameters. These included subject/topic (epidemiology, clinical/intervention/prevention and environmental), geographical region (the Americas, Europe and Australasia) and clinical syndrome (enteric, renal, and sepsis/meningitis). These parameters were plotted in terms of time span to obtain a sense of dynamic change or its absence through the years since the turn of the twentieth century. In terms of region, topic and syndrome, highest meta-analysis productivity was attributed to the Americas, clinical/intervention/prevention and enteric, all of which took place in the last 5 years (2011–2016). Over the combined time span of 16 years, the Americas significantly dominated meta-analysis outputs when compared to Europe and Australasia (P = 0.003). In conclusion, our findings facilitate awareness of the progress in this field wherein the studied parameters were analyzed for patterns over time and differential rates of publication productivity.

Keywords: *Escherichia coli*, meta-analysis

1. Introduction

Published researches on *Escherichia coli* (*E. coli*) have increased in number since the turn of the twentieth century. A search of *E. coli* publications in PubMed reveals an output value of 339,415 (as of July 16, 2016) which when narrowed to *E. coli* in title only, the number is still substantial (96,594). Majority of the *E. coli* publications are primary studies which when addressing the same issue, most often produce contradictory results [1]. Thus when primary studies are reviewed (usually in the narrative style), these contradictions hinder meaningful integration of results. A more systematic way to integrate primary study findings is the use of meta-analysis.

1.1. Meta-analysis defined

Meta-analysis is defined as a statistical analysis of primary study results for the purpose of integrating the findings into a summary effect [2]. Considered at the top of the hierarchy of evidence [3], it is a logically formal and objective technique as well as quantitative mode of summarizing research findings in order to identify genuine associations [1, 4]. Meta-analysis is categorized under the rubric of a systematic review, a process that entails gathering all completed published studies from the primary literature specific to a targeted research question [5]. Meta-analysis opens the possibility to accurately estimate the overall outcome measure, with increased statistical power, than is possible using only a single study [6]. Historical application of meta-analysis in *E. coli* research is relatively extensive as it has addressed key research questions. These include epidemiology, prevention, intervention issues and environmental concerns.

1.2. Importance of meta-analysis

The importance of meta-analysis is best appreciated when compared to the primary study. First, meta-analysis is cheaper, but not necessarily easier to do. Primary studies on the other hand are more expensive and logistically problematic, especially when large [1, 7]. Second, primary studies often do not have enough statistical power to assess relationships between risks (interventions) and outcomes. Being most useful when individual studies are too small to yield valid conclusions, meta-analysis increases power, reduces risk of error and facilitates exploratory analysis to generate hypotheses for future research [8]. The reason for performing a meta-analysis has to do with sample sizes of the studies, when they are large but results conflict, or when they are small, but their positive findings are not consistent [9]. The meta-analysis approach enables its findings to unmask large-scale patterns not obvious in primary studies [10, 11]. This then results in greater statistical precision meriting higher confidence. Thus, meta-analysis findings facilitate more efficient transfer of knowledge from researcher to clinician enabling analyses of important patient subgroups, delineation of high risk factors for infection enough for information to be useful for public health advice in risk for infection. Consequently, meta-analysis lends rigor to better assist health authorities in directing therapeutic decisions to target populations, urgency for health education and control measures [1]. Indeed, in the public health domain, a number of difficult issues that had been repeatedly studied were either resolved or clarified by the application of meta-analysis techniques [12]. This has led some government guidelines to recommend meta-analysis as the preferred method of summarizing evidence of effectiveness and safety of health technologies in the face of multiple study results [13].

1.3. Performing meta-analysis

1.3.1. Literature search and data abstraction

A publishable meta-analysis should have enough primary studies that address a common topic. The published Preferred Reporting Items for Systematic Reviews and Meta-Analyses (PRISMA) statement recommends that a full electronic search strategy for at least one major

http://dx.doi.org/10.5772/67337

database be presented [14], although such an approach is considered insufficient by some [15]. Still a typical search strategy should involve electronic retrieval of all available literature, which includes databases such as PubMed using Medline (http://www.ncbi.nlm.nih.gov/pubmed), ScienceDirect (www.sciencedirect.com), Institute of Scientific Information (ISI) Web of Knowledge (http://www.isiwebofknowledge.com) and Google Scholar (http://scholar.google.com). For greater precision in this step, additional measures to exhaustively identify eligible studies include manual searching of relevant journals, references lists and personal contact with researchers.

1.3.2. Summary effect analysis

Meta-analyses report findings in terms of effect sizes, which provide information about the magnitude of change. The forest plot typifies presentation of meta-analysis results, which are generated by software such as Stata®, Review Manager and Comprehensive Meta-analysis®. The forest plot example [16] in **Figure 1** was generated from Review Manager (Cochrane Collaboration, Oxford, England). The plot is composed of five columns, the leftmost with qualitative data (study, named by last name of first author) and the remaining four with quantitative data. Between columns three and four is the actual forest plot with a solid vertical line (labeled 1 on the x-axis) which corresponds to the null effect. The area to the left of the vertical line indicates decreased risk and to its right increased risk. The two leftmost columns show the raw data (cases/controls) from which the odds ratios (OR) and 95% confidence intervals (CI) (rightmost column) are calculated. The OR and 95% CI express the study-specific findings (there are 18 of them), and a single summary effect that systematically combines the 18 ORs. Significance of the study-specific and summary effects is visually determined when

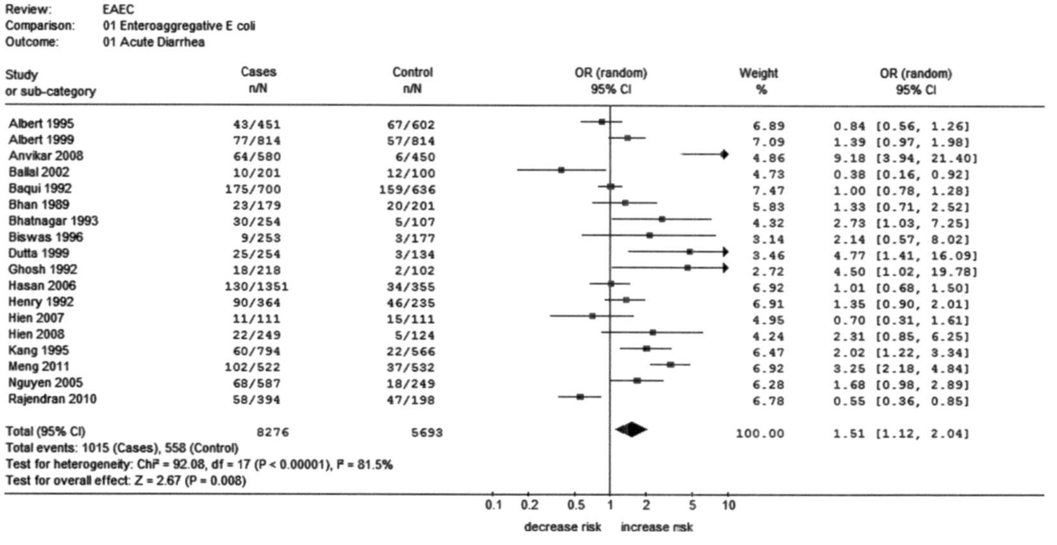

Figure 1. Forest plot for the overall effect of EAEC on acute diarrhea among South-Asian children [16]. EAEC: enteroaggregative *E. coli*; n: affected number; N: total number; OR: odds ratio; CI: confidence interval; df: degree of freedom; I²: measure of variability between studies; P: P value.

the lines associated with the squares and the diamond (◆) touch the vertical line (labeled 1). If the vertical line is touched, the interpretation is non-significant, otherwise it is significant. Numerically, each 95% CI, expressed as decimal, will either pass 1 (non-significant) or not (significant). For significance of the summary effect (◆), this is also determined by the tests generated by the software, results of which are found at the bottom left of the forest plot. The test for overall effect, represented here by the Z-test and its corresponding P value, is 0.008 indicating significance. This graph has been much more explained in detail in two previous papers [1, 16].

1.3.3. Modifier analyses

Standard meta-analysis comprises a set of features that include a summary effect (expressed in various types of statistical metrics). Not being the endpoint, the summary or pooled effect needs to be tested further to ensure rigor of this methodology. An armory of statistical techniques is available to test the stability of this effect. These techniques include subgroup, outlier and sensitivity analyses, collectively known as modifiers. First, modifier analysis could take the forms of subgrouping by categories such as geography, gender and ethnicity. From these categories, one could delineate similar or contrasting effects between the subgroups, along with the precision or lack of it as indicated by the CI. Second, pooled effects could be influenced by outlying studies, and these are determined by the Galbraith plot method [17]. Omission of such studies followed by re-analysis generates one of the two results affecting the original pooled effect: (i) unaltered, indicating stability and (ii) altered in terms of direction of association which indicates instability. In addition, outlier treatment could affect heterogeneity (see below). Finally, summary effects are tested for robustness with sensitivity analysis wherein the studies are serially omitted followed by recalculation to determine deviation or resistance of the pooled effect from the original [18].

1.4. Biases in meta-analysis

Despite the appeal of meta-analysis, it is only as good as the studies used to create it dependent on the experience of the researcher performing it [19]. As in primary studies, meta-analysis is not immune to biases, but the good thing about these limitations is its transparency in admitting their presence. Furthermore, the meta-analysis protocol contains inherent statistical mechanisms to adjust and minimize these biases.

1.4.1. Heterogeneity

Heterogeneity in a broad sense involves clinical, methodological, biological and epidemiological issues and is often topic specific [20]. In this section, we examine statistical heterogeneity, which in the meta-analytical context, is defined as statistical dissimilarity across various studies [1]. Adjusting for heterogeneity involves appropriate use of analysis models. This involves use of the random-effects model [2], which assumes variability across populations usually resulting in a wider CI [21]. However, when component studies in a meta-analysis are similar to each other, this indicates absence of heterogeneity; then, the fixed-effects method of analysis [22] is applied based on the assumption that associations are the same across studies and recognizing that the collection of eligible literature is not heterogeneous. Heterogeneity is statistically estimated using a chi-square–based Q test [23] and quantified with the I^2 metric, which shows what proportion of the total variation across studies is beyond chance [24]. Values of I^2 lie between 0 and 100% where a value >75% may be considered substantially heterogeneous [24]. Heterogeneous results warrant investigation into its sources, either through meta-regression [25] or outlier treatment [17]. The former focuses on covariates and the latter is graphically assessed with the Galbraith plot [17], which is used to detect outlying studies. Exclusion of outliers followed by recalculation either reduces or removes heterogeneity of the original findings.

1.4.2. *Publication bias*

Publication bias [26] occurs when significant findings receive priority in published literature over those whose results are non-significant [18]. This bias is evaluated graphically with the funnel plot (**Figure 2A**). The points with small studies scattered along the length of the x-axis but still centered on the OR estimates from large, more precise studies. This figure shows a symmetrical distribution indicating absence of bias. In contrast, **Figure 2B** shows a simulated funnel plot indicating presence of publication bias, which shows an asymmetrical distribution of the points [1]. The subjectivity in interpreting the funnel plot is overcome with objective statistical tests for publication bias, the Egger's regression asymmetry [21] and Begg's and Mazumdar's rank correlation [27] tests.

1.5. *Escherichia coli*

In this section, we discuss *E. coli* studies as is relevant to the topics addressed by meta-analysis. Meta-analyses have covered *E. coli* topics that included environmental factors such as water quality, clinical aspects, which include intervention/prevention approaches and epidemiological issues which address prevalence factors. *E. coli* is the predominant facultative anaerobe of the human colonic flora that inhabit the gastrointestinal tracts of humans and warm-blooded

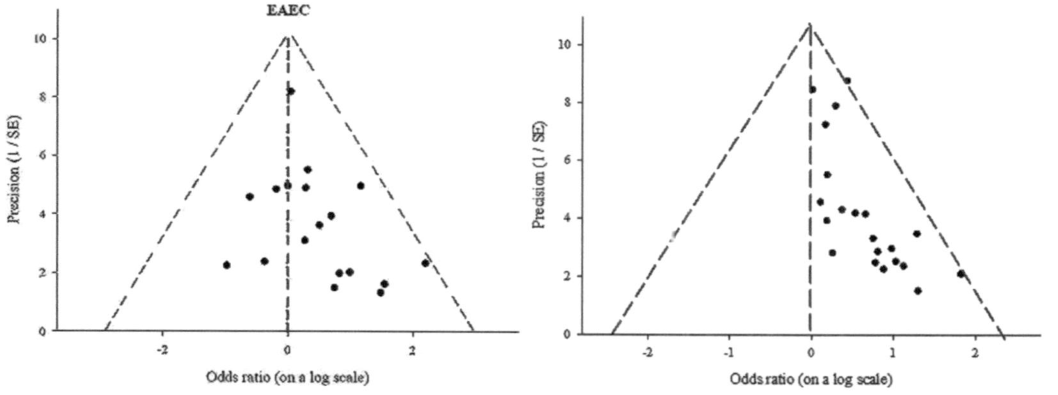

Figure 2. Funnel plot showing absence (A) and presence (B) of publication bias [1]. EAEC: enteroaggregative *E. coli*; SE: standard error; (B) is a simulated funnel plot [1].

animals, as well as one of the most important pathogens [28]. Occupying the mucous layer of the mammalian colon, *E. coli* colonizes this area in infants within hours of life, and thereafter, it usually remains harmlessly confined to the intestinal lumen [29]. As commensal, *E. coli* lives in a mutually beneficial association with hosts and rarely causes disease. Thus, *E. coli* is part of the protective microbial community in the intestine and is essential for general health. The conditions where *E. coli* strains cause disease are among immunocompromised hosts or where the normal gastrointestinal barriers are violated [30]. Infections due to pathogenic *E. coli* may be limited to the mucosal surfaces or can disseminate throughout the body. This spread throughout the body includes the digestive, renal and nervous systems [28, 29, 31]. We use these systems appear in our survey of meta-analysis publications on *E. coli* to track the evolvement and progress in this field.

1.6. Methods used in the survey

To obtain a sense of outputs in *E. coli* meta-analyses, we performed a systematic search of meta-analysis publications using the keywords, "meta-analysis" and "*E. coli*" in PubMed using Medline, Google Scholar and Science Direct in the title/abstract box. If the title did not explicitly indicate the above keywords, we read the abstracts and/or full-text article to determine its study design. Nevertheless, we excluded systematic reviews without the meta-analysis aspect in the article. For articles to be included, meta-analysis and/or *E. coli* should be in the title. If only meta-analysis was in the title, we read the text to determine if the role of *E. coli* was central or marginal. Central role meant that *E. coli* was the focus of the paper. If *E. coli* was among the foci of the paper, findings for *E. coli* should be statistically significant. If otherwise, the paper was relegated to marginal status. We defined marginal as *E. coli* being grouped with other bacteria and/or that *E. coli* findings were non-significant or unassociated with the outcome.

Figure 3 is a flowchart of our literature search of meta-analyses on *E. coli*. Of the 202 citations, 130 were excluded because they were not meta-analyses nor reviews nor about *E. coli*. In addition, many were duplicates of those already found in PubMed. Of the remaining 72 records, 45 had *E. coli* and/or meta-analysis in the title and the other 27 did not. These 27 were then assessed further by reading the full text from which we excluded 14 marginal papers leaving 13 central articles for inclusion in the analysis. These 13 with the 45 titled papers gave a total of 58 articles which we evaluated based on three parameters: (i) subject [epidemiology (EPI), clinical intervention/prevention (CIP), and environmental (ENV)]; (ii) time span (2000–2004, 2005–2010 and 2011–2016) and (iii) region (the Americas, Europe and Australasia). The number of publications was assessed using these parameters. Of the 58 papers, 15 articles could not be categorized into clinical syndromes because they addressed unrelated issues such as water, sanitizing and contamination. The remaining 43 papers were categorized by syndrome wherein the articles were either enteric (ENT), renal (REN), sepsis (SEP) or a combination of these three (MUL for multiple). From these parameters, we generated publication output rates in the following plots: (i) topic spread through time (**Figure 4**); (ii) topic standardized by number of countries per region through time (**Figure 5**); (iii) region through time wherein both were standardized by the number of countries per region (**Figure 6**) and number of years

http://dx.doi.org/10.5772/67337

per time span (**Figure 7**), respectively and (iv) clinical syndrome wherein both were standardized by the number of countries per region (**Figure 8**) and number of years per time span (**Figure 9**), respectively. Visual differences between the parameters were further analyzed statistically.

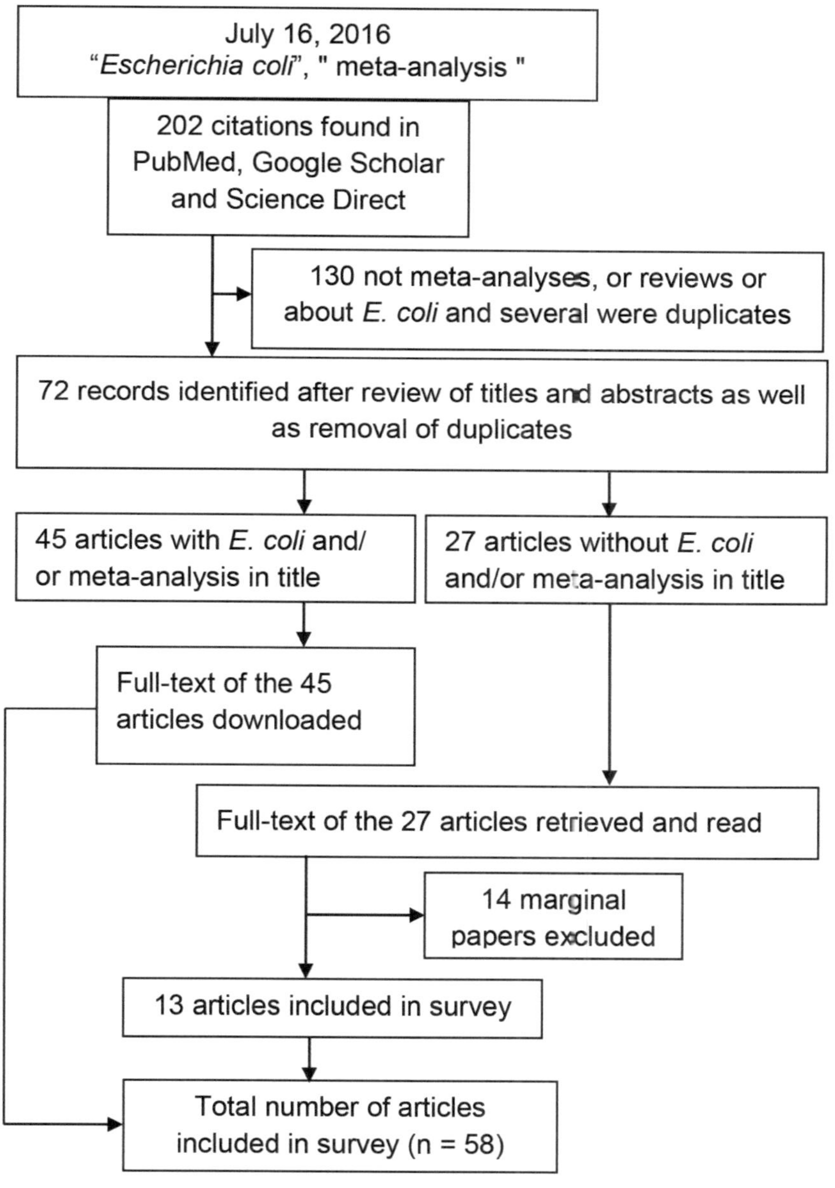

Figure 3. Flowchart of selection of studies for inclusion in the systematic survey.

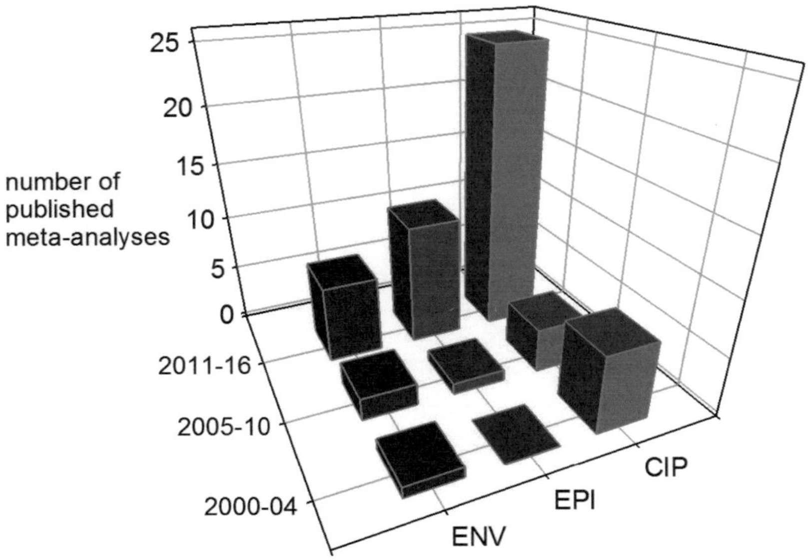

Figure 4. Meta-analysis publication outputs in *E. coli* research by topic. ENV: environmental; EPI: epidemiological; CIP: clinical/intervention/prevention.

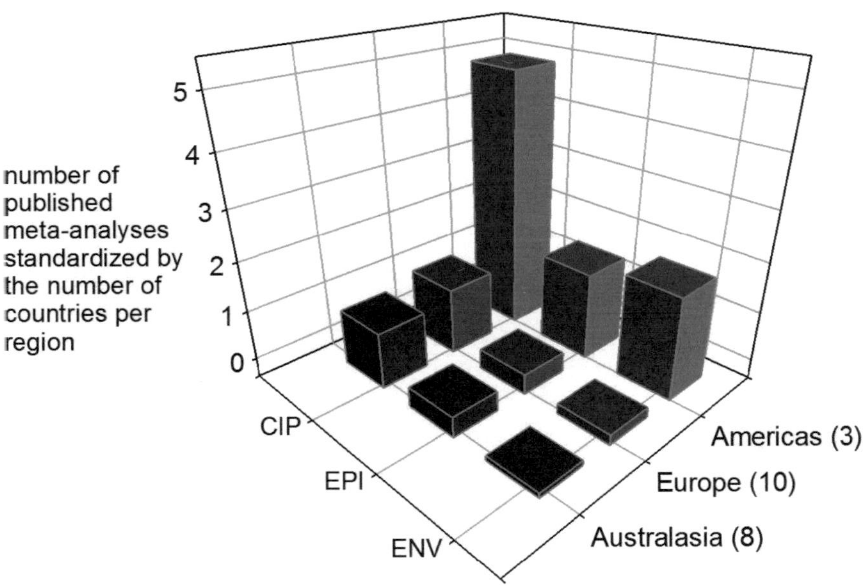

Figure 5. Meta-analysis publication outputs in *E. coli* research of three major world regions categorized by topic. Values in the Y-axis indicate number of meta-analyses divided by the number of countries per region. Numbers in parentheses indicate number of countries comprising the region; ENV: environmental; EPI: epidemiological; CIP: clinical/intervention/prevention.

http://dx.doi.org/10.5772/67337

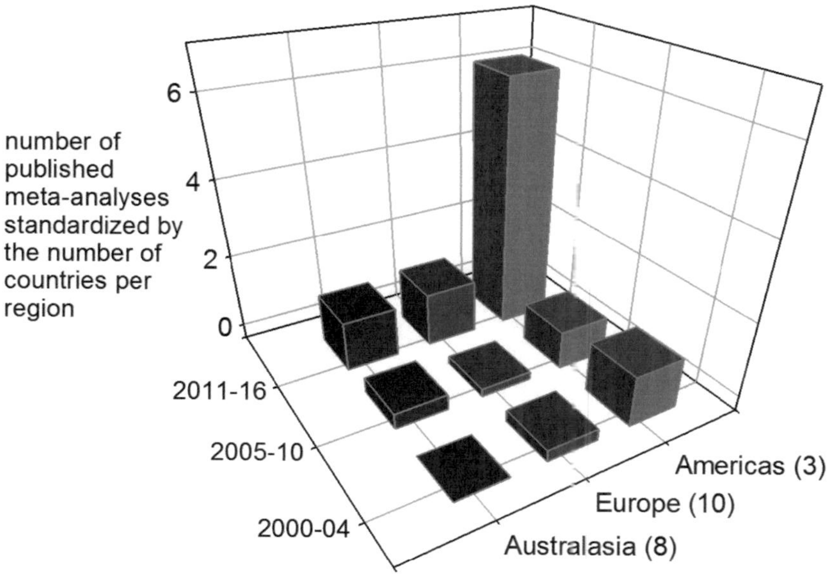

Figure 6. Meta-analysis publication outputs in *E. coli* research standardized by the number of countries per region. Numbers in parentheses indicate number of countries comprising the region.

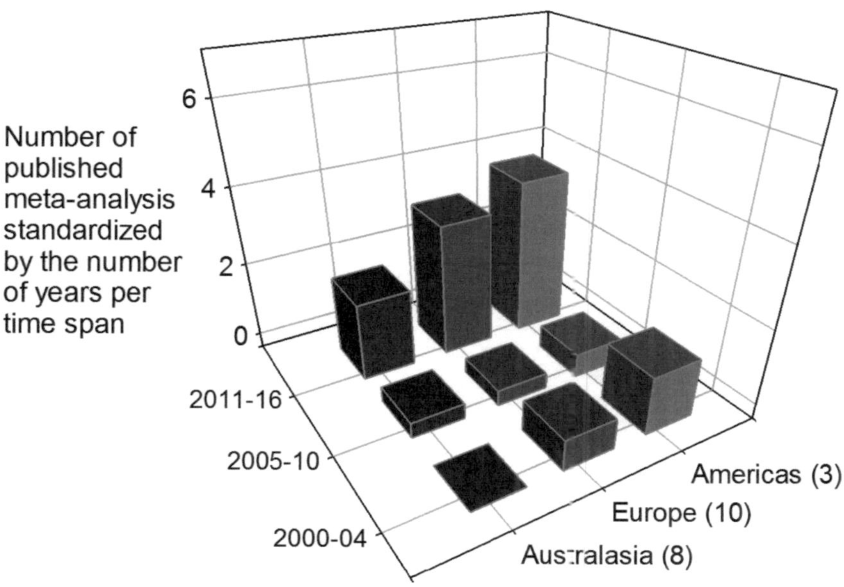

Figure 7. Meta-analysis publication outputs in *E. coli* research standardized by the number of years per time span. Numbers in parentheses indicate number of countries comprising the region.

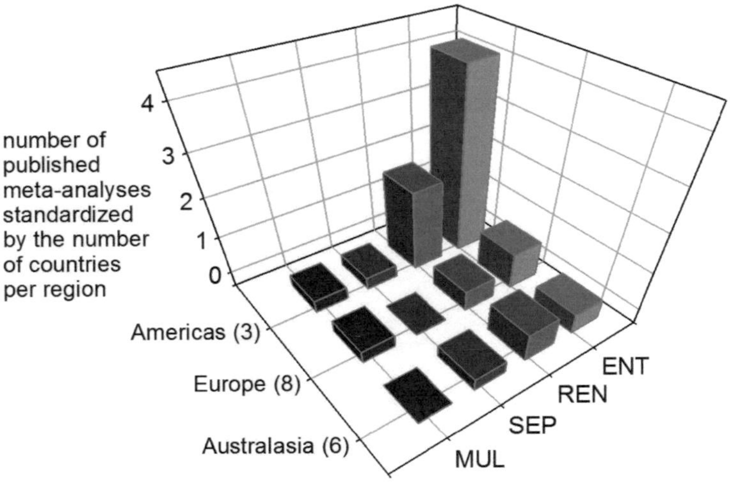

Figure 8. Meta-analysis publication outputs in *E. coli* research by clinical syndrome standardized by the number of countries per region. Numbers in parentheses indicate number of countries comprising the region; MUL: multiple; SEP: sepsis; REN: renal; ENT: enteric.

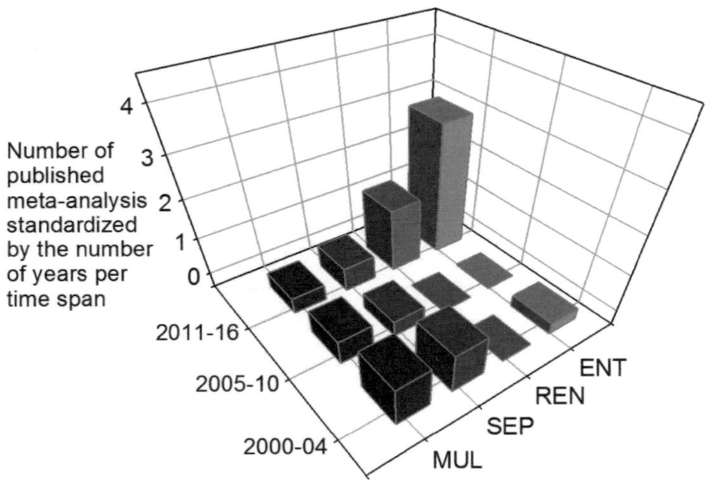

Figure 9. Meta-analysis publication outputs in *E. coli* research by clinical syndrome standardized by the number of years per time span. MUL: multiple; SEP: sepsis; REN: renal; ENT: enteric.

2. Main body

2.1. Review of *E. coli* meta-analyses based on topics

E. coli is responsible for a good number of hospital-acquired and community-acquired infections more than any other single bacterial species. In a wider context, it is responsible for a great deal of infant morbidity and mortality due to its action as a pathogen in the bowel [32].

http://dx.doi.org/10.5772/67337

Studies of *E. coli* in the ENV context have not been well undertaken compared to CIP studies. ENV studies of this pathogen in the meta-analysis context have involved water, which addressed quality [33, 34], contamination [35] and treatment issues [36]. Yet, the importance of this environmental factor related to *E. coli* pathogenicity is relevant to particular regions of the world especially the developing countries. Fecal pollution of natural waters has been increasingly important, and the consequences of discharge of untreated sewage into river estuaries and the sea have been extensively studied [32]. To a lesser degree, soil research has been undertaken to a magnitude that warranted meta-analysis treatment [37]. In general, strategies for prevention and control of the spread of *E. coli* should include access to safe water, good handling practices to reduce the risk of food contamination, sanitation measures, public education and vaccination [38, 39]. *E. coli* in the context of epidemiology as approached from a meta-analysis perspective involves prevalence issues [40, 41] and reviews epidemic potential [42, 43] of this pathogen as well as being a causative factor in diarrheal illness [44]. Given the variety of epidemiological areas of *E. coli* research warranting meta-analysis, it provides a fertile base of future undertakings in this area. Clinical topics addressed with the meta-analysis approach vary depending on subjects involved. These topics provide a sense of the number of primary studies in areas such as infection, treatment and prevention.

2.2. Review of *E. coli* meta-analyses based on clinical syndromes

Enteric/diarrheal diseases involve intestinal pathogens that are spread through the fecal-oral route by ingestion of contaminated food or water [45]. These pathogens termed diarrheagenic *E. coli* (DEC) are differentiated, among others, on the basis of distinct clinical and pathogenic features (pathotypes) [29]. The five pathotypes of DEC are enterotoxigenic *E. coli* (ETEC), enteropathogenic *E. coli* (EPEC), enteroaggregative *E. coli* (EAEC), enterohemorrhagic *E. coli* (EHEC) and enteroinvasive *E. coli* (EIEC). In addition, Shiga Toxin-producing *E. coli* (STEC) are foodborne pathogens that cause human infections acquired through fecal-oral contact with contaminated human and animal feces [46]. Urinary tract infection (UTI) is the most common extra-intestinal *E. coli* infection caused by uropathogenic *E. coli* which when isolated, the condition generally responds rapidly to antibiotic therapy. Sequelae from UTI could complicate pregnancy and target pre-school age children rendering the possibility of chronic renal damage [32]. Related to the renal system is verocytotoxin-producing *E. coli* (VTEC) infection, which could result in hemolytic uremic syndrome; this occurs in up to 15% of cases [47]. An increasingly common cause of extra-intestinal infections is the pathotype responsible for meningitis and sepsis/meningitis-associated *E. coli* [32]. The included meta-analyses here addressed issues with *E. coli* strains such as STEC, VTEC, ETEC and EAEC [16, 40, 44, 47–51]. Two of these strains were addressed with antibiotics [47, 49] Resistance to antibiotics was the subject of five studies [52–56]. Associations of antibiotics with infection were addressed in seven articles [57–63]. The topics of *E. coli* associations with water were addressed in 10 papers [33–37, 64–69]. There were three papers on *E. coli* shedding in cattle [70–72]. Immunology topics were the focus in three papers [73–75]. Although most meta-analyses included here addressed enteric *E. coli* infections, there are papers that addressed renal infections [53, 54, 76] with a fairly good number of *E. coli* meta-analyses and UTI performed in various contexts such as epidemiology [42, 55], intervention [52, 54] and prevention [73]. Meta-analyses of *E. coli* in the context of sepsis/meningitis have so far been confined to mice and infants [58, 77].

2.3. *E. coli* meta-analyses involving non-human animals and plants

Our collection of *E. coli* meta-analyses involved non-human animals and plants, mainly farm animals. These included poultry [78], cattle [41, 69–72, 79–81] and pigs [61, 82]. Non-farm animals where *E. coli* studies have been meta-analyzed were mice [77]. Farmed non-animals where *E. coli* research has been meta-analyzed included fresh-produce studies [68, 83]. *E. coli* infection among pets and wild animals has produced primary studies [32] but not enough of their numbers warranted meta-analysis.

2.4. Assessing *E. coli* meta-analyses by topic

Figure 4 shows the results of *E. coli* meta-analysis productivity in span of 16 years (grouped into three time spans) and across three topics. Between 2000 and 2004, CIP outputs dominated those of EPI and ENV, but between 2005 and 2010, outputs from all three topics were more or less similar. Between 2011 and 2016, CIP outputs dwarfed those of the other two, although EPI outputs were slightly more than those of ENV. The combined data of 16 years between the topics showed non-significant higher CIP outputs than EPI and ENV [one-way analysis of variance (ANOVA): $P = 0.08$].

2.5. Assessing *E. coli* meta-analyses by topic and region

Figure 5 graphs the number of published *E. coli* meta-analyses ordered by topic from the three world regions. Published outputs from the Americas were higher across the topics than Europe and Australasia, but when regionally combined, the higher American productivity was not significant (one-way ANOVA: $P = 0.62$). However, when ordered by topic and analyzed by one-way ANOVA and the Holm-Sidak post-test, CIP productivity was significantly higher than EPI ($P = 0.005$) and ENV ($P = 0.003$) but not between EPI and ENV ($P = 0.63$).

2.6. Assessing *E. coli* meta-analyses by region

Figure 6 shows the number of published meta-analyses which was standardized by region. This figure shows low meta-analysis outputs in the years 2000–2010 from Europe and Australasia compared to the moderate American outputs in the same period. The last 5 years (2011–2016) showed high American output compared to the moderate number of publications from Europe and Australasia. **Figure 7** shows meta-analysis productivity of the three regions standardized by year. Per year output of published meta-analyses on *E. coli* in the first 4 years of the twentieth century was zero for Australasia but moderate for Europe and the Americas. This productivity declined in the following 4 years (2005–2010) for all regions then shot back up to good productivity in between 2011 and 2016. Thus, comparing **Figures 6** and **7**, we observed higher meta-analysis productivity in the Americas per region than that per year. Between 2011 and 2016, Europe and Australasia had higher meta-analysis productivity when standardized by year than that by region. The unadjusted values from **Figures 6** and **7** were subjected to statistical comparison (one-way ANOVA, Holm-Sidak post-test) that combined the data of 16 years. Results showed significantly higher number of published outputs from the Americas than Europe ($P = 0.003$) and Australasia ($P = 0.002$) but not between the latter two ($P = 0.89$).

2.7. Assessing *E. coli* meta-analyses by clinical syndrome

Figure 8 shows the standardized number of meta-analyses from the three regions categorized under the four syndromes. This graph shows American predominance in ENT and REN meta-analysis research compared to the two other regions. Between these two syndromes, ENT had more than twice the output compared to REN. SEP and MUL outputs were flat from all regions. **Figure 9** shows minimal output of REN and ENT meta-analyses between 2000 and 2010 compared to SEP and MUL researches, which were considerably higher in the same time span. Between 2011 and 2016, REN and ENT outputs were up to three times higher than SEP and MUL meta-analyses. The unadjusted values from **Figure 9** of the combined data of 16 years showed non-significant associations between the syndromes over time (one-way ANOVA: $P = 0.20$).

2.8. Summary of *E. coli* meta-analysis publication outputs

Based on the three topics analyzed, increase of CIP meta-analyses indicates *a priori* increase in the number of primary studies (which are requisite to meta-analysis) in a span of 16 years. This increase has probably to do with focus on treating *E. coli* infections given the infrastructure in laboratories that enable such researches. **Table 1** shows that in terms of region, leadership of the Americas, specifically the USA in *E. coli* meta-analysis research seem to have been unchallenged since the turn of the twentieth century. Even when *E. coli* publication outputs were low between 2000 and 2010, the Americas still dominated over Europe and Australasia. This domination is best interpreted in three contexts: (i) only three countries comprise the Americas compared to 10 and eight for the other two regions (**Figure 4** and **Table 1**). (ii) **Table 1** shows the USA output in meta-analysis to be twice that of Canada and eight times that of Brazil. (iii) USA meta-analysis output is four times those of Netherlands and Australia, which both lead Europe and Australasia, respectively (**Table 1**). Given the concentration of developing countries in the Asian region where *E. coli* research would be most useful, such outputs are comparatively low and maybe warrant priority in future research of this pathogen. Our findings suggest that the region with the capabilities to undertake such researches result in higher publication outputs. In terms of outputs per year, Australasia and Europe appear to be catching up in productivity in the last 5 years. Summing the pattern of the graphs (**Figures 4–9**), meta-analysis outputs were highest for CIP, the Americas and ENT, all between 2011 and 2016 where this time span was involved. The lowest meta-analysis outputs were concentrated between 2000 and 2004, specifically in the ENV topic and the Australasian region. The year 2000 showed one published meta-analysis on *E. coli* [75] and none before that.

2.9. Limitations and strengths

One limitation of this undertaking was that we confined our survey to published *E. coli* research from standard databases. There might have been meta-analyses done in government and university settings on *E. coli* but were not included in the databases we searched on. Another limitation is non-inclusion of gray literature in our survey, which by its nature has not been published. However, one strength is that this chapter gave a sense of the direction of

	Europe	N	Americas	N	Australasia	N
1	Netherlands	4	USA	16	Australia	4
2	UK	3	Canada	8	China	3
3	Denmark	2	Brazil	2	Japan	1
4	Germany	4	Total	**26**	Iran	1
5	Poland	1			Pakistan	1
6	Italy	6			Bangladesh	1
7	Sweden	1			Turkey	1
8	Greece	1			Philippines	1
9	France	1			Total	**13**
10	Ireland	1				
11	Portugal	1				
12	Slovenia	1				
	Total	**26**				

N: number of published articles; UK: United Kingdom; USA: United States of America.

Table 1. Countries comprising each of the three world regions and published outputs of *E. coli* research resulting from literature searches in PubMed, Science Direct and Google Scholar.

E. coli research based on previous publications. Because we used parameters such as region, year, topic and clinical syndrome, this provided some measure of direction as to how *E. coli* research was conducted and what areas in this discipline need focusing in the future.

2.10. Conclusions

E. coli meta-analyses in this survey varied in many aspects, not only in geography but also in the topic and syndrome. Most salient was variability in the outcomes and approaches. For outcomes, they ranged from presence to absence of associations and effectivity or absence of treatment. The point of these outcomes is the exposition of magnitude where influence of factors may be great or minimal; all these having been statistically treated. For approaches, subjects range from humans to non-human animals and even plants (fresh produce). This survey of meta-analysis publications indicates areas of discipline that were emphasized and those that were not. *E. coli* research outputs, as in other biomedical disciplines, are increasing at an exponential rate. Because of the critical importance of *E. coli* research findings across populations and geographical regions, objective evaluation of these primary studies may facilitate decision making that impacts upon public health policy. Clinicians, researchers and demographers in this field would likely benefit from the use and interpretation of meta-analysis. The survey in this review delineates a relatively high use of meta-analysis in *E. coli* research in the Americas, where the USA most specifically continues to assert its capability in utilizing outputs from primary *E. coli* studies since the turn of the twentieth century. Of note, the recent years also showed increasing use of *E. coli* meta-analyses from Europe and Australasia. Not only do primary studies addressing the same issue had conflicting results, they also varied in geography, methodology, and sample size-leading to perceived controversy or uncertainty about the pathogenic nature of this organism. Application of systematic statistical approaches allowed confirmation that many strains of *E. coli* cause endpoint diseases. Similar meta-analysis in the larger sphere of microbiology may have the ability to advance our understanding of other emerging and established pathogens.

Of the three *E. coli* topics this chapter has covered, ENV studies have garnered the least attention over the last 16 years compared to EPI and CIP. Even less in magnitude are genetic/genomic issues which were barely covered in this chapter given the paucity of primary studies on this topic. If the past is any guide to future prospects, then it would be judicious to forego what is fashionable in research and begin addressing issues that impact upon the lives of those affected/infected with *E. coli*. The tide of geopolitical forces has given rise to mass migration and exponential increase in world population at the cost of environmental degradation. These global features define regions most susceptible to the ravages of *E. coli* infection. Thus, it seems most suited to emphasize the future in *E. coli* research along these scales in order of priority, ENV, EPI and CIP. However, this is not to de-prioritize the genomic/proteomic approaches as it forms the foundation upon which *E. coli* research achieves milestones. The future of genomic epidemiology is detailed in Eppinger and Cebula's paper where they focus on the EHEC serotype [84].

Acknowledgements

The authors thank our affiliate institution, Angeles University Foundation for infrastructure support.

Appendices and nomenclatures

E. coli	*Escherichia coli*
PRISMA	Preferred Reporting Items for Systematic Reviews and Meta-Analyses
ISI	Institute of Scientific Information
OR	Odds ratio
CI	Confidence interval
CIP	Clinical/intervention/preventive
EPI	Epidemiological
ENV	Environmental
ENT	Enteric or diarrheal
REN	Renal; which includes the term uremic

SEP	Sepsis/meningitis
MUL	Multiple; has the combination of ENT, ENV and/or REN
DEC	Diarrheagenic *E. coli*
EHEC	Enterohemorrhagic *E. coli*
ETEC	Enterotoxigenic *E. coli*
EPEC	Enteropathogenic *E. coli*
EAEC	Enteroaggregative *E. coli*
EIEC	Enteroinvasive *E. coli*
STEC	Shiga toxin-producing *E. coli*
UTI	Urinary tract infection
VTEC	Verocytotoxin-producing *E. coli*
ANOVA	Analysis of variance

Author details

Noel Pabalan[1]*, Eloisa Singian[2], Lani Tabangay[3] and Hamdi Jarjanazi[4]

*Address all correspondence to: npabalan@alumni.yorku.ca

1 Center for Research and Development, Angeles University Foundation, Angeles City, Philippines

2 Department of Medical Technology, College of Allied Medical Professions, Angeles University Foundation, Angeles City, Philippines

3 Department of Biology, Angeles University Foundation, Angeles City, Philippines

4 Environmental Monitoring and Reporting Branch, Ontario Ministry of the Environment and Climate Change, Toronto, ON, Canada

References

[1] Pabalan N, Jarjanazi H, Steiner TS: Meta-analysis in microbiology. Indian J Med Microbiol. 2014. 32:229-35. DOI: 10.4103/0255-0857.136547.

[2] DerSimonian R, Laird N: Meta-analysis in clinical trials. Control Clin Trials. 1986. 7:177-88. DOI: 10.1016/0197-2456(86)90046-2

[3] Yuan Y, Hunt RH: Systematic reviews: the good, the bad, and the ugly. Am J Gastroenterol. 2009. 104:1086-92. DOI: 10.1038/ajg.2009.118.

[4] Egger M, Smith GD, Phillips AN: Meta-analysis: principles and procedures. BMJ. 1997. 315:1533-7. DOI: 10.1136/bmj.315.7121.1533.

[5] Alex J. Sutton, Keith R. Abrams, David R. Jones, Trevor A. Sheldon, Fujian Song. Methods for Meta-analysis in Medical Research. Chichester, UK: John Wiley & Sons, Ltd.; 2000.

[6] Sutton AJ, Abrams KR, Jones DR: An illustrated guide to the methods of meta-analysis. J Eval Clin Pract. 2001. 7:135-48. DOI: 10.1046/j.1365-2753.2001.00281.x.

[7] Egger M, Smith GD: Meta-analysis. Potentials and promise. BMJ. 1997. 315:1371-4. DOI: 10.1136/bmj.315.7119.1371.

[8] Gotzsche PC: Why we need a broad perspective on meta-analysis. It may be crucially important for patients. BMJ. 2000. 321:585-6. DOI: 10.1136/bmj.321.7261.585.

[9] Rowland DY, Debanne SM: Meta-analysis, part I. Gastrointest Endosc. 2002. 55:612-3. DOI: 10.1067/mge.2002.121594.

[10] Buyse M, Piedbois P, Piedbois Y, Carlson RW: Meta-analysis: methods, strengths, and weaknesses. Oncology (Williston Park). 2000. 14:437-43, discussion 44, 47. DOI: n/a.

[11] Egger M, Ebrahim S, Smith GD: Where now for meta-analysis?. Int J Epidemiol. 2002. 31:1-5. DOI: 10.1093/ije/31.1.1

[12] Louis TA, Fineberg HV, Mosteller F: Findings for public health from meta-analyses. Annu Rev Public Health. 1985. 6:1-20. DOI: 10.1146/annurev.pu.06.050185.000245.

[13] NICE. Guide to the Methods of Technology Appraisal. 2008 [Available from: http://www.nice.org.uk/pdf [Last accessed on 2016 July].

[14] Moher D, Liberati A, Tetzlaff J, Altman DG, Group P: Preferred reporting items for systematic reviews and meta-analyses: the PRISMA statement. PLoS Med. 2009. 6:e1000097. DOI: 10.1371/journal.pmed.1000097.

[15] Lemeshow AR, Blum RE, Berlin JA, Stoto MA, Colditz GA: Searching one or two databases was insufficient for meta-analysis of observational studies. J Clin Epidemiol. 2005. 58:867-73. DOI: 10.1016/j.jclinepi.2005.03.004.

[16] Pabalan N, Singian E, Jarjanazi H, Steiner TS: Enteroaggregative *Escherichia coli* and acute diarrhea in children: a meta-analysis of South Asian populations. Eur J Clin Microbiol Infect Dis. 2013. 32:597-607. DOI: 10.1007/s10096-012-1779-3.

[17] Galbraith RF: A note on graphical presentation of estimated odds ratios from several clinical trials. Stat Med. 1988. 7:889-94. DOI: 10.1002/sim.4780070807.

[18] Copas J, Shi JQ: Meta-analysis, funnel plots and sensitivity analysis. Biostatistics. 2000. 1:247-62. DOI: 10.1093/biostatistics/1.3.247.

[19] Verstraete M: Value and limitation of meta-analysis. Pathophysiol Haemost Thromb. 2002. 32:278-81. DOI: 10.1159/000073581.

[20] Ioannidis JP, Patsopoulos NA, Evangelou E: Uncertainty in heterogeneity estimates in meta-analyses. BMJ. 2007. 335:914-6. DOI: 10.1136/bmj 39343.408449.80.

[21] Egger M, Davey Smith G, Schneider M, Minder C: Bias in meta-analysis detected by a simple, graphical test. BMJ. 1997. 315:629-34. DOI: 10.1136/bmj.315.7109.629.

[22] Mantel N, Haenszel W: Statistical aspects of the analysis of data from retrospective studies of disease. J Natl Cancer Inst. 1959. 22:719-48. DOI: 10.1093/jnci/22.4.719

[23] Lau J, Ioannidis JP, Schmid CH: Quantitative synthesis in systematic reviews. Ann Intern Med. 1997. 127:820-6. DOI: 10.7326/0003-4819-127-9-199711010-00008.

[24] Higgins JP, Thompson SG: Quantifying heterogeneity in a meta-analysis. Stat Med. 2002. 21:1539-58. DOI: 10.1002/sim.1186.

[25] Baker WL, White CM, Cappelleri JC, Kluger J, Coleman CI, Health Outcomes P, et al.: Understanding heterogeneity in meta-analysis: the role of meta-regression. Int J Clin Pract. 2009. 63:1426-34. DOI: 10.1111/j.1742-1241.2009.02168.x.

[26] Sterne JA, Egger M, Smith GD: Systematic reviews in health care: investigating and dealing with publication and other biases in meta-analysis. BMJ. 2001. 323:101-5. DOI: 10.1136/bmj.323.7304.101.

[27] Begg CB, Mazumdar M: Operating characteristics of a rank correlation test for publication bias. Biometrics. 1994. 50:1088-101. DOI: 10.2307/2533446

[28] Kaper JB, Nataro JP, Mobley HL: Pathogenic *Escherichia coli*. Nat Rev Microbiol. 2004. 2:123-40. DOI: 10.1038/nrmicro818.

[29] Nataro JP, Kaper JB: Diarrheagenic *Escherichia coli*. Clin Microbiol Rev. 1998. 11:142-201. DOI: n/a.

[30] Drasar BS, Hill MJ. Human Intestinal Flora. London, United Kingdom: Academic Press, Ltd; 1974. 36-43 pp.

[31] Russo TA, Johnson JR: Proposal for a new inclusive designation for extraintestinal pathogenic isolates of *Escherichia coli*: ExPEC. J Infect Dis. 2000. 181:1753-4. DOI: 10.1086/315418.

[32] Cooke EM: *Escherichia coli*--an overview. J Hyg (Lond). 1985. 95:523-30. DOI: n/a.

[33] Arnold BF, Colford JM, Jr.: Treating water with chlorine at point-of-use to improve water quality and reduce child diarrhea in developing countries: a systematic review and meta-analysis. Am J Trop Med Hyg. 2007. 76:354-64. DOI: n/a.

[34] Wade TJ, Pai N, Eisenberg JN, Colford JM, Jr.: Do U.S. Environmental Protection Agency water quality guidelines for recreational waters prevent gastrointestinal illness? A systematic review and meta-analysis. Environ Health Perspect. 2003. 111:1102-9. DOI: 10.1289/ehp.6241.

[35] Williams AR, Bain RE, Fisher MB, Cronk R, Kelly ER, Bartram J: A systematic review and meta-analysis of fecal contamination and inadequate treatment of packaged water. PLoS One. 2015. 10:e0140899. DOI: 10.1371/journal.pone.0140899.

[36] O'Flaherty E. Meta-analysis of the Effect of UV Water Treatment on *Escherichia coli*. UCD Biosystems and Engineering: University College Dublin; Ireland 2016.

[37] Franz E, Schijven J, de Roda Husman AM, Blaak H: Meta-regression analysis of commensal and pathogenic *Escherichia coli* survival in soil and water. Environ Sci Technol. 2014. 48:6763-71. DOI: 10.1021/es501677c.

[38] Mielke M: Prevention and control of nosocomial infections and resistance to antibiotics in Europe - primum non-nocere: elements of successful prevention and control of healthcare-associated infections. Int J Med Microbiol. 2010. 300:346-50. DOI: 10.1016/j.ijmm.2010.04.004.

[39] Seib KL, Zhao X, Rappuoli R: Developing vaccines in the era of genomics: a decade of reverse vaccinology. Clin Microbiol Infect. 2012. 18 Suppl 5:109-16. DOI: 10.1111/j.1469-0691.2012.03939.x.

[40] Dewsbury D. Prevalence of Non-O157 Shiga Toxin-producing *Escherichia coli* (STEC) Serogroups (O26, O45, O103, O111, O121, and O145) and Virulence Genes in Feces, *Escherichia coli*; Kansas State University; Manhattan, Kansas, USA; 2015.

[41] Islam MZ, Musekiwa A, Islam K, Ahmed S, Chowdhury S, Ahad A, et al.: Regional variation in the prevalence of *E. coli* O157 in cattle: a meta-analysis and meta-regression. PLoS One. 2014. 9:e93299. DOI: 10.1371/journal.pone.0093299.

[42] Dautzenberg MJ, Haverkate MR, Bonten MJ, Bootsma MC: Epidemic potential of *Escherichia coli* ST131 and *Klebsiella pneumoniae* ST258: a systematic review and meta-analysis. BMJ Open. 2016. 6:e009971. DOI: 10.1136/bmjopen-2015-009971.

[43] Haverkate M. Epidemic Potential of *Escherichia coli* ST131 and *Klebsiella pneumoniae* ST258: A Systematic Review and Meta-Analysis (Chapter 8). Utrecht, the Netherlands: University Medical Cen; 2016.

[44] Huang DB, Nataro JP, DuPont HL, Kamat PP, Mhatre AD, Okhuysen PC, et al.: Enteroaggregative *Escherichia coli* is a cause of acute diarrheal illness: a meta-analysis. Clin Infect Dis. 2006. 43:556-63. DOI: 10.1086/505869.

[45] Allocati N, Masulli M, Alexeyev MF, Di Ilio C: *Escherichia coli* in Europe: an overview. Int J Environ Res Public Health. 2013. 10:6235-54. DOI: 10.3390/ijerph10126235.

[46] Evans DJ, Evans DG. *Escherichia coli* in diarrheal disease. In: Baron S, editor. Medical Microbiology. 4th ed. Galveston, Texas: University of Texas Medical Branch at Galveston; 1996.

[47] Agger M, Scheutz F, Villumsen S, Molbak K, Petersen AM: Antibiotic treatment of verocytotoxin-producing *Escherichia coli* (VTEC) infection: a systematic review and a proposal. J Antimicrob Chemother. 2015. 70:2440-6. DOI: 10.1093/jac/dkv162.

[48] Ahmed T, Bhuiyan TR, Zaman K, Sinclair D, Qadri F: Vaccines for preventing enterotoxigenic *Escherichia coli* (ETEC) diarrhoea. Cochrane Database Syst Rev. 7:2013. CD009029. DOI: 10.1002/14651858.CD009029.pub2.

[49] Freedman SB, Xie J, Neufeld MS, Hamilton WL, Hartling L, Tarr PI, et al.: Shiga toxin-producing *Escherichia coli* infection, antibiotics, and risk of developing hemolytic uremic syndrome: a meta-analysis. Clin Infect Dis. 2016. 62:1251-8. DOI: 10.1093/cid/ciw099.

[50] Philipsborn R, Ahmed SM, Brosi BJ, Levy K: Climatic drivers of diarrheagenic *Escherichia coli* incidence: a systematic review and meta-analysis. J Infect Dis. 2016. 214:6-15. DOI: 10.1093/infdis/jiw081.

[51] Porter CK, Riddle MS, Tribble DR, Louis Bougeois A, McKenzie R, Isidean SD, et al.: A systematic review of experimental infections with enterotoxigenic *Escherichia coli* (ETEC). Vaccine. 2011. 29:5869-85. DOI: 10.1016/j.vaccine.2011.05.021.

[52] Aykan SB, Ciftci IH: Antibiotic resistance patterns of *Escherichia coli* strains isolated from urine cultures in Turkey: a meta-analysis. Mikrobiyol Bul. 2013. 47:603-18. DOI: 10.5578/mb.6383.

[53] Bryce A, Hay AD, Lane IF, Thornton HV, Wootton M, Costelloe C: Global prevalence of antibiotic resistance in paediatric urinary tract infections caused by *Escherichia coli* and association with routine use of antibiotics in primary care: systematic review and meta-analysis. BMJ. 2016. 352:i939. DOI: 10.1136/bmj.i939.

[54] Fasugba O, Gardner A, Mitchell BG, Mnatzaganian G: Ciprofloxacin resistance in community- and hospital-acquired *Escherichia coli* urinary tract infections: a systematic review and meta-analysis of observational studies. BMC Infect Dis. 2015. 15:545. DOI: 10.1186/s12879-015-1282-4.

[55] Hadifar S, Moghoofei M, Nematollahi S, Ramazanzadeh R, Sedighi M, Salehi-Abargouei A, et al.: Epidemiology of multi drug resistant uropathogenic *Escherichia coli* in Iran: a systematic review and meta-analysis. Jpn J Infect Dis. 2016. 1-26 DOI: 10.7883/yoken.JJID.2015.652.

[56] Penna F: Antimicrobial resistance patterns of *Escherichia coli* in uncomplicated community-acquired urinary tract infections among adults: a meta-analysis. J Urol. 2010. 183:e235. DOI: 10.1016/j.juro.2010.02.911.

[57] Azzopardi EA, Azzopardi E, Camilleri L, Villapalos J, Boyce DE, Dziewulski P, et al.: Gram negative wound infection in hospitalised adult burn patients—systematic review and metanalysis. PLoS One. 2014. 9:e95042. DOI: 10.1371/journal.pone.0095042.

[58] Downie L, Armiento R, Subhi R, Kelly J, Clifford V, Duke T: Community-acquired neonatal and infant sepsis in developing countries: efficacy of WHO's currently recommended antibiotics--systematic review and meta-analysis. Arch Dis Child. 2013. 98:146-54. DOI: 10.1136/archdischild-2012-302033.

[59] Futagami S, Itoh T, Sakamoto C: Systematic review with meta-analysis: post-infectious functional dyspepsia. Aliment Pharmacol Ther. 2015. 41:177-88. DOI: 10.1111/apt.13006.

[60] Ming D.: Classification and distribution of extended-spectrum β-lactamases produced by *Escherichia coli* in China: a meta analysis of their susceptibility. Chin J Nosoconmiol. 2005.

[61] Ščuka L: A meta-analysis and systematic review of the efficacy of enrofloxacin-infections with the bacterium *Escherichia coli* in pigs. Slov Vet Res. 2004. 41:121-7. DOI: n/a.

[62] Vardakas KZ, Tansarli GS, Rafailidis PI, Falagas ME: Carbapenems versus alternative antibiotics for the treatment of bacteraemia due to Enterobacteriaceae producing extended-spectrum beta-lactamases: a systematic review and meta-analysis. J Antimicrob Chemother. 2012. 67:2793-803. DOI: 10.1093/jac/dks301.

[63] Xu QQ, Huang XB, Wang XF, Zhu JC, Liu QW, Zhang ZX, et al.: Prostatic abscess: a report of 2 cases and meta-analysis of domestic literature in recent 10 years. Zhonghua Nan Ke Xue. 2007. 13:903-5. DOI: n/a.

[64] Bain R, Cronk R, Wright J, Yang H, Slaymaker T, Bartram J: Fecal contamination of drinking-water in low- and middle-income countries: a systematic review and meta-analysis. PLoS Med. 2014. 11:e1001644. DOI: 10.1371/journal.pmed.1001644.

[65] Greig J: The efficacy of interventions applied during primary processing on contamination of beef carcasses with *Escherichia coli*: a systematic review-meta-analysis of the published research. Food Control. 2012. 27:385-97. DOI 10.1016/j.foodcont.2012.03.019.

[66] Gruber JS, Ercumen A, Colford JM, Jr.: Coliform bacteria as indicators of diarrheal risk in household drinking water: systematic review and meta-analysis. PLoS One. 2014. 9:e107429. DOI: 10.1371/journal.pone.0107429.

[67] McQuestin OJ, Shadbolt CT, Ross T: Quantification of the relative effects of temperature, pH, and water activity on inactivation of *Escherichia coli* in fermented meat by meta-analysis. Appl Environ Microbiol. 2009. 75:6963-72. DOI: 10.1128/AEM.00291-09.

[68] Prado-Silva L, Cadavez V, Gonzales-Barron U, Rezende AC, Sant'Ana AS: Meta-analysis of the Effects of Sanitizing Treatments on Salmonella, *Escherichia coli* O157:H7, and *Listeria monocytogenes* Inactivation in Fresh Produce. Appl Environ Microbiol. 2015. 81:8008-21. DOI: 10.1128/AEM.02216-15.

[69] Zhilyaev S. Meta-analysis on the effect of interventions used in cattle processing plants to reduce *Escherichia coli* contamination. In: Meeting IA, editor. Diet Intervention Conference Proceedings Portugal; 2016

[70] Ruzante J. The effect of cattle diet on fecal shedding of *Escherichia coli*: a meta-analysis. In: Meeting A, editor. Diet Intervention Conference Proceedings; July 25-28, 2015; North Carolina, USA; 2015.

[71] Snedeker KG, Campbell M, Sargeant JM: A systematic review of vaccinations to reduce the shedding of *Escherichia coli* O157 in the faeces of domestic ruminants. Zoonoses Public Health. 2012. 59:126-38. DOI: 10.1111/j.1863-2378.2011.01426.x.

[72] Wisener LV, Sargeant JM, O'Connor AM, Faires MC, Glass-Kaastra SK: The use of direct-fed microbials to reduce shedding of *Escherichia coli* O157 in beef cattle: a systematic review and meta-analysis. Zoonoses Public Health. 2015. 62:75-89. DOI: 10.1111/zph.12112.

[73] Bauer HW, Rahlfs VW, Lauener PA, Blessmann GS: Prevention of recurrent urinary tract infections with immuno-active *E. coli* fractions: a meta-analysis of five placebo-controlled double-blind studies. Int J Antimicrob Agents. 2002. 19:451-6. DOI: 10.1016/S0924-8579(02)00106-1.

[74] Bolon MK, Wright SB, Gold HS, Carmeli Y: The magnitude of the association between fluoroquinolone use and quinolone-resistant *Escherichia coli* and *Klebsiella pneumoniae* may be lower than previously reported. Antimicrob Agents Chemother. 2004. 48:1934-40. DOI: 10.1128/AAC.48.6.1934-1940.2004.

[75] Huber M, Krauter K, Winkelmann G, Bauer HW, Rahlfs VW, Lauener PA, et al.: Immunostimulation by bacterial components: II. Efficacy studies and meta-analysis of the bacterial extract OM-89. Int J Immunopharmacol. 2000. 22:1103-11. DOI: 10.1016/S0192-0561(00)00070-9.

[76] Taha Neto KA, Nogueira Castilho L, Reis LO: Oral vaccine (OM-89) in the recurrent urinary tract infection prophylaxis: a realistic systematic review with meta-analysis. Actas Urol Esp. 2016. 40:203-8. DOI: 10.1016/j.acuro.2015.04.008.

[77] Li Y, Sun JF, Cui X, Mani H, Danner RL, Li X, et al.: The effect of heparin administration in animal models of sepsis: a prospective study in *Escherichia coli*-challenged mice and a systematic review and metaregression analysis of published studies. Crit Care Med. 2011. 39:1104-12. DOI: 10.1097/CCM.0b013e31820eb718.

[78] S. Belluco, L. Barco, A. Roccato, A. Ricci : *Escherichia coli* and Enterobacteriaceae counts on poultry carcasses along the slaughterline: A systematic review and meta-analysis. Food Control. 2016. 60:269-80. DOI: 10.1016/j.foodcont.2015.07.033.

[79] Kolenda R, Burdukiewicz M, Schierack P: A systematic review and meta-analysis of the epidemiology of pathogenic *Escherichia coli* of calves and the role of calves as reservoirs for human pathogenic *E. coli*. Front Cell Infect Microbiol. 2015. 5:23. DOI: 10.3389/fcimb.2015.00023.

[80] Varela NP, Dick P, Wilson J: Assessing the existing information on the efficacy of bovine vaccination against *Escherichia coli* O157:H7—a systematic review and meta-analysis. Zoonoses Public Health. 2013. 60:253-68. DOI: 10.1111/j.1863-2378.2012.01523.x.

[81] Ison J. A meta-analysis of the association of *Lactobacillus acidophilus* NP51 administration with *Escherichia coli* O157 in feces and on hides of feedlot cattle. J Ison—2013 Texas USA Intervention Thesis. Texas: Texas Tech University; 2013.

[82] Gonzales-Barron U, Cadavez V, Sheridan JJ, Butler F: Modelling the effect of chilling on the occurrence of Salmonella on pig carcasses at study, abattoir and batch levels by meta-analysis. Int J Food Microbiol. 2013. 163:101-13. DOI: 10.1016/j.ijfoodmicro.2013.03.006.

[83] Gonzales-Barron U. A meta-analysis of the effect of sanitizing treatments on *Escherichia coli* O157: H7 counts in fresh produce. In: Meeting A, editor. Diet Intervention Conference Proceedings; July 25-28, 2015; Portugal; 2015

[84] Eppinger M, Cebula TA: Future perspectives, applications and challenges of genomic epidemiology studies for food-borne pathogens: a case study of Enterohemorrhagic *Escherichia coli* (EHEC) of the O157:H7 serotype. Gut Microbes. 2015. 6:194-201. DOI: 10.4161/19490976.2014.969979.

Section 3

Application of E. coli in Biotechnology

Chapter 13

Escherichia coli as a Model Organism and Its Application in Biotechnology

Vargas-Maya Naurú Idalia and Franco Bernardo

Additional information is available at the end of the chapter

http://dx.doi.org/10.5772/67306

Abstract

Without a doubt, in the past 20 or so years, we have achieved the power of biology in different ways. In the present, we have many tools for developing novel technologies and applications for organism modifications that ultimately let us know many aspects of organisms' biology and, therefore, apply that knowledge for technological purposes. Of all the model organisms and tools for genetic modification available, *Escherichia coli* stands out as a model organism and what we would like to call "molecular biologist tool box." In the present chapter, we aim to review our current knowledge regarding genetic modifications and tools for modifying *E. coli* to generate plasmid vectors, single and multiple gene knockouts, whole genome editing, biosensor generation and applications and synthetic gene circuits and genomes.

Keywords: molecular biology tools, synthetic biology, biosensors, plasmids, bioengineerging

1. Introduction

Who in biology has not heard of *Escherichia coli*? Known to many as the fundamental model microbe and perhaps model organism, *E. coli* is the cornerstone of many important findings in molecular biology and other areas of cell physiology. Perhaps even the first chemo-organo-heterotroph had a similar mass composition as *E. coli*, providing the hits necessary to understand the evolution of modern bacteria [1]. Also called the "workhorse" of molecular biology for its fast growing rate in chemically defined media and extensive molecular tools available for different purposes, *E. coli* is considered the most important model organism of them all. Important findings and Nobel Prizes in biology have been developed in *E. coli*. For instance, cracking the genetic code [2], unveiling the nature of DNA replication [3], the groundbreaking advances on gene organization and regulation or as we love to call 'the operon' [4, 5], important evidence for the basis of mutations and ultimately to the evolution of organisms [6, 7], and finally, the achievement of a genetically modified organism [8] that skyrocketed several applications of the enormous capacity for manipulating this organism, rendering *E. coli* as a key player in biotechnology (for an excellent review, see Ref. [9]).

The main reasons why *E. coli* is the organism of choice extends and is not limited to its fast growth in chemically defined media; relative cheap culture media; does not form aggregates; industrial scalability; several molecular tools for manipulation; extensive knowledge of its genetics and genomics; extensive knowledge on its transcriptome, proteome, and metabolome, and several strains are considered biosafety 1, which renders it ideal even for teaching and school demonstrations (for example, Bio-Rad transformation kits, URL: http://www.bio-rad.com/es-mx/category/pglo-plasmid-gfp-kits).

Typical *E. coli,* a Gram-negative bacillus bears a rod-shaped, measures only about 1 μm long by 0.35 μm wide, although this can vary considerably depending on the strain and its conditions, there are studies regarding different mutations that affect its size and length considerably. A recent paper showed that this bacterium can grow up to 750 μm in length. By random Tn10 insertion, they found this particular mutant has an insertion at genes *ybd*N and *ybd*M whose function remains uncertain and another mutation that remains to be identified [10]. Interestingly, this mutant strain gives rise to extremely long cells that are viable (capable of cell division) and retain metabolic activity that can be useful for studies involving intracellular localization or optimize cell-surface contact.

In terms of ecology, *E. coli* is a facultative aerobe (either respiration takes place in the presence of oxygen or fermentation in its absence), which bears a sensor for oxygen presence (redox state in the quinone pool) and can activate or repress the required metabolic enzymes, depending on oxygen levels [11–13]. Also, *E. coli* and other Enterobacteriaceae can be the first organisms to colonize human infant intestine due to this capacity to metabolize oxygen or ferment because this facultative bacteria will consume the remaining oxygen in this environment so that other strict anaerobic bacteria are capable of colonizing the intestine rendering the normal microbiota found in humans and also thrive as part of the normal microbiota [14].

Phylogenetically, *E. coli* is a member of the Enterobacteriaceae and is closely related to pathogens such as *Salmonella, Klebsiella, Serratia,* and the infamous *Yersinia pestis,* which causes plague. Although *E. coli* is mostly harmless, pathogenicity islands have been identified and associated with pathogenesis in *E. coli* resulting in strains that colonize different tissues [15].

The building blocks of *E. coli* consists of about 55% protein, 25% nucleic acids, 9% lipids, 6% cell wall, 2.5% glycogen, and 3% other metabolites [16–18], which for biotechnological applications is important, since carbon flux is often a problematic issue to address in order to generate a novel metabolic pathway or to enhance a current functioning pathway. Also, carbon flux is tightly regulated by sophisticated regulatory networks that require modeling and a basic understanding of the regulatory mechanisms in order to manipulate them and achieve desired goals [19–21].

E. coli is part of the normal microbiota of mammals, rendering the predominant facultative microbe of the gastrointestinal tract and is currently a hot debate on the impact on normal microflora establishment and their role in disease [22].

This organism lacks many interesting features for biotechnology, such as growing at extreme temperatures or pH, the capacity to degrade toxic compounds, pollutants, or difficult to degrade polymers [23]. But as we will see later, this bacterium is capable of doing amazing things and its only limit is our imagination.

E. coli harbors a genome with particular features such as a strikingly organized structure, remnents of many phages, and insertion sequences (IS) and a high transport capacity toward the cytoplasm. In 1997, the complete genome sequence of the K-12 strain was obtained, and a myriad of research was catapulted from that moment on [24]. The complete genome contains a single circular duplex molecule composed of 4,639,221 bp. Regarding its structure, protein-coding regions correspond to 87.8% of the genome, while 0.8% encodes for stable RNAs, and 0.7% consists of noncoding repeats. The remaining 11% encodes for regulatory and other functions. Nevertheless, nearly 34% (1431) proteins are considered orphan or without defined molecular function but in a recent study, it was demonstrated that by homology with distant phylogenetical relationships, they may play a role in defined molecular pathways or processes [25]. From the orphan set in *E. coli*, at least 446 contain some molecular signature that can assess their molecular role. The fact that such a vast portion of the genome remains uncharacterized for defined molecular pathways or roles paves the way for future basic research that may have a strong impact on applied research and development. For biotechnological applications, growth optimization is also a required feature of genetically modified organisms. For *E. coli*, it has been recently shown that growth can be manipulated by removing nonessential genomic sequences that also can lead to the design of important biotechnological strains for industrial purposes [26].

The advancement of genomic, transcriptomic, and proteomic technologies has led to the development of several online resources for the analysis of molecular and physiological aspects of *E. coli*. Some examples are given in **Table 1**.

Escherichia coli **databases**

Name	URL	Description*
EcoCyc: Encyclopedia of *E. coli* Genes and Metabolic Pathways	https://ecocyc.org	A comprehensive database joining together genomic information with biochemical features of *E. coli*
PortEco	http://www.porteco.org	A resource for knowledge and data of the biology of *E. coli* including plasmids, mobile genetic elements, and phages
EcoliWiki	http://ecoliwiki.net/	Community-based pages about everything related to the biology of the nonpathogenic *E. coli*
EcoGen 3.0	http://ecogene.org/	A database dedicated to analyzing and comparing genomic and transcriptomic data

Escherichia coli **databases**		
Name	**URL**	**Description***
Kegg	http://www.genome.jp/kegg-bin/show_organism?org=eco	A powerful resource for understanding molecular datasets in different contexts, also easy access to gene information
RegulonDB	http://regulondb.ccg.unam.mx	Database on transcriptional regulation in *E. coli* K-12 containing knowledge manually curated from original scientific publications, complemented with high throughput datasets and comprehensive computational predictions
E. coli Genetic Stock Center	http://cgsc.biology.yale.edu/	The CGSC Database of *E. coli* genetic information includes genotypes and reference information for the strains in the CGSC collection. An excellent resource for acquiring information and strains for research

**Source*: databases website.

Table 1. Relevant *E. coli* resources and databases.

Recently, using the Genome Conformation Capture technique, it was revealed that the linear organization of the genome is also true for the 3D structure, rendering neighboring genes to form small factories that are coregulated or coexpressed and showed a higher probability of forming protein-protein interactions. This organization represents two important aspects of bacterial genomes, first, the compactness in the 3D space, containing pathways in a nonrandom distribution, and second, genes that are closer to each other tend to be coexpressed and form protein-protein interactions favoring the concept of transcription factor even in microbial cells [27].

In the following sections, we will review what we consider the modern tools for genetic engineering *E. coli*, and the future for this microbe that can be considered the toolbox for molecular biology and may be the answer to many problems that humanity may face in the future.

2. Plasmid and the *E. coli* revolution

Without a doubt, plasmids are the most important tools not only for the manipulation of *E. coli* but also the foundation for the genetic engineering of many organisms, cloning and sequencing, generation of mutants, and many applications in molecular biology. In this section, a brief summary of the myriad of plasmids available will be addressed, providing some of the most important features of plasmids and the up-to-date technologies available for plasmid manipulation and application.

Why plasmids are the basis for genetic engineering? By surveying the literature and commercial sources catalogs, there is a myriad of applications for plasmids: cloning, mutagenesis, protein fusion and overexpression, shuttle vectors from bacteria to a diverse range of hosts, among others. Plasmids must be first presented and then we provide some features that are relevant regarding the importance of plasmids in molecular biology and biotechnology.

Plasmids are extrachromosomal molecules that are self-replicative and sometimes provide interesting features to its host. The term was first coined by Joshua Lederberg in 1952 referring to genetic elements in bacteria that remained as an independent molecule from the chromosome at any stage of their replication cycle [28]. The definition was further refined to all the autonomously replicating DNA molecules to avoid including viruses. These molecules are present not only in eubacteria but also are found in Archea and some lower eukaryotic organisms [29]. In nature, many bacteria contain self-replicating DNA molecules that can be harnessed for molecular biology applications. *E. coli* plasmids were the first ones to be extensively modified for such purposes [30].

In the 1970s, the first generation of cloning plasmids was created, and from that moment on, research in the biological area was enriched with a powerful tool. Plasmids must contain several important features to be used in research: proper size for ease to transform or transfect, selection markers, a replication origin, regulatory elements to control expression, and transcription termination. All features are important when designing a plasmid vector for the desired application, the reader can imagine the goal, and there will always be a way to create the molecular tool for achieving such a goal, and that is possible due to the basic structure of most plasmids used in molecular biology and their modularity [31]. In **Table 2**, we summarize some of the most important features (modules) that plasmids must have in order to serve for different applications. We point out that sequence composition and structure, copy number, selection marker, and special features such as reporter proteins or regulatory elements are the most important features in a plasmid and can influence the outcome of the desired application.

***Escherichia coli* plasmids**		
Name	**Type of element**	**Characteristics**
ColE1	Replication origin	Generates 15–20 copies of each plasmid molecule. Colicin production. Related to plasmids that confer immunity to phage infections [32]. Found in low copy plasmids such as pBR322 [33]. There are mutations in this replication origin that leads to high copy number plasmids, such as pUC series that can render up to 700 copies per cell [34, 35]
p15A	Replication origin	Low copy number replication origin, estimated in 18–22 copies per cell [36]. This type of replication origin is often found in pACYC and its derivative vectors

Escherichia coli plasmids		
Name	**Type of element**	**Characteristics**
pMB1	Replication origin	Versatile replication origin. The original sequence generates 15–20 copies per cell, but a mutant version can lead up to 700 copies per cell [37]. This plasmid contains the *Eco*RI restriction-modification system
pSC101	Replication origin	Five copies per cell [38]
R6K	Replication origin	15–20 copies per cell. Requires the π protein from the gene *pir* for replication [39]. This origin of replication is functional in diverse bacterial species
Amp^r, Kan^r, Cm^r, Tet^r among other	Selection markers	Elements required for the selection and maintenance of plasmids in bacterial hosts. Here are listed the resistance cassettes for Ampicillin, Kanamycin, Chloramphenicol, and Tetracycline, which are the most common selection markers. For additional markers, RAC database contains the information regarding antibiotic resistance traits and their sequence [40] or iGEM website for sequence modules bearing the proper syntax for synthetic constructs
LacZ, CcdB, Green Fluorescent protein (GFP), etc	Additional elements required for positive clone selection, reporter protein fusions among others	Plasmids have been modified so that they contain multiple cloning sites with diverse unique restriction sites, counter selection for positive clone selection. Additional elements such as filamentous origins for single-stranded DNA generation for sequencing of high G+C templates or site-directed mutagenesis

Additional sources: [31], http://blog.addgene.org/plasmid-101-origin-of-replication. https://www.neb.com/, https://www.thermofisher.com/mx/es/home/brands/invitrogen.html, and http://parts.igem.org/Help:Synthetic_Biology, which contains a repository of parts that can be needed for plasmid construction using synthetic methods.

Table 2. Common elements in plasmids used in molecular biology applications.

Some exceptional features of plasmids are they can be used in systems where replication origins (check compatibility first) and selection markers can coexist in the same cell, which can be extremely useful for the coexpression of four different proteins in the same cell (e.g., the four plasmid system developed by Dykxhoorn et al., which are compatible between them [41]); the broad diversity of selection markers and partitioning control elements [30]; cloning capacity [31], which is an important feature for cloning large fragments required for synthetic biology applications or metabolic engineering; reporter proteins useful for selecting positive clones; recombination or assembly technology for easier cloning methods [42, 43], and the

http://dx.doi.org/10.5772/67306

ability to be transferred from one host to another like the case of the OriV from RK2 plasmid [44]. We recommend for further information about replication control of plasmids to refer to del Solar et al. [45].

Linear plasmids are common in bacteria (particularly in actinobacteria), but thus far, only N15 plasmid prophage has been isolated from *E. coli* [46] and is an impediment for generating knockouts using linear DNA (see Section 3). Recently, a linear plasmid was created to clone unstable fragments bearing repetitive sequences without showing size bias during cloning, active promoter sequences, or sequences with A + T content [47].

One of the biggest impediments for plasmid segregation is the insert size. As discussed in Section 5, we are now facing not only the most exciting age of molecular biology but also the most challenging. In order to develop "bugs to the order," i.e., microbes are "trained" to perform specific tasks [48], from simple pathways to synthesize a specific metabolite to complex genetic circuits that can be controlled for novel environmental responses. In all these cases, plasmids play an important role, from generating site-specific integration of chromosomal fusions to large plasmids that can hold complex constructs for further modification. Another challenging area is the generation of strains capable of producing metabolic products required for the pharmaceutical industry, where metabolic pathways and cell metabolism can be a strong impediment for proper synthesis and purification of relevant precursors [49]. *E. coli* renders an important platform for tackling down impediments for the synthesis of novel compounds.

As part of the information needed for plasmid manipulation, databases and repositories are also relevant for the manipulation and selection of the right plasmid for the applications you want to further exploit. Such examples are given: a powerful plasmid repository is Addgene (https://www.addgene.org/vector-database/) where you can get any plasmid in the repository with minimum fees for shipping and handling. This source is important in many aspects; you can gain knowledge about plasmid sequence, special features, creators, and availability to use since you can acquire them with small fees. Also, Harvard University is currently generating a plasmid repository but still under development (https://plasmid.med.harvard.edu/PLASMID/Home.xhtml). These repositories are an excellent option for accelerating research due to finding already generated constructs useful for ongoing projects. Also, *E. coli* Genetic Stock Center (**Table 1**) is a good source of strains and plasmids for different applications. For a small fee, the strains and plasmids can be shipped worldwide and characteristics can be consulted. Also, the American Type Culture Collection (www.atcc.org) is a source for strains with desired characteristics, as well as knowledge on their features. In plasmid biology, strain selection is fundamental for plasmid stability and proper propagation, as well as for the correct function of special features, such as protein expression [50]. For example, DNA methylation is an important impediment in certain applications such as eukaryotic transfection, proper DAM^- and DCM^- strains for plasmid isolation is required. In protein expression experiments, the repertoire for host selection is big. Most applications require lysogen strains harboring the required RNA polymerase. As stated in **Table 2**, some plasmids require the product from the *pir* gene, so careful strain selection must be taken into account so that plasmids replicate efficiently.

Novel methods such as Gibson assembly, Golden Gate assembly, and AQUA (advanced quick assembly) methods [43, 51, 52] have skyrocketed the possibility to assemble any plasmid with the desired characteristics. These methods are based on designed modules that can either be Polymerase Chain Reaction (PCR) amplified or generated as a complete synthetic construct and then assembled in the desired combination either by an enzymatic process (Gibson and Golden gate) or even enzyme-free methods such as AQUA.

Finally, plasmid biology is still under scrutiny, for their involvement in the mobility of traits that are important for human health such as antibiotic resistance, the distribution of pathogenicity islands, and genome evolution. Recently, novel tools for plasmid mining have been developed and uncover from Next Generation Sequencing data that plasmids can be uncovered and analyzed for further characterization [53, 54].

We are still in the process of truly knowing the potential of *E. coli*, novel tools generated through plasmids in combination with other molecular strategies will lead to new discoveries that will render this organism the basis for important discoveries. In the next section, we will discuss some aspects of gene knockouts and the knowledge we have gained from this versatile organism.

3. Genome modifications to understand *E. coli*

One of the basic questions in biology is: what is life? Defining life imposes a challenging burden both intellectual and experimental. Many attempts have been done to answer this. *E. coli* is a model organism that with all the molecular tools available we can get a step closer to provide sufficient information that will lead us to answer the relevance of genomic information and ultimately what is needed to achieve life [55]. In 1997, its genome was fully sequenced, and with all that information (from *E. coli* and all the organisms that have been sequenced thus far), scientists have aimed high to achieve the knowledge of how many genes are needed for life to be sustained. Molecular genetics have provided many tools for understanding gene structure and function, the most fundamentals are gene knockouts and genome deletions. In this section, we provide aspects that are fundamental for understanding genome structure and function taking our knowledge closer to knowing the minimal core genome of bacterial organisms and the optimization of *E. coli* for biotechnology.

In *E. coli*, several tools for genome modification have been developed. Some of the most important methods involve either the generation of deletion mutants by removing specific genes, one outstanding case is the use of the lambda Red system for inhibiting linear DNA degradation and by homologous recombination, the deletion of specific genes using PCR-derived selection marker cassettes with homologous sequences with target gene [56, 57]. Lambda Red-based method have yielded a total of 4288 genes mutated without lethality (Keio collection), 303 genes were unable to be deleted, from which 37 are of unknown function [58]. This experimental evidence has pointed out one very important aspect of genome structure and function. Genome size increase is the result of horizontal gene transfer or DNA fragment retention that somehow is giving some beneficial features to recipient host, apparently an increase in fitness [26]. The function of genes without evident function is still a relevant area of research since

http://dx.doi.org/10.5772/67306

many of them provide support for fitness and evolution has preserved them, therefore full genome engineering is far more complicated than previously thought.

Larger genomic editions are needed to understand how far we can delete redundant or non-essential sequences. By using Cre/lox recombination, substantial genomic fragments can be deleted or sequentially removed, rendering the nonessential regions (regardless the genes present) from the genome [59–61].

Studies regarding genome size analyzed through deletions of specific genes or complete genomic regions have led on thinking about the minimal genome. In the case of *E. coli*, there are several pieces of evidence (reviewed in Ref. [62]) that points out that at least 23% of the genome can be eliminated gaining genomic stability and normal growth. Also, eliminating insertion sequences can enhance the capacity of *E. coli* to synthesize proteins due to the decrease or insertions on plasmids, and strains exhibit normal growth plus increased genome stability [63].

All these methods rely on basic bacterial genetics founded with *E. coli*, such as transposon-based integration of recombination sequences, λ-recombination of PCR products integrating deletion module cassettes, and the gene-specific knockout methods [62]. Mutations can then be transferred from one strain to the other to generate multiple deletions at once, and other technologies are still limited to either whole genome synthesis with previous knowledge on the structure of the genome.

The most relevant study revealed that genome size has an impact on *E. coli* cell growth, where it is shown that apparently dispensable sequences are needed under restrictive conditions, providing a hint of the still far future of fully functioning cells with all the desired characteristics for biotechnological applications [26]. We envision that genome reduction is a worthy effort, regardless of the method used to generate them. Another important aspect that we have to consider is that all conditions of the mutant strains are exposed to laboratory conditions rendering a behavior close to the ancestor or original strains. Nevertheless, there are also hidden features that must be exploited in order to understand fully the behavior of the genome and the essentiality of genes [62]. Thus far, *E. coli* remains restricted to the use of classic genetic tools and transposon or plasmid-based techniques. We encourage *E. coli* research community to join efforts to enter the synthetic biology era toward the generation of a fully synthetic *E. coli*. Our excitement is based on the following:

After 6 years, in 2016, the first bacteria operating under a "minimal chemically synthesized genome" was created after the first fully functioning synthetic genome [64, 65].

This research we believe has an impact in the following areas. First, both studies settled the basis for whole genome synthetic biology, which will lead to important findings in many research areas. Second, the extensive transposon-based mutagenesis studies on the genome of *Mycoplasma mycoides* led to the knowledge of the basis of essential genes or quasi-essential genes that have an important impact on cell fitness. Third, all this knowledge led to the design of a complete chemically synthesized genome with all the basic functions, and we now have the basic information for mining existing genomes to look for core modules in the bacterial genomes and design genomes with specific functions. Taking together all the observations from the synthetic genomes, we envision a bright future for bacterial molecular genetics in many fields of biotechnology, such as the production of molecules for human wellbeing.

E. coli is an extensively studied organism, with all the cumulative data we can ensure that with all this knowledge, we can design tools. In the following section, we comment on the biosensors that are *E. coli*-based.

4. *E. coli*-based biosensors: tools for many applications

In biotechnology, biosensors are broadly defined as any device based on biological part, cell, tissue, or protein complex that are linked to a mechanical sensor or analytical receptor that provides a measurable signal proportional to the analyte in the reaction [66, 67]. *E. coli*-based biosensors using plasmid or chromosomal constructs are useful for the detection of environmental traits or hazards or measuring cellular processes as any standard reporter system [68–70].

In **Figure 1**, we depict the basic design for whole-cell biosensors and some applications. Plasmid vectors with all the possible modifications can lead to almost endless combinations. For practical applications, there are commercial vectors that can be used for such purposes or as mentioned in the previous sections, plasmid methods are powerful enough for fast and robust biosensor design.

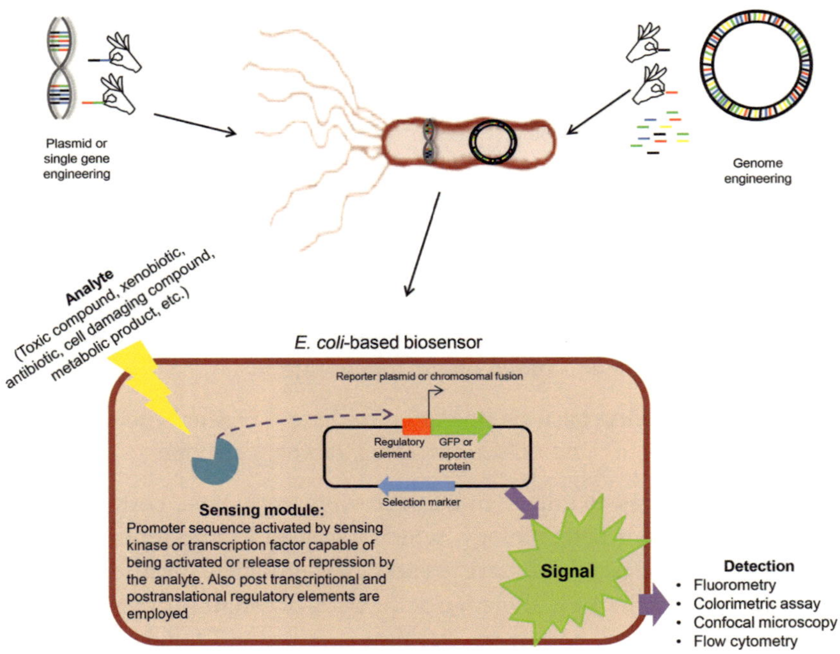

Figure 1. Basic principles for biosensor design. First, the proper design and the experimental creation of reporter strains. With current knowledge, either plasmid creation or whole genome engineering can lead to the creation of a reporter strain. Second, incorporation of such elements into the host cell. Third, sensing module and response measurement. With current reporter proteins and detection technology, it is relatively easy to generate biosensors that can be used in different applications with high sensitivity and selectivity.

The basic design considers the following: copy number, reporter proteins, detection methods, and control elements. The latter is basically the most important feature. As shown in **Table 1**, the available databases provide enough information for promoter selection and design. Bioinformatic tools can make this process easier [71]. Also, generation and detection of this kind of biosensors are cost-effective and easy to generate and reasonably sensitive [71]. In terms of speed, sample analysis with whole-cell biosensors is fast and cheap in comparison with analytical methods. The sensitivity of analytical methods is higher and more accurate, but biosensors are a good alternative for fast detection of hazards. Also, they can be coupled with the controlled production of metabolites of commercial importance.

In the literature, there are several reports where *E. coli*-based biosensors have been successful for detecting different traits: oxidants [72, 73], DNA damaging compounds [74], membrane-damaging compounds [75], protein-damaging compounds [76], aromatic compounds [77–79], xenobiotics [80], antibiotic panels using reporter strains without antibiotic selection [81], etc. The only limitation is the available sensor module and the design. The reporter protein is also important. Stability and reproducibility are two important aspects of biosensor design. In our experience, Green Fluorescent protein (GFP) protein is superior to luciferase, especially that we can detect GFP by various methods (we find flow cytometry, fluorometry, and confocal microscopy our top preferences) without cell lysis or substrate mixtures that are time-consuming [82].

With the improvement of DNA synthesis, recoding protein-coding genes for the desired function is expanding the capabilities of transcription factors, and reporter proteins have created novel sensor modules. For example, XilR recoding has led to a sensor that can detect millimolar concentrations of trinitrotoluene and its derivative compounds [83]. By using shuttle vectors, we can generate biosensors that we can transfer from one host to another, which can provide information about differences in physiological responses during the exposure to a given environmental trait.

E. coli plasticity and tools such as BioBrick building (using standardized DNA fragments with compatible ends for fast assembly) can facilitate plasmid and reporter constructs [84, 85]. Correlations of cell growth and physiology with expression patterns from reporter constructs can expand our knowledge of the impact of exposure to the external stimulus on cell physiology. Biosensors based on whole cells are a cheap alternative and can be coupled to portable devices. Using qualitative reporters can be applied in field research [70]. One good example is the detection of parasites without using cold-protected samples or complicated equipment for the detection process [86].

In the following section, we provide our final overview of the impact of *E. coli* in the synthetic biology future.

5. Genetic engineering and synthetic biology of *E. coli*

With the avenue of *in vitro* DNA synthesis to generate larger fragments with increased fidelity along with novel assembly methods, we are now capable of generating large and custom-made DNA molecules with the desired properties or even without the source of a DNA sample having only the sequence itself. New biological parts (genes, promoter sequence, terminators, etc.), devices (gene networks), and modules (biosynthetic pathways) are only limited by our imagination and the drive to create them. Also, without the advancement of methods for analyzing large amounts of data, bioinformatics, codon optimization software, genome mining, and user-friendly databases, synthetic biology creations are permeating in many laboratories around the world. With this in mind, we will review the current technologies for synthetic genes and genomes, and how this technology can be applied in generating novel regulatory circuits and even whole genomes. In this regard, *E. coli* is the key organism for such endeavors. Why? Well, in this section, we provide some examples that we consider may be helpful in the future of mankind and are in our opinion relevant in the field of genetic engineering and synthetic biology.

Synthetic biology is a relatively new branch of molecular genetics that incorporate engineering principles for modifying several aspects of cell physiology, rewiring genetic circuits, creating novel circuits, and synthesizing custom-made DNA sequences and even genomes [87]. This particular branch of biology needs to be supported by an extensive knowledge of the organism that modifications or even whole genome synthesis is attempted, several novel tools for analyzing big datasets and molecular tools for that particular organism, for the generation of sequences and the computational design of DNA molecules, and a goal that can be achieved with the desired organism. *E. coli* along with *Saccharomyces cerevisiae* are the most studied and well-comprehended organisms in science, and diverse phenotypes have been identified that are helpful for bioengineering [88, 89].

Multiplexing is the novel approach for redesigning organisms to do desired tasks [90]. By cycling through design-build–test framework we can achieve novel features in existing proteins and can further the advancement of genetic engineering. Thus far the most complicated and time-consuming part of this framework is the testing of the novel designs. High-throughput approaches have led to the development of fast and reliable screening methods and advances in this area, such as designed biosensors for the screening of metabolite producing strains or high-throughput methods for product screening, where the use of fluorescent proteins, colorimetric assays, and mass spectrometry are cornerstones for the development of screening methods for assessing success in strain engineering [90, 91]. DNA sequencing and synthesis coupled with good screening methods is the platform for future tools for the development of designed microorganism that can do desired tasks.

With all the technologies available, the advancement of using *E. coli* for biotechnological applications based on synthetic approaches have led to the development of strains capable of synthesizing several novel compounds. In the following lines, we provide some examples that we find important for improving environmental conditions and human well-being.

Synthesis of important metabolites can be difficult, and researchers must face the stubbornness of microorganisms to redirect carbon flux to their own processes, rendering the production of relevant molecules costly and inefficient. But *E. coli* is a flexible platform for the efficient production of molecules for the pharmaceutical industry, metabolites and molecules relevant for food additives, pigments, and more recently complex aliphatic molecules [92].

Several aromatic compounds have been successfully synthesized in *E. coli* due to their biological activities (vitamins and antioxidants, for example), pigmentation (applied in different industrial processes), and fragrance etc. [93]. In the case of the perfume industry, the synthesis of other relevant compounds such as precursors for Ambrox, a highly appreciated odorant for the perfume industry, or the synthesis of Geraniol, a valuable acyclic monoterpene alcohol, is also used in the perfume industry and pharmaceutical applications [94, 95].

Another relevant area was *E. coli* stepping in to biofuel production. The twentieth century is characterized by the human dependence on fossil fuels. They participate in a myriad of processes, and the demand is increasing. In order to alleviate the demand, scientists have turned to the development of novel technologies for biofuel production by the conversion of carbon sources into usable fuel. There are several reports where *E. coli* have been successfully engineered for the synthesis of branched-chain fatty acids or short-chain fatty acids that can ultimately lead to the mass production of fuel precursors or useful materials derived from oil [96–98]. Perhaps, the most promising future is a fully replicated fossil fuel, i.e., a mixture structurally and chemically identical to the fossil fuels that are currently under use, which is a mixture of aliphatic n- and iso-alkanes of various chain lengths [99]. Also, a more complete metabolic atlas of *E. coli* is needed, and recent efforts have mapped the metabolic flux from this bacterium further [100].

Another important field where *E. coli* is making an important contribution powered by synthetic biology is the antibiotic production. From the biomedical standing point of view, increasing antibiotic resistance in pathogens is a burden for humankind, and the discovery of novel compounds is a time-consuming task. Recent efforts with known polyketides have started to give good production rates in *E. coli*, favoring the process of antibiotic production from different sources, eliminating the need for host growth standardization, and inducing conditions [101].

Due to the modularity of polyketide synthases, they are excellent candidates for engineering, for either the production of novel compounds from existing gene clusters (through module shuffling, mutagenesis or deletions), or by the introduction of novel environmentally sequenced gene clusters and heterologous production [102, 103]

Therefore, the production of diverse metabolites or biological or industrially relevant molecules can be successfully achieved in *E. coli*. Success stories have been published more frequently. With the advancement of high-throughput technologies, more sensitive detection, and analytical tools, and better DNA synthesis, the future for *E. coli* is brilliant.

6. Future

With all the research that is currently conducted in *E. coli*, we envision that the future for this versatile microbe is bright. Gained knowledge on *E. coli* is overwhelming, nearly 340,000 research papers with the "*Escherichia coli*" keyword available in Pubmed, versus 115,000 using

"*Saccharomyces cerevisiae*" as a keyword for an example. Several genomes from environmental sources have been sequenced. Thousands of research papers aimed to assess the metabolic and genetic potential of this organism have been published. Now we need to start joining forces for boosting the true potential of this wonder microbe.

With all the data available, we are on the verge of really important findings and novel biotechnological procedures using *E. coli*. Recently, with an extensive analysis of human microbiota, we are approaching exciting times where all the knowledge can be applied to help people during certain diseases related to colon microbiota imbalances [104]. Findings suggest that microbiome can be manipulated to improve certain metabolic pathways [105].

In the rest of the biotechnology fields, we have enough information that suggests *E. coli* will be in the spotlight for quite some time. Even with novel organisms that have been proposed to substitute it, like *Vibrio natriegens*. Recently, Lee and collaborators analyzed the genome sequence and growth properties of the fast-growing bacterium *V. natriegens* [106], where authors created a novel platform for genetic engineering in one of the fastest growing bacteria. In previous reports, it has been shown that *V. natriegens* are capable of being transformed with *E. coli* plasmids [107], rendering that all the molecular tools available thus far may be compatible with this new system. This bacterium as *E. coli* renders only one important drawback: it may be pathogenic to oysters [108]. But as with old *E. coli*, we should be careful when managing genetically modified organisms. With recent efforts to generate lab-contained organisms, *E. coli* mutants that can only survive in the presence of synthetic amino acids have been created [109]. Despite all the molecular tools developed so far for *E. coli*, the future is still open for a novel molecular toolbox. Until a novel toolbox is standardized and incorporated into the everyday life of the laboratories around the world, we will keep exploiting the capabilities of *E. coli*, one wonderful bug.

Acknowledgements

The authors acknowledge the generous support from CONACyT-CIBIOGEM grant CB-4O-040116, CONACyT grant CB-2012-01 182671, and Guanajuato University grant 1081/2016 (DAIP). NVM acknowledge the support from CONACyT for a scholarship grant. We also acknowledge the support from Dr. Felipe Padilla Vaca.

Author details

Naurú Idalia Vargas-Maya* and Bernardo Franco

*Address all correspondence to: naudalia@hotmail.com

Biology Department, Division of Natural and Exact Sciences. University of Guanajuato, México

References

[1] Schönheit P, Buckel W, Martin WF. On the origin of heterotrophy. Trends Microbiol. 2016; **24**:12-25.

[2] Crick FH, Barnett L, Brenner S, Watts-Tobin RJ. General nature of the genetic code for proteins. Nature. 1961; **192**:1227-32.

[3] Lehman IR, Bessman MJ, Simms ES, Kornberg A. Enzymatic synthesis of deoxyribonucleic acid. I. Preparation of substrates and partial purification of an enzyme from *Escherichia coli*. J Biol Chem. 1958; **233**:163-70.

[4] Jacob F, Monod J. Genetic regulatory mechanisms in the synthesis of proteins. J Mol Biol. 1961; **3**:318-56. doi: 10.1016/S0022-2836 (61)80072-7.

[5] Jacob F, Perrin D, Sanchez C, Monod J. L' opéron: groupe de génes à expression coordonnée par un opérateur (The operon: a group of genes whose expression is coordinated by an operator). Comptes Rendus Hebdomadaires Des Séances De l'Acade´mie Des Sciences. 1960; **250**:1727-9. doi: 10.1016/j.crvi.2005.04.005.

[6] Lederberg J, Lederberg E. Replica plating and indirect selection of bacterial mutants. J Bacteriol. 1952; **63**:399-406

[7] Luria SE, Delbrück M. Mutations of bacteria from virus sensitivity to virus resistance. Genetics. 1943; **28**:491-511.

[8] Cohen S, Chang A, Boyer H, Helling R. Construction of biologically functional bacterial plasmids *in vitro*. Proc Natl Acad Sci U S A. 1973; **70**:3240-4. doi: 10.1073/pnas.70.11.3240.

[9] Chen X, Zhou L, Tian K, Kumar A, Singh S, Prior BA, Wang Z. Metabolic engineering of *Escherichia coli*: a sustainable industrial platform for bio-based chemical production. Biotechnol Adv. 2013; **31**:1200-23. doi: 10.1016/j.biotechadv.2013.02.009.

[10] El-Hajj ZW, Newman EB. An *Escherichia coli* mutant that makes exceptionally long cells. J Bacteriol. 2015; **197**:1507-14. doi: 10.1128/JB.00046-15.

[11] Malpica R, Sandoval GR, Rodríguez C, Franco B, Georgellis D. Signaling by the arc two-component system provides a link between the redox state of the quinone pool and gene expression. Antioxid Redox Signal. 2006; **8**:781-95.

[12] Malpica R, Franco B, Rodriguez C, Kwon O, Georgellis D. Identification of a quinone-sensitive redox switch in the ArcB sensor kinase. Proc Natl Acad Sci U S A. 2004; **101**:13318-23.

[13] Georgellis D, Kwon O, Lin EC. Quinones as the redox signal for the arc two-component system of bacteria. Science. 2001; **292**:2314-6.

[14] Palmer C, Bik EM, DiGiulio DB, Relman DA, Brown PO. Development of the human infant intestinal microbiota. PLoS Biol. 2007; **5**:e177.

[15] Garrity G, Brenner DJ, Krieg NR, Staley JR. Bergey's Manual of Systematic Bacteriology, Volume 2. The Proteobacteria, Part B: The Gammaproteobacteria. New York: Springer. pp. 587-850.

[16] Stouthamer AH. A theoretical study on the amount of ATP required for synthesis of microbial cell material. Antonie van Leeuwenhoek. 1973; **39**:545-65.

[17] Lengeler JW, *et al.*, eds Biology of the Prokaryotes, Thieme, 1999. Blackwell Science, Stuttgart.

[18] Neidhardt FC, *et al.*, eds Physiology of the Bacterial Cell, Sinauer Associates, Chicago, 1990.

[19] Romeo T, Vakulskas CA, Babitzke P. Post-transcriptional regulation on a global scale: form and function of Csr/Rsm systems. Environ Microbiol. 2013; **15**:313-24. doi: 10.1111/j.1462-2920.2012.02794.x.

[20] Machado D, Herrgård MJ, Rocha I. Modeling the contribution of allosteric regulation for flux control in the central carbon metabolism of *E. coli*. Front Bioeng Biotechnol. 2015; **3**:154. doi: 10.3389/fbioe.2015.00154.

[21] Romeo T. Post-transcriptional regulation of bacterial carbohydrate metabolism: evidence that the gene product CsrA is a global mRNA decay factor. Res Microbiol. 1996; **147**:505-12.

[22] Conway T, Krogfelt KA, Cohen PS. The life of commensal *Escherichia coli* in the mammalian intestine. EcoSal Plus. 2004; **1**(1). doi: 10.1128/ecosalplus.8.3.1.2.

[23] Blount ZD. The unexhausted potential of *E. coli*. Elife. 2015; **4**. doi: 10.7554/eLife.05826.

[24] Blattner FR, Plunkett G 3rd, Bloch CA, Perna NT, Burland V, Riley M, Collado-Vides J, Glasner JD, Rode CK, Mayhew GF, Gregor J, Davis NW, Kirkpatrick HA, Goeden MA, Rose DJ, Mau B, Shao Y. The complete genome sequence of *Escherichia coli* K-12. Science. 1997; **277**:1453-62.

[25] Hu P, Janga SC, Babu M, Díaz-Mejía JJ, Butland G, Yang W, Pogoutse O, Guo X, Phanse S, Wong P, Chandran S, Christopoulos C, Nazarians-Armavil A, Nasseri NK, Musso G, Ali M, Nazemof N, Eroukova V, Golshani A, Paccanaro A, Greenblatt JF, Moreno-Hagelsieb G, Emili A. Global functional atlas of *Escherichia coli* encompassing previously uncharacterized proteins. PLoS Biol. 2009; **7**:e96. doi: 10.1371/journal.pbio.1000096.

[26] Kurokawa M, Seno S, Matsuda H, Ying BW. Correlation between genome reduction and bacterial growth. DNA Res. 2016. pii: dsw035.

[27] Xie T, Fu LY, Yang QY, Xiong H, Xu H, Ma BG, Zhang HY. Spatial features for *Escherichia coli* genome organization. BMC Genomics. 2015; **16**:37. doi: 10.1186/s12864-015-1258-1.

[28] Lederberg J. Cell genetics and hereditary symbiosis. Physiol Rev. 1952; **32**:403-30.

[29] Summers DK. The Biology of Plasmids, Oxford: Blackwell Science. 1996.

[30] Hayes F. The function and organization of plasmids. Methods Mol Biol. 2003; **235**:1-17.

[31] Preston A. Choosing a cloning vector. Methods Mol Biol. 2003; **235**:19-26.

[32] Chan PT, Ohmori H, Tomizawa J, *et al*. Nucleotide sequence and gene organization of ColE1 DNA. J Biol Chem. 1985; **260**:8925-35.

[33] Bolivar F, Rodriguez RL, Greene PJ, *et al*. Construction and characterization of new cloning vehicles, II: a multipurpose cloning system. Gene. 1977; **2**:95-113.

[34] Lin-Chao S, Chen WT, Wong TT. High copy number of the pUC plasmid results from a Rom/Rop-suppressible point mutation in RNA II. Mol Microbiol. 1992; **6**:3385-93.

[35] Vieira J, Messing J. The pUC plasmids, an M13mp7-derived system for insertion mutagenesis and sequencing with synthetic universal primers. Gene. 1982; **19**:259-68.

[36] Chang AC, Cohen SN. Construction and characterization of amplifiable multicopy DNA cloning vehicles derived from the p15A cryptic miniplasmid. J Bacteriol. 1978; **134**:1141-56.

[37] Betlach M, Hershfield V, Chow L, *et al*. A restriction endonuclease analysis of the bacterial plasmid controlling the *Eco*RI restriction and modification of DNA. Fed Proc. 1976; **35**:2037-43.

[38] Stoker NG, Fairweather NF, Spratt BG. Versatile low-copy-number plasmid vectors for cloning in *Escherichia coli*. Gene. 1982; **18**:335-41.

[39] Kolter R, Inuzuka M, Helinski DR. Trans-complementation-dependent replication of a low molecular weight origin fragment from plasmid R6K. Cell. 1978; **15**:1199-208.

[40] Tsafnat G, Copty J, Partridge SR. RAC: Repository of Antibiotic resistance Cassettes. Database (Oxford). 2011; **2011**:bar054.

[41] Dykxhoorn DM, St Pierre R, Linn T. A set of compatible tac promoter expression vectors. Gene. 1996; **177**:133-6.

[42] Sasaki Y, Sone T, Yoshida S, Yahata K, Hotta J, Chesnut JD, Honda T, Imamoto F. Evidence for high specificity and efficiency of multiple recombination signals in mixed DNA cloning by the Multisite Gateway system. J Biotechnol. 2004; **107**:233-43.

[43] Gibson DG, Young L, Chuang RY, Venter JC, Hutchison CA 3rd, Smith HO. Enzymatic assembly of DNA molecules up to several hundred kilobases. Nat Methods. 2009; **6**:343-5.

[44] Doran KS, Konieczny I, Helinski DR. Replication origin of the broad host range plasmid RK2. Positioning of various motifs is critical for initiation of replication. J Biol Chem. 1998; **273**:8447-53.

[45] del Solar G, Giraldo R, Ruiz-Echevarría MJ, Espinosa M, Díaz-Orejas R. Replication and control of circular bacterial plasmids. Microbiol Mol Biol Rev. 1998; **62**:434-64.

[46] Ravin NV. Replication and maintenance of linear phage-plasmid N15. Microbiol Spectr. 2015; **3**:PLAS-0032-2014. doi: 10.1128/microbiolspec.PLAS-0032-2014.

[47] Godiska R, Mead D, Dhodda V, Wu C, Hochstein R, Karsi A, Usdin K, Entezam A, Ravin N. Linear plasmid vector for cloning of repetitive or unstable sequences in *Escherichia coli*. Nucleic Acids Res. 2010; **38**(6):e88. doi: 10.1093/nar/gkp1181.

[48] Ferber D. Synthetic biology. Microbes made to order. Science. 2004; **9**:158-61.

[49] Baeshen MN, Al-Hejin A, Bora RS, Ahmed MM, Ramadan HA, Saini KS, Baeshen NA, Redwan EM. Production of biopharmaceuticals in *E. coli*: current scenario and future perspectives. J Microbiol Biotechnol. 2015; **28**:953-62.

[50] Casali N. *Escherichia coli* host strains. Methods Mol Biol. 2003; **235**:27-48.

[51] Engler C, Gruetzner R, Kandzia R, Marillonnet S. Golden gate shuffling: a one-pot DNA shuffling method based on type IIs restriction enzymes. PLoS One. 2013; **4**:e5553.

[52] Beyer HM, Gonschorek P, Samodelov SL, Meier M, Weber W, Zurbriggen MD. AQUA cloning: a versatile and simple enzyme-free cloning approach. PLoS One. 2015; **10**(9):e0137652.

[53] de Toro M, Garcilláon-Barcia MP, De La Cruz F. Plasmid diversity and adaptation analyzed by massive sequencing of *Escherichia coli* plasmids. Microbiol Spectr. 2014; **2**(6). doi: 10.1128/microbiolspec.PLAS-0031-2014.

[54] Lanza VF, de Toro M, Garcillán-Barcia MP, Mora A, Blanco J, Coque TM, de la Cruz F. Plasmid flux in *Escherichia coli* ST131 sublineages, analyzed by plasmid constellation network (PLACNET), a new method for plasmid reconstruction from whole genome sequences. PLoS Genet. 2014; **10**(12):e1004766. doi: 10.1371/journal.pgen.1004766.

[55] Padilla-Vaca F, Anaya-Velázquez F, Franco B. Synthetic biology: novel approaches for microbiology. Int Microbiol. 2015; **18**:71-84.

[56] Baba T, Ara T, Hasegawa M, *et al*. Construction of *Escherichia coli* K-12 in-frame, single-gene knockout mutants: the Keio collection. Mol Syst Biol. 2006; **2**:2006 0008.

[57] Yamamoto N, Nakahigashi K, Nakamichi T, *et al*. Update on the Keio collection of *Escherichia coli* single-gene deletion mutants. Mol Syst Biol. 2009; **5**:335.

[58] Yong HT, Yamamoto N, Takeuchi R, Hsieh YJ, Conrad TM, Datsenko KA, Nakayashiki T, Wanner BL, Mori H. Development of a system for discovery of genetic interactions for essential genes in *Escherichia coli* K-12. Genes Genet Syst. 2013; **88**:233-40.

[59] Posfai G, Plunkett G 3rd, Feher T, *et al*. Emergent properties of reduced-genome *Escherichia coli*. Science. 2006; **312**:1044-6.

[60] Kato J, Hashimoto M. Construction of consecutive deletions of the *Escherichia coli* chromosome. Mol Syst Biol. 2007; **3**:132.

[61] Mizoguchi H, Sawano Y, Kato J, Mori H. Superpositioning of deletions promotes growth of *Escherichia coli* with a reduced genome. DNA Res. 2008; **15**:277-84.

[62] Choe D, Cho S, Kim SC, Cho BK. Minimal genome: worthwhile or worthless efforts toward being smaller? Biotechnol J. 2016; **11**(2):199-211.

[63] Park MK, Lee SH, Yang KS, Jung SC, Lee JH, Kim SC. Enhancing recombinant protein production with an *Escherichia coli* host strain lacking insertion sequences. Appl Microbiol Biotechnol. 2014; **98**(15):6701-13. doi: 10.1007/s00253-014-5739-y.

[64] Gibson DG, Glass JI, Lartigue C, Noskov VN, Chuang RY, Algire MA, Benders GA, Montague MG, Ma L, Moodie MM, Merryman C, Vashee S, Krishnakumar R, Assad-Garcia N, Andrews-Pfannkoch C, Denisova EA, Young L, Qi ZQ, Segall-Shapiro TH, Calvey CH, Parmar PP, Hutchison CA 3rd, Smith HO, Venter JC. Creation of a bacterial cell controlled by a chemically synthesized genome. Science. 2010; **329**(5987):52-6.

[65] Hutchison CA 3rd, Chuang RY, Noskov VN, Assad-Garcia N, Deerinck TJ, Ellisman MH, Gill J, Kannan K, Karas BJ, Ma L, Pelletier JF, Qi ZQ, Richter RA, Strychalski EA, Sun L, Suzuki Y, Tsvetanova B, Wise KS, Smith HO, Glass JI, Merryman C, Gibson DG, Venter JC. Design and synthesis of a minimal bacterial genome. Science. 2016; **351**(6280):aad6253.

[66] Bhalla N, Jolly P, Formisano N, Estrela P. Introduction to biosensors. Essays Biochem. 2016; **60**(1):1-8.

[67] Daunert S, Barrett G, Feliciano JS, Shetty RS, Shrestha S, Smith-Spencer W. Genetically engineered whole-cell sensing systems: coupling biological recognition with reporter genes. Chem Rev. 2000; **100**(7):2705-38.

[68] Raut N, O'Connor G, Pasini P, Daunert S. Engineered cells as biosensing systems in biomedical analysis. Anal Bioanal Chem. 2012; **402**:3147-59.

[69] Robbens J, Dardenne F, Devriese L, De Coen W, Blust R. *Escherichia coli* as a bioreporter in ecotoxicology. Appl Microbiol Biotechnol. 2010; **88**(5):1007-25.

[70] Padilla-Martínez F, Carrizosa-Villegas LA, Rangel-Serrano Á, Paramo-Pérez I, Mondragón-Jaimes V, Anaya-Velázquez F, Padilla-Vaca F, Franco B. Cell damage detection using *Escherichia coli* reporter plasmids: fluorescent and colorimetric assays. Arch Microbiol. 2015; **197**(6):815-21.

[71] Ford TJ, Silver PA. Synthetic biology expands chemical control of microorganisms. Curr Opin Chem Biol. 2015; **28**:20-8.

[72] Belkin S, Smulski DR, Vollmer AC, Van Dyk TK, LaRossa RA. Oxidative stress detection with *Escherichia coli* harboring a katG': lux fusion. Appl Environ Microbiol. 1996; **62**:2252-6.

[73] Lu C, Albano CR, Bentley WE, Rao G. Quantitative and kinetic study of oxidative stress regulons using green fluorescent protein. Biotechnol Bioeng. 2005; **89**(5):574-87.

[74] Vollmer AC, Belkin S, Smulski DR, Van Dyk TK, LaRossa RA. Detection of DNA damage by use of *Escherichia coli* carrying *rec*A': *lux*, *uvr*A': *lux*, or alkA': lux reporter plasmids. Appl Environ Microbiol. 1997; **63**:2566-71.

[75] Bechor O, Smulski DR, Van Dyk TK, LaRossa RA, Belkin S. Recombinant microorganisms as environmental biosensors: pollutants detection by *Escherichia coli* bearing *fab*A': *lux* fusions. J Biotechnol. 2002; **94**:125-32.

[76] Van Dyk TK, Majarian WR, Konstantinov KB, Young RM, Dhurjati PS, LaRossa RA. Rapid and sensitive pollutant detection by induction of heat shock gene-bioluminescence gene fusions. Appl Environ Microbiol. 1994; **60**(5):1414-20.

[77] Berno E, Pereira Marcondes DF, Ricci Gamalero S, Eandi M. Recombinant *Escherichia coli* for the biomonitoring of benzene and its derivatives in the air. Ecotoxicol Environ Saf. 2004; **57**(2):118-22.

[78] Vangnai AS, Kataoka N, Soonglerdsongpha S, Kalambaheti C, Tajima T, Kato J. Construction and application of an *Escherichia coli* bioreporter for aniline and chloroaniline detection. J Ind Microbiol Biotechnol. 2012; **39**:1801-10.

[79] Anu Prathap MU, Chaurasia AK, Sawant SN, Apte SK. Polyaniline-based highly sensitive microbial biosensor for selective detection of lindane. Anal Chem. 2012; **84**(15):6672-8.

[80] Truffer F, Buffi N, Merulla D, Beggah S, van Lintel H, Renaud P, van der Meer JR, Geiser M. Compact portable biosensor for arsenic detection in aqueous samples with *Escherichia coli* bioreporter cells. Rev Sci Instrum. 2014; **85**:015120.

[81] Melamed S, Lalush C, Elad T, Yagur-Kroll S, Belkin S, Pedahzur R. A bacterial reporter panel for the detection and classification of antibiotic substances. Microb Biotechnol. 2012; **5**(4):536-48. doi: 10.1111/j.1751-7915.2012.00333.x.

[82] Kohlmeier S, Mancuso M, Tecon R, Harms H, van der Meer JR, Wells M. Bioreporters: gfp versus lux revisited and single-cell response. Biosens Bioelectron. 2007; **22**:1578-85.

[83] Galvão TC, de Lorenzo V. Transcriptional regulators à la carte: engineering new effector specificities in bacterial regulatory proteins. Curr Opin Biotechnol. 2006; **17**(1):34-42.

[84] Røkke G, Korvald E, Pahr J, Oyås O, Lale R. BioBrick assembly standards and techniques and associated software tools. Methods Mol Biol. 2014; **1116**:1-24. doi: 10.1007/978-1-62703-764-8_1.

[85] Sleight SC, Sauro HM. BioBrick™ assembly using the In-Fusion PCR Cloning Kit. Methods Mol Biol. 2013; **1073**:19-30.

[86] Webb AJ, Kelwick R, Doenhoff MJ, Kylilis N, MacDonald JT, Wen KY, McKeown C, Baldwin G, Ellis T, Jensen K, Freemont PS. A protease-based biosensor for the detection of *Schistosome cercariae*. Sci Rep. 2016; **6**:24725. doi: 10.1038/srep24725.

[87] Wang YH, Wei KY, Smolke CD. Synthetic biology: advancing the design of diverse genetic systems. Annu Rev Chem Biomol Eng. 2013; **4**:69-102. doi: 10.1146/annurev-chembioeng-061312-103351.

[88] Cooper GM. The Cell: A Molecular Approach. 2nd edition. Sunderland (MA): Sinauer Associates; 2000. Cells as Experimental Models. Available from: http://www.ncbi.nlm.nih.gov/books/NBK9917/

[89] Davis RH. The age of model organisms. Nat Rev Genet. 2004; **5**(1):69-76.

[90] Rogers JK, Church GM. Multiplexed engineering in biology. Trends Biotechnol. 2016; **34**(3):198-206.

[91] Raman S, Rogers JK, Taylor ND, Church GM. Evolution-guided optimization of biosynthetic pathways. Proc Natl Acad Sci U S A. 2014; **111**(50):17803-8. doi: 10.1073/pnas.1409523111.

[92] Becker J, Wittmann C. Systems metabolic engineering of *Escherichia coli* for the heterologous production of high value molecules-a veteran at new shores. Curr Opin Biotechnol. 2016; **42**:178-88.

[93] Tuli HS, Chaudhary P, Beniwal V, Sharma AK. Microbial pigments as natural color sources: current trends and future perspectives. J Food Sci Technol. 2015; **52**:4669-78.

[94] Liu W, Zhang R, Tian N, Xu X, Cao Y, Xian M, Liu H. Utilization of alkaline phosphatase PhoA in the bioproduction of geraniol by metabolically engineered *Escherichia coli*. Bioengineered. 2015; **6**(5):288-93. doi: 10.1080/21655979.2015.1062188.

[95] Schalk M, Pastore L, Mirata MA, Khim S, Schouwey M, Deguerry F, Pineda V, Rocci L, Daviet L. Toward a biosynthetic route to sclareol and amber odorants. J Am Chem Soc. 2012; **134**(46):18900-3. doi: 10.1021/ja307404u.

[96] Koppolu V, Vasigala VK. Role of *Escherichia coli* in biofuel production. Microbiol Insights. 2016; **9**:29-35.

[97] Bentley GJ, Jiang W, Guamán LP, Xiao Y, Zhang F. Engineering *Escherichia coli* to produce branched-chain fatty acids in high percentages. Metab Eng. 2016; **38**:148-58.

[98] Jawed K, Mattam AJ, Fatma Z, Wajid S, Abdin MZ, Yazdani SS. Engineered production of short chain fatty acid in *Escherichia coli* using fatty acid synthesis pathway. PLoS One. 2016; **11**(7):e0160035.

[99] Howard TP, Middelhaufe S, Moore K, Edner C, Kolak DM, Taylor GN, Parker DA, Lee R, Smirnoff N, Aves SJ, Love J. Synthesis of customized petroleum-replica fuel molecules by targeted modification of free fatty acid pools in *Escherichia coli*. Proc Natl Acad Sci U S A. 2013; **110**(19):7636-41.

[100] Campodonico MA, Andrews BA, Asenjo JA, Palsson BO, Feist AM. Generation of an atlas for commodity chemical production in *Escherichia coli* and a novel pathway prediction algorithm, GEM-Path. Metab Eng. 2014; **25**:140-58.

[101] Yang J, Xiong ZQ, Song SJ, Wang JF, Lv HJ, Wang Y. Improving heterologous polyketide production in *Escherichia coli* by transporter engineering. Appl Microbiol Biotechnol. 2015; **99**(20):8691-700.

[102] Zhang G, Li Y, Fang L, Pfeifer BA. Tailoring pathway modularity in the biosynthesis of erythromycin analogs heterologously engineered in *E. coli*. Sci Adv. 2015; **1**(4):e1500077.

[103] Meng HL, Xiong ZQ, Song SJ, Wang J, Wang Y. Construction of polyketide overproducing *Escherichia coli* strains via synthetic antisense RNAs based on *in silico* fluxome analysis and comparative transcriptome analysis. Biotechnol J. 2016; **11**(4):530-41.

[104] Yaung SJ, Church GM, Wang HH. Recent progress in engineering human-associated microbiomes. Methods Mol Biol. 2014; **1151**:3-25.

[105] Yaung SJ, Deng L, Li N, Braff JL, Church GM, Bry L, Wang HH, Gerber GK. Improving microbial fitness in the mammalian gut by *in vivo* temporal functional metagenomics. Mol Syst Biol. 2015; **11**(1):788.

[106] Lee HH, Ostrov N, Wong BG, Gold MA, Khalil A, Church GM. *Vibrio natriegens*, a new genomic powerhouse. BioRxiv. 2016; 058487. doi: http //dx.doi.org/10.1101/058487.

[107] Simons KL, Thomas SM, Anderson PA. Identification of *Vibrio natriegens uvr*A and *uvr*B genes and analysis of gene regulation using transcriptional reporter plasmids. J Microbiol. 2010; **48**(5):644-56.

[108] Garnier M, Labreuche Y, Garcia C, Robert M, Nicolas JL. Evidence for the involvement of pathogenic bacteria in summer mortalities of the Pacific oyster *Crassostrea gigas*. Microb Ecol. 2007; **53**(2):187-96.

[109] Mandell DJ, Lajoie MJ, Mee MT, Takeuchi R, Kuznetsov G, Norville JE, Gregg CJ, Stoddard BL, Church GM. Biocontainment of genetically modified organisms by synthetic protein design. Nature. 2015; **518**(7537):55-60.

Chapter 14

Biosensor Platforms for Rapid Detection of *E. coli* Bacteria

Rodica Elena Ionescu

Additional information is available at the end of the chapter

http://dx.doi.org/10.5772/67392

Abstract

Risks of contamination with the well-known food pathogen *Escherichia coli* are increasing over the years. Therefore, rapid and portable technologies using different types of advanced devices named biosensors with various transduction capabilities (electrochemical, optical, or acoustic) were developed and seem to offer the most elegant solutions for research communities and final users-humans. Thus, integration of microfluidic biochips/biosensors into smartphones offer the real-time detection of any infection with *E. coli*, helping doctors in proceeding immediately with the clinical treatment. The present chapter will discuss about the analytical performances of biosensors and microfluidics such as selection of substrates, type of (bio)functionalization, low limit of detection, specificity, and response time for monitoring different *E. coli* strains. Thus, it is possible to rapidly identify (30–90 s) very low concentrations of *E. coli* (10^1 CFU/mL) down to a single bacterium in real samples (water, urine, milk, beef-meat) by simple integration of an angle scatter method and microfluidic-cellulosic pads (μPAD) loaded with micro-/nanoparticles functionalized with either polyclonal anti *E. coli* antibodies or with DNA strains into a portable device—a smartphone. Such biosensor configuration can also be used for the detection of other types of microorganisms with potential human and animal health concerns.

Keywords: biosensor platforms, electrode (bio)functionalization, *E. coli*, microfluidics, smartphone

1. Introduction

Coliforms or bacteria are commonly found in the digestive tracts of animals, humans, plants, and soils. Most coliforms do not cause diseases. However, the existences of "coliforms" with four genera (*Escherichia, Citrobacter, Enterobacter,* and *Klebsiella*) are indeed used as indicators to monitor their potential enteric pathogen contamination of waters [1]. One of the hundred strains of the bacterium *Escherichia coli* named *E. coli* O157:H7 is known as one of the most dangerous (for instance, Europe 2011) [2] gram-negative emerging cause of many foodborne and waterborne illnesses [3], bloody diarrhea (hemorrhagic colitis) [4], hemolytic-uremic syndrome (HUS) causing the kidney or renal failure, and hemolytic anemia (loss of red blood cells), which may lead to death, especially in children [5]. *E. coli* microorganisms (width ~ 0.6 μm, length ~ 1.6 μm) [6] produce the Shiga toxin that causes inflammation and secretion of intestinal fluids. Antibiotics and anti diarrheal medicines (such as Imodium) are not recommended for treating *E. coli* O157:H7 pathogenic infections.

Over the years, beside the relatively time-consuming and expensive conventional detection methods (e.g., evaluation of microorganism morphology, counting the bacteria colonies with Violet Red Bile Agar [7] after 72 h, investigations through the polymerase chain reaction (PCR) for amplification of low contents of bacterial nucleic acids), several methodologies with rapid detection using either laboratory instrumental methods (e.g., chromatography, infrared/epi-fluorescence microscopy [8], bioluminescence, flow laser cytometry and immunomagnetic separation [9], fluorimetry [10], etc) or portable, sensitive, and specific devices named biosensors have been reported [11]. Thus, in 1989, Karp's group [12] reported the development of the first biosensor using stable-light-emitting *E. coli* cells. Technically, a biosensor is a self-contained integrated device, which is capable of providing specific quantitative or semi-quantitative analytical information using a biological recognition element (biochemical receptor), which is in direct spatial contact with a transducer element [13]. Today, on the ISI Web of Science are reported more than 1220 publications about different biosensor configurations for the specific and selective detection of *E. coli* bacterial cells.

Biosensors are classified either as bioaffinity sensors when the biological recognition entity is an antigen/antibody (named immunosensors) [14] or a single strain DNA or ssDNA/RNA sequences (named DNA-/RNA sensors) immobilized onto a solid support via a linker molecule [15] that interact specifically with a target (named the complementary ssDNA-sequence to the ssDNA-probe), enzyme sensors, receptor ligand-binding sensors [16], and whole cell biosensors (named microbial sensors); or in function of the type of used physical transducer in electrochemical, optical, piezoelectric, and calorimetric (bio) sensors.

On the other hand, since early 1997 [17] bioluminescent genetically engineered *E. coli* microorganisms were intensively used as sensitive and friendly bioreporter's tools for screening the genotoxicity and cytotoxicity of various classes of water pollutants, endocrine disruptor's compounds, explosives [17, 18], and nanoparticles [19–22].

This chapter presents the latest developments for the detection of *E. coli* strains using electrochemical, optical, and acoustic biosensors and their integration in microfluidic platforms as well as the next generation of portable biosensors using smartphones (**Figure 1**, **Table 1**).

http://dx.doi.org/10.5772/67392

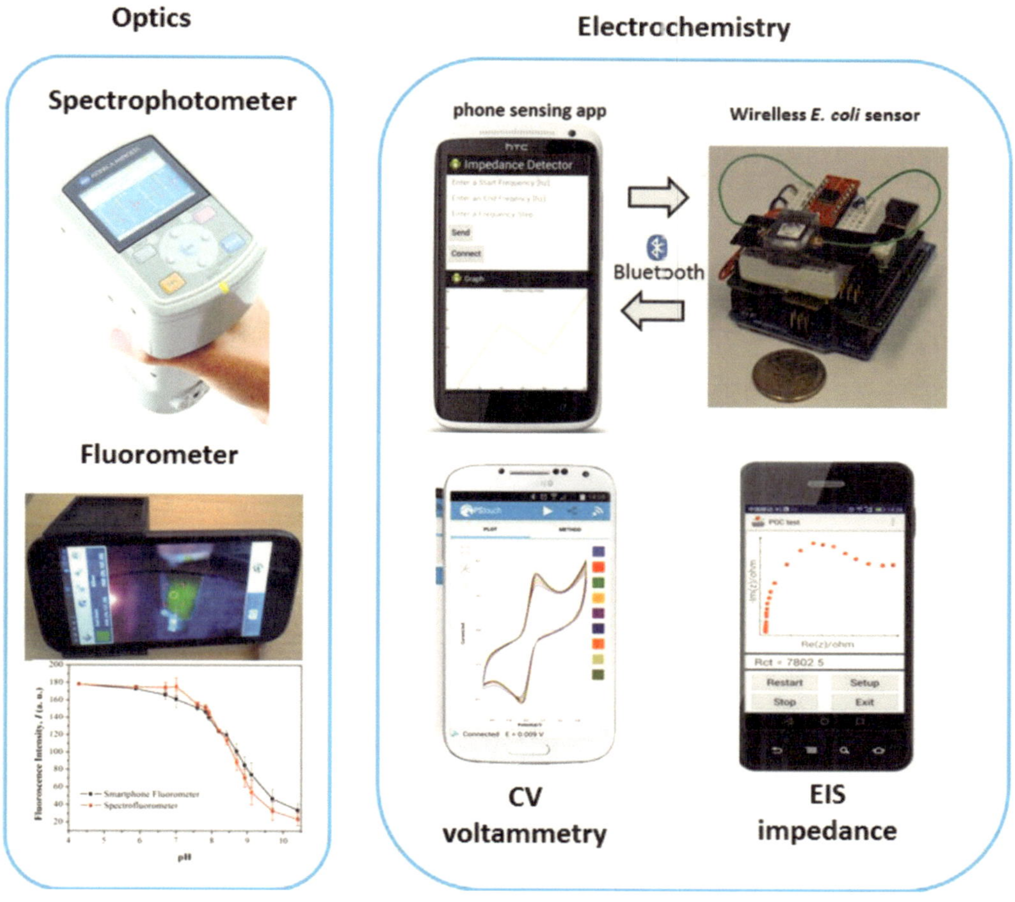

Figure 1. Optics and electrochemistry connected to smartphones for the detection of *E. coli* bacteria. For instance, an electrochemical system includes an Android cellphone (HTC ONE X), a Bluetooth shield (Seeed SLD63030P), a micro controller (Arduino), a chip for impedance converter network analyzer (AD 5933), and packaged sensor [66]. Also an Xcode (Apple, CA, USA), which allows users to take pictures at the four specific angles of scatter detection (15°, 30°, 45°, and 60°) at a fixed distance is reported [62]. CV—cyclic voltammetry, EIS—electrochemical impedance spectroscopy.

2. Biosensor platforms for the quantification of *E. coli*

Optical-based surface plasmon resonance and acoustic quartz crystal microbalance biosensors are known for their analytical performances in terms of label free and real-time detection capabilities, fast and stable response time, and target low detection limits. Furthermore, electrochemical impedance spectroscopy (EIS) label free biosensors are suitable for electrical characterization (such as double layer capacitance, solution resistance, electron transfer resistance, and Warburg impedance) of biocatalytic transformations on electrode surfaces after each biofunctionalization step [23].

Transduction method	Biofunctionalization	Strain of *E. coli* (analyte)	Media	LOD/range (CFU/mL)	Ref
Electrochemical					
	Polyclonal-antibodies 10 μg mL^{-1} for 1 h, RT/DTSSP for overnight, 4°C/AuSPEs *(Configuration 1)* Thiolated-polyclonal anti *E. coli* antibodies 200 μg mL^{-1} overnight, 4°C/AuSPEs *(Configuration 2)*	Wild-type *E. coli* (CECT 515)	PBS buffer + redox probe	3.3 ($5.0–1.0 \times 10^8$)	[24]
EIS	Biotinylated Con A-*E. coli*/Au-SPE	Wild type *E. coli* (CECT 515)	PBS buffer + redox probe	5.0×10^3 (5.0×10^3–5.0×10^7)	[25]
	Antibodies (24 h, 4°C)/indium-tin oxide (ITO)—interdigitated glass array microelectrode	*E. coli* O157:H7 (ATCC 43888)	PBS buffer + redox probe	1.0×10^6 (4.36×10^5–4.36×10^8)	[26]
	Antibodies (1 mg/ml, moisture chamber 24 h, 4°C)/GPTRES/ indium-tin oxide (ITO)—glass	*E. coli* O157: H7	PBSM buffer	6×10^5 cells/ml	[27]
	Monoclonal antibodies, 24 h, 4°C/ EDC-NHS/MPA-SAM/Au-glass *(Substrate preparation)* Bacteria + Biotinylated-*E. coli* polyclonal antibody/streptavidin superparamagnetic beads (*Fluid preparation*) (syringe pump, 20 min incubation time for immunocomplexes formation)	*E. coli* O157:H7 (strain B1409) (Prajna Biology Technique Shanghai)	PBS buffer	50 (50–500)	[56]
FET	0.1% Tween20/Ethanolamine/ Polyclonal Antibodies/ PBSE-linker/Graphene	*E. coli* K12 ER2925	PBS buffer + traces of LB medium	1.6×10^7	[40]
Optical					
SPR	UV-light, 20 min, RT/Bacteria + Mixture of (HEMA/EGDMA/ deionized water/MAH/the initiator AIBN)Dry bacteria/GA/ APTES/Glass-slide (20 min, flow measurements)	*E. coli* (Sigma-Aldrich)	Aqueous solutions	1.54×10^6 (0.5–4.0 McFarland*)	[52]

http://dx.doi.org/10.5772/67392

Transduction method	Biofunctionalization	Strain of *E. coli* (analyte)	Media	LOD/range (CFU/mL)	Ref
Reflectivity	*E. coli* suspensions or lysates, 1 h/K-7α12/OAK/MPTMS/ $PSiO_2$-wafer	*E. coli*, ATCC 8739	Saline solution	10^3 cells/mL (10^3–10^5 cells/mL)	[28]
Chrono-fluorimetry	ssDNA 25 mer of 0.1 μM + EB/ Ether wash/DMT-HEG, RT, 4 h/ GPTES under argon at 80°C, 24 h/ Silica optical fiber (10 min, flow measurements, response speed of 20–40 s 40°C)	*E. coli* K12	PBS solution	10 pmol cDNA	[1]
Prism	NH_2-ssDNA of 100 μM, 1 h at 37°C//HEPES, 10 min/PDC, 2 h/10 min at 100°C/APTES in water + ethanol, 20 min/ SiO_2-TiO_2—15 layers (air measurements after hybridization at 37°C for 2 h)	*E. coli* O157 : H7 of Gene ID: 957271	Air	8.13 μM DNA	[29]
FT-RIS	Antibodies 40 ng/mL, 24 h at 4°C/GA RT, 2.5 h/APTES 1.5 h/ NaOH/Oxidized pSi-wafer (flow measurements, 15 min, dark conditions)	*E. coli*	MHB solution	10^3 (10^3–10^7)	[30]
Acoustic					
	Antibodies/Protein A/SAM/ QCM-crystal	*E. coli* O157: H7		10^3–10^8 (CFU within 30–50 min)	[31]
	Iron magnetite-NPs coated with Streptavidin and polyclonal biotinylated antibodies/*E. coli* cells/Antibodies/ProteinA/QCM-crystal (7.99 MHz, NPs = 145 nm, 30 min stop-peristaltic flow measurements)	*E. coli* O157: H7	PBS buffer	10^8	[32]

Transduction method	Biofunctionalization	Strain of *E. coli* (analyte)	Media	LOD/range (CFU/mL)	Ref
	Fe_3O_4—NPs coated BSA-Steptavidin/Biotinylated-DNA/BSA-blocker/ssDNA-thiol/QCM-crystal (8 MHz, NPs = 145 nm, flow measurements)	*E. coli* O157: H7	PBS buffer	2.67 x 10^{-2} and 10^{-12} M DNA	[33]
	Ethanolamine/Polyclonal Antibodies/MUA-SAM/QCM-D (peristaltic flow measurements)	*E. coli* MRE 162	Air + PBS	2.4 × 10^7	[34]
	Biotinylated polyclonal IgG antibodies/Avidin/NHS-PEG-biotin/Cysteamine/Au/Cr/LGS-crystal (syringe pump flow measurements at RT)	Fluorescent labeled *E. coli* O157:H7	PBS + BSA	~10^6 cells/mL	[35]
QCM	Mixture of twice heated *E. coli* (first at 60°C for 30 min and second at 37°C prior use) and solute lyophilized TAL/Ag-QCM-crystal (9 MHz, peristaltic flow measurements at 37°C)	*E. coli* in mixture with *TAL*	Culture medium	~10 cells/mL	[51]
	Imprinting the bacteria on overoxidazed polypyrrole film/QCM-AT-crystal	*E. coli* (Japan)	Sterilized water	10^3–10^9	[6]
	0.1% SDS Wash/Polymerization/Bacteria/Pre-Polymerization at 70°C, 15 min/DMMP-MIP (~300–400 nm) spin-coated onto QCM-sides with screen-printed dual electrode structures (10 MHz, peristaltic flow measurements at RT)	*E. coli* strains b and w (Sigma)	Aqueous solution	0.1 mg/mL (0.1–5 mg/mL)	[36]

Transduction method	Biofunctionalization	Strain of *E. coli* (analyte)	Media	LOD/range (CFU/mL)	Ref
	UV-light 20 min, RT/ Bacteria+Mixture of (HEMA/ EGDMA/deionized water/MAH/ the initiator AIBN)/Dry/Rinse-PEA/AM 12 h/QCM-crystal (7 min, flow measurements)	*E. coli* (Sigma-Aldrich)	Aqueous solutions	3.72×10^5 (0.5–3.0 McFarland*)	[52]

Legend: MPA-Mercaptopropionic acid MPA; GPTRES-(3-glycidoxypropyl)trimethoxysilane: PBSM-6.7 mM $[Fe(CN)6]^{3-/4-}$ (1:1 mixture), $MgCl_2$ and 3 mM 5-bromo-4-chloro-3-indolyl phosphate disodium salt hydrate; Con A-concavalin A; AuSPEs-gold screen printed electrodes; DTSSP-3,3′-dithiobis[sulfosuccinimidylpropionate]; PDC-diisothiocyanate; HEPES-4-(2-hydroxyethyl)-1-piperazineethanesulfonic acid; EB-ethidium bromide intercalator; DMT-HEG-dimethoxytrityl hexaethylene glycol; $PSiO_2$-oxidized porous silicon nanostructure; OAKs-oligomers of acylated lysines; K-7α12 - synthetic antimicrobial peptide with similar name K-$[C_{12}K]_7$, where K-lysine; MPTMS-mercaptopropyltrimethoxysilane; MES-morpholinoethanesulfonic acid; AEE-2-(2-aminoethoxy)ethanol; GPTES-3-Glycidoxy-propyldimethoxymethylsilane; CFU-Colony Forming Units; SAM-self-assembled monolayer; MUA, 11-mercaptoundecanoic acid, QCM-D, quartz crystal microbalance with dissipation shifts capability; BSA-bovine serum albumin; TAL-tachypleus amebocyte lysate; PBSE-1-pyrenebutanoic acid succinimidyl ester in dimethylformamide (DMF); LB-Luria Bertani medium; MIP-molecular imprinted polymer; DMMP-dimethyl methyl phosphonate; RT-room temperature; SDS-sodium dodecyl sulfate solution; AM-allyl mercaptan; PEA-pure ethyl alcohol; GA-glutaraldehyde; APTES-(3-Aminopropyl)-trimethoxysilane; HEMA-2-hydroxyethyl methacrylate; EGDMA-ethylene glycol dimethacrylate; AIBN-α,α'-azoisobutyronitrile; FT-RIS-Fourier Transformed Reflectometric Interference Spectroscopy; MHB-Mueller-Hinton broth; *MsFarland-McFarland Equivalence Standards [37]-units for adjusting densities of bacterial suspensions: 1.5–12 x 10^8 cells (SPR) and 1.5–3 x 10^8 cells (QCM)range (for Ref. [52]); PBS solution of pH 7.4 containing 10 mM $[Fe(CN)6]^{3-/4-}$ (1:1) for Interdigitated array (IDA) microelectrode (1.4 cm x 0.5 cm)-each electrode had 25 digital pairs with 15 μm digit width, 15 μm interdigit space, and a digit length of 2985 μm.

Table 1. Different biosensor platforms for detection of *E. coli* bacteria.

2.1. Electrochemical biosensors

In January 2016, it has been reported for the first time an amperometric detection of PCR products (longer DNA chain's) by using three modified magneto working electrodes (m-GEC) with silica magnetic beads (0.05 mg) functionalized with either digoxigenin-tagged amplicon of the *eaeA* gene for *E. coli* (151 bp), fluorescein-tagged amplicon of the *invA gene for Salmonella enterica* (278 bp) or streptavidin-tagged amplicon of the *pfrA gene for Listeria monocytogenes* (217 bp) as specific carriers for independent magneto-genosensing amperometric investigations of single-tagged amplicons originated from three bacteria strains: *E. coli* K12, *S. enterica* Typhimurium LT2 and *L. monocytogenes* DSM20600 (DSMZ), respectively. Such amperometric magneto-silica beads platform was using HRP-labeled antibodies and the same redox mediator (HQ-hydroquinone) and substrate (H_2O_2) (**Figure 2**) in a unique electrochemical cell connected to a multichannel potentiostat and was able to identify 0.04, 0.13, and 0.05 ng/μL DNA of *S. enterica, L. monocytogenes,* and *E. coli,* respectively, in about 3 h, including PCR amplification time [38].

Label-free impedimetric immunosensors-based ITO substrates modified with epoxysilane and anti *E. coli* antibodies were used for detection of *E. coli* O157:H7 over a large linear working range (10–10^6 CPU/mL) with a limit of detection (LOD) of 1 CPU/mL were also reported. Moreover, the authors demonstrated the specific binding of *E. coli* O157:H7 to the antibody-patterned surface (only 20% of non specific bacteria) (**Figure 3**) using control bacteria strains such as *Salmonella typhimurium* and *E. coli K12* [39].

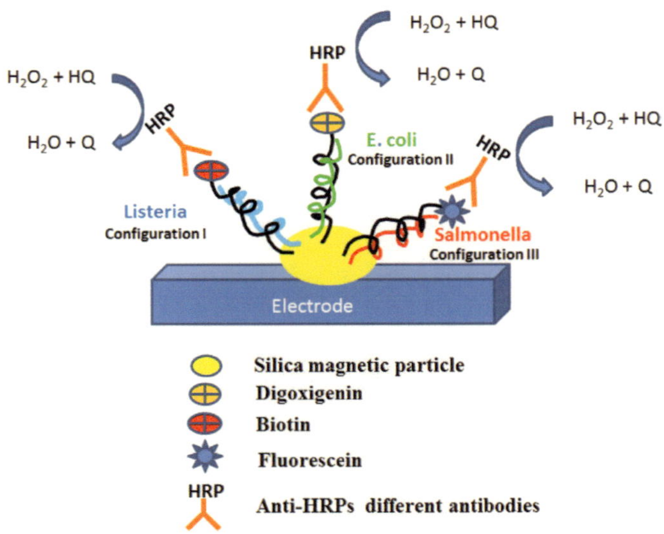

Figure 2. The construction of three configurations of DNA-amperometric magneto-genosensors for the independent detection of *S. enterica* Typhimurium LT2, *L. monocytogenes* DSM20600, and *E. coli* K12 strains. Type of used antibodies: AntiFlu-HRP (Anti-Fluorescein-Fab fragments), Strep-HRP (Streptavidin-POD conjugate), and AntiDig-HRP (Anti-Digoxigenin-POD Fab fragments). HQ-hydroquinone; Q-quinone. All bacterial strains were grown in Luria Bertani (LB) broth or agar plates for 18 h at 37°C.

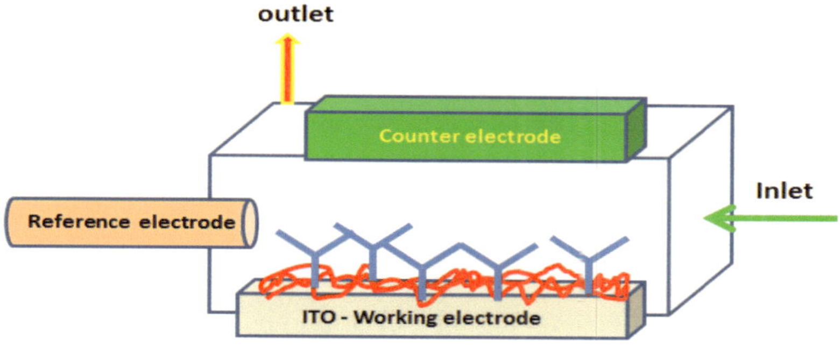

Figure 3. Electrochemical cell I using silanized ITO-electrodes and antibodies for specific detection of *S. typhimurium* and *E. coli K12* strains.

Impedimetric gold screen printed electrodes (AuSPEs) modified with thiolated *E. coli* antibodies were fabricated for the detection of *E. coli* at 10 CFU/mL level in river and tap water samples [24]. Another example of using EIS principles for specific detection of *E. coli* O157:H7 on ITO-based interdigitated microelectrode array in the presence of ($[Fe(CN)6]^{3-/4}$) electroactive redox probe (**Figure 4**) was also reported. Thus, it was found a direct correlation between the electron transfer resistance of the electrode (27.8%) and the concentration of *E. coli* cells (2.6 x 10^7 cells) upon their binding onto antibodies-based ITO array [26].

In another work, epoxysilanized ITO glass-modified with anti *E. coli* antibodies were used for EIS and atomic force microscopy (AFM) detection and topography investigations in the presence of different concentrations of *E. coli*. The research team found that *E. coli* cells and insoluble

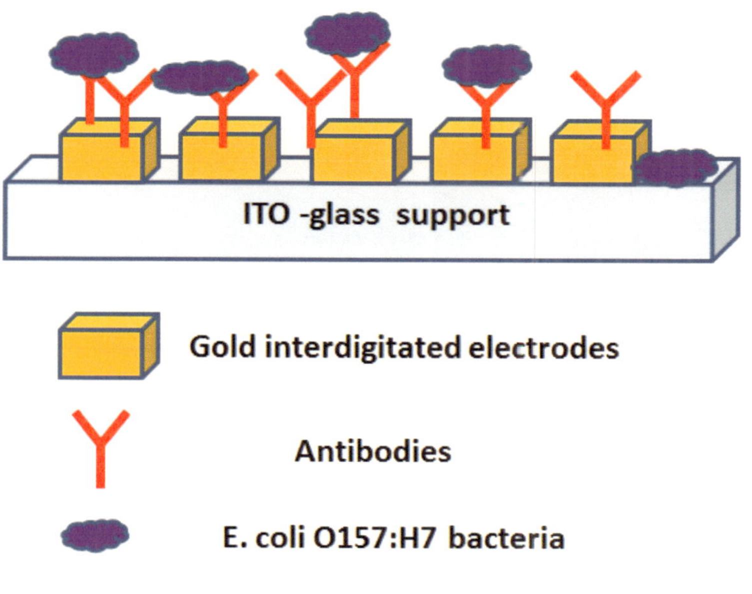

Figure 4. Direct impedance measurements using interdigitated immunosensors on ITO-glass support in the presence of ($[Fe(CN)6]^{3-/4}$) redox probe for the detection of *E. coli* O157:H7 cells.

precipitate mainly affected the electron transfer resistance and Warburg impedance even though the (3-glycidoxypropyl)trimethoxysilane chemical formed after immersion protocol over night at room temperature was uniform, dense, and homogeneous SAM monolayer onto ITO substrate. In this study, an enzyme labeled secondary antibodies namely alkaline phosphatase labeled secondary antibodies and its specific substrate 5-bromo-4-chloro-3-indolyl phosphate disodium were used for signal amplification of antibody bacterial interactions (**Figure 5**) [27].

Recently, homemade graphene-based field effect transistor (FET) Si/SiO_2—sensors for recording in real-time the proportional bias current signal responses in the presence of three different concentrations (1.6×10^7 CFU/mL, 1.67×10^7 CFU/mL, and 1.7×10^7 CFU/mL, respectively) of a nonpathogenic strain *E. coli* K12 ER2925 were reported [40]. Graphene FET biosensors were also developed to detect *E. coli* by recording the proportional increases in conductance

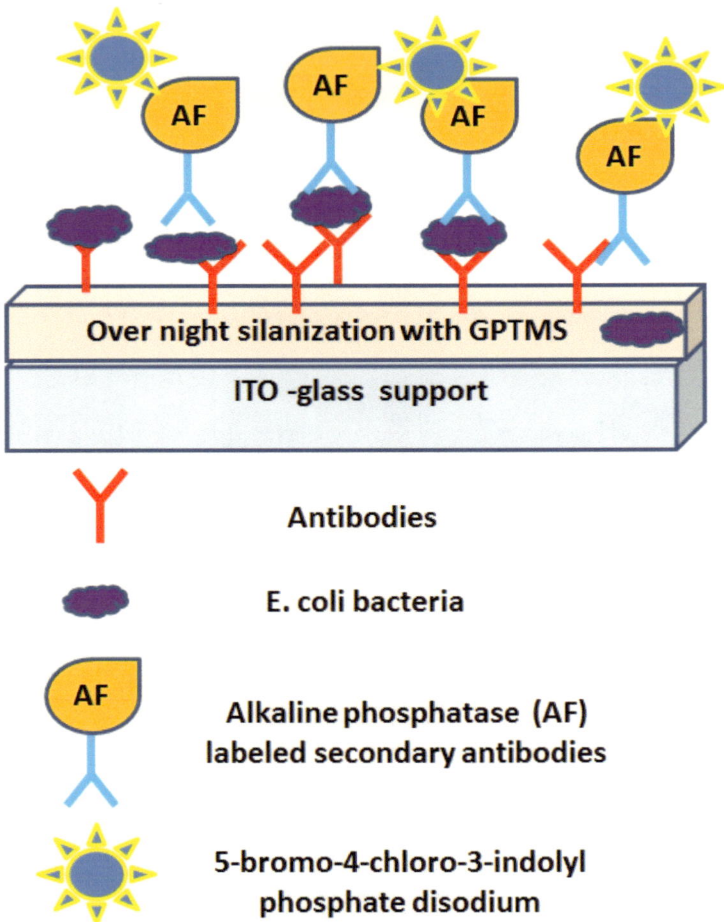

Figure 5. Silanization of ITO substrates with 3-glycidoxypropyl)trimethoxysilane (GPTMS) for further biofunctionalization with anti-*E. coli* antibodies.

values for different bacteria concentrations ranging from 0 to 10^5 CFU/mL. Artificial neural network and support vector regression algorithms have also been proposed for the *I-V* characteristics [41].

2.2. Optical biosensors

Fluorescence detection of several biomolecules in parallel using a sheath flow device with one inlet and five outlets has been reported [42]. On the other hand, it has been reported on the successful use of annealed (150°C for 4 h)/ultrasonicated mixtures of aqueous solutions of gold nanoparticles (Au-NPs ranging from 40 to 100 nM), and oxidized multi-walled carbon nanotubes (MWCNTs) for bacterial adhesion investigations of four different concentrations of *E. coli* namely 10^2, 10^3, 10^4, and 10^5/mL, respectively. The authors concluded that for increased contents of Au-NPs in composites, the Raman signals for higher *E. coli* concentrations improved, as bacteria have more Au-NPs to attach due to the transfer of its negative charge to MWCNTs [43]. Interestingly, bacterial anti-adhesive materials named "Rice leaf-like surfaces" (RLLS) (**Figure 6**) inspired by the hollowed morphology of rice leaves (*Oryza sativa* L. ssp. *japonica* cv. Calmati-202) were prepared on SiO_2-quartz glasses by a templateless, self-masking reactive ion etching approach with high optical-grade transparency properties (i.e., ≥92% transmission). The anti-adhesion property of *E. coli* O157:H7 during the dynamic flow conditions onto RLLS substrates was validated through fluidic channels at low flow (shear) rates and transmission spectra investigations at a wavelength range of 400–800 nm [44].

Label-free optical biosensors based on nanostructured (~50–100 nm) porous silicon ($PSiO_2$) thin films modified with synthetic peptide sequence K-7α12 OAKs (similar name K-$[C_{12}K]_7$, with K-lysine, and oligomers of acylated lysines-K) as a novel capture probe for whole bacteria *E. coli* ATCC 8739 and its lysates detection were reported [28] (**Figure 7**). Control experiments with neat and thiol-modified $PSiO_2$ (with no OAKs) exposed to lysate suspension of *Listeria innocua* and *Erwinia carotovora* (10^5 cells/mL) were also conducted to eliminate the possibility of non specific adsorption of bacterial lysate to the silicon-based surface. The same research team concluded that with K-7α12 OAK-tethered $PSiO_2$ substrates was possible to

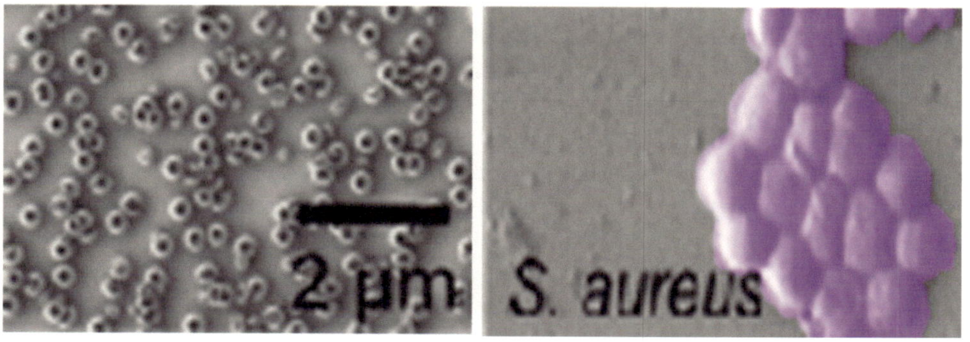

Figure 6. Bacterial (anti)adhesion on RLSS—substrates (a) and bacterial (*S. aureus*) adhesion on hydrophobic quartz (b). Reprinted with permission from Ref. [44] Copyright (2015) American Chemical Society.

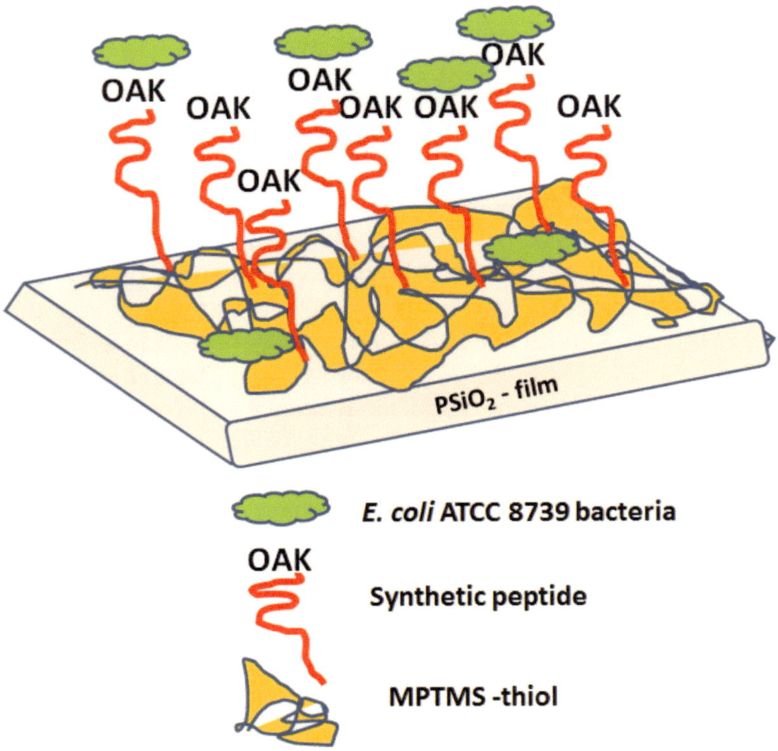

Figure 7. OAK-modified porous silicon ($PSiO_2$) modified with the synthetic peptide sequence K-7α12 OAK for the detection of *E. coli* ATCC 8739 and its lysates. MPTMS - mercaptopropyltrimethoxysilane.

achieve one order of magnitude improvement in the low detection limit in comparison with a previous team studies using monoclonal antibodies [45].

The ability of ssDNA probe for the *lacZ* gene of *E. coli* K12 (25 mer) covalently immobilized onto HEG/GOPS-silanized fused silica optical fiber (400 μm i.d. × 48 mm length) with a strong hybridization in the presence of its fully complementary target 10 pmol cDNA *E. coli* (25 mer *lac*Z), and ethidium bromide intercalator was reported. For systematic (bio)functionalization steps, the fibers were inserted into a holder system with cylindrical bores that accommodated maximum eight fibers at the time. Moreover, PCR amplicons of 100 m length containing the fragment of the *lac*Z sequence, and genomic DNA from *E. coli* were optically investigated. However, the authors mentioned that the optical system was not optimized for sensitivity whereas a significantly faster rate of non selective adsorption of non complementary oligonucleotides (25 mer to approximately 600 mer—ncDNA) than hybridization of complementary oligomers (cDNA) was recorded [1].

2.3. Acoustic biosensors

Commonly used acoustic wave biosensors are based on a thickness share mode (TSM) device [46] known as quartz crystal microbalance (QCM), which are classified as bulk acoustic wave (BAW) devices. Thus, since 1980, various chemical and biological BAW sensors for the detection of either organic solvents or biomolecules have been reported [47]. Moreover, shear horizontal surface acoustic wave (SH-SAW), surface transverse wave (STW), love wave (LW), flexural plate wave (FPW), shear horizontal acoustic plate mode (SH-APM), and layered guided acoustic plate mode (LG-APM) have demonstrated a high sensitivity in the detection of biomolecules in liquid media [48]. *E. coli* O157:H7 cells were also detected using shear horizontal surface acoustic wave IDTs sensors connected to a computer aid design (CAD) software [49].

A functional mannose self-assembled monolayer in combination with lectin concanavalin A (Con A) for the detection of *E. coli* W1485 using a QCM as transducer was reported [50]. The multivalent binding of Con A to the *E. coli* surface O-antigen favors the strong adhesion of the bacteria to the mannose-modified QCM surface. The minimal detection threshold was 7.5×10^2 CFU/mL.

Air samples containing four biological warfare agents including *E. coli* MRE 162 (collected using a "cyclone" sampler (Biotrace International, UK) and concentrated in collecting buffer PBS Tween—0.01% v/v) were detected in parallel using a flow-through system with four piezoelectric QCM crystals biofunctionalized with polyclonal antibodies located in separate fluidic chambers in the first attempt to determine the low level of detection as well as the specificity of each agent binding to its specific immobilized antibodies [34].

SH-SAW devices fabricated on langasite (LGS, $La_3Ga_5SiO_{14}$) - crystal sputtered with chromium/gold layers accommodated interdigitated transducers (each IDT consisted of 240 electrodes) and a gold platform region for subsequent (bio)functionalization steps with cysteamine/NHS-PEG-biotin/Avidin/Biotinylated polyclonal rabbit immunoglobulin G (IgG) antibody directed against fluorescently labeled *E. coli* were imaged with a cooled CCD camera on a BX51 fluorescence microscope. Furthermore, The MetaMorph software was used for counting the cells and analyzing their selective binding to anti-O157:H7 LGS-slide versus non selective binding to an anti- trinitrophenyl hapten modified LGS-slide (control experiments) [35].

A simple and rapid method (less than 90 min) that combined the bulk acoustic wave (BAW) technique based on Ag-plated AT cut 9 MHz quartz crystal (diameter 12.5 mm) with the gelation reaction of *tachypleus* amebocyte lysate (TAL), was used for viscosity and density measurement, of *Escherichia coliform* in very small mixed volumes (100 μL) was reported. A thermostat was used to control the reaction temperature at 37°C through a thermostatic water jacket. Thus, the frequency decreases very slowly after an initial lag time according to the progress of gelation of TAL, then drops quickly and a sudden change (its mechanism is still under investigation) followed, with finally a constant value after the completion of the gelation. *E. coli* of unknown concentration was determined using a regression equation. The linear range of detected *E. coli* was recorded for 2.7×10^4–2.7×10^8 cells/mL [51].

Microcontact imprinted QCM crystal and SPR glass with *E. coli* cells were obtained by a sandwich approach based on HEMA/EGDMA/deionized water/MAH/the initiator AIBN containing stock monomer solution. A 3 μL aliquot was taken from the stock monomer solution and dropped onto the allyl mercaptan modified SPR and QCM chips. Thus, the limit of detection (LOD) and the limit of quantification (LOQ) were found as 3.72×10^5 CFU/mL and 1.24×10^6

CFU/mL with QCM system whereas 1.54 × 10^6 CFU/mL and 5.13 × 10^6 CFU/mL with SPR system (**Figure 8**). The microcontact imprinted QCM crystal and SPR glass selectivity and specificity were proved in the presence of *Bacillus* and *Streptococcus* of 0.5 McFarland (1.5 x 10^8 cells). *Bacillus* was selected due to its morphological similarity to *E. coli* whereas *Streptococcus* as a gram-positive bacteria. The authors concluded that both sensor surfaces have the ability to recognize *E. coli* with high affinity due to the obtained recognition cavities via microcontact imprinted glass with *E. coli* [52].

2.4. Microfluidic biochips

From the beginning, microfluidic biochips or lab-on-chip biosensors strongly attract interest of different research communities (physics, chemistry, biology, and business entrepreneurs) due to their undeniable advantages in terms of measurements in real environments of tested biomolecules, low volumes of bioreagents, small variations of temperature, and low cost of fabrication of flow cell usually based on poly(dimethylsiloxane) (PDMS) material that can be disposable. Several biological applications have been reported based on microfluidics including studies. Some are discussed in this section.

Poly(lactic acid) (PLA)/PLA-PEG–based electrospun nanofibers (NFs) and K3-Brij76 (KB) polymer were used for colorimetric single-step paper-based lateral flow assays (LFA) for the rapid detection of 1.9 × 10^4 cells *E. coli* O157:H7 bacteria through a well-known sandwich configuration: HRP-labeled secondary antibodies/streptavidin-conjugated sulforhodamine B (SRB)–encapsulating liposomes/anti *E. coli* captured antibodies adsorbed onto PLA-PEG NFs (**Figure 9**) [53].

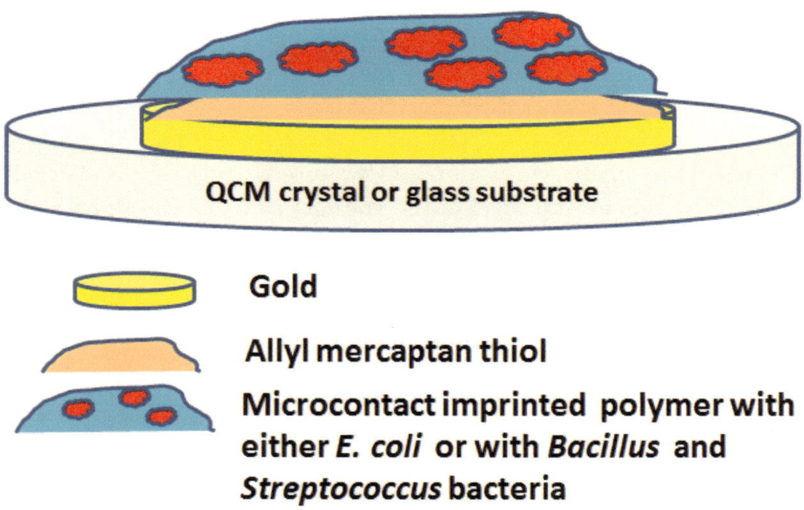

Figure 8. Surface plasmon resonance (SPR) and quartz crystal microbalance (QCM) sensors using microcontact imprinted polymer with either *E. coli* (for specific detection) or *Bacillus* and *Streptococcus* (for non-specific detection).

http://dx.doi.org/10.5772/67392

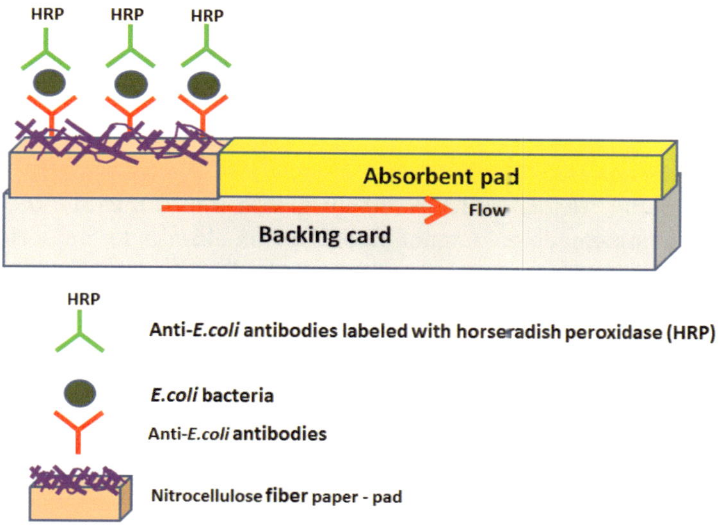

Figure 9. Colorimetric detection of *E. coli* bacteria using lateral flow (LFA) principles on nitrocellulose paper. In the absence of *E. coli*, the HRP antibodies flow through the nanofiber pad and no optical signal is observed.

A high-throughput PDMS microfluidic system with seven parallel channels (each channel contains 32 square-shaped microchambers) was employed for long-term growth monitoring of *E. coli HB101* (2.0×10^9 CFU/mL) growth monitoring and for the studies of inhibitory effects of various concentrations of two antibiotics (tetracycline and erythromycin at 0–4 μg/mL and 0–8 μg/mL, respectively) over bacterial cells. For flow antibiotic (**Figure 10**) sequential measurements were used bacterial suspensions at their stationary-growth phase. It was found that in the presence of at least 3 μg/mL tetracycline or erythromycin, the *E. coli* morphology remained similar to that of normal bacterial growth states cultured

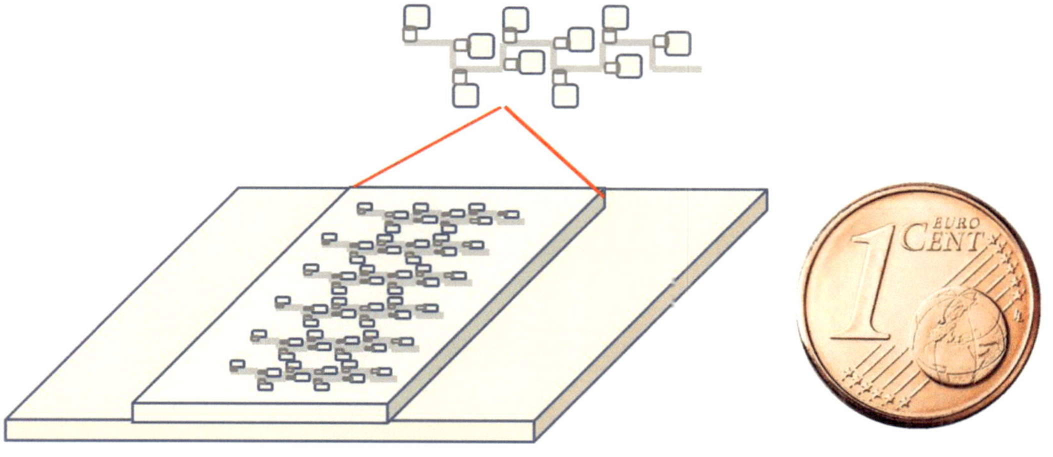

Figure 10. Configuration of the microfluidic device with multichannels.

in the absence of antibiotics, whereas in the presence of 3 μg/mL tetracycline for 8 h bacteria became filamentous [54]. Moreover, the mechanism of formation of long filamentous bacteria in the presence of cephalexin antibiotic was also studied with molecular biology techniques [55].

In June 2016, it was reported the fabrication of tortuous-shaped giant magnetoimpedance (GMI) sensor (working frequency 2.2 MHz) integrated into a microfluidic device (MFD) (**Figure 11**) using a homemade gold nanofilm biofunctionalized with monoclonal anti *E. coli* antibodies, *E. coli* bacteria/biotinylated polyclonal antibodies/streptavidin-labeled superparamagnetic beads (2.8 μm) and sensitive and specific detection of different concentrations of *E. coli* O157:H7 (50–500 CFU/mL) [54].

Electrochemically etched porous silicon (pSi) with ordered nanopore array integrated into a microfluidic PDMS channel was used for reflectivity effective optical thickness/fluorescence detection of specific *(E. coli,* ranging from 10^3 to 10^7 CFU/mL) and non specific (NOX and P17 strains) bacteria after their staining with a mixed solution of SYTO9 and propidium iodide, and confirmed by a significant pore blockage (specific) or any pore blockage (non specific) effects [30].

Sputtered nanofibers (NFs) of different densities (one layer sparse or larger pore sizes, one layer dense or smaller pore sizes, two layer sparse, two layer dense, three layer sparse, and three layer dense) with either positive or negative charge were tested for maximizing the amount of *E. coli K12* cells retained. For microfluidic investigations, nanofiber multilayers

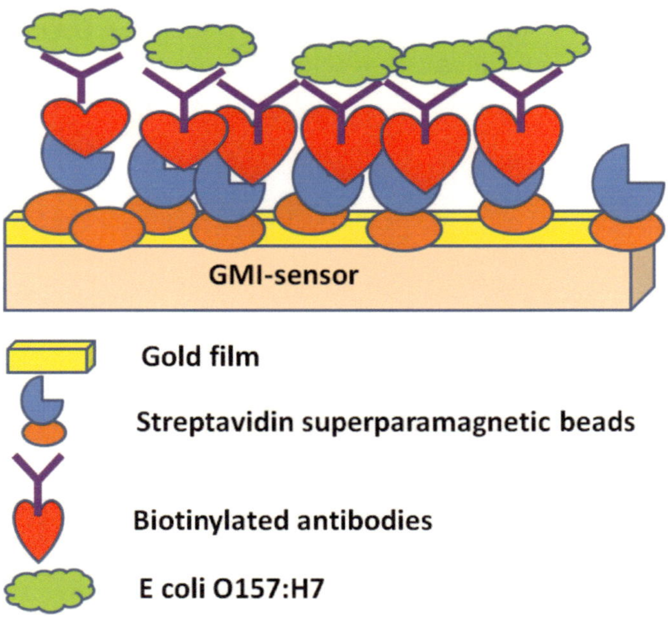

Figure 11. Tortuous-shaped giant magnetoimpedance (GMI) gold based-sensor for microfluidic detection of *E. coli.*

proved more homogeneous morphologies and were subsequently transferred onto poly(methyl methacrylate) (PMMA) films. Experimentally, negatively charged fibers spun with poly(methyl vinyl ether-alt-maleic anhydride) [PVApoly(MVE/MA)] of 300–400 nm and positively charged nanofibers of 450–550 nm have been employed. It was found that three layers sparse negatively charged NFs significantly reduced the non specific analyte (bacteria) retention (17%), whereas positive charged NFs were used for the detection of different concentrations of *E. coli K12* (87%). For this work, polyclonal anti *E. coli* antibodies were immobilized via EDC/sulfo-NHS chemistry on negatively charged NFs in order to selectively capture the negatively charged *E. coli* cells over 60 min using a syringe flow system and counted the number of colonies in the resulted effluent (low—average number of colonies in inlet solution was 62 CFU/mL) [57].

3. Conclusions

Paper microfluidics and smartphone technology were used for the detection of *E. coli* in real water sample using beads functionalized with anti *E. coli* antibodies predeposited in two out of a three channel paper device. It was found that by integration an internal gyroscope into a smartphone at an optimized angle of scatter detection, the presence of a single cell level in 90 s was possible [58]. Furthermore, a droplet-based, multiplexed fluorescence/light scatter submicron polystyrene particles functionalized with rabbit polyclonal anti K12 antibodies using nanofibrous substrate for the detection of 10^2 CFU/mL *E. coli* K-12 and *T. S. typhimurium* were reported in 2015. For experiments, all reagents were preimmobilized at fixed locations and included into two smartphones with necessary filters: one for incidence and the other for detection, positioned at 90° angle [59]. A microfluidic-cellulosic pad (μPAD) was loaded with polystyrene particles functionalized with polyclonal anti *E. coli* K12 antibodies and used for the detection of 10 CFU/mL *E. coli* K-12 in the human urine in about 30 s with a smartphone [60]. *E. coli* K-12 (10^1 CFU/mL) was detected in water sample (30 s) using also the principles of a μPAD-pad modified with antibodies coated particles and scattering intensity recorded by a smartphone with an autoexposure and autofocus locked on the central paper channel surface at 65° [61]. Identification of contaminated ground beef meat with various concentration of *E. coli* was possible without the need of functionalized particles with antibodies just by recording the resulted scattering light values at different angles with a smartphone after exposure to a perpendicular irradiation at 880 nm NIR-LED system. Therefore, different low detection limits were recorded: 10^1 CFU/mL at 45° and 10^2 CFU/mL at 30° and 60°. However, this method suffers from impossibility of distinguishing between different similar bacteria species (e.g., *E. coli* and *Salmonella* spp.) [62]. Moreover, the development of the first integrated paper-based DNA genosensor including nucleic acid extraction, amplification, and visual detection in about 1 h of *E. coli* (10–1000 CFU/mL) in spiked drinking water, milk, blood, and spinach using a smartphone was reported [63].

In conclusion, biosensors [62, 64, 65] and microfluidics [66] in combination with smartphone technology hold great hope that *E. coli* and various other coliforms may be detected in real time avoiding human suffering and save lives.

Author details

Rodica Elena Ionescu

Address all correspondence to: elena_rodica.ionescu@utt.fr

Laboratory of Nanotechnology, Instrumentation and Optics, UMR-CNRS 6281, Institute Charles Delaunay, University of Champagne, University of Technology of Troyes, Troyes CEDEX, France

References

[1] Almadidy A, Watterson J, Piunno PAE, Raha S, Foulds IV, Horgen PA, Castle A, Krull U. Direct selective detection of genomic DNA from coliform using a fiber optic biosensor. Analytica Chimica Acta. 2002;**461**:37-47. DOI: 10.1016/S0003-2670(02)00243-X

[2] Roda A, Mirasoli M, Roda B, Bonvicini F, Colliva C, Reschiglian P. Recent developments in rapid multiplexed bioanalytical methods for foodborne pathogenic bacteria detection. Microchimica Acta. 2012;**178**:7-28. DOI: 10.1007/s00604-012-0824-3

[3] https://www.epa.gov/region8-waterops/epa-region-8-drinking-water-unit-tech-tips-follow-unsafetotal-coliform-positive. 1-4 [Accessed 2016-10-12]

[4] Buchanan RL, Doly MP. Foodborne disease significance of *Escherichia coli* O157:H7 and other enterohemorrhagic *E. coli*. Food Technology. 1997;**51**:69-76.

[5] Rowe PC, Orrbine E, Wells GA, McLaine PN. Epidemiology of hemolytic-uremic syndrome in Canadian children from 1986 to 1988. The Journal of Pediatrics. 1991;**119**:218-224. DOI: 10.1016/S0022-3476(05)80730-9

[6] Tokonami S, Nakadoi Y, Takahashi M, Ikemizu M, Kadoma T, Saimatsu K, Dung LQ, Shiigi H, Nagaoka T. Label-free and selective bacteria detection using a film with transferred bacterial configuration. Analytical Chemistry. 2013;**85**:4925-4929. DOI: 10.1021/ac3034618

[7] Speak ML, Compendium of Methods for the Microbiological Examination of Foods, American Public Health Association, Washington, DC, 1976.

[8] Pyle BH, Broadaway SC, McFetters GA. A rapid, direct method for enumerating respiring enterohemorrhagic *Escherichia coli* O157:H7 in water. Applied and Environmental Microbiology. 1995;**61**:2614-2619.

[9] Pyle BH, Broadaway SC, McFetters GA. Sensitive detection of *Escherichia coli* O157:H7 in food and water by immunomagnetic separation and solid-phase laser cytometry. Applied and Environmental Microbiology. 1999;**65**:1966-1972.

[10] McFeters GA, Pyle BH, Lisle JT, Broadaway SC. Rapid direct methods for enumeration of specific, active bacteria in water and biofilms. Journal of Applied Microbiology Symposium Supplement. 1999;**85**:193s–200s. DOI: 10.1111/j.1365-2672.1998.tb05299.x

[11] Ivnitski D, Abdel-Hamid I, Atanasov P, Wilkins E. Biosensors for detection of pathogenic bacteria. Biosensors and Bioelectronics. 1999;**14**:599-624. DOI: 10.1016/S0956-5663(99)00039-1

[12] Korpela M, Mantsala P, Lilius EM, Karp M. Stable-light-emitting *Escherichia coli* as a biosensor. Journal of Bioluminescence and Chemiluminescence. 1989;**4**:551-554. DOI: 10.1002/bio.1170040172.

[13] Thevenot DR, Toth K, Durst RA, Wilson GS. Electrochemical biosensors: Recommended definitions and classification. Pure and Applied Chemistry. 1999;**7**:2333-2348. https://hal-enpc.archives-ouvertes.fr/hal-00862855

[14] Salgado AM, Silva LM, Melo AF. Biosensor for environmental applications. In: Vernon Somerset. Environmental Biosensors: InTech. 2011. pp. 1-16. DOI: 10.5772/20154

[15] Watterson JH, Piunno PAE, Wust CC, Raha S, Krull UJ. Influences of non-selective interactions of nucleic acids on response rates of nucleic acid fiber optic biosensors. Fresenius Journal of Analytical Chemistry. 2001;**369**:601-608. DOI: 10.1007/s002160000683

[16] de Jong LA, Uges DR, Franke JP, Bischoff R. Receptor–ligand binding assays: Technologies and applications. Journal of Chromatography B. 2005;**829**:1-25. DOI: 10.1016/j.jchromb.2005.10.002

[17] Burlage RS, Patek DR, Everman KR. Method for detection of buried explosives using a biosensor U.S. Patent No. 5,972,638. Washington, DC: U.S. Patent and Trademark Office. 1997.

[18] Tan J, Kan N, Wang W, Ling J, Qu G, Jin J, Shao Y, Liu G, Chen H. Construction of 2,4,6-trinitrotoluene biosensors with novel sensing elements from *Escherichia coli* K-12 MG1655. Cell Biochemistry and Biophysics. 2015;**72**:417-428. DOI: 10.1007/s12013-014-0481-8

[19] Jia K, Ionescu RE. Measurement of bacterial bioluminescence intensity and spectrum: Current physical techniques and principles. Advances in Biochemical Engineering/Biotechnology. 2016;**154**:19-45. DOI: 10.1007/10_2015_32

[20] Jia K, Eltzov E, Toury T, Marks RS, Ionescu RE. A lower limit of detection for atrazine was obtained using bioluminescent reporter bacteria via a lower incubation temperature. Ecotoxicity and Environmental Safety. 2012;**84**:221-226. DOI: 10.1016/j.ecoenv.2012.07.009

[21] Jia K, Eltzov E, Marks RS, Ionescu RE. Bioluminescence enhancement through an added washing protocol enabling a greater sensitivity to carbofuran toxicity. Ecotoxicity and Environmental Safety. 2013;**96**:61-66. DOI: 10.1016/j.ecoenv.2013.06.013

[22] Jia K, Marks RS, Ionescu RE. Influence of carbon-based nanomaterials on lux-bioreporter *Escherichia coli*. Talanta. 2014;**126**:208-213. DOI: 10.1016/j.talanta.2014.03.024

[23] Maalouf CR, Coste J, Fournier-Wirth R, Chebib H, Saïkali Y, Vittori O, Errachid A, Cloarec J-P, Martelet C, Jaffrezic-Renault N. Label-free detection of bacteria by electrochemical impedance spectroscopy: Comparison to surface plasmon resonance. Analytical Chemistry. 2007;**79**:4879-4886. DOI: 10.1021/ac070085n

[24] Escamilla-Gomez V, Campuzano S, Pedrero M, Pingarron JM. Gold screen-printed-based impedimetric immunobiosensors for direct and sensitive *Escherichia coli* quantisation. Biosensors and Bioelectronics. 2009;**24**:3365-3371. DOI: 10.1016/j.bios.2009.04.047

[25] Gamella M, Campuzano S, Parrado C, Reviejo AJ, Pingarron JM. Microorganisms recognition and quantification by lectin adsorptive affinity impedance. Talanta. 2009;**78**:1303-1309. DOI: 10.1016/j.talanta.2009.01.059

[26] Yang LJ, Li YB, Erf GF. Interdigitated array microelectrode-based electrochemical impedance immunosensor for detection of *Escherichia coli* O157:H7. Analytical Chemistry. 2004;**76**:1107-1113. DOI: 10.1021/ac0352575

[27] Yang L, Li Y. AFM and impedance spectroscopy characterization of the immobilization of antibodies on indium–tin oxide electrode through self-assembled monolayer of epoxysilane and their capture of *Escherichia coli* O157:H7. Biosensors and Bioelectronics. 2005;**20**:1407-1416. DOI: 10.1016/j.bios.2004.06.024.

[28] Tenenbaum E, Segal E. Optical biosensors for bacteria detection by a peptidomimetic antimicrobial compound. Analyst. 2015;**140**:7726-7733. DOI: 10.1039/c5an01717c

[29] Bahşi ZB, Büyükaksoy A, Ölmezcan SM, Şimşek F, Aslan MH, Oral AY. A novel label-free optical biosensor using synthetic oligonucleotides from *E. coli* O157:H7: Elementary sensitivity tests. Sensors. 2009;**9**:4890-4900. DOI: 10.3390/s90604890

[30] Tang YY, Li Z, Luo QH, Liu JQ, Wu JW. Bacteria detection based on its blockage effect on silicon nanopore array. Biosensors and Bioelectronics. 2016;**79**:715-720. DOI: 10.1016/j.bios.2015.12.109.

[31] Su XL, Li Y. A QCM immunosensor for Salmonella detection with simultaneous measurements of resonant frequency and motional resistance. Biosensors and Bioelectronics. 2004;**19**:563-574. DOI: 10.1016/S0956-5663(03)00254-9

[32] Liu F, Li Y, Su XL, Slavik MF, Ying Y, Wang J. QCM immunosensor with nanoparticle amplification for detection of *Escherichia coli* O157:H7. Sensing and Instrumentation for Food Quality and Safety. 2007;**1**:161-168. DOI: 10.1007/s11694-007-9021-1

[33] Mao X, Yang L, Su XL, Li Y. A nanoparticle amplification based quartz crystal microbalance DNA sensor for detection of *Escherichia coli* O157:H7. Biosensors and Bioelectronics. 2006;**21**:1178-1185. DOI: 10.1016/j.bios.2005.04.021

[34] Lava T, Berthet-Duroure N, Ayela C, Trevisiol E, Pugniere M, Morel Y, Rameil P, Nicu L. Parallel acoustic detection of biological warfare agents surrogates by means of piezoelectric immunochips. Sensors and Actuators B-Chemical. 2009;**138**:532-538. DOI: 10.1016/j.snb.2009.02.060

[35] Berkenpas E, Millard P, Pereira da Cunha M. Detection of *Escherichia coli* O157:H7 with langasite pure shear horizontal surface acoustic wave sensors. Biosensors and Bioelectronics. 2006;**21**:2255-2262. DOI: 10.1016/j.bios.2005.11.005

[36] Findeisen A, Wackerlig J, Samardzic R, Pitkänen J, Anttalainen O, Dickert FL, Lieberzeit PA, Artificial receptor layers for detecting chemical and biological agent mimics. Sensors and Actuators B-Chemical. 2012;**170**:196-200. DOI: 10.1016/j.snb.2011.08.025

[37] http://pro-lab.com/inserts/McFarland.pdf [Accessed 2016-10-12]

[38] Liébana S, Brandão D, Cortés P, Campoy S, Alegret S, Pividori MI. Electrochemical genosensing of *Salmonella, Listeria* and *Escherichia coli* on silica magnetic particles. Analytica Chimica Acta. 2016;**904**:1-9. DOI: 10.1016/j.aca.2015.09.044

[39] Barreiros dos Santos M, Azevedo S, Agusil JP, Prieto-Simón B, Sporer C, Torrents E, Juárez A, Teixeira V, Samitier J. Label-free ITO-based immunosensor for the detection of very low concentrations of pathogenic bacteria. Bioelectrochemistry. 2014;**101**:146-152. DOI: 10.1016/j.bioelechem.2014.09.002

[40] Zhu JY, Niu FZ, Zhu CA, Yang J, Xi N. Graphene-based FET detector for *E. coli* K12 real-time monitoring and its theoretical analysis. Journal of Sensors. 2016;ID 4641398:1-9. DOI: 10.1155/2016/4641398

[41] Akbari E, Buntat Z, Afroozeh A, Zeinalinezhad A, Nikoukar A. *Escherichia coli* bacteria detection by using graphene-based biosensor. IET Nanobiotechnology. 2015;**9**:273-279. DOI: 10.1049/iet-nbt.2015.0010

[42] Ozaki K, Sugino H, Arakawa T, Shirasaki Y, Funatsu T, Shoji S. High performance multiple *E. coli* cell sorting system using thermosensitive hydrogel and fluorescence spectrum detection. In: Proceedings 13th International Conference on Miniaturized Systems for Chemistry and Life Sciences (mTAS'09); 1-5 November 2009; Korea; Jeju. 2006. pp. 1856-1858

[43] Mehmood S, Naeem A, Sabahat S, Ciancio R, Carlino E, Bhopal MF, Bhatti AS. Modified structural and optical characteristics of Au-NPs-MWCNTs nanohybrids. Superlattices and Microstructures. 2015;**81**:248-264. DOI: 10.1016/j.spmi.2015.01.020

[44] Oh JK, Lu X, Min YJ, Cisneros-Zevallos L, Akbulut M. Bacterially antiadhesive, optically transparent surfaces inspired from rice leaves. ACS Applied Materials & Interfaces. 2015;**7**:19274-19281. DOI: 10.1021/acsami.5b05198

[45] Massad-Ivanir N, Shtenberg G, Tzur A, Krepker MA, Segal E. Engineering nanostructured porous SiO_2 surfaces for bacteria detection via "direct cell capture". Analytical Chemistry. 2011;**83**:3282-3289. DOI: 10.1021/ac200407w

[46] Kogai T, Yatsuda H. 3F-3 Liquid sensor using SAW and SH-SAW on quartz. IEEE Ultrasonics Symposium. 2006:552-555. DOI: 10.1109/ULTSYM.2006.143

[47] Yao SZ, Zhou TA. Dependence of the oscillation frequency of a piezoelectric crystal on the physical parameters of liquid. Analytica Chimica Acta. 1988;**212**:61-72. DOI: 10.1016/S0003-2670(00)84129-X

[48] Rocha-Gaso MI, March-Iborra C, Montoya-Baides A, Arnau-Vives A. Surface generated acoustic wave biosensors for the detection of pathogens: A review. Sensors. 2009;**9**:5740-5769. DOI: 10.3390/s90705740

[49] Ten ST, Hashim U, Sudin A, Liu WW, Foo KL, Salleh NHM, Hisham H, Nazwa T. Design development of acoustic waves based sensitive sensors for *Escherichia coli* O157:H7 detection. In: Proceedings of the Joint International Conference on Nanoscience, Engineering and Management (BOND21); 19-21 August 2013; Malaysia. Penang. Micro/Nano Science and Engineering. 2014, **925.** pp. 590-594.

[50] Shen Z, Huang M, Xiao C, Zhang Y, Zeng X, Wang PG. Nonlabeled quartz crystal microbalance biosensor for bacterial detection using carbohydrate and lectin recognitions. Analytical Chemistry. 2007;**79**:2312-2319. DOI: 10.1021/ac061986j

[51] Qu X, Bao LL, Su X, Wei W. Rapid detection of *Escherichia coliform* with a bulk acoustic wave sensor based on the gelation of *Tachypleus* amebocyte lysate. Talanta. 1998;**47**:285-290. DOI: 10.1016/S0039-9140(98)00136-2

[52] Yilmaz E, Majidi D, Ozgur Denizli E. An whole cell imprinting based *Escherichia coli* sensors: A study for SPR and QCM. Sensors and Actuators B-Chemical. 2015;**209**:714-721. DOI: 10.1016/j.snb.2014.12.032

[53] Reinholt SJ, Sonnenfeldt A, Naik A, Frey MW, Baeumner AJ. Developing new materials for paper-based diagnostics using electrospun nanofibers. Analytica Bioanalytical Chemistry. 2014;**406**:3297-3304. DOI: 10.1007/s00216-013-7372-5

[54] Suna P, Liua Y, Shaa J, Zhanga Z, Tua Q, Chenc P, Wanga J. High-throughput microfluidic system for long-term bacterial colony monitoring and antibiotic testing in zero-flow environments. Biosensors and Bioelectronics. 2011;**26**:1993-1999. DOI: 10.1016/j.bios.2010.08.062

[55] Nelson DE, Young KD. Penicillin binding protein 5 affects cell diameter, contour, and morphology of *Escherichia coli*. Journal of Bacteriology. 2000;**182**:1714-1721. DOI: 10.1128/JB.182.6.1714-1721.2000

[56] Yang Z, Liu Y, Lei C, Sun XC, Zhou Y. Ultrasensitive detection and quantification of *E. coli* O157:H7 using a giant magnetoimpedance sensor in an open-surface microfluidic cavity covered with an antibody-modified gold surface. Microchimica Acta. 2016;**183**:1831-1837. DOI: 10.1007/s00604-016-1818-3

[57] Matlock-Colangelo L, Coon B, Pitner CL, Frey MW. Functionalized electrospun poly(vinyl alcohol) nanofibers for on-chip concentration of *E. coli* cells. Analytical and Bioanalytical Chemistry. 2016;**408**:1327-1334. DOI: 10.1007/s00216-015-9112-5

[58] Park TS, Yoon JY. Smartphone detection of *Escherichia coli* from field water samples on paper microfluidics. IEEE Sensors Journal. 2015;**15**:1902-1907. DOI: 10.1109/JSEN.2014.2367039

[59] Nicolini AM, Fronczek CF, Yoon JY. Droplet-based immunoassay on a 'sticky' nanofibrous surface for multiplexed and dual detection of bacteria using smartphones. Biosensors and Bioelectronics. 2015;**67**:560-569. DOI: 10.1016/j.bios.2014.09.040

[60] Cho S, Park TS, Nahapetian TG, Yoon JY. Smartphone-based, sensitive RAD detection of urinary tract infection and gonorrhea. Biosensors and Bioelectronics. 2015;**74**:601-611. DOI: 10.1016/j.bios.2015.07.014

[61] McCracken KE, Angus SV, Reynolds KA, Yoon JY. Multimodal imaging and lighting bias correction for improved mu PAD-based water quality monitoring via smartphones. Scientific Reports. 2016;**6**:1-13. DOI: 10.1038/srep27529

[62] Liang PS, Park TS, Yoon JY. Rapid and reagentless detection of microbial contamination within meat utilizing a smartphone-based biosensor. Scientific Reports. 2014;**4**:1-8. DOI: 10.1038/srep05953

[63] Choi JR, Hu J, Tang RH, Gong YY, Feng SS, Ren H, Wen T, Li XJ, Abas WAW, Pingguan-Murphy B, Xi F. An integrated paper-based sample-to-answer biosensor for nucleic acid testing at the point of care. Lab-on-Chip. 2016;**16**:611-621. DOI: 10.1039/c5lc01388g

[64] Zhang D, Lu Y, Zhang Q, Liu L, Li S, Jiang J, Liu GL, Liu Q. Protein detecting with smartphone-controlled electrochemical impedance spectroscopy for point-of-care applications. Sensors and Actuators B: Chemical. 2016;**222**:994-1002. DOI: 10.1016/j.snb.2015.09.041

[65] Zhang D, Liu Q. Biosensors and bioelectronics on smartphone for portable biochemical detection. Biosensors and Bioelectronics. 2016;**75**:273-284. DOI: 10.1016/j.bios.2015.08.037

[66] Jiang J, Wang X, Chao R, Ren Y, Hu C, Xu Z, Liu GL. Smartphone based portable bacteria pre-concentrating microfluidic sensor and impedance sensing system. Sensors and Actuators B: Chemical. 2014;**193**:653-659. DOI: 10.1016/j.snb.2013.11.103

Chapter 15

Essential Oils: The Ultimate Solution to Antimicrobial Resistance in *Escherichia coli*?

Polly Soo Xi Yap, Shun Kai Yang, Kok Song Lai and Swee Hua Erin Lim

Additional information is available at the end of the chapter

http://dx.doi.org/10.5772/67776

Abstract

Antimicrobial resistance (AMR) is on the rise; the only solution for overcoming this is through accelerated drug discovery. At current, bacterial evolutionary rates is still clearly the undisputed winner in this war. To circumvent this, evolution of resistance need to be curbed and this can only be effective via novel approaches, one of which includes the use of a resistance modifying agent. The criterion to qualify as a resistance modifier necessitates the co-administration of the agent with an inhibitor that deactivates the bacterial resistance mechanism, restoring its original effectiveness. Natural products such as plant extracts and essential oils (EOs) have been viewed as a privileged group for investigation of their potential roles to combat antibiotic resistance, due to their compositions of active chemical compounds. The route for multidrug resistance development in Gram-negative bacteria is primarily mediated by the sophisticated inner and outer membrane barriers, which function to protect the cell against external toxic compounds; hence, bypass of these bacterial membranes would successfully restore or improve efficacy of the antimicrobials. The aim of this chapter is to concisely describe some examples for recent strategies used in the screening of possible resistance modifiers from essential oils specifically against MDR *Escherichia coli*.

Keywords: essential oils, combination therapy, drug synergism, resistance modifying, membrane permeability

1. Introduction

Antimicrobial resistance is an especially pressing problem in the clinical setting today. The pinnacle of secondary infections due to convergence between communicable disease

(CD) and noncommunicable diseases (NCD) further complicates the problem [1]. There is a two-sided role for antibiotics; and although their uncontested and unquestionable role was recognized to significantly reduce the statistics of the infectious diseases burden worldwide, their rampant use also contributed to the unexpected emergence of antibiotic resistant microorganisms attributed to over-prescription and misuse, hence, the emergence of the multidrug resistant Enterobacteriaceae, especially *Escherichia coli* (*E. coli*). Adversely, the last line of antibiotics, colistin, which had only been recently revived since 1959 amidst the fairly new emergence of carbapenem-resistant *Enterobacteriaceae*, had been reported by Chinese researchers to be inefficacious against *E. coli* recently, in infected pigs from a farm near Shanghai, and the spread of colistin resistance had increased significantly especially in the agriculture industry over time, which may be escalated to a global scale [2, 3]. With the establishment of new resistance, the Chinese authors have emphasized the urgent need for coordinated global action in the fight against pan-drug-resistant Gram-negative bacteria and one of these strategies proposed included investigation into natural products, in this case, essential oils. This chapter aims to introduce the usage of synergistic combinatorial therapy between different classes of antibiotics and essential oils against multidrug resistant *E. coli* (MDR *E. coli*) and to detail the methodologies used to establish synergism as well as the mechanisms involved.

2. Antibiotic classes and multidrug-resistant *E. coli*

2.1. Antibiotic classes and their respective natures

From the discovery of penicillin by Alexander Fleming in the early nineteenth century, approximately 20 classes of antibiotic have been discovered in time. However, only antibiotic classes that are effective against *E. coli* would be thoroughly discussed in this subsection.

2.1.1. β-lactam antibiotics

β-Lactam antibiotics are one of the most common yet diverse classes of antibiotics and are the first class of antibiotics discovered in the 1930s. They were effective against both Gram-positive and Gram-negative bacteria and were categorized into four main groups, carbapenems, cephalosporins, monobactams, and penicillins, with each group sharing structural similarity in the β-lactam ring within the antibiotic molecule [4]. The β-lactam antibiotics mainly target the bacterial cell wall synthesis pathway, and are thus termed "broad spectrum antibiotics." Under normal physiological conditions, bacteria constantly renew their cell wall in order to replace broken ones. A unit of peptidoglycan cell wall consists of two subunits, the alternating *N*-acetylglucosamine and *N*-acetylmuramic acid. Each subunit contains an identical pentapeptide chain, which links both subunits together via the action of a transpeptidase, penicillin-binding protein (PBP) [5, 6]. β-Lactam antibiotics would act as an irreversible inhibitor toward PBP. The β-lactam ring of the antibiotic mimics the structure of the pentapeptide chain and thus is able to bind with PBP, acylating it's active site and rendering it inactive [7, 8]. Hence, the action of β-lactam antibiotic halts cell wall synthesis of bacteria, which eventually compromises the rigidity of the cell wall, leading to cell lysis.

2.1.2. *Fluoroquinolone*

Fluoroquinolones is another class of antibiotics that exert their effect on both Gram-positive and -negative bacteria. The main structural feature of this particular antibiotic class is the presence of the fluorine atom within these antibiotics. It exhibits a broad spectrum activity against a large panel of bacteria as this group of antibiotic inhibits DNA synthesis by locking both the DNA gyrase and topoisomerase IV with the DNA strand during DNA replication. This prevents the action of other enzymes such as the RNA polymerase and DNA helicase for normal DNA replication, which eventually leads to cell death [9, 10]. Commonly prescribed fluoroquinolones include ciprofloxacin, gemifloxacin, levofloxacin, and moxifloxacin, which had relatively low adverse effects.

2.1.3. *Aminoglycosides*

Aminoglycoside is another major group of antibiotics showing enhanced potency toward Gram-negative bacteria. As the name suggests, this compound comprises of sugar units bounded to an amino group. Aminoglycosides exhibit high potency as well as a broad spectrum of action as it disrupts protein synthesis by binding only to the prokaryotic 30S ribosomal subunit, which then impairs the proofreading mechanism during protein translation [11, 12]. This disruption produces dysfunctional proteins, either due to misreading or premature termination, and eventually causes cell death. Even though aminoglycosides are specific toward prokaryotic ribosome, toxicity had been observed and reported in mammalian cells when a high dosage was applied [13]. Hence, aminoglycosides are only prescribed during life-threatening infections. Commonly prescribed aminoglycosides includes amikacin, gentamicin, and streptomycin.

2.1.4. *Nitrofurans*

Nitrofurans are a highly potent antibiotic class, which contain a furan ring and a nitro group. They are only used against urinary tract infections, especially when the infection is caused by an antibiotic-resistant pathogen. This is due to the high metabolism rate of the liver in partially breaking down the ingested nitrofuran. The remaining nitrofuran is then concentrated in the urinary bladder and thus suitable to be used in urinary tract infection, enabling targeted delivery [14]. High potency of nitrofuran is contributed by its diverse mode of actions when used against bacteria. In the presence of bacterial nitroreductases, nitrofuran is converted into reactive intermediates such as peroxynitrite and nitric oxide, which attack the bacterial ribosome, thus halting the protein synthesis in bacteria [15]. It was also reported that these reactive intermediates of nitrofuran can attack bacterial DNA as well as acting as a quorum sensing inhibitor [16, 17]. Due to the attribute of their multiple-action mode, resistance toward nitrofurans has yet to be observed in pathogens. Nonetheless, the exact mechanism of nitrofuran has yet to be fully understood. Nitrofurantoin is the common form of nitrofuran, which is prescribed generally.

2.1.5. Polymyxin

Polymyxin is a lipopeptide antibiotic that had been sidelined previously due to its high toxicity against mammalian cells. However, the emergence of multidrug-resistant pathogens has caused a resurgence in the use of polymyxin in treatments for bacterial infections as last resort. Polymyxin consists of a cyclic peptide bounded to a long hydrophobic fatty acid tail and it targets mainly Gram-negative bacteria [18, 19]. Potency is only targeted toward Gram-negative bacteria due to their mode of action, whereby the fatty acid tail of the antibiotic specifically targets and binds to the lipid moiety of a lipopolysaccharide, Lipid A that can only be found in Gram-negative bacteria. This results in the insertion the cyclic peptide of the antibiotic into the cell membrane, thus compromising its integrity and increasing the permeability of the cell membrane. This eventually causes cytoplasmic leakage and leads to cell death [20–22]. Commonly prescribed polymyxin includes colistin and Polymyxin B.

2.2. Antibiotic resistance mechanisms in MDR *E. coli*

The introduction of antibiotics as therapeutic agents to treat bacterial infection or as a growth promoter in molecular engineering had adversely propelled bacterial evolution, forcing bacteria to develop resistance mechanisms in order to survive within an antibiotic-filled environment. This gave rise to multidrug-resistant (MDR) pathogens, especially *E. coli* as they are commensal microorganisms and often used as the model bacteria in research. The emergence of MDR *E. coli* has posed a great threat toward the survivability of mankind, thus, the in-depth understanding of the strategies used by MDR *E. coli* to bypass antibiotic treatment is necessary to address this issue.

MDR *E. coli* exhibits the ability to resist multiple antibiotics simultaneously due to the acquisition of several genes that confer abilities such as antibiotic inactivation, multidrug efflux pump, target modification, or overproduction and reduction of cell membrane permeability. The multidrug efflux pumps are energy-dependent and have been reported to be overexpressed in the presence of antibiotics, helping it to expel antibiotics that had successfully permeated into the cell [23]. The multidrug efflux pumps indicated low specificity enabling the removal of antibiotics beyond the same class, rendering the antibiotics ineffective. For instance, efflux pump AcrAB-TolC of RND family is able to expel β-lactam antibiotic, fluoroquinolones, tetracycline, and glycylcycline [23–26]. Furthermore, MDR *E. coli* can alter their outer membrane permeability by modifying the structure of porins and/or reduce or stop their expression, which would be ultimately responsible for antibiotic access into the cell [27]. It has been reported that porins observed in MDR *E. coli* had narrower channels when compared to normal strains, which prevents the antibiotics from entering the cell [28]. MDR *E. coli* had been reported to be able to deactivate antibiotic with the production of antibiotic-targeting enzymes. β-Lactamase is one example of enzymes produced by MDR

http://dx.doi.org/10.5772/67776

E. coli, which has the ability to cleave β-lactam antibiotic, rendering it nonfunctional [29]. Antibiotic target modification had also been observed in MDR *E. coli*. Penicillin-binding protein (PBP), a transpeptidase, which links peptidoglycan subunit together, is the main target of the β-lactam antibiotic. It has been observed that isolated PBP from MDR *E. coli* had conformational differences when compared to nonresistant strains of *E. coli*. This slight conformational change prevents effective binding of β-lactam antibiotic but allows the transpeptidase to carry out its normal physiological function [30].

3. Synergistic potential of essential oils and antibiotics: challenges

The emergence of multidrug-resistant pathogens, especially *E. coli*, have caused an interest shift from the onerous development of novel classes of antibiotics to the more straightforward application of synergism or combinatory therapy in the hope of reviving the efficacy and effectiveness of existing antibiotics. Quite a number of publications regarding the usage of essential oils and antibiotics as a combinatory therapy have indicated great success, with significant reductions in the dosage of antibiotics required to completely annihilate multidrug-resistant pathogens [31–36]. Despite this, the usage of essential oils as a component for combinatory treatment posed a few challenges in its application. For instance, solubility of the hydrophobic essential oil in the aqueous medium is one of the greatest challenges faced. To solve this problem, emulsifiers such as dimethyl sulfoxide (DMSO) and polysorbate 80 (Tween 80) had been used to increase the solubility of essential oils in the aqueous medium. This would ensure maximum contact between the test organism as well as the test compound used throughout the experiment [37]. The concentration of such emulsifiers should also be taken into consideration as high concentration would cause toxicity to the test organism, resulting in false positivity during testing. For example, usage of DMSO at a concentration of more than 4% would reduce the viability of *Salmonella paratyphi* A, *Staphylococcus epidermis*, *Shigella flexneri*, *Vibrio cholerae*, and *Pseudomonas oleovorans* to less than 50% [38]. To better address the solubility issue, there is need to standardize the method used to determine synergism. The broth microdilution method has been shown to be the most accurate when compared to other susceptibility tests such as the disk diffusion and agar dilution methods, which are less informative [39]. In order to further maximize solubility, the incubation parameter should be standardized to shake at 200 rpm to ensure the formation of consistent emulsion, a crucial attribute in indicating the solubility of essential oils.

Another challenge faced when using essential oils in combinatorial therapy would be the volatility of essential oils. It has been well documented that essential oils consist of 20–60 compounds, which are highly volatile, but none of which are actually lipid in nature [40]. Thus, with the solubility problem solved, volatility of essential oils is the next problem to tackle in order to achieve accurate determination of synergism in combinatorial therapy. Volatility of essential oils can be affected by several factors. For instance, exposure to light can accelerate the degradation as well as volatility of essential oils. It has been demonstrated that in the presence of light, the autoxidation process of essential oil was accelerated, leading to the loss of several compounds within the essential oil itself [41, 42]. Another factor that can affect the volatility of essential oils would be the temperature. As temperatures increases, the autoxidation and degradation process of essential oils are markedly increased [43]. However, little can be done about the temperature factor as heat is still required for the test organism to grow optimally. At the least, testing should be carried out with minimal light to reduce the autoxidation and degradation of the essential oils.

4. Establishment of synergism

In combination therapy, synergy is said to occur when the combined effect of two agents is greater than the sum of the individual effects. Currently there is no clear standardization or regulation of the methodology in combination therapy [44], further complicated by different test methods, different EOs extraction methods and test assays. The most widely used techniques to detect synergy are the checkerboard and time-kill curve methods [33, 45–48]. In checkerboard assay, in which two test agents are tested individually in serial dilutions and in all combinations of these dilutions together to find the concentration of each test agent, both alone and in combination, that produce some specific antimicrobial effects i.e., minimal inhibitory concentration (MIC). In antibiotics and EOs synergistic testing, the combined effects of the antibiotics and EOs are calculated and expressed in its fractional inhibitory concentration (FIC) using the following formula:

$$\text{FIC} = \frac{\text{MIC of EOs or antibiotic in combination}}{\text{MIC of EO or antibiotic alone}} \tag{1}$$

The sum of these fractions is expressed as fractional inhibitory concentration index (FICI) where:

$$\text{FICI} = \text{FIC of EO} + \text{FIC of antibiotic} \tag{2}$$

When FICI is less than or equal to 0.5, the combination is said to be synergistic; when FICI is between 0.5 and 4.0, the combination is said to have no interaction while FICI is more than 4.0, the combination is antagonistic [49]. Although checkerboard assay is by far one of the most reliable methods for demonstrating synergy, culture conditions predominantly influence the outcome of the study hence determinant factors should be precisely reported in manuscripts to better facilitate reproducibility of these experiments.

4.1. Investigations into membrane-specific effects in combination therapy

Bacterial peptidoglycan/ cell wall disruption remains one of the most promising approaches for EO-mediated cell death. Numerous data are already available on membrane disruptive effects of EOs against the Gram-negative bacteria including *E. coli* [50–54]. In our previous work, several encouraging synergistic combinations of EOs and antibiotics against beta-lactam resistant *E. coli* were obtained. Our understanding of how EOs synergies antibiotic action and induce bacterial cell death is focused on the generalized membrane disruptive effects of the EOs.

http://dx.doi.org/10.5772/67776

4.1.1. Assessing bacterial surface charge using zeta potential measurement

The zeta potential is a consequence of the existence of surface charge; it provides the information on the electrophoretic mobility of the dispersed particles. Zeta potential measurement can be used to investigate the membrane potential, which reflects the inherent metabolic state of the bacteria. Zeta potential reflects the electrical potential interface between the aqueous solution and the layer of such fluid attached to the bacterial cell, suggesting that loss of bacterial cell charge is related to the metabolic energy loss [55]. It has been found that the values are more negative at higher growth rates [56, 57]. The bacterial cell surfaces are negatively charged under normal physiological conditions, owing to the presence of anionic groups such as carboxyl and phosphate in their membranes. The magnitude of the charge varies between species and it fluctuates in response to various culture conditions such as the pH and ionic strength of the culture [58, 59]. More recently, we have employed technology using a Nano Zetasizer (Malvern Instruments, UK) to investigate the influence of antibiotic-EO combinations on the cell surface physiology of *E. coli*. Different concentrations of piperacillin exerted different degree of zeta potential reduction in *E. coli* J53 R1. It has been observed that when the concentration of the antibiotic increased, the cells became less negatively charged (**Figure 1**). The cells' zeta potential also responded differently to different types of EOs treatments at different test concentrations (**Figure 2**). The technique of electrophoretic light scattering offers advantages on the study of membrane potential with accuracy, measurement time and ease of use [60]. The work of Halder et al. further validated the use of zeta potential measurement as a measurable variable for membrane permeability studies [61].

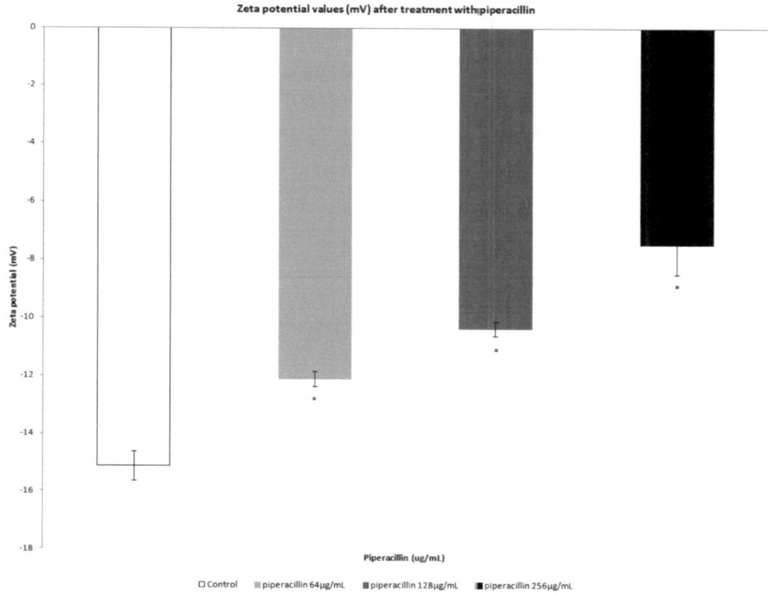

Figure 1. Zeta potential values (mV) of suspensions of *E. coli* J53 R1 when exposed to different concentrations of piperacillin treatments. File represents: (□) control; (□) piperacillin (64 µg/mL); (■) piperacillin (128 µg/mL); (■) piperacillin (256 µg/mL). The mean ± SD for three replicates is illustrated. Data were analyzed by one-way analysis of variance with *$P < 0.05$ being significant different from the control.

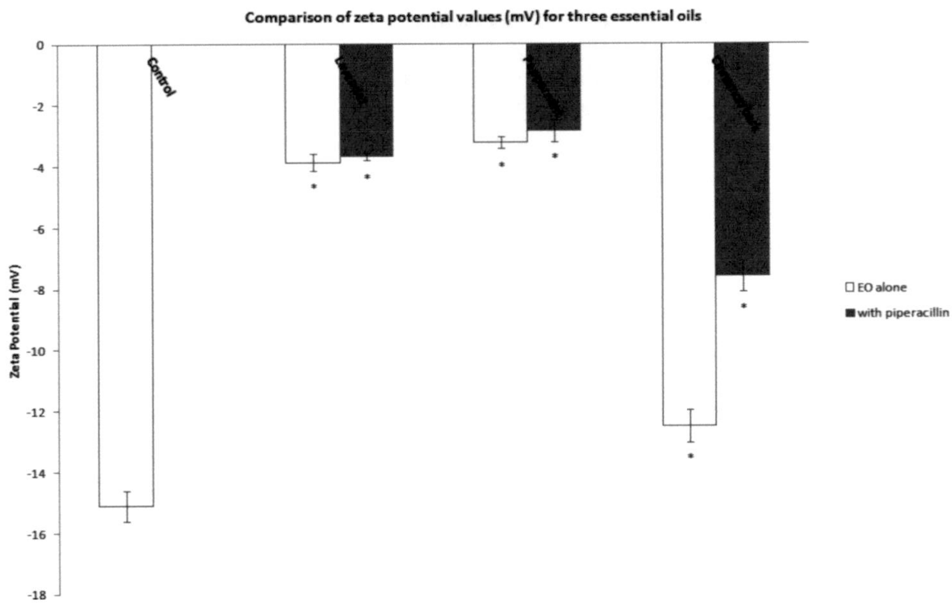

Figure 2. Zeta potential values (mV) of suspension *E. coli* J53 R1 when exposed to different EOs alone (□) or in combination with antibiotic (■). The mean ± SD for three replicates is illustrated. Data were analyzed by one-way analysis of variance with $^*P < 0.05$ being significant different from the control.

4.1.2. Illustrations of cell physical changes using electron microscopy

In the study of membrane-active mechanisms, scanning electron microscope (SEM) is employed to directly observe cell morphological changes after treatments. In our work, we observed the morphological changes of *E. coli* after treatment with EOs, namely peppermint, lavender, and cinnamon bark. In the nontreated cells, a rod-shape morphology that is characteristic of *E. coli* was observed (**Figure 3**); and cells treated with beta-lactam antibiotic at different concentrations did not show any observable alterations in size, shape, and surface morphology (**Figure 4**). Interestingly, cells treated with cinnamon bark EO were observed to show surface irregularities and corrugation, as is similar to the cells treated with lavender and peppermint EOs (**Figure 5**). It is important to note that a disturbed cell membrane system would affect other cellular structures in a cascade type action. In addition to SEM, transmission electron microscope (TEM) is also often employed to study the membrane integrity and intracellular alteration of the bacterial cells before and after treatments.

4.2. Investigations on antiquorum sensing properties of EOs

N-acyl-L-homoserine lactone (AHL)-mediated quorum sensing is a widespread system of stimuli and responses, which regulates the virulent determinants in most Gram-negative bacteria [62]. Antiquorum sensing antimicrobials are unlikely to contribute to the development of

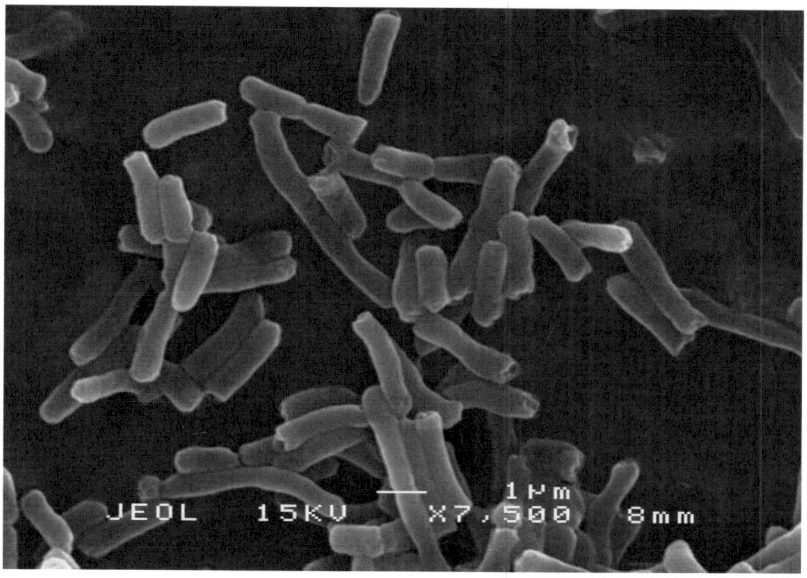

Figure 3. Scanning electron micrograph of the untreated *E. coli* J53 R1.

multidrug-resistant pathogens since it does not impose any selection pressure. Consequently, quorum sensing has been viewed as an attractive alternative strategy used to combat bacterial antibiotic resistance. The lack of AHL synthase-encoding gene, which should be naturally occurring of *E. coli* has made this variant a suitable biosensor for the screening of AHL synthase inhibitors. Experimentally, external AHLs are supplied exogenously to induce quantifiable quorum sensing traits such as bioluminescence. The antiquorum sensing ability of the test compounds are then measured by the significance of light inhibition [63]. In our previous work, we have employed *E. coli* [pSB401] and [pSB1075], which produce bioluminescence in response to short and long chain AHL respectively as the biosensors [64]. *Lavandula angustifolia* and *Cinnamomum verum* bark essential oils were found to significantly inhibit the light production of the biosensors, indicating the possibility of these EOs as quorum-sensing inhibitors [31, 32].

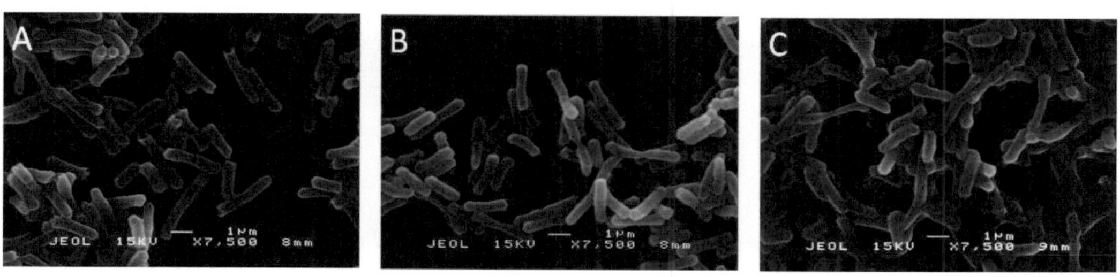

Figure 4. Scanning electron micrographs of *E. coli* J53 R1 after treatment of piperacillin at (a) 64 μg/mL, (b) 128 μg/mL, and (c) 256 μg/mL.

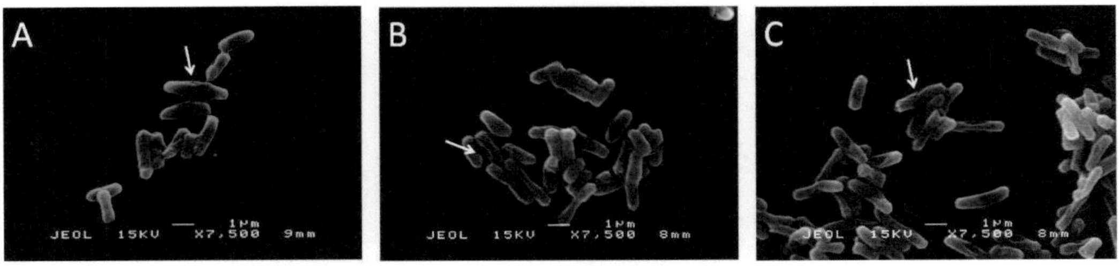

Figure 5. Scanning electron micrographs of *E. coli* J53 R1 after (a) peppermint, (b) lavender, and (c) cinnamon bark essential oils treatment.

5. Moving forward: present and future prospects

The exploitation of EOs has shed new light on antimicrobial therapeutics research and also the resurgence in the use of herbal medicine worldwide. Although possibilities of combination therapy appear to be extensive, the mode of interaction between two antimicrobials is extremely crucial. One of the challenges encountered in the *in vitro* study on a particular antibiotic is that despite proven synergism, it does not guarantee the success of the clinical use of the therapeutic agent. A major issue to be addressed is the pharmacology aspects of the membrane active properties of the EOs as a candidate therapeutic agent and their precise condition of use. Thus, in line with *in vitro* susceptibility testing, *in vivo* experiments are needed in tandem to provide sufficient supporting evidence to serve as a basis for new antimicrobials to survive through the phases of clinical trials.

In view of current efforts in developing alternative strategies by combining antibiotics with other compounds (antibiotic or nonantibiotic) —following the encouraging paradigm in Augmentin, this approach needs to be intensified. Besides inhibiting the effector molecules such as β-lactamase or DNA replication, supplementary compounds that interfere with regulatory mechanisms such as virulence genes or cell physiology have shown great potential. Furthermore, targeting nonessential bacterial pathways is also an alternative and very possible strategy employed to reduce the risk of developing resistance. Ultimately, just because bacteria can evolve in various ways to resist antibiotics at the rate that is insurmountable by new antibiotic development, it would be imperative for medical researchers to employ multiple strategies in the combat of antibiotic resistance. There is no single "magic bullet" to adequately address the phenomenon of multidrug resistance evolution.

Acknowledgements

This study was funded by the Fundamental Research Grant Scheme (FRGS) from the Ministry of Higher Education (MOHE), Malaysia, under the grant number FRGS/1/2011/SKK/IMU/03/3. The bacterial strains were a kind gift from Dr George A. Jacoby.

http://dx.doi.org/10.5772/67776

Author details

Polly Soo Xi Yap[1], Shun Kai Yang[2], Kok Song Lai[3] and Swee Hua Erin Lim[4]*

*Address all correspondence to: erinlimsh@gmail.com

1 School of Postgraduate Studies and Research, International Medical University, Kuala Lumpur, Malaysia

2 School of Graduate Studies, Universiti Putra Malaysia, Selangor, Malaysia

3 Department of Cell and Molecular Biology, Faculty of Biotechnology and Biomolecular Sciences, Universiti Putra Malaysia, Selangor, Malaysia

4 Perdana University-Royal College of Surgeons in Ireland (PU-RCSI), Perdana University, Selangor, Malaysia

References

[1] Kelley PW. Antimicrobial resistance in the age of noncommunicable diseases. Rev Panam Salud Publica. 2011;30(6):515-8.

[2] Durkin M. Hospitalists on high alert as colistin resistance spreads Pennsylvania: American College of Physicians; 2016 [Available from: http://www.acphospitalist.org/archives/2016/09/colistin-resistance.htm].

[3] Liu Y-Y, Wang Y, Walsh TR, Yi L-X, Zhang R, Spencer J, et al. Emergence of plasmid-mediated colistin resistance mechanism MCR-1 in animals and human beings in China: a microbiological and molecular biological study. Lancet Infect Dis.16(2):161-8.

[4] Kong KF, Schneper L, Mathee K. Beta-lactam antibiotics: from antibiosis to resistance and bacteriology. APMIS. 2010;118(1):1-36.

[5] Goffin C, Ghuysen JM. Multimodular penicillin-binding proteins: an enigmatic family of orthologs and paralogs. Microbiol Mol Biol Rev. 1998;62(4):1079-93.

[6] Sauvage E, Kerff F, Terrak M, Ayala JA, Charlier P. The penicillin-binding proteins: structure and role in peptidoglycan biosynthesis. FEMS Microbiol Rev. 2008;32(2):234-58.

[7] Fisher JF, Mobashery S. Three decades of the class A beta-lactamase acyl-enzyme. Current protein & peptide science. 2009;10(5):401-7.

[8] Zapun A, Contreras-Martel C, Vernet T. Penicillin-binding proteins and beta-lactam resistance. FEMS Microbiol Rev. 2008;32(2):361-85.

[9] Shea ME, Hiasa H. Interactions between DNA helicases and frozen topoisomerase IV-quinolone-DNA ternary complexes. J Biol Chem. 1999;274(32):22747-54.

[10] Willmott CJ, Critchlow SE, Eperon IC, Maxwell A. The complex of DNA gyrase and quinolone drugs with DNA forms a barrier to transcription by RNA polymerase. J Mol Biol. 1994;242(4):351-63.

[11] Lortholary O, Tod M, Cohen Y, Petitjean O. Aminoglycosides. Med Clin North Am. 1995; 79(4):761-87.

[12] Melancon P, Tapprich WE, Brakier-Gingras L. Single-base mutations at position 2661 of *Escherichia coli* 23S rRNA increase efficiency of translational proofreading. J Bacteriol. 1992;174(24):7896-901.

[13] Takano M, Okuda M, Yasuhara M, Hori R. Cellular toxicity of aminoglycoside antibiotics in G418-sensitive and -resistant LLC-PK1 cells. Pharm Res. 1994;11(5):609-15.

[14] Shah RR, Wade G. Reappraisal of the risk/benefit of nitrofurantoin: review of toxicity and efficacy. Adverse Drug React Acute Poisoning Rev. 1989;8(4):183-201.

[15] McOsker CC, Fitzpatrick PM. Nitrofurantoin: mechanism of action and implications for resistance development in common uropathogens. J Antimicrob Chemother. 1994;33 (Suppl A):23-30.

[16] McCalla DR. Nitrofurans. In: Hahn FE, editor. Mechanism of Action of Antibacterial Agents. Berlin, Heidelberg: Springer Berlin Heidelberg; 1979. pp. 176-213.

[17] Zaitseva J, Granik V, Belik A, Koksharova O, Khmel I. Effect of nitrofurans and NO generators on biofilm formation by Pseudomonas aeruginosa PAO1 and Burkholderia cenocepacia 370. Res Microbiol. 2009;160(5):353-7.

[18] Orwa JA, Govaerts C, Busson R, Roets E, Van Schepdael A, Hoogmartens J. Isolation and structural characterization of colistin components. J Antibiot (Tokyo). 2001;54(7):595-9.

[19] Orwa JA, Govaerts C, Busson R, Roets E, Van Schepdael A, Hoogmartens J. Isolation and structural characterization of polymyxin B components. J Chromatogr A. 2001;912 (2):369-73.

[20] Groisman EA, Kayser J, Soncini FC. Regulation of polymyxin resistance and adaptation to low-Mg^{2+} environments. J Bacteriol. 1997;179(22):7040-5.

[21] Hermsen ED, Sullivan CJ, Rotschafer JC. Polymyxins: pharmacology, pharmacokinetics, pharmacodynamics, and clinical applications. Infect Dis Clin North Am. 2003;17 (3):545-62.

[22] Tam VH, Schilling AN, Vo G, Kabbara S, Kwa AL, Wiederhold NP, et al. Pharmacodynamics of polymyxin B against Pseudomonas aeruginosa. Antimicrob Agents Chemother. 2005;49(9):3624-30.

[23] Wang H, Dzink-Fox JL, Chen M, Levy SB. Genetic characterization of highly fluoroquinolone-resistant clinical *Escherichia coli* strains from China: role of acrR mutations. Antimicrob Agents Chemother. 2001;45(5):1515-21.

[24] Perreten V, Schwarz FV, Teuber M, Levy SB. Mdt(A), a new efflux protein conferring multiple antibiotic resistance in Lactococcus lactis and *Escherichia coli*. Antimicrob Agents Chemother. 2001;45(4):1109-14.

[25] Rahmati S, Yang S, Davidson AL, Zechiedrich EL. Control of the AcrAB multidrug efflux pump by quorum-sensing regulator SdiA. Mol Microbiol. 2002;43(3):677-85.

[26] Hirata T, Saito A, Nishino K, Tamura N, Yamaguchi A. Effects of efflux transporter genes on susceptibility of *Escherichia coli* to tigecycline (GAR-936). Antimicrob Agents Chemother. 2004;48(6):2179-84.

[27] Masi M, Pages JM. Structure, function and regulation of outer membrane proteins involved in drug transport in enterobactericeae: the OmpF/C – TolC case. Open Microbiol J. 2013;7:22-33.

[28] De E, Basle A, Jaquinod M, Saint N, Mallea M, Molle G, et al. A new mechanism of antibiotic resistance in Enterobacteriaceae induced by a structural modification of the major porin. Mol Microbiol. 2001;41(1):189-98.

[29] Poole K. Mechanisms of bacterial biocide and antibiotic resistance. Symp Ser Soc Appl Microbiol. 2002(31):55S–64S.

[30] Macheboeuf P, Di Guilmi AM, Job V, Vernet T, Dideberg O, Dessen A. Active site restructuring regulates ligand recognition in class A penicillin-binding proteins. Proc Natl Acad Sci U S A. 2005;102(3):577-82.

[31] Yap PS, Krishnan T, Chan KG, Lim SH. Antibacterial mode of action of cinnamomum verum bark essential oil, alone and in combination with piperacillin, against a multi-drug-resistant *Escherichia coli* strain. J Microbiol Biotechnol. 2015;25(8):1299-306.

[32] Yap PS, Krishnan T, Yiap BC, Hu CP, Chan KG, Lim SH. Membrane disruption and anti-quorum sensing effects of synergistic interaction between Lavandula angustifolia (lavender oil) in combination with antibiotic against plasmid-conferred multi-drug-resistant *Escherichia coli*. J Appl Microbiol. 2014;116(5):1119-28.

[33] Yap PS, Lim SH, Hu CP, Yiap BC. Combination of essential oils and antibiotics reduce antibiotic resistance in plasmid-conferred multidrug resistant bacteria. Phytomedicine. 2013;20(8-9):710-3.

[34] Duarte A, Ferreira S, Silva F, Domingues FC. Synergistic activity of coriander oil and conventional antibiotics against Acinetobacter baumannii. Phytomedicine. 2012;19 (3-4):236-8.

[35] Lorenzi V, Muselli A, Bernardini AF, Berti L, Pages JM, Amaral L, et al. Geraniol restores antibiotic activities against multidrug-resistant isolates from gram-negative species. Antimicrob Agents Chemother. 2009;53(5):2209-11.

[36] Rosato A, Piarulli M, Corbo F, Muraglia M, Carone A, Vitali ME, et al. In vitro synergistic antibacterial action of certain combinations of gentamicin and essential oils. Curr Med Chem. 2010;17(28):3289-95.

[37] Mann CM, Markham JL. A new method for determining the minimum inhibitory concentration of essential oils. J Appl Microbiol. 1998;84(4):538-44.

[38] Wadhwani T, Desai K, Patel D, Lawani D, Bahaley P, Joshi P, et al. Effect of various solvents on bacterial growth in context of determining MIC of various antimicrobials. Internet J Microbiol. 2008;7(1).

[39] Hood JR, Wilkinson JM, Cavanagh HMA. Evaluation of common antibacterial screening methods utilized in essential oil research. J Essent Oil Res. 2003;15(6):428-33.

[40] Belanche A, Ramos-Morales E, Newbold CJ. In vitro screening of natural feed additives from crustaceans, diatoms, seaweeds and plant extracts to manipulate rumen fermentation. J Sci Food Agric. 2016;96(9):3069-78.

[41] Choe E, Min D. Mechanisms and factors for edible oil oxidation. Comprehensive Reviews in Food Science and Food Safety. 2006;5(17):168-186.

[42] Misharina TA, Polshkov AN. Antioxidant properties of essential oils: autoxidation of essential oils from laurel and fennel and effects of mixing with essential oil from coriander. Prikladnaia biokhimiia i mikrobiologiia. 2005;41(6):693-702.

[43] Atkinson R, Arey J. Atmospheric Chemistry of Biogenic Organic Compounds. Accounts of Chemical Research. 1998;31(9):574-83.

[44] Bassolé IHN, Juliani HR. Essential oils in combination and their antimicrobial properties. Molecules. 2012;17:3989-4006.

[45] Palaniappan K, Holley RA. Use of natural antimicrobials to increase antibiotic susceptibility of drug resistant bacteria. Int J Food Microbiol. 2010;140(2-3):164-8.

[46] Magi G, Marini E, Facinelli B. Antimicrobial activity of essential oils and carvacrol, and synergy of carvacrol and erythromycin, against clinical, erythromycin-resistant Group A Streptococci. Front Microbiol. 2015;6:165.

[47] Utchariyakiat I, Surassmo S, Jaturanpinyo M, Khuntayaporn P, Chomnawang MT. Efficacy of cinnamon bark oil and cinnamaldehyde on anti-multidrug resistant Pseudomonas aeruginosa and the synergistic effects in combination with other antimicrobial agents. BMC Complement Altern Med. 2016;16:158.

[48] D'Arrigo M, Ginestra G, Mandalari G, Furneri PM, Bisignano G. Synergism and postantibiotic effect of tobramycin and Melaleuca alternifolia (tea tree) oil against Staphylococcus aureus and *Escherichia coli*. Phytomedicine. 2010;17(5):317-22.

[49] Odds FC. Synergy, antagonism, and what the chequerboard puts between them. J Antimicrob Chemother. 2003;52(1):1.

[50] Souren P, Dubey RC, Maheswari DK, Kang SC. *Trachyspermum ammi* (L.) fruit essential oil influencing on membrane permeability and surface characteristics in inhibiting foodborne pathogens. Food Control. 2011;22:725-31.

[51] Devi KP, Nisha SA, Sakthivel R, Pandian SK. Eugenol (an essential oil of clove) acts as an antibacterial agent against Salmonella typhi by disrupting the cellular membrane. J Ethnopharmacol. 2010;130(1):107-15.

[52] Diao WR, Hu QP, Feng SS, Li WQ, Xu JG. Chemical composition and antibacterial activity of the essential oil from green huajiao (zanthoxylum schinifolium) against selected foodborne pathogens. J Agric Food Chem. 2013;61(25):6044-49.

[53] La Storia A, Ercolini D, Marinello F, Di Pasqua R, Villani F, Mauriello G. Atomic force microscopy analysis shows surface structure changes in carvacrol-treated bacterial cells. Res Microbiol. 2011;162(2):164-72.

[54] Bajpai VK, Sharma A, Baek K, H. Antibacterial mode of action of Cudrania tricuspidata fruit essential oil, affecting membrane permeability and surface characteristics of food-borne pathogens. Food Control. 2013;32(2):582-90.

[55] Kłodziń ska E, Szumski M, Dziubakiewicz E, Hrynkiewicz K, Skwarek E, Janusz W, et al. Effect of zeta potential value on bacterial behaviour during electrophoretic separation. Electrophoresis. 2010;31:1590-6.

[56] Tymczyszyn EE, del Rosario Diaz M, Gomez-Zavaglia A, Disalvo EA. Volume recovery, surface properties and membrane integrity of Lactobacillus delbrueckii subsp. bulgaricus dehydrated in the presence of trehalose or sucrose. J Appl Microbiol. 2007;103(6):2410-9.

[57] van der Mei HC, de Vries J, Busscher HJ. Hydrophobic and electrostatic cell surface properties of thermophilic dairy streptococci. Appl Environ Microbiol. 1993;59(12):4305-12.

[58] Gilbert P, Evans DJ, Evans E, Duguid IG, Brown MR. Surface characteristics and adhesion of *Escherichia coli* and Staphylococcus epidermidis. J Appl Bacteriol. 1991;71(1):72-7.

[59] Palmer J, Flint S, Brooks J. Bacterial cell attachment, the beginning of a biofilm. J Ind Microbiol Biotechnol. 2007;34(9):577-88.

[60] Wilson WW, Wade MM, Holman SC, Champlin FR. Status of methods for assessing bacterial cell surface charge properties based on zeta potential measurements. J Microbiol Methods. 2001;43(3):153-64.

[61] Halder S, Yadav KK, Sarkar R, Mukherjee S, Saha P, Haldar S, et al. Alteration of Zeta potential and membrane permeability in bacteria: a study with cationic agents. SpringerPlus. 2015;4:672.

[62] Van Houdt R, Aertsen A, Moons P, Vanoirbeek K, Michiels CW. N-acyl-L-homoserine lactone signal interception by *Escherichia coli*. FEMS Microbiol Lett. 2006;256(1):83-9.

[63] Krishnan T, Yin WF, Chan KG. Inhibition of quorum sensing-controlled virulence factor production in Pseudomonas aeruginosa PAO1 by Ayurveda spice clove (Syzygium aromaticum) bud extract. Sensors (Basel). 2012;12(4):4016-30.

[64] Winson MK, Swift S, Fish L, Throup JP, Jorgensen F, Chhabra SR, et al. Construction and analysis of luxCDABE-based plasmid sensors for investigating N-acyl homoserine lactone-mediated quorum sensing. FEMS Microbiol Lett. 1998;163(2):185-92.

Section 4

E. coli as a Model in Physiology and Cell Biology

Chapter 16

Horizontal Gene Transfer and the Diversity of *Escherichia coli*

Maryam Javadi, Saeid Bouzari and Mana Oloomi

Additional information is available at the end of the chapter

http://dx.doi.org/10.5772/intechopen.68307

Abstract

Escherichia coli (E. coli) strains are normal flora of human gastrointestinal tract. The evolution encoded by horizontally-transferred genetic (HGT) elements has been perceived in several species. E. coli strains have acquired virulence potential factors by attainment of particular loci through HGT, transposons or phages. The heterogeneous nature of these strains is because of HGT through mobile genetic elements. These genetic exchanges that occur in bacteria provide the genetic diversity.

A diverse enterobacterial species of E. coli is classified into (i) commensal nonpathogenic, (ii) intestinal and (iii) extraintestinal pathogenic strains. This is related to the presence or absence of regions which are associated with certain pathotypes. The genetic information belongs to the flexible E. coli genome and it has been horizontally acquired by plasmids, bacteriophages and genomic islands. The rapid evolution of E. coli variants results from the genomic regions, contribute to frequently rearrangements, excision and transfer as well as acquisition of additional genome thus resulting to the creation of new (pathogenic) variants.

HGT is a key step in the evolution of bacterial pathogens. This study is focused on determining the common virulence factors as a signature at the genetic level to use for classification, diversity and evolution of E. coli.

Keywords: *Escherichia coli* (*E. coli*), horizontal gene transfer (HGT), pathogenicity islands (PAIs), evolution, bacteriophages

1. Introduction

Escherichia coli (*E. coli*) are commensal organisms and are a part of human and animal microflora. Although most strains of *E. coli* are harmless, some isolates have the potential to cause severe diseases. Among the various nonpathogenic *E. coli* strains, some are able to acquire virulence determinants through the horizontal transfer of virulence genes. Based on the site of the infection and disease caused by *E. coli*, pathogenic strains are divided into major groups: extraintestinal pathogenic *E. coli* (ExPEC) and intestinal pathogenic *E. coli* (InPEC). This variability and adaptability reinforces the necessity of novel approaches to overcome pathogenic *E. coli*. Antibiotic resistance among pathogenic strains is considerable and is due to uncontrolled usage of antibiotics in human and veterinary field. Consequently, focus on modern and reverse vaccination, besides comparative genome analysis, is the most useful approach to control disease [1].

Genome evolution is the process by which the content and organization of genetic information of a species change over time. This process includes different forms of changes: point mutation and gene conversions, rearrangement (inversion or translocation), and deletion and insertion of foreign DNA (plasmid integration and transposition). These mechanisms seem to be the primary forces behind the genetic adaptation of bacterial organisms to novel environments and by which bacterial populations diverge and form separate, evolutionarily distinct species. Mechanisms of horizontal gene flux include the transmission of mobile genetic elements such as conjugative plasmids, bacteriophages, transposons, insertion elements, and genomic islands, as well as the mechanism of recombination of foreign DNA into host DNA [2].

Point mutations and genetic rearrangements only lead to evolutionary development, primarily without creation of novel genetic determinants, while horizontal gene transfer (HGT) produces extremely dynamic genomes. Thus, HGT can effectively alter the life-style of bacterial species. This is particularly true for bacterial pathogens, where virulence is linked to acquisition of virulence determinants by HGT [3].

A major driving force of evolution and diversification in pathogenic bacteria compared with modification of the existing DNA is the acquisition of virulence determinants through successive horizontal gene transfer [4]. The evolution of pathogenic bacteria with a strong lineage dependency often results from integration, retention, and expression of foreign DNA with a specific genomic background. In fact, parallel evolution from strains with the same genomic pathotype has occasionally emerged from multiple lineages, although the genetic mechanisms are not fully understood [4].

The modification of old functions and the development of new ones are required for bacterial evolution. The most frequent events are nucleotide exchange, insertion, and deletion. Mutation rates, per nucleotide per generation, are generally in the range of 10^{-6}–10^{-9} in bacteria. Moreover, gene disruption, deletions, and module exchange between different genes occur at appreciable frequency. These mechanisms are common in all living organisms. They allow modification of existing functions for optimizing in a niche or adapting to a new niche. Bacteria have no sexual life cycles, in contrast to higher organisms, to facilitate the exchange of alleles within a population. This function is fulfilled by horizontal gene transfer in bacteria; in this way the entire functional genomic unit can be imported from other sources that are not restricted by species. The DNA is transferred from less than 1 to more than 100 kb, in size. It can encode entire metabolic pathways or complex surface structures. These genes can be taken up as naked DNA or transferred in the form of plasmids, transposons, or phages [5].

2. Horizontal gene transfer (HGT)

2.1. Horizontal gene transfer (HGT) and pathogenicity islands

Subgroups of genomic islands which have a pivotal role in HGT are pathogenicity islands (PAIs). The concept of PAI was founded in the late 1980s by Jörg Hacker and colleagues in Werner Goebel's group at the University of Würzburg, Germany [2, 3].

2.1.1. The genetic features of PAIs

One or more virulence genes are carried by PAIs. There are also genomic or metabolic islands with genomic elements and characteristics similar to PAI, but lacking virulence genes. They are not present in the genome of a nonpathogenic species or a closely related species, but they are present in the genome of the same pathogenic bacterium [3].

Large genomic regions are relatively occupied by PAIs. They often differ from the core genome and the majority of PAIs are in the range of 10–200 kb in their base compositions and they also show different codon usage. It is considered that the horizontally acquired PAI still has the base composition of the donor species. On the other hand, it is also observed that the horizontally acquired DNA base composition will tend to the base composition of the recipient's genome during evolution. Further factors such as DNA topology or specific codon usage of the virulence genes in PAI may also account for the maintenance of the divergent base composition [3].

PAIs are frequently adjacent to tRNA genes. tRNA genes serve as anchor points for insertion of foreign DNA that has been acquired by horizontal gene transfer through recombination process. They are frequently associated with mobile genetic elements and they are often flanked by direct repeat (DR) sequences. PAIs delete with distinct frequencies and they are often unstable. PAI virulence functions are lost with a frequency higher than the normal rate of mutation. Integrases, transposases, and insertion sequence (IS) elements have been identified as elements that contribute to the mobilization and instability of PAIs [2].

PAIs often represent mosaic-like structures rather than the homogeneous nature of horizontally acquired DNA [2].

The islands are divided into different subtypes based on their genetic composition and also on their effects in a specific ecological niche, within a particular organism. Therefore, the same islands may have different functions [2].

2.1.2. Evolution, transfer, regulation, and integration sites of PAIs

The observation that important virulence factors are present in very similar forms in different bacteria may be explained by horizontal gene transfer. PAIs transfer via three major paths, including (i) natural transformation, (ii) plasmids, and (iii) transduction. PAI integration into the bacterial chromosome is a site-specific process. PAIs are mostly inserted at the 3′ end of tRNA loci. Furthermore, phage attachment sites are frequently located in this region. Specific genes and intergenic regions have been used by PAIs, in operons. For instance, *selC* locus is an insertion site frequently used by *E. coli* [3].

PAI genes respond to environmental signals by gene expression. PAIs are part of complex regulatory networks that include regulators encoded by the PAI itself or by other PAIs, and other global regulators elsewhere in the chromosome or by plasmids. PAI regulators can be involved in the regulation of genes located outside the PAI. Regulators mostly belong to the AraC/XylS family or to the two-component response family [2].

2.2. Horizontal gene transfer and transduction by phages

2.2.1. Evolution of bacterial pathogens by phages

Phages play an important role in the evolution and virulence of many pathogens. From common virulence factors encoded by phages in *E. coli* strains, we could mention Shiga toxin, enterohemolysin, cytolethal distending toxin, superoxide dismutase, and some outer membrane protein (OMP) [5].

The analysis of bacterial genome sequencing revealed that phages affect the bacterial genome architecture [5]. In addition, phages are important vehicles for horizontal gene exchange between different bacterial species and account for a good share of the strain-to-strain differences within the same bacterial species. In fact, two-third of gamma proteobacteria and low G+C Gram-positive bacteria harbor prophages [4, 5].

The early studies had indicated that some prophages carry additional cargo genes (lysogenic conversion genes) which are not required for the phage life cycle. Instead, a lot of DNA from phages or morons (more DNA) from prophages in pathogenic bacteria encode virulence factors. Lysogenic conversion is thought to have a great impact on the evolution of pathogenic bacteria and results in a very interesting situation of bacterium-phage coevolution.

2.2.2. Phage-mediated gene transfer

Phage-mediated horizontal gene transfer occurs via transduction or lysogenic conversion. In addition, bacterial gene disruption can occur by prophage integration into the bacterial genome.

2.2.2.1. Transduction

The phage DNA must be packed, after the phage heads are completed. In a limited frequency, DNA fragments of the host genome are packed instead of the phage DNA; however, the transduction process is quite accurate. In this process, fully functional phage particles can result, which in return deliver the packed DNA into other suitable bacteria. On the one side of transduction, the absence of phage DNA does not harm the bacterium. Instead, the injected foreign bacterial DNA can be incorporated into the genome. This is a typical example of phage-mediated horizontal gene transfer. These phages have been observed in many bacteria, for instance *Salmonella spp* [5].

2.2.2.2. Lysogenic conversion

Phages can play an important role in the emergence of new pathogens. This was recognized for Shiga toxin of *E. coli,* which is phage-encoded. Moron genes are thought to enhance phage replication when the temperate phage is residing as a prophage in the chromosome of a bacterium [5]. Moron-encoded functions enhance the fitness of the lysogen and improve the fitness of the phage. Phage-mediated horizontal transfer of virulence factors between bacteria is a very significant mechanism for evolutionary pathways. Several investigations indicate that pathogenic *E. coli* strains harbor different prophages, including P2, Mu, and lambda prophages. In comparison, phage-possessing strains grow quicker than non-lysogenic *E. coli* [5].

2.2.2.3. Gene disruption

Acquiring virulence genes is not the only mechanism by which pathogenicity develops. Pathogenic bacteria also develop from commensal bacteria by loss of genes. *Shigella* is an example of virulence by loss of *E. coli*-specific genes, including flagellar genes and *cadA*. On a small scale, prophage can cause single-gene loss when integrated into host genes. A common locus for prophage integration evolves from the tRNA genes [5].

2.3. Phages, PAIs, and plasmids in the evolution of pathogenic *E. coli* through horizontal gene transfer (HGT)

2.3.1. PAIs and E. coli pathotypes

The best understood genomic islands are PAIs, to date, which carry a cluster of virulence genes. The virulence gene products contribute to the pathogenicity of bacterium. In the case of *E. coli,* bacteria have adopted pathogenic islands to cause disease in specific environments by acquiring a foreign DNA from ancient nonpathogenic *E. coli* strains (e.g., a normal inhabitant of the gut). In enterohaemorrhagic *E. coli* (EHEC), due to the specific adaptation to different environments, a virulence-associated plasmid, one Stx-converting phage, and several PAIs have been acquired and maintained. Genomic islands may be involved in the development of specific diseases, such as diarrhea and hemolytic-uremic syndrome in a specific environment. For instance, colonization in the large intestine (EHEC), watery diarrhea in small intestine (enteropathogenic *E. coli,* EPEC), and survival and colonization in the bladder (uropathogenic

E. coli, UPEC). Such events probably led to the development of specific pathotypes of *E. coli* as mentioned above. In the case of EHEC, *stx* gene (transfer by phages), OI (O-island), and LEE (PAI) were acquired through HGT [6]. The acquisition of LEE island and *espC* gene (*E. coli* secreted protease gene) by ancient core genome led to the emergence of EPEC pathotype. Several PAIs, such as PAI-I, -II, -III, and -IV are present in the UPEC genome, indicating the occurrence of horizontal gene transfer in distinct evolutionary pathways in this particular pathotype [2].

LEE (the locus of enterocyte effacement) was initially described in EPEC strains, the causative agents of infant diarrhea in developing and industrial countries. EPEC strains are able to cause attaching-and-effacing (A/E) lesions of the microvillus brush border of enterocytes [6]. All of the genes necessary for this phenotype are located on a PAI, termed LEE. LEE is horizontally transferred and contains 41 ORFs, integrated adjacent to either the *selC*, *pheU*, or *pheV* loci. EHEC strains also possess a LEE which has 54 ORFs; 41 are common to the LEE of both EPEC and EHEC. The remaining 13 ORFs belong to a putative prophage, designated 933L (P4-like prophage), which is located close to the *selC* locus [7]. In contrast to the LEE of EPEC, cloned EHEC LEE is not able to induce A/E lesions. It has been suggested that the different phenotypes produced by LEE of EPEC and EHEC are based on natural selection for adaptation with the host microenvironment or for evasion of the host immune system [2, 6].

HPI (high pathogenicity island) was first described in *Yersinia spp*. Then it was shown in enteroinvasive (EIEC), enterotoxigenic (ETEC), enteropathogenic (EPEC), and Shiga toxin-producing (STEC) *E. coli* and extraintestinal *E. coli*. The widespread presence of HPI in different species and pathotypes also implies an efficient mechanism of horizontal transfer [6].

E. coli is the most prevalent bacterial causative agent of urinary tract infection (UTI). UPEC strains also express an array of virulence factors, which are often encoded by PAI. Alpha-hemolysin belongs to the RTX toxins with pore-forming activities in erythrocytes and other eukaryotic cells. The alpha-hemolysin operon (*hly* gene) of UPEC can be located either on a plasmid or on the chromosome [7].

In the *E. coli* species, CFT073, 536 (O6: K15), J96 (O4: K6) strains can cause urinary tract infection. When related PAI encoding alpha-hemolysin is deleted, it can lead to nonpathogenic strains from pathogenic ones. In the case of *E. coli* C5, *hly* loci is located on PAI-I and inserted in *leuX* loci. However, in other UPEC strains, several PAIs including PAI-I, PAI-II, PAI-IV, and PAI-V could harbor *hly* genes [7, 8].

Regions encoding hemolysin and P-fimbriae are named as PAI-I, -II, which are located at centisomes 82 and 97 in *E. coli* chromosome. Moreover, tRNA loci *leuX* and *selC* are also located in this region. Direct repeats (DR) 16 and 18 are adjacent to these PAIs [9]. In *E. coli* strains, besides hemolysin toxin, there is another toxin named as enterohemolysin which is encoded by a large virulence plasmid. Both of the related operons contain *hlyA*, *hlyB*, *hlyC*, and *hlyD* genes. Hemolysin and enterohemolysin are different toxins in terms of the genes that encode them and in terms of their immunological features. In contrast to hemolysin, enterohemolysin is a cell-associated toxin and it is also a member of pore-forming toxin family [9].

Since most virulence factors must be exposed on the surface of a bacterium or be secreted, many bacteria develop secretion pathways. An example of a T1SS (type 1 secretion system) encoded by a PAI is the *hly* operon of UPEC which is responsible for synthesis, activation, and transport of α-hemolysin. Genes encoding the T2SS (type 2 secretion system) belong to the core gene set; however, a large number of substrate proteins for T2SS are encoded by genes within PAI. Some of these proteins are important for pathogenesis. The gene cluster encoding T3SS (type 3 secretion system) can be found on virulence plasmid. PAI encoding T3SS includes LEE in enteropathogenic *E. coli*. Various passenger domains secreted by T5SS (type V secretion system) are referred to as autotransporters, e.g., the immunoglobulin G proteases and the VacA toxin. Examples of T5SS encoded by PAI are LPA and the EspC PAI of pathogenic *E. coli* [9].

Finally, there are many identified PAIs in different *E. coli* pathoypes which could transfer via horizontal gene transfer process and consequently led to emergence of new clinical isolates with distinct characteristics [2].

2.3.2. *The role of phages in E. coli pathogenicity and evolution*

Phages were acquired through horizontal gene transfer by an old nonpathogenic *E. coli* strain and led to the development of specific pathotypes. However, the genomic background has a pivotal role in evolutionary pathways. Pathogenic *E. coli* strains are classified based on repertoires of virulence factors and the most common diseases associated with them [10].

2.3.2.1. *Shiga toxins*

Shiga toxins (Stxs) are a family of related toxins with two major groups, Stx1 and Stx2, which are expressed by genes considered to be horizontally acquired by bacteriophages. Shiga toxin encoded by *stx1* and *stx2* genes is an A-B type toxin that inhibits protein synthesis and causes hemorrhagic colitis and hemolytic-uremic syndrome. The *stx* genes are located in the genome of heterogeneous lytic (*stx2*) or cryptic (*stx1*) lambdoid phages.

E. coli strain O157:H7 is a very prominent example of phage acquisition. *E. coli* O157:H7 is a mucosal pathogen and produces numerous pathogenic factors, of which the most significant one is phage-encoded Shiga toxin [10].

The second important factor is T3SS encoded by LEE, a PAI which is adjacent to 933L prophage. Shiga toxin is a causative agent of severe diarrhea, hemorrhagic colitis syndrome (HC), and hemolytic-uremic syndrome (HUS) in STEC strains. The Shiga toxin released by bacteria residing in the intestinal lumen is thought to be responsible for all of these symptoms. The toxin crosses the intestinal epithelial barrier, and then enters the bloodstream, damages colon vascular cells, kidneys, and the central nervous system [5, 10].

O157:H7 *E. coli* is a group of closely related strains which has diverged from enteropathogenic *E. coli* O55: H7 during the evolutionary process. The current model of emergence of toxigenic *E. coli* O157:H7 from its non-toxigenic, less virulent progenitor, *E. coli* O55:H7 relies on a number of genetic events. Key events in this process were the replacement of the *rfb* gene region, followed by the sequential acquisition of first bacteriophage *stx2* and then phage *stx1*. Genome diversity occurred through random drift and bacteriophage-mediated events. Many strains possess only the *stx2* prophage. The *rfb* region encodes the enzymes necessary for the synthesis of the O side chains of the bacterial lipopolysaccharides. *rfb* locus is the target for frequent recombination and horizontal gene transfer [5, 11].

A large number of STEC serotypes are known. Although O157:H7 is the most important, four non-O157 STEC serotypes such as O26:H11, O103:H2, O145:H28, and O111:H8, have emerged as leading causes of infection. The major virulence factor of STEC is Shiga toxins (Stxs). STEC strains carry Stx1, Stx2, or both. Stx1 and Stx2 are divided into three (a, c, and d) and seven (a–g) subtypes, respectively. Stx phages can insert their DNA into specific chromosomal sites during infection of *E. coli* cells. They remain silent, allowing their bacterial hosts to survive as lysogenic strains [11].

Stx phages' insertion of DNA into genes can be in the basic genetic elements of the *E. coli* chromosome, in contrast to many genetic elements that are frequently integrated within tRNA genes. Nine Stx phage-insertion sites have been described. *wrbA*, codes for a tryptophan repressor-binding protein; *yehV*, which codes for a transcriptional regulator; *yecE*, whose function is unknown; *sbcB*, produces an exonuclease; *Z2577*, which codes for an oxidoreductase; *ssrA*, a tmRNA; *prfC*, that encodes peptide chain release factor 3; *argW*, a tRNA-Arg; and *torS-torT*, which is the intergenic region. The *ssrA* gene is also carries type III effector for EspK-encoding gene, which is an insertion site for EspK phages [12].

Prophages of non-O157 EHEC strains were also shown to be remarkably divergent in their structure and integration sites from those of EHEC O157 (Sakai strain). Consequently, among STEC O26:H11 strains isolated from dairy products, cattle, and human patients, a diverse range of genetic patterns was observed. Different *stx* subtypes and various insertion sites were identified among the Stx phages. Lysogenic STEC O26:H11, between human strains and strains from food and cattle was observed with some differences. These results confirm the existence of different clones of STEC O26:H11 with various levels of pathogenicity [12].

Some outbreaks in the world were noticeable because they highlighted the potential contributions of rapid whole-genome sequencing for understanding the phylogenetic origins of a new pathogen, its transmission and epidemiology, and the genetic basis for its pathogenicity. One of them is related to *E. coli* O104:H4, which ended in early July 2011 after the O104:H4 outbreak; sporadic diarrhea/HUS cases linked to *E. coli* O104:H4 have been reported. It is unknown whether these sporadic cases are derived from the new outbreak strain or it is continued transmission which was indicated. Variation in the panel of virulence factors can appear even in closely related *E. coli*. For instance, it is not clear that the pathogenicity of the O104:H4 outbreak is contributed to what extent by shared virulence factors of the sporadic isolates. Some isolates from HUS patients were compared and the most significant differences in their mobile elements were indicated. Besides variation in plasmid content, there is also substantial variation in the number and content of the prophages and genomic islands. The number of predicted prophages varies across the O104:H4 isolates, illustrating the dynamics of phage gain and loss over the relatively short evolutionary time. A key event in the evolution of fully virulent *E. coli* O104:H4 capable of causing HUS was acquisition of O104:H4-G (the *stx2*-containing prophage). Moreover, there is a unique antibiotic resistance profile in each isolate [13].

On the whole, investigations have indicated that, the Stx phages provide an example of the rapid exchange of moron cassettes between phages from different *E. coli* strains. The two sequenced O157 strains, Sakai and EDL933, are closely related on the DNA sequence organization of the Stx2 phages, sp5 and 933W, respectively. The genome organization of phage lambda is integrated into the same chromosomal site, *wrbA*. In contrast, the Stx1 phages, sp15 and 933V from the two sequenced O157 strains, share DNA sequence only across the non-structural genes. The Stx2-encoding bacteriophage P27 from a clinical *E. coli* isolate clearly differs from the corresponding prophages in the Sakai and EDL933 strains, and it was integrated into a different *E. coli* gene *yecE*. In fact, the Stx phages provide strong evidence for the shuffling of phage modules and morons between phages from different *E. coli* strains [12].

2.3.2.2. Cytolethal distending toxins (CDTs)

First, CDTs were recognized as bacterial toxins that block the eukaryotic cell cycle, suppress cell proliferation, and eventually lead to cell death [14]. The holotoxin is a heterotrimer of three protein subunits, CdtA, CdtB, and CdtC. These are encoded by three adjacent and sometimes overlapping genes. CdtB is the active subunit, possessing DNase activity and sharing homology with the mammalian DNaseI. Genes encoding CDTs are widely disseminated among Gram-negative pathogenic bacteria, including *E. coli* strains. The production of CDTs has been associated with several pathotypes, for instance enterohemorrhagic *E. coli* (EHEC) and enteropathogenic *E. coli* (EPEC) [15].

Five different CDTs (I–V) have been reported for *E. coli* so far, and they were designated in order of publication. CDT production has been associated with pathogenic *E. coli*. *cdt-III* gene is localized into a large conjugative virulence plasmid (pVir). *cdt-I* and *cdt-IV* are encoded by lambdoid prophages, while the *cdt-V* operon is flanked by P2-like phage sequences: *repA* (replication gene A) and *Q* (a capsid gene) [16].

CDT-I and CDT-II were identified in EPEC serotype O86:H34 and O128: NM strains, respectively. CDT-III was detected in *E. coli* O15:H21 [14].

CDT-IV was detected in human and animal pathogenic *E. coli* strains of intestinal and extraintestinal origin (*E. coli* 28C, APEC O1). *cdt*-IV operon of strain 28C is flanked on both sides by prophage-related ORFs that was indicated by a DNA homology search and it encodes putative prophage-related proteins. Phage putative proteins include a lambdoid prophage host-specificity protein (*orf1*), a Lom-like protein (*orf2*), a putative tail fiber protein (*orf3*), a putative CP-933-like protease (*rorf1*), and a putative OmpT-like outer membrane protease (*rorf2*) [17]. The genome sequence of APECO1 strain revealed that the *cdt*-IV operon is framed by two prophages and pathogenicity island-associated DNA sequences, including integrase and tRNA genes. Also, genetic mosaic organization among the sequenced *cdt*-I and *cdt*-IV alleles was observed [16]. The phenomenon could also be a result of extensive genetic exchanges among different phages, which might even occur in the mammalian intestine. Similar to virulence genes, morons such as orf4, orf5, orf6, *cdt*, rorf1, and rorf2 might have spread by horizontal gene transfer [17]. *cdt*-I and *cdt*-IV genes might have been acquired by phage transduction from a common ancestor and evolution of the CDT-encoding phages in different bacterial host-generated differences in the *cdt* genes and their flanking DNA contents [16].

The presence of CDT-V in Shiga-toxigenic *E. coli* (STEC) strains of various serotypes has been reported with clinical and nonclinical origin. CDT-V has also been associated with other strains in different serotypes and pathotypes associated with human diarrhea. The P2-like prophage sequences seem to be characteristic for the CDT-V-positive strains, with few differences that can be attributed to the adaptation processes in various hosts. The common acquisition of the *cdt*-V operon in O157: NM EHEC strains has been proposed by the presence of P2-like phage sequences after lineage divergence from the O157:H7 strains. However, there is a strong association between the presence of CDT-V and O157: NM strains [14].

These findings indicate that during evolution, while the *cdt-V* genes are rather conserved and the carrier P2-like phages became diverse, in most cases it may have resulted in loss of their mobility. Therefore, the evolutionary history of the *cdt-V* operon and its P2-like carrying prophages is proposed. Within more variable and potentially inactivated bacteriophage genomes, the highly conserved *cdt-V* operon may cause selective pressure to maintain a functional *cdt* gene cluster. Stabilization of this cargo determinant was done by inactivation of this bacteriophage genome. It is clear that further investigations of flanking regions and P2-like prophage sequences in CDT-V-positive strains will help to clarify the evolutionary background of the distribution of these variants [14–17].

The presence of *cdt* genes in different bacterial species and the analysis of DNA in the vicinity of the *cdt* genes suggest that the toxin has been acquired from heterogenic species by horizontal gene transfer. However, the probable phylogenetic origin (or ancestor) has still remained elusive. Interestingly, the phage and the corresponding insertion sequence remnants were found nearby the *E. coli cdt* genes. All these data suggest that *cdt* genes were acquired by horizontal transfer events and evolved separately since then. *stx* gene, and some types of *cdt* genes are the examples of horizontally acquired genes by phages in *E. coli*. CDT production which has been associated with some pathogenic *E. coli*, isolated from clinical diarrheal patients, suggests that the *cdt* genes are acquired independently in a number of *E. coli* lineages, possibly as a result of HGT.

2.3.3. HGT and plasmids harboring virulence genes in pathogenic E. coli

It is now evident that some virulent genes are located on a large plasmid (pO157) in pathogenic *E. coli*. Some of these genes are the extracellular serine protease gene (*espP*), catalase-peroxidase gene (*katP*), and type II secretion pathway protein D (*etpD*). Different sizes of this plasmid were reported that may contain some of these three genes. pO157 plasmid is mainly associated with EHEC and ETEC strains. In fact, pO157 plasmid was detected in clinical EHEC O157 isolates in 1983 for the first time. This plasmid could be detected in other atypical human EPEC. Atypical EPEC strain lacks EAF plasmid and *bfp* gene. In addition, the genome content of this plasmid in Shiga toxin-producing strains is quite divergent. However, virulence-associated genes' profile is serotype dependent [18].

EspP can be grouped into the autotransporter proteins family and characterized by catalytically active serine residue in the active center. EspP cleaves pepsin and human coagulation factor V. EspP was detected in EHEC O157 and O26 strains. Catalase-peroxidase gene (*katP*) encodes a protein which shows bi-functional catalase and peroxidase activity. This enzyme is expressed by pathogenic strains, and has been thought to protect these pathogens from oxidative damage caused by reactive oxygen molecules produced by phagocytes or other host cells during the infection process. Type II secretion pathway protein D, encoded by *etpD* gene, is another pathogenic factor encoded on the mentioned plasmid. Analysis of ~14 kb DNA derived from plasmid pO157 of EHEC strain EDL933 has indicated 13 ORFs (*etpC-etpO*) operon which had great similarity to type II secretion pathway. *etp* genes are separated from the EHEC-*hlyC* genes with an *IS911*-like insertion element. The existence of IS elements indicates that *etp* gene cluster could be exchangeable between EHEC plasmids [18].

In pathogenic bacteria, there are S-fimbriae and P-fimbriae as different types of fimbriae in uropathogenic *E. coli,* which can cause attachment to host cells. The *pap* gene cluster includes 14 genes encoding P-fimbriae. A cluster of six genes, termed *sfp* including *sfpA* gene, is located on a large plasmid, pSFO157, in some of the pathogenic *E. coli* strains. This genomic cluster mediates mannose-resistant hemagglutination and expression of a novel type of fimbriae, Sfp fimbriae, which is 3–5 nm in diameter, the major subunit of which is SfpA. Sorbitol-fermenting (SF) EHEC O157: H^{-}, which is one of the HUS disease agents, harbors pSFO157 plasmid. The *sfp* gene cluster is surrounded by IS elements, and the origin of plasmid replication proves that these genes might be acquired by HGT. There are nine ORFs (open Reading frames) in the *sfp* gene cluster. The upstream region of *sfpA* is homologous to *IS*1294 and *IS*2 insertion sequences besides Tn2501-like sequence and *IS*100, which is integrated in *IS*3. Moreover, in iso-*IS*1-like sequence, *IS*3 and *IS*100 regions possess DR (directed repeat) sequences indicating the regular transposition process in plasmids [18–21].

3. Diversity of *E. coli* strains

The coevolution of bacterial pathogens related to genetic elements, including pathogenicity islands and phages encoding virulence factors, has been observed in several species. *E. coli* is a member of the normal intestinal microflora of humans and animals. However, certain *E. coli* strains have acquired virulence-associated factors via horizontal gene transfer, enabling the bacteria to colonize its host and cause disease. Pathogenic *E. coli* utilize particular strategies to penetrate into host cells and tissues. Special enzymes and pathogenic factors are known as unique virulence determinants of each bacterium. However, each bacterium has a unique genomic background of its own chromosome, such as *fliC* and *fimH* genes that encode the main subunit of flagella and fimbriae type I, respectively. Both of them are known as virulence-associated factors and interfere in pathogenicity of *E. coli* [19].

Investigations have revealed, *hly* gene which is located on a PAI and encodes alpha-hemolysin, is frequently detected in *cdt*-III- and *cdt*-IV-producing human and animal pathogenic *E. coli* strains.

The prevalence of *hly* gene in *cdt*-type III, IV, and V was more than other isolates. These results demonstrate that, possibly, there could be a relationship between the existence of *hly* gene and the type of *cdt* gene in clinical *E. coli* isolates. *fliC* and *fim* are two chromosomally located genes that can be defined as the genomic background of *E. coli* strains. The *fliC* gene encodes the flagellin subunit; type 1 fimbriae are also encoded by the chromosomally located *fim* gene cluster. The presence of *fim* DNA sequences is common among *E. coli* strains. In fact, the majority of clinical isolates, both virulent and non-virulent, could be induced to express type 1 fimbriae [19].

Among pathogenic *E. coli*, the existence of a large virulent plasmid (pO157) has also been observed. The *etpD, katP*, and *espP* genes are located on this plasmid. The pO157 plasmid is mainly associated with EHEC and ETEC strains. There is a relation between the occurrence of *stx* genes and these virulent plasmid-associated genes. Moreover, PCR analysis revealed a close relationship between the occurrence of plasmid-born *katP* gene and *stx* gene in pathogenic *E. coli.* Most of the *katP*+ strains belong to Shiga toxin-producing *E. coli.* The *katP* gene is mostly present in CDT-I- and CDT-II-producing strains. EspP, which possesses human coagulation factor V and pepsin A proteolytic activity, is a significant marker of virulence in Shiga toxin-producing strains. In CDT-III-producing isolates, high frequency of *espP gene* is considerable. Alpha-hemolysin is frequently associated with human uropathogenic *E. coli* (UPEC); furthermore, related encoding PAI is also unstable and the operon could be located on either a plasmid or the chromosome. Besides, urinary tract infection (UTI) is caused predominantly by type 1fimbriated UPEC and initial binding is mediated by the FimH adhesin of the mentioned fimbriae. Investigation showed that most of the hly^{+} strains harbor *fimH* gene. In addition, all hly^{+} strains possess one or more of plasmid pO157 genes, including *etpD, katP*, and *espP*. These genes plus the *stx* gene are among the EHEC and STEC characteristics, although the *espP* gene is common in EPEC and EHEC. Simultaneous presence of these genes indicates that clinical isolates obtain *hly* operon and relevant PAI. In addition, in evolutionary pathways, isolates improve their pathogenicity by achieving the *cdt* genes. Studies demonstrate that virulence genes from CDT-producing strains belong to the heterogeneous group. Strains which are clustered as particular groups have similar characteristics, while possessing their own unique genotype and genomic content. For instance, each distinct *cdt*-type group, by possessing a particular *cdt* gene as genomic backbone, has an approximately similar pattern based on other virulence genes [19].

This evidence further confirms that horizontal gene transfer could occur among pathogenic strains. Moreover, findings indicate that CDT-producing strains may have originated from a common ancestor during their evolution by HGT, and they departed from each other [17].

CDT-producer strains did not show particular phylogenomic relation and pattern. Indeed, they might carry the same or similar virulence gene sets, but remarkably possess their own divergent genomic structure. This is probably because of their complex and distinct evolutionary pathways, indicating independent acquisition of mobile genetic elements that have driven from their evolution [19]. Furthermore, it was shown that there are different types of CDTs that are encoded by prophages, plasmids, and/or pathogenicity islands that result in different types of CDTs through HGT in different origins [7, 17, 19, 22].

http://dx.doi.org/10.5772/intechopen.68307

In the recent years, whole-genome sequences for many bacteria have become accessible. It improves our understanding about virulence-associated genes and horizontal gene transfer from the emergence of new pathogens aspects. Some pathogens like *E. coli* could acquire virulence genes via HGT. On the other hand, from the diagnostic point of view, virulent gene examination could improve our knowledge about different pathotypes' detection and classification.

Phage-related and virulence-associated factors transferred by phages were found to be prevalent signature proteins. The signature proteins identified include several individual phage proteins (holins, nucleases, terminases, and transferases) and multiple members of different protein families (the lambda family, phage-integrase family, phage-tail tape protein family, putative membrane proteins, regulatory proteins, restriction-modification system proteins, tail fiber-assembly proteins, base plate-assembly proteins, and other prophage tail-related proteins).

4. Conclusions and the way forward

The heterogeneous nature of strains could be because of the HGT through mobile genetic elements. The genetic exchanges that occur in bacteria provide genetic diversity and versatility. Plasmids, bacteriophages, and genomic islands belong to the flexible *E. coli* genome and their genetic information can be horizontally acquired. The rapid evolution of *E. coli* variants contributes to these genomic regions as they are subject to rearrangements, excision, and transfer frequently. The creation of new pathogenic variants is the result of further acquisition of additional genome.

The accumulating amount of sequence information generated in the era of "genomics" helps to increase our understanding of factors and mechanisms that are involved in diversification of this new bacterial species, as well as in those that may direct host-specificity. From a comparative genomic aspect, a significant challenge is to utilize bulky amount of datasets to distinguish and conceptualize specific sequence signatures that scientifically or diagnostically are applicable traits. By comparing more sequence data from different strains, new signature biomarkers will be recognized for use as vaccines or as diagnostic factors in future. Signature conserved proteins in a wide range of pathogenic bacterial strains can potentially be used in modern vaccine-design strategies.

Author details

Maryam Javadi, Saeid Bouzari and Mana Oloomi*

*Address all correspondence to: manaoloomi@yahoo.com

Molecular Biology Department, Pasteur Institute of Iran, Tehran, Iran

References

[1] Moriel DG, Rosini R, Seib KL, Serino L, Pizza M, Rappuoli R. *Escherichia coli*: Great diversity around a common core. MBio. 2012;**3**(3):e00118-12

[2] Schmidt H, Hensel M. Pathogenicity islands in bacterial pathogenesis. Clinical Microbiology Reviews. 2004;**17**(1):14-56

[3] Schubert S, Darlu P, Clermont O, Wieser A, Magistro G, Hoffmann C, Weinert K, Tenaillon O, Matic I, Denamur E. Role of intraspecies recombination in the spread of pathogenicity islands within the *Escherichia coli* species. PLoS Pathogens. 2009;**5**(1):e1000257

[4] Ogura Y, Ooka T, Iguchi A, Toh H, Asadulghani M, Oshima K, Kodama T, Abe H, Nakayama K, Kurokawa K, Tobe T, Hattori M, Hayashi T. Comparative genomics reveal the mechanism of the parallel evolution of O157 and non-O157 enterohemorrhagic *Escherichia coli*. Proceedings of the National Academy of Sciences of the United States of America. 2009;**106**(42):17939-17944

[5] Brüssow H, Canchaya C, Hardt WD. Phages and the evolution of bacterial pathogens: From genomic rearrangements to lysogenic conversion. Microbiology and Molecular Biology Reviews. 2004;**68**(3):560-602

[6] Mohammadzadeh M, Oloomi M, Bouzari S. Genetic evaluation of locus of enterocyte effacement pathogenicity island (LEE) in enteropathogenic *Escherichia coli* isolates (EPEC). Iran Journal of Microbiology. 2013;**5**(4):345-349

[7] Oloomi M, Bouzari S. Molecular profile and genetic diversity of cytolethal distending toxin (CDT)-producing *Escherichia coli* isolates from diarrheal patients. APMIS. 2008;**116**(2):125-132

[8] Bidet P, Bonacorsi S, Clermont O, De Montille C, Brahimi N, Bingen E. Multiple insertional events, restricted by the genetic background, have led to acquisition of pathogenicity island IIJ96-like domains among *Escherichia coli* strains of different clinical origins. Infection and Immunity. 2005;**73**(7):4081-4087

[9] Taneike I, Zhang HM, Wakisaka-Saito N, Yamamoto T. Enterohemolysin operon of Shiga toxin-producing *Escherichia coli*: A virulence function of inflammatory cytokine production from human monocytes. FEBS Letters. 2002;**524**(1-3):219-224

[10] Gyles CL. Shiga toxin-producing *Escherichia coli*: An overview. Journal of Animal Sciences. 2007;**85**(13 Suppl):E45-62

[11] Kyle JL, Cummings CA, Parker CT, Quiñones B, Vatta P, Newton E, Huynh S, Swimley M, Degoricija L, Barker M, Fontanoz S, Nguyen K, Patel R, Fang R, Tebbs R, Petrauskene O, Furtado M, Mandrell RE. *Escherichia coli* serotype O55:H7 diversity supports parallel acquisition of bacteriophage at Shiga toxin phage insertion sites during evolution of the O157:H7 lineage. Journal of Bacteriology. 2012;**194**(8):1885-1896

[12] Bonanno L, Loukiadis E, Mariani-Kurkdjian P, Oswald E, Garnier L, Michel V, Auvray F. Diversity of Shiga toxin-producing *Escherichia coli* (STEC) O26:H11 strains examined via Stx subtypes and insertion sites of Stx and EspK bacteriophages. Applied Environmental Microbiology. 2015;**81**(11):3712-3721

[13] Grad YH, Godfrey P, Cerquiera GC, Mariani-Kurkdjian P, Gouali M, Bingen E, Shea TP, Haas BJ, Griggs A, Young S, Zeng Q, Lipsitch M, Waldor MK, Weill FX, Wortman JR, Hanage WP. Comparative genomics of recent Shiga toxin-producing *Escherichia coli* O104:H4: Short-term evolution of an emerging pathogen. MBio. 2013;**4**(1):e00452-12

[14] Sváb D, Horváth B, Maróti G, Dobrindt U, Tóth I. Sequence variability of P2-like prophage genomes carrying the cytolethal distending toxin V operon in *Escherichia coli* O157. Applied Environmental Microbiology. 2013;**79**(16):4958-4964

[15] Tóth I, Nougayrède JP, Dobrindt U, Ledger TN, Boury M, Morabito S, Fujiwara T, Sugai M, Hacker J, Oswald E. Cytolethal distending toxin type I and type IV genes are framed with lambdoid prophage genes in extraintestinal pathogenic *Escherichia coli*. Infection and Immunity. 2009;**77**(1):492-500

[16] Asakura M, Hinenoya A, Alam MS, Shima K, Zahid SH, Shi L, Sugimoto N, Ghosh AN, Ramamurthy T, Faruque SM, Nair GB, Yamasaki S. An inducible lambdoid prophage encoding cytolethal distending toxin (Cdt-I) and a type III effector protein in enteropathogenic *Escherichia coli*. Proceedings of the National Academy of Sciences of the United States of America. 2007;**104**(36):14483-14488

[17] Javadi M, Oloomi M, Bouzari S. Genotype cluster analysis in pathogenic *Escherichia coli* isolates producing different CDT types. Journal of Pathogens. 2016;**2016**:9237127

[18] Brunder W, Khan AS, Hacker J, Karch H. Novel type of fimbriae encoded by the large plasmid of sorbitol-fermenting enterohemorrhagic *Escherichia coli* O157:H(−). Infections and Immunity. 2001;**69**(7):4447-4457

[19] Oloomi M, Javadi M, Bouzari S. Presence of pathogenicity island-related and plasmid encoded virulence genes in cytolethal distending toxin producing *Escherichia coli* isolates from diarrheal cases. International Journal of Applied Basic Medical Research. 2015;**5**(3):181-186

[20] Brunder W, Schmidt H, Karch H. KatP, a novel catalase-peroxidase encoded by the large plasmid of enterohaemorrhagic *Escherichia coli* O157:H7. Microbiology. 1996;**142**(Pt11):3305-3315

[21] Brunder W, Schmidt H, Karch H. EspP, a novel extracellular serine protease of enterohaemorrhagic *Escherichia coli* O157:H7 cleaves human coagulation factor V. Molecular Microbiology. 1997;**4**(4):767-778

[22] Bouzari S, Oloomi M, Oswald E. Detection of the cytolethal distending toxin locus cdtB among diarrheagenic *Escherichia coli* isolates from humans in Iran. Research in Microbiology. 2005;**156**(2):137-144

Chapter 17

Molecular Mechanisms of Phosphate Homeostasis in *Escherichia coli*

William R. McCleary

Additional information is available at the end of the chapter

http://dx.doi.org/10.5772/67283

Abstract

Life's processes absolutely require inorganic phosphate for structural and energetic purposes. *Escherichia coli* has developed sophisticated mechanisms to acquire phosphate and to maintain intracellular amounts at optimal levels. The processes by which these simple cells maintain stable intracellular concentrations of phosphate are termed phosphate homeostasis, which involves mechanisms to balance the import, assimilation, sequestration, and export of phosphate. This chapter introduces the proteins involved in phosphate homeostasis and reviews information concerning the multiple phosphate transporters and the mechanisms by which they are regulated. It also introduces new concepts of how this bacterium responds to elevated extracellular levels of phosphate and presents a model for the integration of all of these processes to achieve homeostasis. The predominant importers are PitA, PitB, and the PstSCAB complex. Assimilation, or the incorporation of Pi into organic molecules, occurs primarily through the formation of ATP. Gene regulation relies on the PhoB/PhoR two-component system and the formation of a signaling complex at the membrane. The amount of intracellular phosphate can be fine-tuned through the formation or degradation of polyphosphate. Polyphosphate formation requires adequate supplies of ATP. In addition, when intracellular phosphate levels become too high, phosphate can be exported through PitA, PitB, or the YjbB transporters.

Keywords: phosphate homeostasis, ABC transporter, phosphate transporter, polyphosphate, two-component signal transduction

1. Introduction

Inorganic phosphate (Pi) is essential for life. For example, it is found in the hydrophilic ends of the amphipathic lipids in the cellular membranes that define the boundaries of a cell. Together with the sugars ribose or deoxyribose, it makes up the structural backbone of DNA or RNA through its phosphodiester bonds. The cell's energy currency is based upon the energy released from the hydrolysis of the phosphoanhydride bonds between the phosphates of ATP or of the other nucleotides. Moreover, the biochemical activities of many proteins are regulated by the phosphorylation of specific amino acids—histidine and aspartate in bacteria, as well as serine, threonine, and tyrosine.

Because of its essential roles, cells must maintain intracellular Pi pools at optimal levels. In bacteria, such as *Escherichia coli,* this is believed to be between 1 and 10 mM [1–3]. Pi is assimilated into biological molecules through the synthesis of ATP from ADP and Pi. The mechanisms to control intracellular Pi levels include multiple transport proteins with characteristic patterns of expression, different affinities for Pi, and rates of Pi transport [4]. *E. coli* cells also employ a well-studied sensory transduction system that monitors extracellular Pi levels to control the expression of genes for scavenging Pi under limiting conditions and to utilize alternate phosphorous sources. Additionally, there are also metabolic reactions that control the amount of polyphosphate, a Pi storage compound.

The primary Pi importers in *E. coli* are PitA, PitB, and PstSCAB [5]. PitA and PitB are secondary transporters that bring neutral metal-Pi complexes into the cell at the expense of a proton [6, 7]. PstSCAB is a Pi-specific ABC transporter that imports Pi at the expense of ATP hydrolysis [8, 9]. Proteins that export Pi include PitA, PitB, and GlpT, which is a glycerol-3-phosphate:Pi antiporter [10], UhpT, which is a hexose-6-phosphate:Pi antiporter [11], and potentially YjbB, which has been suggested to be a Pi exporter [12]. The signal transduction system that controls gene expression in response to limiting extracellular Pi levels has at its heart the histidine kinase PhoR and the response regulator PhoB [4, 13]. When PhoB receives a phosphoryl group from PhoR, it binds to DNA and activates the transcription of a number of genes for the high-affinity acquisition of Pi (including the PstSCAB transporter) and the utilization of alternate sources of phosphorous [14–17]. At least 31 genes have been shown to be directly controlled and positively regulated by PhoB. They are called the Pho regulon and include *phoA,* which encodes the periplasmic enzyme alkaline phosphatase, *pstSCAB, phoB,* and *phoR* [4]. Alkaline phosphatase removes phosphoryl groups from organophosphate molecules. The members of the Pho regulon that are involved in utilizing alternate phosphorous sources are *ugpBAECQ,* which encodes a glycerol-3-phosphate ABC transporter and a phosphodiesterase and *phnCDEFGHIJKLMNOP,* which encodes a phosphonate transporter and enzymes of a C-P lyase complex that produces a phosphoribosyl product from imported phosphonate. Phosphonates are compounds that contain a carbon-phosphorous bond. In addition to the 31 genes that have been demonstrated to be directly controlled by PhoB [4, 18], 2D-polyacrylamide gels and computational methods suggest that possibly 400 proteins may be controlled directly or indirectly by PhoB [19, 20]. These include genes that are both up- and down-regulated.

http://dx.doi.org/10.5772/67283

The presence of the PhoBR signal transduction system underscores the need for maintaining a minimal intracellular level of Pi when extracellular Pi is limiting. That too much intracellular Pi can also be a problem is underscored by the phenotype of a *phoU* mutant [21]. *phoU* is the fifth gene in the *pstSCAB-phoU* operon and its function is to control the activity and the amount of the PstSCAB transporter [22]. It has been shown that *phoU* mutations cause a severe growth defect, probably because these cells become poisoned by too much intracellular Pi [21, 23, 24]. Taken together, these observations suggest that *E. coli* cells possess homeostatic mechanisms that maintain intracellular Pi levels within an optimal range. It is the purpose of this chapter to introduce the reader to the principle players involved in Pi homeostasis and to highlight advances in our understanding of the mechanisms involved.

2. The multiple Pi importers

E. coli is capable of using multiple transporters to bring Pi into cells. Three of them, PitA, PitB, and PstSCAB, are individually capable of supporting growth with Pi as the only source of phosphorous [6]. The others, GlpT, UhpT, and PhnCDE, are capable of secondarily importing Pi but are not able to support growth when the sole source of phosphorous is Pi [5]. GlpT primarily transports glycerol-3-phosphate, UhpT transports hexose-6-phosphates and PhnCDE brings phosphonates into the cell. Complicating many of the early studies on Pi transport was the use of the K10 strain of *E. coli*, which harbored a G220D mutation in the *pitA* gene [25]. The interpretations of some of the genetic and biochemical studies of Pi transport in these strains are therefore difficult because many early strains contained compensatory mutations in other genes that restored growth on Pi [21].

2.1. PitA and PitB—the low-affinity Pi importers

The low-affinity PitA and PitB transporters utilize the energy stored in the proton-motive force to bring neutral metal-Pi complexes into the cell [6, 25, 26]. These homologous proteins each contain 499 amino acid residues and show 80.8 and 89.8% sequence identity and similarity, respectively (see **Figure 1A**). Amino acid identities between the two proteins are indicated by vertical lines and similarities are indicated with two dots. A membrane topology model for these two proteins was created using the SCAMPI2 web server [27] and is shown in **Figure 1B**. This model predicts that PitA and PitB have 10 transmembrane helices with the N- and C-termini facing the periplasm. The sequences of the predicted transmembrane helices are surrounded by green boxes in **Figure 1A**. Support for this N_{out}-C_{out} topology model comes from a recent paper in which the authors tagged the C-termini of 601 inner membrane proteins from *E. coli* with alkaline phosphatase and green fluorescent proteins (GFPs) [28]. Because alkaline phosphatase is only active in the periplasm and GFP is only fluorescent in the cytoplasm, they concluded that PitA and PitB have a C_{out} topology [28]. These two proteins show very high levels of amino acid identity and similarity within the predicted 10 transmembrane segments (91.4 and 96.7%, respectively). The greatest degree of divergence is found in a putative 127-amino acid cytoplasmic loop domain (L7) located between helices 7 and 8. This loop shows 59.1% identity and 75.6% similarity between the two proteins suggesting that it may contribute to differences in protein stability, potential binding partners, or means of regulation.

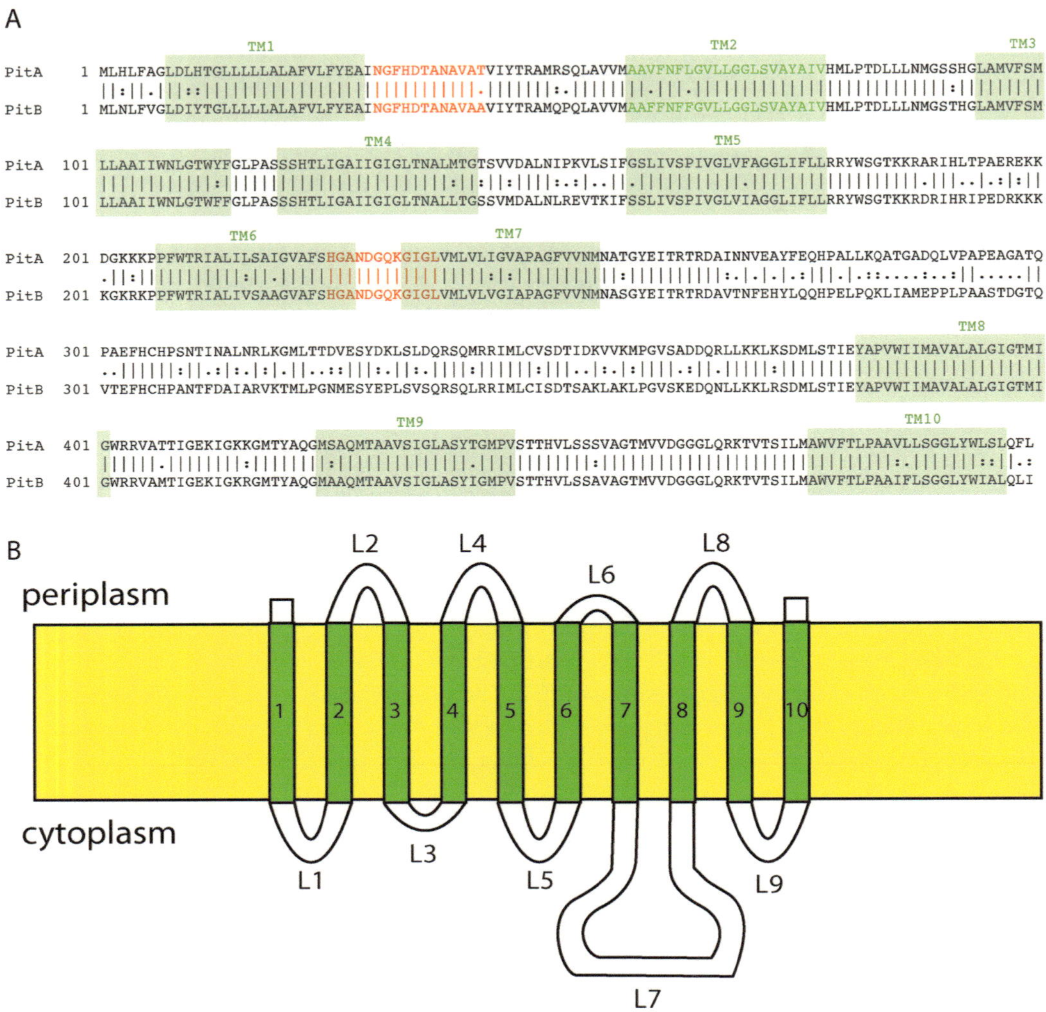

Figure 1. Sequence alignments of PitA and PitB with an accompanying topology model. (A) PitA and PitB amino acid sequences are given in one-letter code and are aligned. The alignment was made using the European Molecular Biology Open Software Suite (EMBOSS) [29]. Predicted transmembrane helices are boxed in green and the conserved signature motifs are marked with a red font. (B) Topology model of PitA and PitB. The model includes an N_{out}-C_{out} topology. The predicted transmembrane helices are labeled TM1–TM10 and the connecting loops are labeled L1–L9.

Analysis of the kinetic properties of Pi uptake in whole cells where *pitA* and *pitB* were expressed from the pBR322 plasmid showed that the PitA protein has a K_m^{app} of 1.9 μM and a V_{max}^{app} of 58 nmol of Pi minute^{-1} milligram (dry weight)$^{-1}$, whereas the values for PitB are 6 μM and 67 nanomoles of Pi minute^{-1} milligram (dry weight)$^{-1}$ [6].

It was originally thought that *pitA* expression was constitutive, but it has recently been shown that it is positively regulated by the availability of Zn(II) and also by limiting Pi [7]. *pitB* expression appears to be repressed when cells are grown in limiting Pi conditions [25], so its

http://dx.doi.org/10.5772/67283

function may be more important during growth in Pi-replete environments. The mechanisms for the regulation of these genes are not known.

PitA and PitB are members of the PiT family of Pi transporters within the transporter classification database (TC #2.A.20) [30] and the PHO4 family within the Pfam database [31]. These families include bacterial, archaeal, and eukaryotic members, suggesting that these Pi transporters developed early in evolution and that they continue to play important functions in all domains of life. A conserved signature sequence has been identified in both the N- and C-terminal ends of these transporters that has the common core sequence of **G**(**A**FGST)(**N**H)(**D**N)(**V**ATIG)(**A**QSG)(**N**KA)(**A**STG)(IMVF)(GAS)(TPIL), with the bolded amino acids representing the most common amino acids at that position. This signature sequence is highlighted with red letters in **Figure 1A**. The human proteins from this family are thought to be involved in housekeeping functions and are called PiT1 and PiT2, whereas the *Neurospora crassa* and *Saccharomyces cerevisiae* members are called Pho-4 and Pho89, respectively [32, 33]. Mutations in the signature sequence of the PiT2 protein block Pi transport [34]. In addition to their role in Pi transport, the PiT1 and PiT2 proteins are also receptors for the gamma-retroviruses [32]. This protein family includes both Na^+-dependent and H^+-dependent Pi symporters. PiT1, PiT2, Pho-4, and Pho89 are sodium-dependent transporters, whereas PitA, PitB, and the Pht2_1 proteins from *Arabidopsis thaliana* are proton-dependent Pi symporter [35].

It has recently been suggested that neither PitA nor PitB play primary roles in Pi transport, but function instead for the purpose of metal ion transport [4]. However, considering the homologies between PitA and PitB with other Pi transporters from other organisms, it seems unlikely that they are retained in this genome primarily to function as transporters of divalent metal cations, which have their own primary transporters, as well [36]. Clearly, further work is needed to better understand the roles of PitA and PitB in Pi homeostasis.

2.2. PstSCAB—the high-affinity Pi importer

The PstSCAB protein is a high-affinity Pi transporter that has a K_m of 0.4 μM Pi and a V_{max} of 16 nmol Pi mg (dry weight)$^{-1}$ min^{-1} [37]. It is a member of the ATP-binding cassette (ABC) superfamily from the transporter classification and Pfam databases [30, 31]. This protein superfamily employs the hydrolysis of ATP to bring a variety of substrates across biological membranes, both as importers and as exporters [38]. Members of this protein superfamily are found among the bacteria, archaea, and eukaryotes. Prokaryotic importers, such as the PstSCAB protein, utilize an extra-cytoplasmic substrate-binding protein that binds substrates and presents them to their membrane-spanning proteins [39]. PstS is the periplasmic substrate-binding protein. PstC and PstA compose the membrane-spanning components of the transporter [40, 41]. The most highly conserved feature within the superfamily is the nucleotide-binding domain, also called the ATP-binding cassette, which binds ATP, hydrolyzes it, and then releases it in order to provide the energy for transport [42]. PstB contains the nucleotide-binding domain for this transporter [43]. The crystal structures of several ABC importers have been solved, which has shed some light onto the mechanisms of transport [44]. Of particular note is the structure of the putative molybdate transporter, called ModABC, from the archaeon *Archaeoglobus fulgidus* [45]. Like the PstSCAB transporter, this protein also imports an oxyanion. A clue to understanding the mechanisms of Pi transport through the PstSCAB protein comes from sequence similarities between the molybdate, sulfate, and Pi transporters. The most highly conserved sequences within this group are found in a region of the protein that creates a cavity within the membrane-spanning region and a gate that most likely represents the pathway through which the substrate must pass. The published ModABC structure is of the protein in a nucleotide-free conformation and shows 12 transmembrane helices situated in an inward-facing conformation with the gate at the periplasmic surface of the membrane. It has been proposed that PstSCAB, like other transporters in this superfamily, utilizes an alternating access mechanism to transport their substrates in which they alternate between inward- and outward-facing states that are driven by substrate binding, ATP hydrolysis, ADP release, and subsequent ATP binding (see **Figure 2**) [44]. ATP binding across the PstB dimer interface would be predicted to close the cavity and lead to an outward-facing structure that can receive Pi from the substrate-loaded, periplasmic PstS protein. This event would trigger ATP hydrolysis that would flip the outward-facing transmembrane components to an inward-facing conformation, thereby opening the gate and allowing Pi to gain access to the cytoplasm. The cycle would be continued as ADP is released and ATP is rebound.

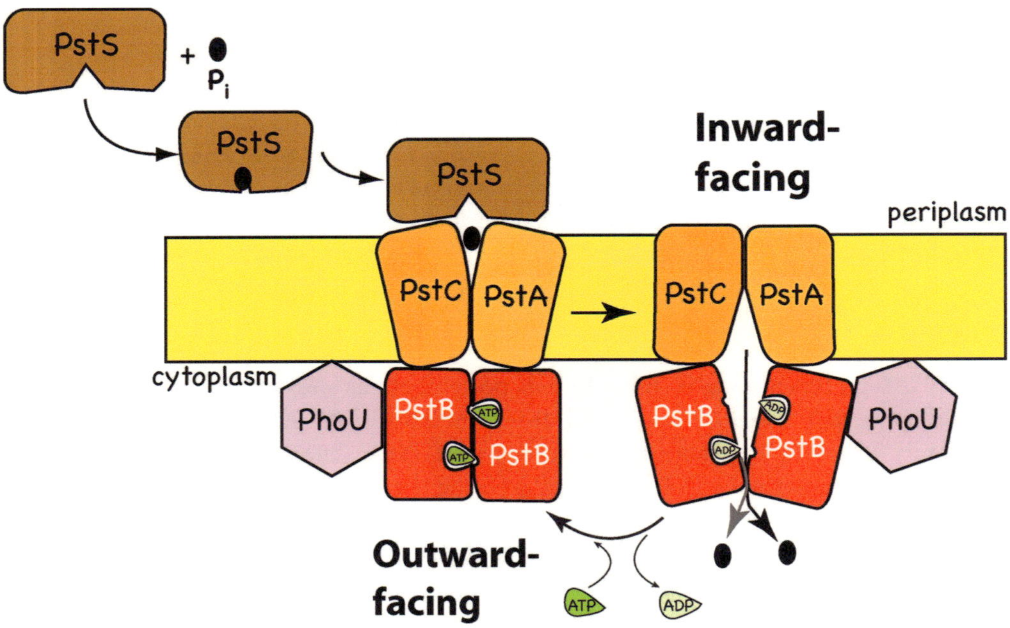

Figure 2. Model of the mechanism of Pi import through the PstSCAB transporter. Free Pi is bound within the periplasm and presented to the outward-facing PstCAB proteins. This docking triggers ATP hydrolysis, which causes a conformational change that triggers the adoption of an inward-facing conformation. The transported Pi is then released into the cytoplasm, as well as the Pi from the hydrolysis of ATP. The transporter is reset as PstB binds ATP again. The PhoU protein interacts with the PstB protein and slows transport when cytoplasmic Pi concentrations are high.

The Pst transporter is most highly expressed when environmental Pi levels are low. For this reason, it was assumed that it played its most important role in Pi transport under those conditions. More recently, it has been proposed that it plays the primary role in Pi transport

http://dx.doi.org/10.5772/67283

under all conditions [4]. The expression of the *pstSCAB* genes is controlled by the PhoBR two-component system described below. The primary promoter for this operon, and the one which is regulated by Pi levels, is found upstream of the *pstS* gene [46]. Other promoters that are internal to the operon have been identified upstream of the *pstC, pstB,* and *phoU* genes and are rather weak; but they may play a role in maintaining a basal level of the PstSCAB transporter under Pi-replete conditions [47].

3. The two-component signal transduction system for Pi homeostasis

Two-component-signaling systems constitute the most common signaling pathways in bacteria [48]. These pathways regulate many important cellular processes ranging from cell development and virulence, to motility and metabolism, and most species have over 10–20 different two-component systems [49]. Most frequently, they are composed of receptors on the cell periphery and signal-processing components and targets in the interior of the cell. These pathways rely on a phospho-transfer reaction between the histidine residues of sensor kinases, which generally receive input from the cell surface, and a conserved aspartate residue within the response regulators, which are located in the cytoplasm [50]. Response regulators are most frequently, but not always, transcription factors that interact with RNA polymerase [51].

3.1. PhoB and PhoR—the transcription factor and the histidine kinase

In *E. coli*, gene regulation in response to limiting Pi concentrations depends on the function of seven proteins: the two-component regulatory proteins PhoB and PhoR, as well as the Pst transporter, PstSCAB, and an auxiliary protein PhoU [4]. The hub of this signaling pathway consists of the PhoB and PhoR proteins. PhoB is the response regulator that has an N-terminal receiver domain (Pfam: PF00072, response_reg) and a C-terminal DNA-binding domain (Pfam: PF00486, trans_reg_c). This particular domain architecture represents the largest group of response regulators [31]. The receiver domain has a doubly wound α/β-fold with a central five-stranded beta-sheet [52]. This domain contains the site of aspartyl phosphorylation, which in PhoB is Asp53. The receiver domain of PhoB contains the necessary catalytic residues to transfer a phosphoryl group from the phospho-histidine residue of phospho-PhoR [17]. The C-terminal DNA-binding domain has a winged-helix structure [53]. When PhoB becomes phosphorylated, it forms a dimer that binds to DNA sequences, called pho boxes [17, 53–55]. These short sequences are located upstream of Pho regulon genes to recruit RNA polymerase and initiate transcription by remodeling the RNA polymerase holoenzyme-DNA complex [53, 54, 56].

PhoR is a homodimeric, bifunctional histidine autokinase/phospho-PhoB phosphatase. When environmental Pi is limiting, it autophosphorylates on a conserved histidine residue and subsequently donates this phosphoryl group to PhoB, but when Pi is plentiful, it removes the phosphoryl group from phospho-PhoB [57, 58]. PhoR is an integral membrane protein that is not predicted to contain a significant periplasmic domain but does contain a membrane-spanning region, a cytoplasmic charged region, a Per-ARNT-Sim (PAS) domain (Pfam: PF00989, PAS) [59], and prototypical dimerization/histidine phosphorylation (DHp; Pfam:

PF06580, His_kinase) and catalytic ATP-binding (CA; Pfam: PF02518, HATPase_c) domains at its C-terminus (see **Figure 3**) [57]. PAS domains generally function in signal perception activities [60]. Since PhoR does not contain a significant periplasmic sensory domain, it is assumed that its PAS domain senses a cytoplasmic signal that reflects extracellular Pi concentrations, but the nature of the signal is not completely known. The CA domain harbors the enzymatic activity for transferring a phosphoryl group from ATP to the conserved histidine residue of the DHp domain. The DHp domain consists of a four-helix bundle with the conserved phospho-accepting histidine residue being positioned midway on one face of one of the helices. It has been shown that phosphorylation of PhoR occurs in cis, where the CA domain of one of the monomers phosphorylates the His residue of the same polypeptide chain [61]. The DHp domain also contains all of the residues necessary for phospho-PhoB phosphatase activity [57]. We propose that the control of the opposing kinase and phosphatase activities of PhoR involves the constraint of the CA domains to prevent their access to the DHp domain and simultaneously exposing the residues of the DHp domain that are required for phosphatase function (see **Figure 3**). If this proposal is correct, then how are the interactions between the different PhoR domains controlled?

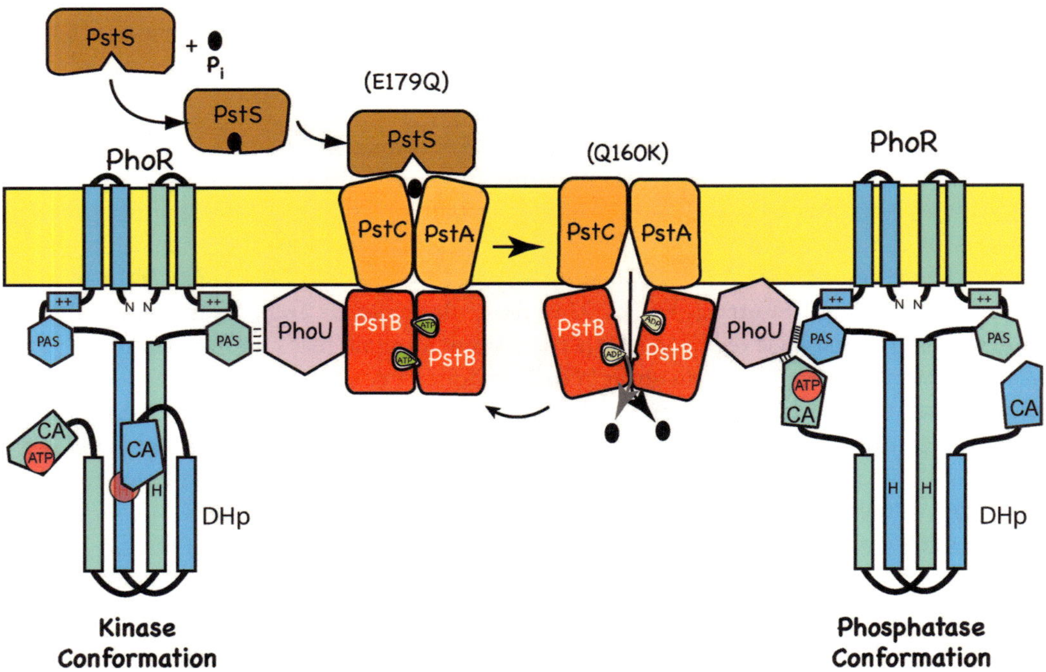

Figure 3. A signaling model involving different conformations of PstSCAB and PhoR. As the Pst transporter switches between its inward- and outward-facing conformations during Pi transport, it interacts differently with PhoR, depending upon its conformation. This interaction is mediated by PhoU. The inward-facing conformation, which is stabilized by the *pstB*Q160K mutation, interacts with PhoR to constrain its CA domain in order to stabilize the phosphatase conformation of PhoR. The outward conformation, which is stabilized by the *pstB*E179Q mutation, does not interact with the CA domain and favors the kinase conformation of PhoR, which allows the CA domain to bind ATP and autophosphorylate its DHp domain.

3.2. PstSCAB—the sensor of extracellular Pi

In addition to its role in Pi transport, the Pst transporter is also required for signal transduction. Because PhoR does not have a periplasmic domain, it has been assumed that this transporter is the ultimate sensor of extracellular Pi [5]. In fact, if any of the Pst proteins are absent, the Pho regulon becomes unregulated, leading to the overexpression of Pho regulon genes [5]. Thus, the default biochemical activity of PhoR is an autokinase and the role of the Pst transporter is to negatively regulate this activity and to stimulate its phospho-PhoB phosphatase activity. There are two possibilities for how the Pst protein may function to control the activity of PhoR. The first is by controlling intracellular Pi levels. If PhoR senses intracellular Pi, most likely through its PAS domain, then the Pst system may function by controlling the amount of Pi within the cell. This model seems unlikely for two reasons. Intracellular Pi has been measured by phosphorous nuclear magnetic resonance (^{31}P NMR) and has been shown to be constant under conditions in which the Pho regulon is both repressed and derepressed [2]. Also, there are several mutations in *pstC* and *pstA* that lead to defective transporters, but that retain their signaling capacity, that is, they can still stimulate the phospho-PhoB phosphatase activity of PhoR [40, 41]. The second model for how the Pst transporter functions in signal transduction is that PhoR may somehow sense its transport activity [62]. That is to say, it is not the intracellular level of Pi that is sensed, but how active the transporter is. Support for this model is provided below.

3.3. PhoU—the adaptor protein

In addition to the PstSCAB protein, PhoU is also required for Pi-signal transduction, but not for transport through the complex [21]. When *phoU* is mutated or deleted, PhoR is constitutively active as an autokinase leading to high-level expression of Pho regulon genes. *phoU* mutants show poor growth and frequently accumulate compensatory mutations in *phoR*, *phoB*, or the *pstSCAB* genes [21, 23, 24]. PhoU is a peripheral membrane protein that modulates Pi transport through the PstSCAB complex [22–24]. When Pi is plentiful, PhoU acts like a brake to prevent too much Pi import, with its accompanying ATP hydrolysis [23]. Multiple crystal structures have been reported for PhoU proteins from various organisms [63–65]. PhoU consists of two symmetric, three alpha-helix bundles and metal ions are found associated with two of these structures. The metals are coordinated by highly conserved amino acid residues that are found in each three-helix bundle. PhoU from *Thermotoga maritima* coordinates iron clusters [63], while PhoU from *Streptococcus pneumoniae* shows zinc ions bound [64]. Gardner et al. have recently shown that the soluble form of PhoU from *E. coli* is a dimer that binds manganese or magnesium [66]. Mutagenesis experiments demonstrated that these divalent metals are bound by the same conserved amino acid residues that bind the iron and zinc ions in the two crystal structures. It was also suggested in this study that metal binding may be important for PhoU interactions with the membrane. Alternatively, PhoU may bind Pi through its interactions with these metals.

Two general classes of models have been previously suggested for how PhoU participates in the signaling pathway. It may mediate the formation of a signaling complex between the PstSCAB transporter and PhoR [5, 64] or it may produce a soluble messenger that is recognized by the cytoplasmic domains of PhoR (consistent with observations reported by Hoffer and Tommassen [67] and by Rao and Torriani [68]). The following section presents new evidence in favor of the Pi-signaling complex model.

3.4. Protein interactions within the Pi-signaling complex

It has recently been demonstrated through bacterial two-hybrid analysis and through co-elution experiments that PhoU interacts with both the PhoR protein and PstB [66]. The two-hybrid experiments used the BACTH system [69]. Adenylate cyclase from *Bordetella pertussis* can be genetically divided into nonfunctional T18 and T25 fragments. The enzyme can be reconstituted in vivo and cAMP can be produced when the two fragments are brought into physical proximity within the cell by fusing interacting proteins with either the T18 or T25 fragments and monitoring cAMP production. Gardner et al. fused various parts of PhoR, or the PstB protein, to the T25 fragment and PhoU to the T18 fragment and indirectly monitored cAMP production by assaying the cAMP-dependent gene β-galactosidase [66]. They found that the interaction between PhoR and PhoU occurred through its PAS domain and that the PstB-PhoU interaction was weaker than the PhoR-PhoU interaction. They then employed a complementary co-elution method by using His-tagged versions of either PstB or PhoR and showed by Western blotting that PhoU was retained on a nickel column in a PstB- or PhoR-dependent manner. In a subsequent paper, Gardner et al. were able to further localize the sites on PhoR and PhoU that are important for the formation of the signaling complex [70]. They knew that the phenotype of a mutant containing the *phoU35* allele was unlike that of a *phoU* deletion mutation. Neither the *phoU35* nor the *phoU* deletion mutants could signal Pi sufficiency and they both constitutively expressed alkaline phosphatase. However, the *phoU35* mutant did not have a severe growth defect [71]. Since the *phoU35* allele encoded a change from alanine at position 147 to glutamic acid (A147E) [72], Gardner et al. hypothesized that the *phoU*35 mutation may disrupt PhoU's interaction with PhoR, preventing the signal for the switch to PhoR phosphatase activity, but that it maintained its interaction with PstB, limiting excess transport of Pi into the cell during Pi-replete conditions. From this assumption, they were able to identify the surface residues Ala147 and Arg148 of PhoU as being important for the interaction with PhoR. Moreover, they employed a scanning mutagenesis approach to identify a surface on the PAS domain of PhoR that is essential for the interaction. Every two amino acids within the PAS domain were sequentially mutated and then tested using the BACTH assay for interactions with PhoU. They identified residues 141–146, 157–162, and 169–176 of PhoR as important for the interaction with PhoU. By using these genetic constraints, they were able to build a plausible three-dimensional model of the docked proteins. This model was then supported by using a bioinformatic method, called direct-coupling analysis that identifies residues from one sequence that tend to co-evolve with residues from another sequence. Proteins that physically interact co-evolve with each other. These analyses supported a model in which PhoU interacts with both the PAS and CA domains of PhoR. Gardner et al. proposed the existence of a Pi-signaling complex in which under high-Pi growth conditions PhoU interacts with PhoR to constrain its CA domain and inhibit its kinase activity and promote its phosphatase activity.

http://dx.doi.org/10.5772/67283

3.5. Conformational signaling model

To answer the question of how PhoR senses the signaling activity of the Pst transporter, we propose that PhoR interacts differently with the alternate outward- and inward-facing conformations of the transporter that are sampled throughout the transport cycle. When Pi is limiting, the transporters are not actively importing Pi and reside primarily in the outward-facing conformation. We propose that this conformation contacts PhoU in such a manner that it does not interact with both the PAS and CA domains of PhoR, which promotes its autokinase activity. It is only under Pi-replete environments when Pi import is occurring that the Pst transporter adopts the inward-facing conformation. We propose that in this conformation, it interacts with PhoU in such a manner to constrain the CA domain of PhoR so that its phosphatase activity is stimulated.

To test this model, we have recently created two *pst3* mutations that are predicted to lock the transporter into these alternate conformations (Vuppada and McCleary, manuscript in preparation). Based upon work with the homologous maltose transporter [73], an E179Q mutation in *pstB* should lock the transporter into an outward-facing conformation because it cannot hydrolyze ATP and a Q160K mutation should lock it into an inward-facing conformation because it does not bind ATP. The *pstSCAB-phoU* genes were cloned onto a medium-copy number plasmid and were introduced into a Δ*pstSCAB-phoU* strain of *E. coli* to confirm that the plasmid could complement the deletion mutation. Mutations were then introduced into the plasmid by site-directed mutagenesis and confirmed by DNA sequencing. Neither the E179Q nor the Q160K mutants showed high-affinity Pi transport, showing that the transporters were dead. By using alkaline phosphatase expression as a reporter of the Pho regulon, we observed that the E179Q mutant constitutively signaled Pistarvation, whether the cells were grown in Pi-replete or Pi-starvation media. We also observed that the Q160K mutant always signaled Pisufficiency. In other words, these cells always expressed low levels of alkaline phosphatase, presumably resulting from the activation of the phosphatase activity of PhoR. These results support the model in which the inward-facing form of the Pst transporter interacts with PhoU and PhoR in a manner that stimulates the phospho-PhoB phosphatase activity of PhoR. This signaling output of the PhoBR pathway reduces the expression of the PstSCAB transporter when low-level expression is sufficient for maximal growth. It also downregulates other genes whose expression would be wasteful in times of Pi sufficiency.

4. The response to high levels of extracellular Pi

Clues to understanding how *E. coli* and other bacteria cope with high levels of extracellular Pi came from studies on Pi remediation [12, 74, 75]. Excess Pi in natural water sources is a major cause of eutrophication [76]. Toxic cyanobacterial blooms are frequently attributed to Pi accumulation in water sources resulting from agricultural runoff [77]. Normally, Pi is removed from wastewaters by chemical precipitation, which is an expensive process [78]. Biological Pi removal is an alternative to chemical treatments in which bacteria accumulate excess Pi as polyphosphate (polyP) [79, 80]. The bacteria can then be retained as sludge, which can be separated from the wastewater, which now has a much reduced phosphorous concentration.

PolyP is found in all kingdoms of life [81, 82]. It is a linear chain of variable length of Pi residues that are linked by phosphoanhydride bonds. The cellular amounts of polyP are controlled through its polymerization and depolymerization, presumably to meet cellular needs for free Pi. PolyP can be synthesized from ATP by polyP kinase, encoded by the *ppk* gene [83]. It is degraded by exopolyphosphatase, encoded by the *ppx* gene. The Ppk reaction is fully reversible and cells can also use polyP to synthesize ATP.

To enhance biological removal of Pi from wastewater, Kato et al. cloned the *pstSCAB* and *ppk* genes on plasmids [74]. They found that an *E. coli* strain harboring these plasmids could accumulate up to 16% of their dry weight as phosphorus with over 60% of the cellular phosphorous stored as polyP. They also noted that these strains grew very poorly. Subsequent work from this group showed that *phoU* mutants also accumulated high levels of polyP [75]. It was known that *phoU* mutants expressed the transporter at high levels, even when environmental Pi levels were high. As an additional contribution to understanding the phenotype of a *phoU* mutant, our group showed that PhoU also negatively regulates the activity of the Pst transporter [23]. Those experiments were performed by uncoupling expression of the Pst transporter from its normal PhoB-dependent mechanism through a technique called promoter swapping [84]. We felt that it was important to keep the *pstSCAB-phoU* operon at its normal location in the *E. coli* chromosome, so we developed a technique using Lambda-Red recombineering methodology to swap the P_{tac} promoter for the wild-type P_{pstS} promoter [85]. As we held expression levels constant with an exogenous promoter, we demonstrated that a *phoU* deletion mutant accumulated Pi at a higher rate than cells expressing the *pstSCAB* genes and *phoU*. Other ABC transporters, such as the methionine transporter, have regulatory domains that respond to the cytoplasmic concentrations of transported substrates and function as sites of allosteric inhibition of transport [86–88]. We proposed that PhoU plays a similar role for Pi transport in *E. coli*. We learned from these observations that *E. coli* cells tightly control the amounts of the Pst transporter as well as its activity. When intracellular amounts of Pi become too high,*E. coli* cells store excess Pi as polyP.

In addition to its role as a Pi and energy store, PolyP has many other important functions in *E. coli* [89]. For example, it is involved in metal detoxification and can function as a primitive chaperone to protect against oxidative damage [90–92]. Of importance to our discussion here, Keasling hypothesized that *E. coli* cells could detoxify metals by sequestering them with intracellular polyP. Following hydrolysis of polyP to Pi, the metal/Pi complexes would be exported through the Pit transporters. PolyP is also involved in cell signaling, respiratory chain gene expression, bacterial persistence, and in stress response networks [93–96]. It has recently been shown that when external Pi levels are very high, polyP can even activate PhoB during the stationary phase of growth through the small molecule acetyl phosphate [97]. It is then postulated that phospho-PhoB inhibits the synthesis of c-di-GMP, blocking the production of AI-2, leading to the inhibition of biofilm formation.

http://dx.doi.org/10.5772/67283

4.1. The Tn-seq experiment—identifying the players of the high-Pi response

In order to further investigate cellular processes involved in Pi homeostasis when cells are grown in conditions of high environmental Pi, we performed a Tn-seq experiment. Tn-seq relies on the ability to saturate a bacterial genome by transposon mutagenesis. Cells are grown in a selective environment and individual transposon insertions are mapped using next-generation-sequencing protocols. The frequency of insertions in each gene is used to analyze the importance of each gene under those growth conditions. Those genes that receive few or no insertions are identified as essential (no insertions under any conditions), conditionally essential (no or few insertions under one condition), or conditionally important for fitness (reduced insertion frequency under one particular condition) (see **Figure 4**).

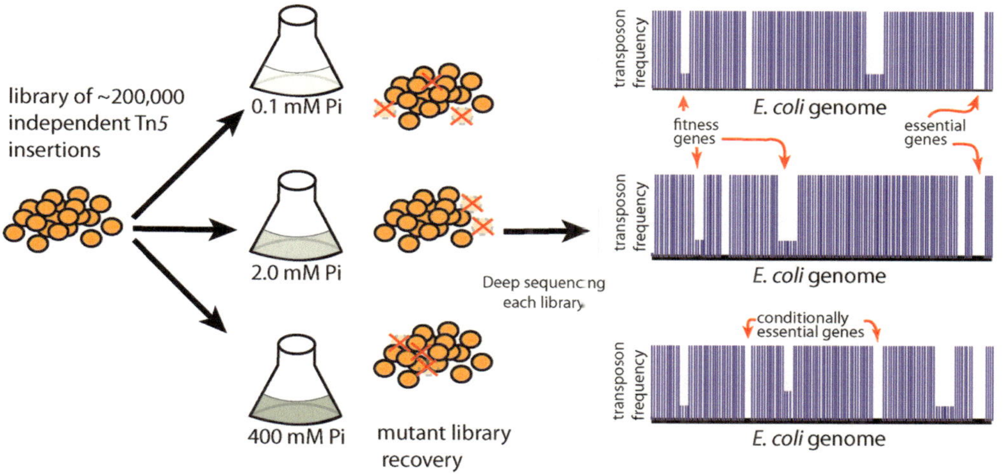

Figure 4. The design of a Tn-seq experiment. A library of transposon insertion mutants was grown in duplicate in liquid cultures containing either 0.1 mM Pi, 2.0 mM Pi, or 400 mM Pi. Chromosomal DNA was prepared from each sample for deep sequencing to identify the sites of insertion and their frequencies. If an insertion does not affect the growth of a strain, then it is assumed that that gene is not required for growth. Genes with no insertions under any conditions were classified as essential genes. Genes with no or very few insertions under one condition were classified as conditionally essential and those with reduced frequency were classified as important for fitness.

Wild-type *E. coli* strain MG1655 that harbors a *rpsL* mutation conferring streptomycin resistance was mutagenized with a mini-Tn*5* transposon delivered from a conjugative plasmid that required the lambda Π protein for replication. The donor strain could be counter-selected because it contained a mutation in the *dapA* gene and required supplementation with diaminopimelic acid. By selecting transconjugants that were kanamycin-resistant and that did not require diaminopimelic acid we were able to obtain a library of about 200,000 independent mutants. Such a library would be predicted to give about 30–50 random insertions per gene. This mutant library was then grown in duplicate in one of three different defined media containing variable Pi concentrations. We used media containing 0.1, 2.0, and 400 mM Pi. Preliminary experiments showed that growth of the wild-type strain in 400 mM Pi was significantly slower than in the other media. This high-Pi medium was also of a significantly higher osmolarity than the other two media. After growing cells until stationary phase, the cultures were harvested and DNA extractions were performed. The chromosomal DNA was then enzymatically fragmented and a polyC tail was then added to these DNA fragments using terminal transferase. Polymerase chain reactions (PCRs) were then performed using transposon-specific and polyG primers to amply DNA where transposons had inserted. A second round of PCR was then used to add primers for Illumina sequencing. The reads were mapped to the published MG1655 genome and the number of reads was normalized to 4×10^6 reads per sample.

To identify genes that are important for growth in high-Pigrowth conditions, we sorted from low to high each of the genes based upon the quotient of the number of hits in high-Pi media divided by the total number of hits in all three media. We were particularly interested in genes with few hits in the high-Pi medium and were able to identify many genes whose functions are important for fitness under these growth conditions. As mentioned above, the high-Pi growth medium that we employed was also high in osmolarity. As an internal control to identify genes that were important for this growth condition, we were able to identify many top hits as occurring in genes that are known to be important in a high osmolarity response, such as*ompR*, *envZ*, *galU*, *otsB*, *hupA*, *cpxR*, and *hupB* [98–100]. OmpR and EnvZ are two-component regulators that respond to changes in osmolarity. GalU and OtsB are involved in the synthesis of trehalose, a compatible solute, that is produced under high osmolarity growth conditions. *hupA* encodes for a component of the HU protein, which is a small DNA-binding protein that helps regulate the expression of the osmoresponsive gene *proU* [101]. CpxR is a response regulator that responds to cell envelope damage and it is known that it participates in the regulation of gene expression in response to osmolarity [99].

We also identified genes that are known to be involved in the control of the Pho regulon, for example, each of the *pstSCAB* genes was found near the top of the list. Mutations in any of these genes lead to elevated expression of the entire Pho regulon, whose genes are involved in the high-affinity acquisition of Pi and the utilization of alternate Pi sources. It is easy to hypothesize why the expression of these genes would be deleterious when Pi levels are very high. With the Pho regulon fully expressed, Pi may be imported through the phosphonate or other transporters without the requisite expression of genes to accommodate the increased Pi. Another common class of genes that had few transposon insertions under high Pi conditions was genes involved in central metabolism of glucose and most importantly in ATP production (*ptsG*, *pykF*, *ackA*, *zwf*, *pta*, and *sdhBCD*). PstG is the enzyme IIBC component of the phosphotransferase system for glucose uptake [102]. PykF is pyruvate kinase from glycolysis and synthesizes ATP from ADP and phospho*enol*pyruvate. Zwf is glucose-6-phosphate-1-dehydrogenase, which catalyzes the first steps in the Enter Doudoroff or oxidative pentose phosphate pathways [103, 104]. AckA and Pta are acetate kinase and phosphotransacetylase, respectively, and are involved in ATP production, acetyl phosphate synthesis, and acetate secretion [105]. SdhBCD are subunits of succinate dehydrogenase, which is part of the TCA cycle. It is interesting to note that these genes are repressed during growth on glucose [106], so it is unclear why mutations in these genes lower the fitness of *E. coli* grown on glucose high-Pi medium. It is also important to note that there were very few hits under

http://dx.doi.org/10.5772/67283

any condition in the *ppk* gene, suggesting that it was an essential gene under these defined growth conditions, as well as in the genes for ATP synthase. Another intriguing class of genes with low frequency of transposon insertions included genes of unknown function, such as *ydhP, yodD, yniC,* and *glcG*. We conclude from these results that when placed in very high Pi environments cells need to regulate Pi import and continue to synthesize ATP at high rates for the production of polyP. We expect that there are some previously unknown functions that are necessary to deal with high-Pi stresses that are represented by the "y" genes. These may include other transporters, regulators of transporters, or genes for metabolic functions.

4.2. Pi homeostasis model and questions for further research

E. coli inhabits environments with widely ranging Pi concentrations. It is often limiting in environmental conditions and can be quite high in the intestinal lumen of a healthy human [96]. Pi homeostasis is a balancing act of import, export, utilization, and sequestration (see **Figure 5**). Pi can be imported through the secondary transporters PitA and PitB or through the PstSCAB ABC transporter. The multiple transporters that import Pi have various specificities and expression patterns, which allow them to be used primarily under conditions when they are most needed, but which also permits a considerable amount of redundancy in function. Of primary importance in Pi homeostasis is the ability to increase transcription of genes when environmental Pi levels are low for the high-affinity acquisition of Pi and for the utilization of alternate sources of phosphorous. To monitor extracellular Pi, *E. coli* utilizes a Pi-signaling complex consisting of the PstSCAB transporter, PhoU and PhoR. In its two states, it can either activate or deactivate the response regulator PhoB. We propose that the signaling complex does not directly sense extracellular Pi, but senses the activity of the Pst transporter by recognizing its alternate conformational states. It is the inward-facing conformation of the Pst transporter that represents Pi-sufficient environments because it is only formed when Pi is actively transported. Once imported, Pi becomes part of an intracellular pool and can be incorporated into ATP through substrate-level phosphorylation or through oxidative phosphorylation. From ATP or its equivalents, the phosphoryl groups are transferred to all other phosphorylated intermediates of the cell. Cellular growth is inhibited when intracellular Pi levels become too elevated, so cells must have mechanisms to control this parameter also. To maintain its intracellular Pi levels near 10 mM, *E. coli* can either export excess Pi or it can sequester it through the synthesis of PolyP. PitA and PitB are known metal-Pi exporters and rely on high intracellular Pi levels and metals, such as Mg^{2+}, Mn^{2+}, Ca^{2+}, Zn^{2+}, and Co^{2+} for Pi export [7, 107]. Pi export through the Pit proteins contributes to the generation of a proton-motive force. It has also been suggested that YjbB plays a role in Pi export [12]. This protein is very interesting because it consists of two segments, a hydrophobic N-terminal half with sequence similarity to Na^+/Pi transporters and a C-terminal half with sequence similarity to PhoU. Motomura et al. showed that overexpression of YjbB resulted in lower intracellular polyP levels and that it released significant amounts of Pi into the medium. These results are consistent with YjbB being a Pi exporter. PolyP serves as a Pi buffer to fine-tune intracellular Pi levels.

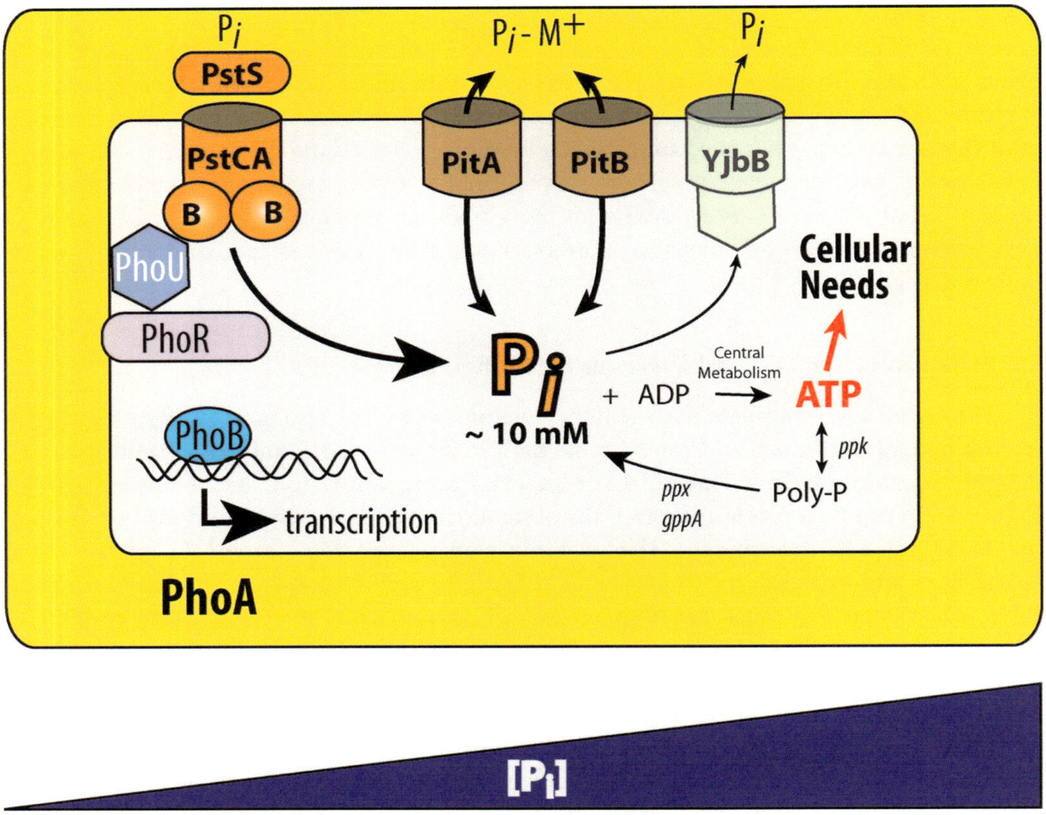

Figure 5. Model for Pi homeostasis in *E. coli*. Intracellular amounts of Pi are maintained within a modest range around 10 mM. The mechanisms for this homeostatic maintenance include the use of multiple Pi importers with variable affinities and rates of Pi transport. Cells also utilize the sophisticated PhoBR two-component-signaling mechanism that directly controls the expression of genes for high-affinity Pi acquisition and for the use of alternate sources of phosphorous. In addition, when Pi levels become too high, the cells sequester Pi by accumulating polyP, which is produced from ATP by the enzyme Ppk or they export it.

While the general outlines of Pi homeostasis have begun to be filled in, there are still important questions that remain. How do cells sense intracellular levels of Pi to control polyP synthesis/degradation and Pi export? What are the roles of the genes that are repressed by the PhoBR system? What are the functions of the unknown genes that were identified by Tn-seq to be important for fitness in very high levels of environmental Pi? What are the control mechanisms for the expression of PitA and PitB? Why does *E. coli* retain both the *pitA* and *pitB* genes? What are their differential functions? What effects does the stoichiometry of PstSCAB, PhoU, PhoR, and PhoB have on signaling, especially at the level of the single cell? Knowledge gained in studying Pi homeostasis will continue to be important in understanding global regulatory mechanisms, as Pi is involved in so many cellular processes. It will also be important in the engineering of organisms for improved Pi bioremediation.

http://dx.doi.org/10.5772/67283

5. Conclusion

Pi homeostasis is essential for life's basic processes. Without the ability to control intracellular levels of Pi within optimal levels, cells would be unable to maintain energy stores, synthesize nucleic acids and phospholipids, or carry out central metabolic pathways. The molecular mechanisms by which *E. coli* cells maintain intracellular Pi levels include utilizing multiple importers with characteristic patterns of expression, affinities for Pi and rates of Pi import [4]. These cells also employ a highly characterized signal transduction system that monitors extracellular Pi levels through the conformational states of the high-affinity Pi importer to control gene expression for scavenging Pi and utilizing alternate phosphorous sources. In addition, polyphosphate plays an important role in fine-tuning the amounts of free intracellular Pi. Understanding these mechanisms is important because this knowledge can be used to design organisms and pathways for the remediation of phosphate pollution. Moreover, the expression of virulence genes in many organisms is controlled by the PhoBR signal transduction system.

Acknowledgements

I thank Ramesh Vuppada, a Master's student in our laboratory, who provided the preliminary results about the signaling states of the alternate conformations of PstB and Tanner Robinson, an undergraduate student, for the preliminary Tn-seq results. I also thank the many undergraduate and graduate students who have contributed to the ongoing work and discussions in the laboratory. Work from our laboratory was supported by Public Health Service grant R15GM96222 from the National Institute of General Medical Sciences.

Author details

William R. McCleary

Address all correspondence to: bill_mccleary@byu.edu

Microbiology and Molecular Biology Department, Brigham Young University, Provo, UT, USA

References

[1] Shulman RG, Brown TR, Ugurbil K, Ogawa S, Cohen SM, den Hollander JA. Cellular applications of ^{31}P and ^{13}C nuclear magnetic resonance. Science. 1979;**205**:160–166. DOI: 10.1126/science.36664

[2] Rao NN, Roberts MF, Torriani A, Yashphe J. Effect of *glpT* and *glpD* mutations on expression of the *phoA* gene in *Escherichia coli*. J Bacteriol. 1993;**175**:74–79.

[3] Xavier KB, Kossmann M, Santos H, Boos W. Kinetic analysis by in vivo 31P nuclear magnetic resonance of internal Pi during the uptake of sn-glycerol-3-phosphate by the *pho* regulon-dependent Ugp system and the *glp* regulon-dependent GlpT system. J Bacteriol. 1995;**177**:699–704.

[4] Hsieh YJ, Wanner BL. Global regulation by the seven-component P_i signaling system. Curr Opin Microbiol. 2010;**13**:198–203. DOI: 10.1016/j.mib.2010.01.014

[5] Wanner BL. Phosphorous assimilation and control of the phosphate regulon. In: Neidhardt FC, Curtiss III R, Ingraham JL, Lin ECC, Low KB, Magasanik B, et al., editors. *Escherichia coli* and *Salmonella*: cellular and molecular biology. 2nd ed. Washington, D.C.: ASM Press; 1996. p. 1357–1381.

[6] Harris RM, Webb DC, Howitt SM, Cox GB. Characterization of PitA and PitB from *Escherichia coli*. J Bacteriol. 2001;**183**:5008–5014. DOI: 10.1128/JB.183.17.5008-5014.2001

[7] Jackson RJ, Binet MR, Lee LJ, Ma R, Graham AI, McLeod CW, et al. Expression of the PitA phosphate/metal transporter of Escherichia coli is responsive to zinc and inorganic phosphate levels. FEMS Microbiol Lett. 2008;**289**:219–224. DOI: 10.1111/j.1574-6968.2008.01386.x

[8] Rosenberg H. Phosphate transport in prokaryotes. In: Rosen BP, Silver S, editors. Ion Transport in Prokaryotes. San Diego: Academic Press, Inc; 1987. p. 205–248.

[9] Webb DC, Rosenberg H, Cox GB. Mutational analysis of the *Escherichia coli* phosphate-specific transport system, a member of the traffic ATPase (or ABC) family of membrane transporters. J Biol Chem. 1992;**267**:24661–24668.

[10] Elvin CM, Hardy CM, Rosenberg H. Pi exchange mediated by the GlpT-dependent sn-glycerol-3-phosphate transport system in *Escherichia coli*. J Bacteriol. 1985;**161**:1054–1058.

[11] Ambudkar SV, Anantharam V, Maloney PC. UhpT, the sugar phosphate antiporter of *Escherichia coli*, functions as a monomer. J Biol Chem. 1990;**265**:12287–12292.

[12] Motomura K, Hirota R, Ohnaka N, Okada M, Ikeda T, Morohoshi T, et al. Overproduction of YjbB reduces the level of polyphosphate in Escherichia coli: a hypothetical role of YjbB in phosphate export and polyphosphate accumulation. FEMS Microbiol Lett. 2011;**320**:25–32. DOI: 10.1111/j.1574-6968.2011.02285.x

[13] Santos-Beneit F. The Pho regulon: a huge regulatory network in bacteria. Front Microbiol. 2015;**6**:402. DOI: 10.3389/fmicb.2015.00402

[14] Bachhawat P, Swapna GV, Montelione GT, Stock AM. Mechanism of activation for transcription factor PhoB suggested by different modes of dimerization in the inactive and active states. Structure. 2005;**13**:1353–1363. DOI: 10.1016/j.str.2005.06.006

[15] Makino K, Amemura M, Kim SK, Nakata A, Shinagawa H. Role of the sigma 70 subunit of RNA polymerase in transcriptional activation by activator protein PhoB in Escherichia coli. Genes Dev. 1993;**7**:149–160. DOI: 10.1101/gad.7.1.149

[16] Makino K, Shinagawa H, Amemura M, Nakata A. Nucleotide sequence of the *phoB* gene, the positive regulatory gene for the phosphate regulon of *Escherichia coli* K-12. J Mol Biol. 1986;**190**:37–44. DOI: 10.1016/0022-2836(86)90073-2

[17] McCleary WR. The activation of PhoB by acetylphosphate. Mol Microbiol. 1996;**20**:1155–1163. DOI: 10.1111/j.1365-2958.1996.tb02636.x

[18] Baek JH, Lee SY. Novel gene members in the Pho regulon of Escherichia coli. FEMS Microbiol Lett. 2006;**264**:104–109. DOI: 10.1111/j.1574-6968.2006.00440.x

[19] VanBogelen RA, Olson ER, Wanner BL, Neidhardt FC. Global analysis of proteins synthesized during phosphorus restriction in *Escherichia coli*. J Bacteriol. 1996;**178**:4344–4366.

[20] Yuan ZC, Zaheer R, Morton R, Finan TM. Genome prediction of PhoB regulated promoters in Sinorhizobium meliloti and twelve proteobacteria. Nucleic Acids Res. 2006;**34**:2686–2697. DOI: 10.1093/nar/gkl365

[21] Steed PM, Wanner BL. Use of the *rep* technique for allele replacement to construct mutants with deletions of the *pstSCAB-phoU* operon: evidence of a new role for the PhoU protein in the phosphate regulon. J Bacteriol. 1993;**175**:6797–6809.

[22] Surin BP, Rosenberg H, Cox GB. Phosphate-specific transport system of *Escherichia coli*: nucleotide sequence and gene-polypeptide relationships. J Bacteriol. 1985;**161**:189–198.

[23] Rice CD, Pollard JE, Lewis ZT, McCleary WR. Employment of a promoter-swapping technique shows that PhoU modulates the activity of the $PstSCAB_2$ ABC transporter in *Escherichia coli*. Appl Environ Microbiol. 2009;**75**:573–582. DOI: 10.1128/AEM.01046-08

[24] Haldimann A, Daniels LL, Wanner BL. Use of new methods for construction of tightly regulated arabinose and rhamnose promoter fusions in studies of the *Escherichia coli* phosphate regulon. J Bacteriol. 1998;**180**:1277–1286.

[25] Hoffer SM, Schoondermark P, van Veen HW, Tommassen J. Activation by gene amplification of pitB, encoding a third phosphate transporter of Escherichia coli K-12. J Bacteriol. 2001;**183**:4659–4663. DOI: 10.1128/JB.183.15.4659-4663.2001

[26] van Veen HW, Abee T, Kortstee GJ, Konings WN, Zehnder AJ. Translocation of metal phosphate via the phosphate inorganic transport system of Escherichia coli. Biochemistry. 1994;**33**:1766–1770. DOI: 10.1021/bi00173a020

[27] Peters C, Tsirigos KD, Shu N, Elofsson A. Improved topology prediction using the terminal hydrophobic helices rule. Bioinformatics. 2016;**32**:1158–1162. DOI: 10.1093/bioinformatics/btv709

[28] Daley DO, Rapp M, Granseth E, Melen K, Drew D, von Heijne G. Global topology analysis of the Escherichia coli inner membrane proteome. Science. 2005;**308**:1321–1323. DOI: 10.1126/science.1109730

[29] Rice P, Longden I, Bleasby A. EMBOSS: the European Molecular Biology Open Software Suite. Trends Genet. 2000;**16**:276–277. DOI: 10.1016/S0168-9525(00)02024-2

[30] Saier MH, Jr., Reddy VS, Tsu BV, Ahmed MS, Li C, Moreno-Hagelsieb G. The Transporter Classification Database (TCDB): recent advances. Nucleic Acids Res. 2016;**44**:D372–379. DOI: 10.1093/nar/gkv1103

[31] Finn RD, Coggill P, Eberhardt RY, Eddy SR, Mistry J, Mitchell AL, et al. The Pfam protein families database: towards a more sustainable future. Nucleic Acids Res. 2016;**44**:D279–285. DOI: 10.1093/nar/gkv1344

[32] Bottger P, Pedersen L. Evolutionary and experimental analyses of inorganic phosphate transporter PiT family reveals two related signature sequences harboring highly conserved aspartic acids critical for sodium-dependent phosphate transport function of human PiT2. FEBS J. 2005;**272**:3060–3074. DOI: 10.1111/j.1742-4658.2005.04720.x

[33] Dick CF, Dos-Santos AL, Meyer-Fernandes JR. Inorganic phosphate uptake in unicellular eukaryotes. Biochim Biophys Acta. 2014;**1840**:2123–2127. DOI: 10.1016/j.bbagen.2014.03.014

[34] Bottger P, Pedersen L. Mapping of the minimal inorganic phosphate transporting unit of human PiT2 suggests a structure universal to PiT-related proteins from all kingdoms of life. BMC Biochem. 2011;**12**:21. DOI: 10.1186/1471-2091-12-21

[35] Daram P, Brunner S, Rausch C, Steiner C, Amrhein N, Bucher M. Pht2;1 encodes a low-affinity phosphate transporter from Arabidopsis. Plant Cell. 1999;**11**:2153–2166. DOI: 10.2307/3871016

[36] Patzer SI, Hantke K. The ZnuABC high-affinity zinc uptake system and its regulator Zur in Escherichia coli. Mol Microbiol. 1998;**28**:1199–1210. DOI: 10.1046/j.1365-2958.1998.00883.x

[37] Willsky GR, Malamy MH. Characterization of two genetically separable inorganic phosphate transport systems in Escherichia coli. J Bacteriol. 1980;**144**:356–365.

[38] Davidson AL, Dassa E, Orelle C, Chen J. Structure, function, and evolution of bacterial ATP-binding cassette systems. Microbiol Mol Biol Rev. 2008;**72**:317–364. DOI: 10.1128/MMBR.00031-07

[39] Quiocho FA, Ledvina PS. Atomic structure and specificity of bacterial periplasmic receptors for active transport and chemotaxis: variation of common themes. Mol Microbiol. 1996;**20**:17–25. DOI: 10.1111/j.1365-2958.1996.tb02484.x

[40] Cox GB, Webb D, Godovac-Zimmermann J, Rosenberg H. Arg-220 of the PstA protein is required for phosphate transport through the phosphate-specific transport system in *Escherichia coli* but not for alkaline phosphatase repression. J Bacteriol. 1988;**170**:2283–2286.

[41] Cox GB, Webb D, Rosenberg H. Specific amino acid residues in both the PstB and PstC proteins are required for phosphate transport by the *Escherichia coli* Pst system. J Bacteriol. 1989;**171**:1531–1534.

[42] Rees DC, Johnson E, Lewinson O. ABC transporters: the power to change. Nat Rev Mol Cell Biol. 2009;**10**:218–227. DOI: 10.1038/nrm2646

[43] Chan FY, Torriani A. PstB protein of the phosphate-specific transport system of *Escherichia coli* is an ATPase. J Bacteriol. 1996;**178**:3974–3977.

[44] Beis K. Structural basis for the mechanism of ABC transporters. Biochem Soc Trans. 2015;**43**:889–893. DOI: 10.1042/BST20150047

[45] Hollenstein K, Frei DC, Locher KP. Structure of an ABC transporter in complex with its binding protein. Nature. 2007;**446**:213–216. DOI: 10.1038/nature05626

[46] Kimura S, Makino K, Shinagawa H, Amemura M, Nakata A. Regulation of the phosphate regulon of *Escherichia coli*: characterization of the promoter of the *pstS* gene. Mol Gen Genet. 1989;**215**:374–380.

[47] Spira B, Aguena M, de Castro Oliveira JV, Yagil E. Alternative promoters in the pst operon of *Escherichia coli*. Mol Genet Genomics. 2010;**284**:489–498.

[48] Capra EJ, Laub MT. Evolution of two-component signal transduction systems. Annu Rev Microbiol. 2012;**66**:325–347. DOI: 10.1146/annurev-micro-092611-150039

[49] Stock AM, Robinson VL, Goudreau PN. Two-component signal transduction. Annu Rev Biochem. 2000;**69**:183–215. DOI: 10.1146/annurev.biochem.69.1.183

[50] Gao R, Stock AM. Biological insights from structures of two-component proteins. Annu Rev Microbiol. 2009;**63**:133–154. DOI: 10.1146/annurev.micro.091208.073214

[51] Galperin MY. Diversity of structure and function of response regulator output domains. Curr Opin Microbiol. 2010;**13**:150–159. DOI: 10.1016/j.mib.2010.01.005

[52] Sola M, Gomis-Ruth FX, Serrano L, Gonzalez A, Coll M. Three-dimensional crystal structure of the transcription factor PhoB receiver domain. J Mol Biol. 1999;**285**:675–687. DOI: 10.1006/jmbi.1998.2326

[53] Blanco AG, Sola M, Gomis-Ruth FX, Coll M. Tandem DNA recognition by PhoB, a two-component signal transduction transcriptional activator. Structure (Camb). 2002;**10**:701–713. DOI: 10.1016/S0969-2126(02)00761-X

[54] Makino K, Shinagawa H, Amemura M, Kimura S, Nakata A, Ishihama A. Regulation of the phosphate regulon of Escherichia coli. Activation of pstS transcription by PhoB protein in vitro. J Mol Biol. 1988;**203**:85–95. DOI: 10.1016/0022-2836(88)90093-9

[55] Blanco AG, Canals A, Coll M. PhoB transcriptional activator binds hierarchically to pho box promoters. Biol Chem. 2012;**393**:1165–1171. DOI: 10.1515/hsz-2012-0230

[56] Canals A, Blanco AG, Coll M. sigma70 and PhoB activator: getting a better grip. Transcription. 2012;**3**:160–164. DOI: 10.4161/trns.20444

[57] Carmany DO, Hollingsworth K, McCleary WR. Genetic and biochemical studies of phosphatase activity of PhoR. J Bacteriol. 2003;**185**:1112–1115. DOI: 10.1128/JB.185.3.1112-1115.2003

[58] Shinagawa H, Makino K, Yamada M, Amemura M, Sato T, Nakata A. Signal transduction in the phosphate regulon of *Escherichia coli*: dual functions of PhoR as a protein kinase and a protein phosphatase. In: Torriani-Gorini A, Yagil E, Silver S, editors. Phosphate in Microorganisms: Cellular and Molecular Biology. Washington, DC: American Society for Microbiology; 1994. p. 285–289.

[59] Etzkorn M, Kneuper H, Dunnwald P, Vijayan V, Kramer J, Griesinger C, et al. Plasticity of the PAS domain and a potential role for signal transduction in the histidine kinase DcuS. Nat Struct Mol Biol. 2008;**15**:1031–1039. DOI: 10.1038/nsmb.1493

[60] Moglich A, Ayers RA, Moffat K. Structure and signaling mechanism of Per-ARNT-Sim domains. Structure. 2009;**17**:1282–1294. DOI: 10.1016/j.str.2009.08.011

[61] Ashenberg O, Keating AE, Laub MT. Helix bundle loops determine whether histidine kinases autophosphorylate in cis or in trans. J Mol Biol. 2013;**425**:1198–1209. DOI: 10.1016/j.jmb.2013.01.011

[62] Peterson CN, Mandel MJ, Silhavy TJ. *Escherichia coli* starvation diets: essential nutrients weigh in distinctly. J Bacteriol. 2005;**187**:7549–7553. DOI: 10.1128/JB.187.22.7549-7553.2005

[63] Liu J, Lou Y, Yokota H, Adams PD, Kim R, Kim SH. Crystal structure of a PhoU protein homologue: a new class of metalloprotein containing multinuclear iron clusters. J Biol Chem. 2005;**280**:15960–15966. DOI: 10.1074/jbc.M414117200

[64] Oganesyan V, Oganesyan N, Adams PD, Jancarik J, Yokota HA, Kim R, et al. Crystal structure of the "PhoU-like" phosphate uptake regulator from *Aquifex aeolicus*. J Bacteriol. 2005;**187**:4238–4244. DOI: 10.1128/JB.187.12.4238-4244.2005

[65] Lee SJ, Park YS, Kim SJ, Lee BJ, Suh SW. Crystal structure of PhoU from Pseudomonas aeruginosa, a negative regulator of the Pho regulon. J Struct Biol. 2014;**188**:22–29. DOI: 10.1016/j.jsb.2014.08.010

[66] Gardner SG, Johns KD, Tanner R, McCleary WR. The PhoU protein from *Escherichia coli* interacts with PhoR, PstB, and metals to form a phosphate-signaling complex at the membrane. J Bacteriol. 2014;**196**:1741–1752. DOI: 10.1128/JB.00029-14

[67] Hoffer SM, Tommassen J. The phosphate-binding protein of *Escherichia coli* is not essential for P_i-regulated expression of the *pho* regulon. J Bacteriol. 2001;**183**:5768–5771. DOI: 10.1128/JB.183.19.5768-5771.2001

[68] Rao NN, Wang E, Yashphe J, Torriani A. Nucleotide pool in pho regulon mutants and alkaline phosphatase synthesis in *E. coli*. J Bacteriol. 1986;**166**:205–211.

[69] Battesti A, Bouveret E. The bacterial two-hybrid system based on adenylate cyclase reconstitution in *Escherichia coli*. Methods. 2012;**58**:325–334. DOI: 10.1016/j.ymeth.2012.07.018

[70] Gardner SG, Miller JB, Dean T, Robinson T, Erickson M, Ridge PG, et al. Genetic analysis, structural modeling, and direct coupling analysis suggest a mechanism for phosphate signaling in Escherichia coli. BMC Genet. 2015;**16 Suppl 2**:S2. DOI: 10.1186/1471-2156-16-S2-S2

[71] Amemura M, Shinagawa H, Makino K, Otsuji N, Nakata A. Cloning of and complementation tests with alkaline phosphatase regulatory genes (*phoS* and *phoT*) of *Escherichia coli*. J Bacteriol. 1982;**152**:692–701.

[72] Muda M, Rao NN, Torriani A. Role of PhoU in phosphate transport and alkaline phosphatase regulation. J Bacteriol. 1992;**174**:8057–8064.

[73] Daus ML, Grote M, Muller P, Doebber M, Herrmann A, Steinhoff HJ, et al. ATP-driven MalK dimer closure and reopening and conformational changes of the "EAA" motifs are crucial for function of the maltose ATP-binding cassette transporter (MalFGK2). J Biol Chem. 2007;**282**:22387–22396. DOI: 10.1074/jbc.M701979200

[74] Kato J, Yamada K, Muramatsu A, Hardoyo, Ohtake H. Genetic improvement of Escherichia coli for enhanced biological removal of phosphate from wastewater. Appl Environ Microbiol. 1993;**59**:3744–3749.

[75] Morohoshi T, Maruo T, Shirai Y, Kato J, Ikeda T, Takiguchi N, et al. Accumulation of inorganic polyphosphate in phoU mutants of Escherichia coli and Synechocystis sp. strain PCC6803. Appl Environ Microbiol. 2002;**68**:4107–4110. DOI: 10.1128/AEM.68.8.4107-4110.2002

[76] Zamparas M, Zacharias I. Restoration of eutrophic freshwater by managing internal nutrient loads. A review. Sci Total Environ. 2014;**496**:551–562. DOI: 10.1016/j.scitotenv.2014.07.076

[77] Rastogi RP, Madamwar D, Incharoensakdi A. Bloom dynamics of cyanobacteria and their toxins: environmental health impacts and mitigation strategies. Front Microbiol. 2015;**6**:1254. DOI: 10.3389/fmicb.2015.01254

[78] de-Bashan LE, Bashan Y. Recent advances in removing phosphorus from wastewater and its future use as fertilizer (1997–2003). Water Res. 2004;**38**:4222–4246. DOI: 10.1016/j.watres.2004.07.014

[79] Gebremariam SY, Beutel MW, Christian D, Hess TF. Research advances and challenges in the microbiology of enhanced biological phosphorus removal—a critical review. Water Environ Res. 2011;**83**:195–219.

[80] Shen N, Zhou Y. Enhanced biological phosphorus removal with different carbon sources. Appl Microbiol Biotechnol. 2016;**100**:4735–4745. DOI: 10.1007/s00253-016-7518-4

[81] Brown MR, Kornberg A. Inorganic polyphosphate in the origin and survival of species. Proc Natl Acad Sci U S A. 2004;**101**:16085–16087. DOI: 10.1073/pnas.0406909101

[82] Jimenez J, Bru S, Ribeiro MP, Clotet J. Polyphosphate: popping up from oblivion. Curr Genet. 2016. DOI: 10.1007/s00294-016-0611-5

[83] Rao NN, Liu S, Kornberg A. Inorganic polyphosphate in *Escherichia coli*: the phosphate regulon and the stringent response. J Bacteriol. 1998;**180**:2186–2193.

[84] McCleary WR. Application of promoter swapping techniques to control expression of chromosomal genes. Appl Microbiol Biotechnol. 2009;**84**:641–648. DOI: 10.1007/s00253-009-2137-y

[85] Datsenko KA, Wanner BL. One-step inactivation of chromosomal genes in *Escherichia coli* K-12 using PCR products. Proc Natl Acad Sci USA. 2000;**97**:6640–6645. DOI: 10.1073/pnas.120163297

[86] Kadaba NS, Kaiser JT, Johnson E, Lee A, Rees DC. The high-affinity E. coli methionine ABC transporter: structure and allosteric regulation. Science. 2008;**321**:250–253. DOI: 10.1126/science.1157987

[87] Liu CE, Ames GF. Characterization of transport through the periplasmic histidine permease using proteoliposomes reconstituted by dialysis. J Biol Chem. 1997;**272**:859–866. DOI: 10.1074/jbc.272.2.859

[88] Yang JG, Rees DC. The allosteric regulatory mechanism of the Escherichia coli MetNI methionine ATP binding cassette (ABC) transporter. J Biol Chem. 2015;**290**:9135–9140. DOI: 10.1074/jbc.M114.603365

[89] Albi T, Serrano A. Inorganic polyphosphate in the microbial world. Emerging roles for a multifaceted biopolymer. World J Microbiol Biotechnol. 2016;**32**:27. DOI: 10.1007/s11274-015-1983-2

[90] Keasling JD, Van Dien SJ, Pramanik J. Engineering polyphosphate metabolism in Escherichia coli: implications for bioremediation of inorganic contaminants. Biotechnol Bioeng. 1998;**58**:231–239.

[91] Gray MJ, Wholey WY, Wagner NO, Cremers CM, Mueller-Schickert A, Hock NT, et al. Polyphosphate is a primordial chaperone. Mol Cell. 2014;**53**:689–699. DOI: 10.1016/j.molcel.2014.01.012

[92] Grillo-Puertas M, Schurig-Briccio LA, Rodriguez-Montelongo L, Rintoul MR, Rapisarda VA. Copper tolerance mediated by polyphosphate degradation and low-affinity inorganic phosphate transport system in Escherichia coli. BMC Microbiol. 2014;**14**:72. DOI: 10.1186/1471-2180-14-72

[93] Kuroda A, Murphy H, Cashel M, Kornberg A. Guanosine tetra- and pentaphosphate promote accumulation of inorganic polyphosphate in Escherichia coli. J Biol Chem. 1997;**272**:21240–21243. DOI: 10.1074/jbc.272.34.21240

[94] Maisonneuve E, Castro-Camargo M, Gerdes K. (p)ppGpp controls bacterial persistence by stochastic induction of toxin-antitoxin activity. Cell. 2013;**154**:1140–1150. DOI: 10.1016/j.cell.2013.07.048

[95] Schurig-Briccio LA, Rintoul MR, Volentini SI, Farias RN, Baldoma L, Badia J, et al. A critical phosphate concentration in the stationary phase maintains ndh gene expression and aerobic respiratory chain activity in Escherichia coli. FEMS Microbiol Lett. 2008;**284**:76–83. DOI: 10.1111/j.1574-6968.2008.01188.x

[96] Schurig-Briccio LA, Farias RN, Rintoul MR, Rapisarda VA. Phosphate-enhanced stationary-phase fitness of *Escherichia coli* is related to inorganic polyphosphate level. J Bacteriol. 2009;**191**:4478–4481. DOI: 10.1128/JB.00082-09

[97] Grillo-Puertas M, Rintoul MR, Rapisarda VA. PhoB activation in non-limiting phosphate condition by the maintenance of high polyphosphate levels in the stationary phase inhibits biofilm formation in Escherichia coli. Microbiology. 2016;**162**:1000–1008. DOI: 10.1099/mic.0.000281

[98] Wood JM. Osmosensing by bacteria: signals and membrane-based sensors. Microbiol Mol Biol Rev. 1999;**63**:230–262.

[99] Jubelin G, Vianney A, Beloin C, Ghigo JM, Lazzaroni JC, Lejeune P, et al. CpxR/OmpR interplay regulates curli gene expression in response to osmolarity in *Escherichia coli*. J Bacteriol. 2005;**187**:2038–2049. DOI: 10.1128/JB.187.6.2038-2049.2005

[100] Oberto J, Nabti S, Jooste V, Mignot H, Rouviere-Yaniv J. The HU regulon is composed of genes responding to anaerobiosis, acid stress, high osmolarity and SOS induction. PLoS One. 2009;**4**:e4367. DOI: 10.1371/journal.pone.0004367

[101] Manna D, Gowrishankar J. Evidence for involvement of proteins HU and RpoS in transcription of the osmoresponsive *proU* operon in *Escherichia coli*. J Bacteriol. 1994;**176**:5378–5384.

[102] Bouma CL, Meadow ND, Stover EW, Roseman S. II-BGlc, a glucose receptor of the bacterial phosphotransferase system: molecular cloning of ptsG and purification of the receptor from an overproducing strain of *Escherichia coli*. Proc Natl Acad Sci USA. 1987;**84**:930–934. DOI: 10.1073/pnas.84.4.930

[103] Fraenkel DG, Banerjee S. Deletion mapping of zwf, the gene for a constitutive enzyme, glucose 6-phosphate dehydrogenase in Escherichia coli. Genetics. 1972;**71**:481–489.

[104] Banerjee S, Fraenkel DG. Glucose-6-phosphate dehydrogenase from Escherichia coli and from a "high-level" mutant. J Bacteriol. 1972;**110**:155–160.

[105] McCleary WR, Stock JB, Ninfa AJ. Is acetyl phosphate a global signal in *Escherichia coli*. J Bacteriol. 1993;**175**:2793–2798.

[106] Wilde RJ, Guest JR. Transcript analysis of the citrate synthase and succinate dehydrogenase genes of Escherichia coli K12. J Gen Microbiol. 1986;**132**:3239–3251. DOI: 10.1099/00221287-132-12-3239

[107] Keasling JD. Regulation of intracellular toxic metals and other cations by hydrolysis of polyphosphate. Ann N Y Acad Sci. 1997;**829**:242–249. DOI: 10.1111/j.1749-6632.1997.tb48579.x

Chapter 18

From Biology to Biotechnology: Disulfide Bond Formation in *Escherichia coli*

Bradley J. Landgraf, Guoping Ren, Thorsten Masuch,
Dana Boyd and Mehmet Berkmen

Additional information is available at the end of the chapter

http://dx.doi.org/10.5772/67393

Abstract

Disulfide bonds formed between a pair of oxidized cysteines are important to the structural integrity and proper folding of many proteins. Accordingly, Nature has evolved several systems for the genesis and maintenance of such bonds. Beginning with the discovery of protein disulfide isomerase, which provided the first evidence for enzyme-catalyzed disulfide-bond formation, many years of research have resulted in the explication of the complex network of electron transport pathways needed for this process. Herein, we take a historical approach in describing the elucidation of disulfide-bond formation in E. coli. We frame this topic in the context of genome sequencing eras. The first section describes the discovery of eukaryotic protein disulfide isomerase and the subsequent research that followed from the early 1960s to the early 1990s, a time period we have named the pre-genomic sequencing era. The second section details the renaissance in research on disulfide-bond formation in the periplasm of prokaryotes, fueled by bacterial genetic screens and the development of genomic sequencing technology. Accordingly, we have named this section the genomic sequencing era, which ranges from the early 1990s to approximately 2010. The final section outlines the use of bacterial genetic screens to select for new oxidoreductase enzymes and their potential uses in biotechnological and pharmaceutical applications. This era we have dubbed the post-genomic sequencing era, and we envision it to represent the future of research on oxidative folding.

Keywords: disulfide bond, thiol, redox, oxidation, reduction, Dsb, SHuffle

1. Introduction: covalent bonds in proteins

The amino acids comprising a protein are covalently linked by peptide bonds, which collectively form the "backbone" of the protein. These bonds are the most prevalent covalent links between amino acids in proteins and form the foundations that support protein secondary and tertiary structures. In addition to peptide bonds, disulfide bonds are the second most common covalent bonds between amino acids. Disulfide bonds are sulfur-sulfur bonds formed within a protein when the thiol (-SH) groups of two cysteine residues are each oxidized, resulting in the net loss of two electrons to an oxidizing agent. Other names for these bonds include S-S bonds, disulfide bridges, disulfide crosslinks, and simply disulfides/disulphides. Disulfide bonds play three main roles in proteins as signal relays (signaling disulfide bonds), as active site residues in enzymatic catalysis (catalytic disulfide bonds), and as structural supports (structural disulfide bonds). Signaling disulfide bonds act as environmental redox readouts, such as those observed in the OxyR transcription factor (reactive oxygen species sensing), the ArcAB system (senses changes in respiratory growth conditions), and the antisigma factor RsrA (activates cytoplasmic oxidative stress response) [1–3]. Catalytic disulfide bonds act as active site residues in oxidoreductases such as DsbA and DsbC, which catalyze the oxidation and isomerization of disulfide bonds, respectively [4–6]. While signaling and catalytic disulfide bonds are important, the primary functions of structural disulfide bonds are to facilitate protein folding and to stabilize protein tertiary structure, which will be the focus of this chapter.

2. Disulfide-bond research during the pre-genomic sequencing era

The pre-genomic sequencing era focuses on the research surrounding disulfide-bond formation conducted in the early 1960s through the early 1980s. The work of Anfinsen, Straub, and others on the disulfide-bond formation in Ribonuclease A (RNase A) provided the initial impetus behind studying this process and is described below.

The roles of structural disulfide bonds in protein folding and stability are well exemplified and characterized in the protein RNase A, which contains a total of four disulfide bonds (Cys26-Cys84, Cys40-Cys95, Cys58-Cys110, and Cys65-Cys74) that contribute to the "legendary" stability of RNase A [7]. Indeed, the classic isolation and purification protocol of active RNase A from bovine pancreas calls for extremely harsh conditions in the context of proteins: treatment of pancreatic tissue with 0.25 *N* sulfuric acid at 5°C for 1 day, followed by ammonium sulfate precipitation and boiling in 20% saturated ammonium sulfate at pH 3.0 for 5–10 min [8]. While these purification conditions disrupt noncovalent interactions, the covalent nature of disulfide bonds allows them to survive such treatments, thereby imparting structural stability to the protein. Disulfide bonds also constrain the number of conformations an unfolded protein can adopt, which destabilizes the unfolded state relative to the folded state [9]. In fact, the stability of properly folded RNase A has been estimated to be 8 kcal/mol greater than the unfolded state [10], and the four disulfide bonds collectively contribute an estimated 19 kcal/mol to this stability [11]. While it is clear that structural disulfide bonds play important roles in maintaining the overall integrity of a protein, especially in the case of RNase A, they also serve to aid in the initial folding and refolding of a protein.

Seminal experiments conducted in the early 1960s on RNase A led to the idea that all of the information required to form the correct structures and disulfide bonds of small, globular proteins is contained within its amino acid sequence [12–17]. Evidence supporting this idea—now known as Anfinsen's dogma—was obtained from *in vitro* experiments in which RNase A was denatured and completely reduced to yield an unstructured polypeptide chain containing eight cysteine residues. Removal of denaturant and reducing agent and subsequent incubation of the enzyme open to atmosphere resulted in relatively rapid and spontaneous formation of disulfide bonds—formed by oxidation via molecular oxygen—followed by much slower recovery of RNase activity. Under optimized conditions, the halftime required for recovery of RNase activity was 20 min. This apparent lag phase between disulfide-bond formation and recovery of activity suggested that spontaneous disulfide-bond formation resulted in incorrect cysteine pairing and that the recovery of activity required additional time for disulfide interchange and proper formation to occur [16]. This also suggested that a system for oxidizing and reshuffling disulfide bonds existed *in vivo*, since the 20-min recovery of activity observed *in vitro* was far too slow to be operative in the cell.

Shortly after demonstrating the spontaneous formation of disulfide bonds in reduced RNase A, Anfinsen and colleagues identified an enzyme, isolated from rat liver microsomes, that stimulated RNase A reactivation, with recovery of activity requiring a halftime of 4.5 min. This discovery confirmed the existence of an *in vivo* system capable of catalyzing the formation of the correct disulfide bonds to yield the active enzyme [18]. In addition to the rat liver, the same enzyme had been identified by Venetianer and Straub in chicken, pig, and pigeon pancreatic tissue [17]. Further studies in which the microsomal enzyme was incubated with reduced egg white lysozyme as a substrate—which contains four disulfide bonds required for its activity—demonstrated similar recovery of activity. Due to the recovery of activity in RNase A from both bovine pancreas and rat liver and in egg white lysozyme, the substrate specificity of the enzyme appeared to be rather low. As a result, this enzyme was speculated to be a general mediator of "sulfhydryl-disulfide exchange" *in vivo*. The catalyzed reaction is driven by the release of free energy attained upon folding substrates from unorganized conformations to their more stable native structures [18–20]. Furthermore, the enzyme catalyzing sulfhydryl-disulfide exchange enzyme was shown to possess a DTT-sensitive disulfide bond that was likely to be involved in catalysis [19]. In 1973, nearly 6 years after its identification, the microsome-associated enzyme that catalyzed sulfhydryl-disulfide exchange was given a name: protein disulfide isomerase (PDI).

In the early 1980s, several studies demonstrated a correlation between PDI activity and the synthesis of disulfide-bond containing proteins in specialized cells and tissues [21, 22]. However, it was not until 1983—nearly 10 years after its naming—that PDI was purified to homogeneity and biochemically characterized [23]. Homogenous PDI was shown to catalyze the reduction of disulfide bonds in insulin *in vitro*. This result demonstrated that PDI could catalyze both disulfide-bond formation and reduction, and led some to question whether the name 'protein disulfide isomerase' was a misnomer. Based on the physiological evidence surrounding PDI—its distribution in tissue with great abundance of disulfide-bonded proteins [22]; its localization in the endoplasmic reticulum, where many disulfide-bonded proteins are synthesized; and its broad substrate specificity—in conjunction with findings showing PDI to be a relatively poor reductase, the name PDI was retained and is still in use [24].

The advent of genome sequencing and PCR in the later 1980s caused a shift from eukaryotic PDI studies to research centered on bacterial disulfide-bond formation, which is detailed in the following section. It should be noted that Anfinsen's idea that the amino acid sequence of a protein encodes all of the information necessary for its proper folding was not fully correct. Even though Anfinsen shared the 1972 Nobel Prize in Chemistry with Stanford Moore and William H. Stein, the following decades of his and others' research showed that disulfide-bond formation and protein folding are, in fact, catalyzed processes *in vivo*. The work surrounding RNase A refolding and the elucidation of PDI serves as an example wherein the true answers to fundamental questions often require far more research to unravel their complexities.

3. Genome sequencing enables a great leap forward in bacterial redox biology research

The eponymous Sanger DNA sequencing method was developed by Frederick Sanger and colleagues in 1977 [25]. This method is based on selective incorporation of chain-terminating dideoxynucleotides by DNA polymerases during *in vitro* DNA replication [26]. Sanger sequencing was the most widely utilized DNA sequencing technology until relatively recently. Gene sequencing became reasonably attainable with the 1986 release of a fully automated DNA sequencer made by Applied Biosystems. Around the same time, Kary Mullis of Cetus Corporation developed polymerase chain reaction (PCR) technology, which led to the first commercial PCR enzyme and thermal cycler systems available to scientists in 1987 [27]. Together, Sanger sequencing and the development of PCR technology ushered in the gene sequencing era and revolutionized molecular biology.

With the ability to sequence genes, in conjunction with the already rich field of bacterial genetics and its corresponding techniques, the stage was set for identifying genes involved in redox biology. Along these lines, a genetic selection in *Escherichia coli* designed to identify factors involved in protein translocation led to the serendipitous discovery of mutations in the *dsbA* gene that affected disulfide-bond formation [28]. The DsbA protein was isolated and demonstrated to catalyze disulfide-bond reduction using insulin as a substrate *in vitro* [28, 29]. Later studies revealed DsbA to be a potent and sequential oxidant [30]. Specifically, DsbA forms disulfide bonds between sequential cysteines in proteins as they are translocated to the periplasm [31] (**Figure 1**). Collectively, these studies identified DsbA as the first periplasmic protein involved in disulfide-bond formation and paved the way for elucidating the disulfide-bond forming machinery in *E. coli*.

A second protein involved in disulfide-bond formation was identified through genetic screens of resistance or sensitivity to strong reducing agents. In these screens, Tn*10* insertion mutants sensitive to DTT and benzylpenicillin were mapped to a second gene, which was named *dsbB* [30, 32]. The *dsbB* gene product was later confirmed to specifically oxidize DsbA [33]. Since then, research in several laboratories has elucidated the electron transfer pathway through which approximately 40% of cell envelope proteins in *E. coli* obtain disulfide bonds [34–38]

http://dx.doi.org/10.5772/67393

(see **Figure 1**). Specifically, the DsbA protein transfers disulfide bonds to substrate proteins in the periplasm by accepting electrons from the substrate's cysteine residues. As a result, the cysteine residues of DsbA become reduced and the protein must be oxidized for it to catalyze another round of disulfide bond transfer [28, 29]. This oxidation reaction is carried out by DsbB, an inner membrane protein with two pairs of redox-active cysteines [30, 32]. The electrons received by DsbB in its oxidation of DsbA are transferred to the pool of quinones within the inner membrane [37, 39–43]. Then, the reduced quinones are recycled by cytochrome and terminal oxidases of the electron transport chain [42, 44–46]. Together, DsbA and DsbB act as the oxidation system for disulfide-bond formation in the periplasm (**Figure 1**). These two proteins form one part of the periplasmic disulfide-bond forming pathway; additional proteins, DsbC and DsbD, among others, play downstream roles in the fidelity of native disulfide bonds.

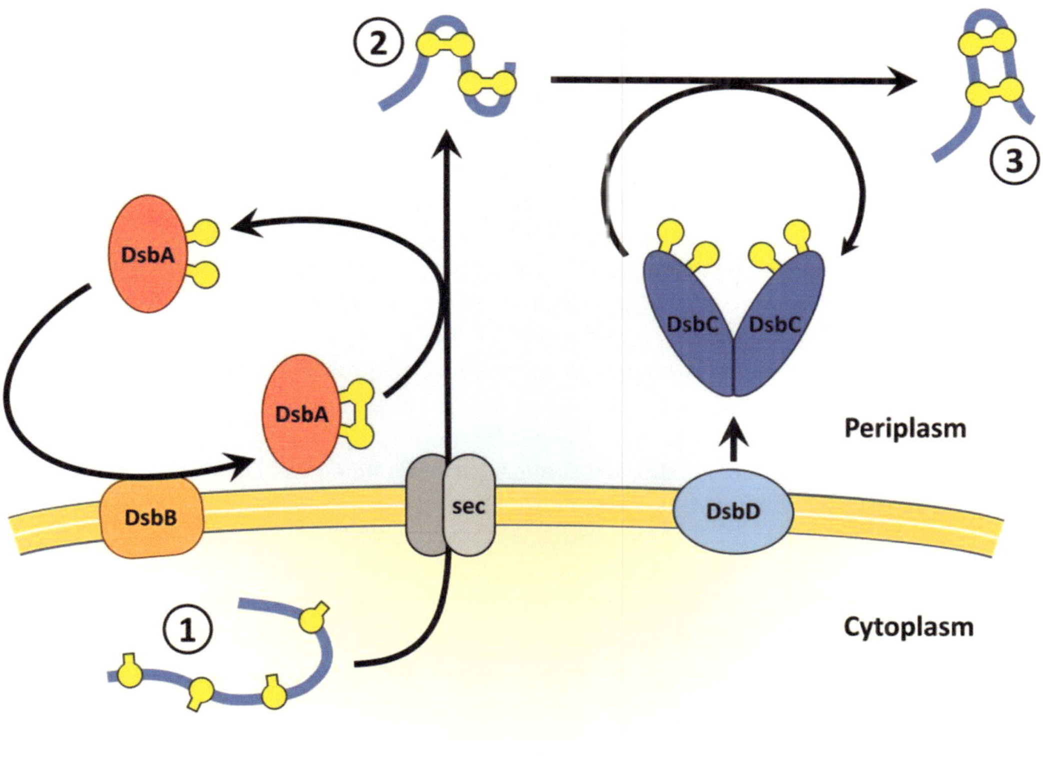

Figure 1. The disulfide-bond-forming pathways in the periplasm of E. coli. A protein containing four cysteines in their reduced (free thiol) states is translocated into the periplasm by the SecYEG translocon. (1). Oxidized DsbA catalyzes disulfide-bond formation either as the protein is translocated or after, resulting in sequential disulfide bonds in this protein. DsbA is then oxidized to its active state by DsbB. DsbB is oxidized by ubiquinone or menaquinone under aerobic or anaerobic conditions, respectively (not shown). (2). If the disulfide bonds formed by DsbA are misoxidized, reduced DsbC catalyzes their isomerization to yield the properly folded protein. (3). DsbD then reduces DsbC to its active state. DsbD is reduced by an electron cascade originating from NADPH and mediated by thioredoxin reductase and thioredoxin in the cytoplasm (not shown).

The misoxidation of substrates by DsbA necessitates the existence of a system capable of isomerizing incorrect disulfide bonds to their correct linkages in prokaryotes. In *E. coli*, the isomerization of disulfide bonds in proteins is catalyzed by DsbC. The *dsbC* gene was discovered in 1994, shortly after the discovery of the *dsbB* gene, using the same genetic selection approach [47]. The *dsbC* gene product was characterized and was shown to contain two cysteines that reside in the CXXC motif generally found in oxidoreductases. Subsequently, DsbC was demonstrated to catalyze disulfide-bond isomerization of substrates containing nonconsecutive disulfide bonds [48–51] (**Figure 1**). This substrate preference of DsbC was illustrated with two nearly identical *E. coli* proteins, phytase (AppA) and glucose-1-phosphatase (Agp), which differ by the former containing a nonconsecutive disulfide bond, while the latter has only consecutive disulfide bonds. AppA was shown to be dependent on DsbC for proper folding into its active conformation, whereas Agp exhibited no dependence on DsbC until a nonconsecutive disulfide bond placed similarly as that found in phytase was introduced [48]. To date, no exceptions to the substrate preference of DsbC have been found. Taken together, these results suggested that DsbC is a protein disulfide isomerase that catalyzes the rearrangement of misoxidized disulfide bonds, in particular, the rearrangement of nonconsecutive disulfide bonds. Thus, DsbA and DsbC work in parallel in maintaining the correct disulfide bonds in the periplasmic *E. coli* proteome. DsbA catalyzes disulfide-bond formation as the protein is translocated into the periplasm, resulting in the formation of consecutive disulfide bonds. In those proteins requiring nonconsecutive disulfide bonds, DsbC catalyzes the isomerization of misoxidized bonds to yield active enzymes. The exact details of substrate recognition and the *in vivo* mechanism of isomerization catalyzed by DsbC have yet to be elucidated. However, preliminary evidence suggests that certain correctly oxidized proteins may result not only from oxidation and isomerization but also from iterative cycles of reduction and oxidation by DsbA and DsbC [52]. Another protein, DsbG, shares 28% sequence identity with DsbC and exhibits protein disulfide isomerase activity, albeit on a more narrow scope of yet-to-be-identified substrates [5, 53, 54].

Like DsbA, DsbC has a dedicated redox protein partner, named DsbD, which is responsible for maintaining it in its reduced state (**Figure 1**). The *dsbD* gene was discovered using the same genetic screens that led to the discoveries of both DsbB and DsbC [55]. The *dsbD* gene product consists of three domains: an N-terminal periplasmic domain, a transmembrane domain, and a C-terminal periplasmic thioredoxin-like domain that shares approximately 45% sequence homology with eukaryotic PDIs [56]. Each of the domains of DsbD contains a pair of conserved cysteine residues that are redox active and essential for its function [56]. To maintain DsbC in its reduced state, DsbD channels reducing equivalents that are mediated through a cascade of disulfide-bond reductions starting with the reduction of thioredoxin reductase by NADPH [57, 58]. Thioredoxin reductase reduces thioredoxin, which then reduces the cysteine pair in the transmembrane domain of DsbD [58, 59]. This reduced cysteine pair initiates the sequential reduction of disulfide bonds in the C-terminal and N-terminal DsbD domains, respectively [59]. The reduced N-terminal domain cysteines then reduce DsbC (**Figure 1**). Reduction of DsbC occurs only when it is dimeric [60, 61]. This substrate preference likely stems from the tertiary structure of the N-terminal domain of DsbD, which adopts a immunoglobulin-like fold and places the active site in the antigen-binding-like region [62]. The tertiary

http://dx.doi.org/10.5772/67393

structure promotes the binding of the DsbC dimer and occludes the binding of the monomeric DsbA and DsbB proteins, thereby separating the oxidative and reductive pathways [63].

The formation of disulfide bonds is essential to the structural integrity and folding of proteins that are vital in many biological processes. *E. coli* and other prokaryotes have evolved a complex network of electron transport chains and quality control systems to facilitate and ensure proper disulfide-bond formation in the form of the Dsb proteins described above. The discovery of these Dsb proteins, and the subsequent revival of interest in disulfide-bond formation in eukaryotes, would not have been realized without the powerful combination of well-designed, selective genetic screens to produce mutants and the ability to sequence the resulting mutated genes. With the advent of next-generation sequencing, we should expect further elucidation of the biological and chemical processes that we do not yet understand or have yet to be discovered.

4. Disulfide-bond research in the post-genomic sequencing era

Since 2008, the cost of genome sequencing has declined faster than predicted by Moore's Law [64]. Currently, the cost of sequencing a genome is ~$1500, and the lofty $1000/genome goal is within reach. Due to the radical drop in DNA sequencing costs, a multitude of laboratories and private and government institutions have completed the sequencing of approximately 30,000 bacterial genomes [65]. This wealth of data is currently being used for a variety of biotechnological and clinical purposes including diagnostics, public health benefits, and biosurveillance/epidemiological studies [66, 67]. Accordingly, we have termed this time period as the "post-genomic sequencing era" to represent research that uses sequenced genomes, metagenomes, and environmental samples to search for novel enzymes and pathways and to predict the redox biology of bacteria.

4.1. Hunting for new disulfide-bond forming enzymes in the genomic landscape

One of the first examples of the use of sequenced genomes to predict and identify novel disulfide-bond forming pathways was conducted by Todd Yeates and colleagues [68–70]. They hypothesized that organisms rich in disulfide-bonded proteins would have a propensity to encode for proteins with an even number of cysteine residues, since an odd number might cause formation of aberrant disulfide bonds. This conjecture was based on the observation that the predicted open reading frames (ORFs) of the hyperthermophilic *Pyrobaculum aerophilum* and *Aeropyrum pernix* species are strongly biased toward an even number of cysteines [70]. Since then, they have expanded their analysis to show that hyperthermophilic members of the Crenarchaeota branch all contain a multitude of disulfide-bonded proteins [68]. Mass spectrometric analysis of the proteome of *Sulfolobus solfataricus* revealed the majority of cysteines to be disulfide bonded [71], and several disulfide-bonded proteins were identified using 2D gel analysis of lysates of *P. aerophilum* [72]. The presence of a high number of disulfide bond-containing proteins in hyperthermophilic Crenarchaeota suggested these bacteria possess an undiscovered method of disulfide-bond maintenance. Indeed, experimental evidence of such a system was obtained from the *in vitro* characterization of protein disulfide oxidoreductases (PDO) from *Pyrococcus furiosus* [73], *Aquifex aeolicus* [74], *A. pernix* [75], and *S. solfataricus* [76]. PDOs have been shown to be functional homologs of PDI and DsbC, that exhibit reduction, oxidation, and isomerization of disulfide bonds. Although there is growing evidence that the cytoplasm of Crenarchaeota is more amenable to disulfide-bond formation, the exact mechanism and the enzymes involved remain to be elucidated *in vivo*.

The method of predicting redox biology of organisms by simply analyzing the cysteine content of the predicted ORFs from sequenced genomes was expanded to all prokaryotic organisms with known genome sequences. By separating the predicted proteome into two subgroups—proteins predicted to be exported and those that remained in the cytoplasm—this bioinformatic method was further developed to predict whether the periplasmic space was oxidizing or reducing [77]. This method led to the observation that some bacteria predicted to have an oxidizing periplasm encode a homolog of DsbA but lack a homolog of its partner DsbB. A closer look at these strains revealed that the DsbA homolog in *Mycobacterium* was a fusion protein to vitamin K epoxide reductase (VKOR) [77]. Characterization of bacterial VKOR homologs confirmed that VKOR can indeed functionally replace DsbB in certain organisms [78, 79]. To our knowledge, this was the first use of genomic data to mine for new oxidoreductases, leading to the discovery of VKOR as a functional homolog of DsbB.

4.2. Selecting for new oxidoreductases using living bacteria

The advent of modern biomolecular tools, in conjunction with classical bacterial genetic screens, has led to the discovery of novel enzymes, yielded many new insights into biochemical pathways, and elucidated molecular mechanisms. The discovery that disulfide bonds are not formed spontaneously but are, in fact, formed catalytically by the enzyme DsbA was a serendipitous discovery using a blue/white screen for secretion defects [28]. The malF-lacZ fusion has been used to not only discover DsbA [28] but also mutants of DsbA with various kinetic properties [31]. Since then, many other genetic screens have been developed to specifically detect the activity of an oxidoreductase in *E. coli*. These screens, described briefly below, allow for the selection of gene products whose activities permit the growth of strains in the absence of a *dsb* component. Characterization of mutant strains revealed insight into the molecular machinery of disulfide-bond formation and highlighted the plasticity of the dsb machinery. A few key mutations could convert a dedicated reductase into an oxidase or create novel pathways to maintain cell viability.

FlgI is a protein component of the flagellar machinery and requires a disulfide bond for its correct folding and activity [80]. Strains that have a functional disulfide-bond forming pathway are motile, while those with defects in disulfide-bond formation are not. By simply spotting bacteria incapable of forming disulfide bonds on dilute agar, researchers are able to screen and select for bacteria that have gained the ability to form disulfide bonds, since they become motile and swim away from the center. This phenotype has been used to characterize and select for new disulfide bond oxidases, such as selecting for mutant thioredoxins possessing a new mechanism of disulfide-bond formation in the periplasm [81]. In another approach, researchers screened a multicopy plasmid library of *E. coli* and selected a rhodanese protein

http://dx.doi.org/10.5772/67393

(PspE) with a single cysteine that can promote disulfide-bond formation in a strain completely lacking the *dsb* pathway [82].

Heavy metals such as copper or cadmium can oxidize thiol groups in periplasmic proteins, resulting in misfolding of proteins containing cysteines and, in some cases, leading to death [83]. DsbC can reduce and refold proteins that were misoxidized by such metals and is therefore necessary to protect cells from copper and cadmium-induced oxidative damage. This phenotype was used to select for strains containing mutant DsbG proteins that have gained the ability to isomerize misoxidized proteins [84]. In another heavy metal screen, cells lacking the *dsbA* gene were screened for cadmium resistance to select for mutant DsbB that can bypass the need for DsbA [85]. The mutant DsbB proteins were able to oxidize DsbC and thus promote disulfide-bond formation.

A blue/white screen was developed using a mutant alkaline phosphatase (*phoA**) that required DsbC for its correct folding and activity. Unlike DsbC, DsbG cannot isomerize misoxidized PhoA*. Mutants of *dsbG* were selected for their gained ability to isomerize PhoA*, resulting in the first *in vivo* screen that directly detected disulfide-bond isomerization of a single protein. This screen permitted the identification of key residues that converted a sulfenic acid reductase (DsbG) into a disulfide-bond isomerase whose activity increased the cells' resistance to copper. Searching the genomes of sequenced prokaryotes, homologs of DsbG were discovered to naturally have the key residues identified through the *phoA** screen. Interestingly, these naturally existing homologs were also capable of protecting cells against copper toxicity. Thus, through the identification of these key residues, activities of homologs can be predicted and tested [86].

The study of disulfide-bond formation has grown and matured significantly since the discovery of DsbA in 1991 [28]. Subsequently, the Dsb pathway in the model organism *E. coli* has been studied in great detail both *in vivo* and *in vitro,* and many novel and interesting mutants and suppressors have been identified using various *in vivo* screens. These new enzymes should have applications in both biotechnology and the pharmaceutical industry as detailed in the next section.

4.3. Biotechnological applications of disulfide-bonded proteins

Both the pharmaceutical and the biotechnological industries are extremely interested in disulfide-bonded proteins. Most eukaryotic cell surface and secreted proteins are rich in disulfide bonds due to the increased stability they confer, making these proteins attractive candidates as therapeutics (also known as biologics). For example, the first recombinant biologic was the hormone insulin, which was introduced by Eli Lilly in 1982, and the most profitable biologic is the antibody Humira (adalimumab), both of which are disulfide-bonded proteins [87]. Between 1982 and 2013, approximately 100 recombinant protein therapeutics have been approved by the FDA, of which more than one-third are disulfide-bonded proteins (in particular monoclonal antibodies) [88].

Currently, antibodies represent the fastest growing category of biologics. Their specificity to therapeutic targets, ability to induce or inhibit immune response, and favorable pharmacokinetic profiles within the human body make them attractive therapeutics. The first therapeutic monoclonal antibody product, Orthoclone OKT3 (muromonab-CD3), was FDA approved in 1986. Since then, research and development of biologics has led to many successful therapeutics, with projected sales expected to reach nearly $125 billion by 2020 [89] (see **Table 1** for top 11 best-selling biologics in 2013 [90]). The production of antibodies for therapeutic applications is a well-established pipeline dominated by the use of Chinese hamster ovary (CHO) cells or hybridomas. However, identifying, characterizing, and engineering therapeutic antibodies are still expensive, time-consuming, and effortful endeavors, leaving room for these aspects of biologic development to be streamlined.

Name	Lead company	Molecule type	Approved indication(s)	2013 worldwide sales ($ millions)
Humira *(adalimumab)*	AbbVie	mAb	RA, juvenile RA, Crohn's disease, PA, psoriasis, ankylosing spondylitis, UC	10,659
Enbrel *(etanercept)*	Amgen	Protein	RA, psoriasis, ankylosing spondylitis, PA juvenile RA	8739
Lantus (*insulin glargine*)	Sanofi	Peptide	Diabetes mellitus type I, diabetes mellitus type II	7593
Rituxan (*rituximab*)	Roche	mAb	RA, chronic, lymphocytic leukemia/small cell lymphocytic lymphoma, non-Hodgkin's lymphoma, antineutrophil cytoplasmic antibodies-associated vasculitis, indolent non-Hodgkin's lymphoma, diffuse large B-cell lymphoma	7500
Remicade (*infliximab*)	Johnson & Johnson	mAb	RA, Crohn's disease, psoriasis, UC, ankylosing spondylitis, PA	6962
Avastin (*bevacizumab*)	Roche	mAb	Colorectal cancer, non-small cell lung cancer, renal cell cancer, brain cancer (malignant glioma; AA and GBM)	6747
Herceptin (*trastuzumab*)	Roche	mAb	Breast cancer, gastric cancer	6558
Gleevec (*imatinib*)	Novartis	Small molecule	Chronic myelogenous leukemia, gastrointestinal stromal tumor, acute lymphocytic leukemia, hypereosinophilic syndrome, mastocytosis, dermatofibrosarcoma protuberans, myelodysplastic syndrome, myeloproliferative disorders	4693
Neulasta (*pegfilgrastim*)	Amgen	Protein	Neutropenia/leukopenia	4392
Copaxone (*glatiramer acetate*)	Teva Pharmaceutical	Peptide	Multiple sclerosis	4356
Revlimid (*lenalidomide*)	Celgene	Small molecule	Multiple myeloma, myelodysplastic syndrome, mantle cell lymphoma	4281

Abbreviations: mAb, monoclonal antibody; RA, rheumatoid arthritis; PA, psoriatic arthritis; UC, ulcerative colitis; AA, anaplastic astrocytoma; GBM, glioblastoma multiforme. Adapted from Ref. [90].

Table 1. The top 10 best selling biologics in 2013. Of these 11 biologics, five are antibody-based therapeutics, indicated by the mAb under molecule type.

http://dx.doi.org/10.5772/67393

The use of *E. coli* as the most popular host for recombinant engineering of proteins stems from the bevy of powerful genetic tools available, its cost effectiveness, and the short time frames required for both its growth and genetic experiments. The periplasm, where conditions favor oxidized proteins, was the clear compartment to express various antibody fragments, including full-length antibodies, versus the reducing conditions of the cytoplasm [91, 92]. The periplasmic space remains an attractive alternative for the production of disulfide-bonded proteins whose presence/activities may be toxic when expressed in the cytoplasm [93]. However, translocation of the target protein across the inner membrane to the periplasm can be problematic and may require extensive optimization of both the expression conditions and the targeting signal sequence. Furthermore, the lack of ATP in the periplasm makes it an energy-poor environment for proteins that require ATP-dependent chaperones for their folding. The cytoplasm is therefore a more suitable compartment for high-yielding protein production. It also obviates the problem of crossing the membrane and is rich in ATP, chaperones, and folding factors.

With the introduction of the Δ*trxB*, *gor* engineered strains of *E. coli* [94, 95], it is now possible to not only express various antibody fragments but also full-length antibodies in the cytoplasm [96]. Yet, the lack of N-linked glycosylation in *E. coli* has hampered its use in the production of therapeutic immunoglobulins (IgGs), although a few examples of *E. coli*-produced therapeutic antibody fragments can be found, such as the Fab' fragment named Lucentis (ranibizumab) against age-related macular degeneration [97]. The discovery of mutations in the Fc portion of IgG that circumvent the dependency on glycosylation for effective interaction with its cognate Fcγ receptor [98] opened the path to potential therapeutic applications of *E. coli*-expressed IgG [96]. Though *E. coli* is currently not as established as CHO or hybridoma cell lines for the production of therapeutic IgG, it is slowly becoming a more common host for the production of antibodies. Other *E. coli*-based technologies, such as phage display, have had extensive use in the discovery and engineering of antibodies, both for the biotech and the pharmaceutical industries. The use of phage display technology to identify novel antibodies of therapeutic targets, such as the HIV virus coat protein, was first described in 1991 [99]. Since then, phage display has been used to develop novel antibody-based applications. For example, the antibody Humira went through extensive engineering using this technique to create an effective biologic [100].

4.4. Engineering disulfide bonds

One key feature of disulfide bonds is their ability to increase the thermostability of proteins by decreasing the number of conformations a protein can attain and thus lowering the conformational entropy of a protein. Secreted proteins leave the protective environment of the cell cytoplasm, and they are rich in disulfide bonds which help to increase their extracellular half-lives. These enzymes are of significant utility in the biotech industry where high-temperature processes are often used. In some cases, disulfide bonds have been introduced into such enzymes to increase their thermostability [101]. Early investigations into the effects of engineered disulfide bonds were performed on phage lambda repressor [102], T4 lysozyme [103], and subtilisin [104], and later were expanded to antibodies [105] and other proteins used in the biotechnology industry. For example, the disulfide bond engineered into the extracellular ribonuclease (barnase) from *Bacillus amyloliquefaciens* unfolds 20 times slower than wild type and 170 times slower than the reduced protein [106]. It is also possible to engineer an interchain disulfide bond within two subunits to bring together the activities of two distinct enzymes [107].

In addition to engineering disulfide bonds into proteins, the reactivity of disulfide-bond forming proteins can also be altered to provide new functionalities. For example, chimeras were created by fusing the disulfide-bond oxidase DsbA to the dimerization domain and α-helical linker derived from the bacterial proline *cis/trans* isomerase FkpA. These chimeras were capable of catalyzing the *in vivo* isomerization of misoxidized disulfide bonds with similar efficiency as that of DsbC [108]. The DsbA-FkpA chimeras also conferred modest resistance to $CuCl_2$, which is dependent on disulfide-bond isomerization. This resistance allowed for the selection of DsbA-FkpA mutants which were found to contain a single amino acid variation in the active site of DsbA from CPHC to CPYC. Substitution of histidine with tyrosine made the active site more DsbC-like (CGYC), which could partially explain the gain of DsbC-like isomerization activity. Interestingly, DsbC is not a substrate for the DsbA-DsbB oxidation system and does not exhibit disulfide-bond oxidase activity. However, the DsbA-FkpA chimeras exhibited both oxidase and isomerization functionalities, and *dsbA* deletion strains were partially complemented by the presence of the DsbB-dependent DsbA-FkpA chimeras [108].

4.5. Dsb enzymes as novel antimicrobial targets

Many pathogenic bacteria, including *Vibrio cholerae, Pseudomonas aeruginosa, Salmonella enterica, Helicobacter pylori, Bordetella pertussis,* and *E. coli,* among others, make use of periplasmic disulfide-bonded proteins that act as virulence factors or function in processes related to their pathogenicity [109–114]. These virulence factors and pathogenic functions rely on the Dsb proteins, in particular DsbA, for proper folding. As a consequence, disruptions in the redox and isomerization activities of the dsb system partially or fully attenuate the pathogenicity of these bacterial species [115]. Specifically, maturation of toxins of *V. cholerae, B. pertussis,* and *E. coli* requires the formation of DsbA-dependent disulfide bonds [109, 113, 116, 117]. Strains of these bacteria lacking *dsbA* synthesize misfolded, misassembled, and/or unstable toxin proteins that are severely impaired or nonfunctional. Along these lines, Δ*dsbA* strains of *S. enterica* and *E. coli* lack the flagellin (FliC) protein, which is a primary constituent of the filaments of their flagella. FliC does not contain any disulfide bonds. However, due to the hierarchical assembly of the flagellum machinery, which requires several proteins with disulfide bonds to precede FliC in its biogenesis, it is thought that FliC simply is not translated or that it cannot be assembled into the organelle due to the missing disulfide bonds and/or disulfide-bonded proteins [50, 118]. As a result, these Δ*dsbA* strains of *S. enterica* and *E. coli* bacteria are nonmotile and their pathogenicity is severely attenuated. Additionally, the loss of disulfide bonds in Δ*dsbA* strains of *V. cholerae* and *E. coli* affects their ability to adhere to eukaryotic cells and/or form biofilms due to defects in their pili, thereby limiting their infectivity [109, 119, 120]. All together, these studies showed that the Dsb enzymes, especially DsbA, play crucial roles in the pathogenicity of several species of bacteria, making these enzymes logical targets for novel antibiotic development.

Indeed, some research has focused on the development of small molecule inhibitors of Dsb enzymes and their homologs (reviewed in Refs. [121, 122]). In humans, blood coagulation

http://dx.doi.org/10.5772/67393

involves the activity of the enzyme vitamin K epoxide reductase (VKOR), which is inhibited by the anticoagulant drug warfarin (Coumadin). Interestingly, *Mycobacterium tuberculosis (Mtb)* and other bacteria do not encode for a DsbB protein, but instead encode a homolog of VKOR. Although DsbB and VKOR exhibit little sequence similarity, they appear to be functionally similar, since VKOR can replace DsbB in both *E. coli* and cyanobacterial *ΔdsbB* strains [77, 123]. Warfarin was shown to both inhibit *Mtb*VKOR activity and bacterial growth. Furthermore, mutations in the VKOR protein from warfarin-resistant *Mtb* mutants were mapped to nearly identical locations in mutant VKORs from patients who require higher effective doses of warfarin, indicating the drug likely inhibits bacterial and human VKORs in similar manners [34]. These findings, in conjunction with the severe growth defects observed in *Mtb*VKOR homolog deletion strains, suggested that stronger inhibitors of *Mtb*VKOR could be used as effective antituberculosis agents [34].

Promising small molecule inhibitors of bacterial Dsb proteins have been identified using fragment-based lead discovery (FBLD) [124]. FBLD identifies small molecule fragments that weakly bind to a target of interest. Through many rounds of iterative combinations of such fragments and high-throughput screening, candidate molecules with higher binding affinities for the target are created, leading to possible drug candidates. Using a detergent-solubilized *Ec*DsbB immobilized onto sepharose resin and ^{1}H NMR, 1071 fragments were tested for both binding to and inhibition of *Ec*DsbB, yielding eight fragments exhibiting IC_{50} values of 7–170 μM. The eight fragments were divided into two groups based on their molecular scaffolds and hypothesized mechanisms of inhibition: blocking of quinone binding and blocking of both quinone and *Ec*DsbA binding to DsbB [124]. A further study improved the IC_{50} value of a candidate molecule to 1.1 μM through additional rounds of FBLD. This molecule inhibited both *Ec*DsbA and DsbB through covalent modification of active site cysteine residue in each protein with a propionyl group, thereby abrogating their ability to form disulfide bonds. The molecule also exhibited a degree of selectivity for DsbA and DsbB proteins, since it was shown to have no effect on human thioredoxin activity [125].

Through the use of high-throughput blue/white screening, six additional small molecule inhibitors of *Ec*DsbB were identified from a pool of approximately 52,000 compounds. These six molecules all contained a pyridazinone ring and exhibited a degree of selectivity for *Ec*DsbB, since they were unable to inhibit the *Mtb*VKOR homolog described above. Interestingly, the molecules inhibited DsbB enzymes from other Gram-negative pathogens, including *V. cholerae, Haemophilus influenzae, Salmonella typhimurium, Klebsiella pneumoniae, Francisella tularensis, Acinetobacter baumannii*, and *P. aeruginosa*, to varying degrees [126].

In addition to small molecules, larger peptides capable of inhibiting the formation of the DsbA-DsbB complex have been developed. Using the crystal structure of the DsbA-DsbB complex [127], a peptide of seven amino acids corresponding to a loop of DsbB involved in docking with DsbA was identified and found to bind to *Ec*DsbA with low micromolar affinity (K_d = 13.1 ± 0.4 μM). Further engineering of this peptide resulted in a new peptide with greater affinity (K_d = 5.7 ± 0.4 μM) that also exhibited fairly potent inhibition of *Ec*DsbA oxidase activity (IC_{50} = 8.8 ± 1.1 μM) [128]. The studies described herein clearly show that the DsbA-DsbB protein system is an attractive and tractable target for novel antibiotic development. While the inhibitors described above exhibit relatively weak binding affinities, the resulting phenotypes observed support their disruption of disulfide-bond formation in the cell. These "first-generation" molecules can serve as a foundation from which more potent compounds can be identified and developed.

5. Future directions

There are 4306 predicted *E. coli* K12 protein sequences present in the UniProt proteome database (http://www.uniprot.org/proteomes/) [129]. An initial analysis of their compartmentalization within the cell using the prediction software TOPCONS2 (http://topcons.cbr.su.se/pred/) [130] allowed us to putatively assign each of these proteins to one of three subcellular compartments: cytoplasmic, transmembrane in the inner membrane (referred to as transmembrane hereafter), or secreted. To hone in on proteins exhibiting possible oxidoreductase activity, the CXXC motif was used as a signature to identify 406 proteins, which showed that approximately 10% of all predicted *E. coli* proteins contain this motif, thereby demonstrating its relative ubiquity. Of these 406 proteins, ~75% are cytoplasmic, ~18% are transmembrane, and ~7% are secreted (see **Table 2**). The pool of non-CXXC-containing proteins comprises the remaining 3900 proteins, of which ~63% are cytoplasmic, ~23% are transmembrane, and ~14% are secreted (omitted from **Table 2**). The transmembrane and secreted compartments have a lower fraction of CXXC-containing proteins in keeping with the exclusion of cysteine residues from these compartments in aerobes [77]. A comparison of the non-CXXC sequence pool with the CXXC sequence pool shows a slight enrichment of CXXC proteins in the cytoplasm (~75%) versus non-CXXC cytoplasmic proteins (~63%). The distribution of CXXC and non-CXXC proteins in the transmembrane is similar (18 and 23%, respectively); however, about twice as many non-CXXC proteins are secreted (14%) compared to CXXC proteins. Approximately 22% (90 of 406) of CXXC proteins are annotated in the UniProt data as binding metal ions or as iron-sulfur cluster-containing proteins. While 46% of all CXXC proteins have been functionally characterized, the remaining majority (54%) should be characterized to develop a better understanding of the reactions they catalyze, how those identified to be oxidoreductases may contribute to the redox biology of bacteria, and to identify novel targets for therapeutics.

Compartment	Number of proteins		Contain CXXC		Known function		Unknown function		Metal binding	
Cytoplasm	2755	64%	305	75%	147	78%	158	72%	79	88%
Transmembrane	970	23%	72	18%	33	18%	39	18%	7	8%
Secreted	581	13%	29	7%	8	4%	21	10%	4	4%
Total	4306	100%	406	100%	188	100%	218	100%	90	100%

Secreted refers to proteins in the periplasm and secreted outside of the cell. Compartment location was predicted using topological and signal sequence input data on the TOPCONS server. Gene ontology (GO) codes EXP and IDA were used to identify proteins with experimentally verified function from the UniProt database; those lacking these codes were defined as having unknown function. GO codes were also used to identify CXXC proteins annotated to bind metals [129].

Table 2. The *E. coli* proteome separated by compartment, the presence of CXXC motifs, and known function.

http://dx.doi.org/10.5772/67393

6. Conclusions

While more than 20 years of research have elucidated many of the Dsb proteins and their functions, more questions surrounding these proteins remain to be answered: What are the precise mechanisms by which PDI and DsbC catalyze disulfide-bond isomerization *in vivo*? How are electrons transported across the inner membrane by DsbD? What are the redox states and midpoint potentials of the cytoplasm of Crenarchaeota? Additionally, most of the characterization of Dsb proteins has been done in *E. coli*, which is not an appropriate model for all bacteria, e.g., *M. tuberculosis, Staphylococcus aureus,* and *Listeria monocytogenes*, so further characterization of the Dsb protein networks in other organisms is needed. Along these lines, Dsb proteins from pathogenic bacteria represent possible targets for antibiotic/vaccine development. Since several Dsb proteins have been structurally characterized, it is now possible to develop antibiotics by structure-guided design. While broad-spectrum antibiotic molecules are unlikely to be developed, again due to the diversity of Dsb proteins/networks within bacterial species, those targeting specific pathogenic species are not out of reach.

As more disulfide-bonded proteins are characterized, our knowledge of the stability and structures these bonds confer, their likelihood of scrambling in mulitply disulfide-bonded proteins, and their relative redox potentials will grow. This will allow researchers to better predict native disulfide bonds from sequence data and better engineer disulfide bonds in proteins for desirable physicochemical properties, which will benefit both the biotechnological and pharmaceutical industries, especially in the development and production of antibodies. Ideally, both industries should aim to produce antibodies as quickly, cheaply, and effectively as possible. The engineering of bacterial strains to overproduce correctly folded antibodies and/or engineering antibodies themselves for desired properties represents a technically challenging but incredibly useful advancement in the field of oxidative protein folding. Future research in these areas should lead to great innovations in both the biotechnological and pharmaceutical industries that will improve the health and increase the knowledge of humankind.

Author details

Bradley J. Landgraf[1], Guoping Ren[1], Thorsten Masuch[1], Dana Boyd[2] and Mehmet Berkmen[1*]

*Address all correspondence to: berkmen@neb.com

1 New England Biolabs / Ruhr-Universität Bochum, Germany

2 Department of Microbiology and Immunology, Harvard Medical School, Boston, MA, USA

References

[1] Lee C, Lee SM, Mukhopadhyay P, Kim SJ, Lee SC, et al. 2004. Redox regulation of OxyR requires specific disulfide bond formation involving a rapid kinetic reaction path. Nat. Struct. Mol. Biol. 11: 1179-85.

[2] Alvarez FA, Georgellis D. 2010. *In vitro* and *in vivo* analysis of the ArcB/A redox signaling pathway. Methods Enzymol. 471: 205-26.

[3] Kang JG, Paget MS, Seok YJ, Hahn MY, Bae JB, et al. 1999. RsrA, an anti-sigma factor regulated by redox change. EMBO J. 18: 4292-8.

[4] Jander G, Martin NL, Beckwith J. 1994. Two cysteines in each periplasmic domain of the membrane protein DsbB are required for its function in protein disulfide bond formation. EMBO J. 13: 5121-7.

[5] Andersen CL, Matthey-Dupraz A, Missiakas D, Raina S. 1997. A new *Escherichia coli* gene, *dsbG*, encodes a periplasmic protein involved in disulphide bond formation, required for recycling DsbA/DsbB and DsbC redox proteins. Mol. Microbiol. 26: 121-32.

[6] Gon S, Faulkner MJ, Beckwith J. 2006. *In vivo* requirement for glutaredoxins and thioredoxins in the reduction of the ribonucleotide reductases of *Escherichia coli*. Antioxid. Redox Signal. 8: 735-42.

[7] Klink TA, Woycechowsky KJ, Taylor KM, Raines RT. 2000. Contribution of disulfide bonds to the conformational stability and catalytic activity of ribonuclease A. Eur. J. Biochem. 267: 566-72.

[8] Kunitz M, McDonald MR. 1953. Biochem. Prep. 3: 9.

[9] Flory PJ. 1956. Theory of elastic mechanisms in fibrous proteins. J. Am. Chem. Soc. 78: 5222-35.

[10] Pfeil W. 1981. The problem of the stability of globular proteins Mol. Cell. Biochem. 40: 3-28.

[11] Konishi Y, Ooi T, Scheraga HA. 1982. Regeneration of ribonuclease A from the reduced protein. 2. Energetic analysis. Biochemistry 21: 4741-8.

[12] White FH, Jr. 1960. Regeneration of enzymatic activity by air oxidation of reduced ribonuclease with observations on thiolation during reduction with thioglycolate. J. Biol. Chem. 235: 383-9.

[13] Haber E, Anfinsen CB. 1961. Regeneration of enzyme activity by air oxidation of reduced subtilisin-modified ribonuclease. J. Biol. Chem. 236: 422-4.

[14] Anfinsen CB, Haber E. 1961. Studies on the reduction and re-formation of protein disulfide bonds. J. Biol. Chem. 236: 1361-3.

[15] Anfinsen CB, Haber E, Sela M, White FH, Jr. 1961. The kinetics of formation of native ribonuclease during oxidation of the reduced polypeptide chain. Proc. Natl. Acad. Sci. U. S. A. 47: 1309-14.

[16] Goldberger RF, Epstein CJ, Anfinsen CB. 1963. Acceleration of reactivation of reduced bovine pancreatic ribonuclease by a microsomal system from rat liver. J. Biol. Chem. 238: 628-35.

[17] Venetianer P, Straub FB. 1963. The enzymic reactivation of reduced ribonuclease. Biochim. Biophys. Acta (BBA) Spec. Sec. Enzymol. Subj. 67: 166-8.

http://dx.doi.org/10.5772/67393

[18] Goldberger RF, Epstein CJ, Anfinsen CB. 1964. Purification and properties of a microsomal enzyme system catalyzing the reactivation of reduced ribonuclease and lysozyme. J. Biol. Chem. 239: 1406-10.

[19] De Lorenzo F, Goldberger RF, Steers E, Jr., Givol D, Anfinsen B. 1966. Purification and properties of an enzyme from beef liver which catalyzes sulfhydryl-disulfide interchange in proteins. J. Biol. Chem. 241: 1562-7.

[20] Fuchs S, De Lorenzo F, Anfinsen CB. 1967. Studies on the mechanism of the enzymic catalysis of disulfide interchange in proteins. J. Biol. Chem. 242: 398-402.

[21] Brockway BE, Forster SJ, Freedman RB. 1980. Protein disulphide-isomerase activity in chick-embryo tissues. Correlation with the biosynthesis of procollagen. Biochem. J. 191: 873-6.

[22] Roth RA, Koshland ME. 1981. Role of disulfide interchange enzyme in immunoglobulin synthesis. Biochemistry 20: 6594-9.

[23] Lambert N, Freedman RB. 1983. Structural properties of homogeneous protein disulphide-isomerase from bovine liver purified by a rapid high-yielding procedure. Biochem. J. 213: 225-34.

[24] Lambert N, Freedman RB. 1983. Kinetics and specificity of homogeneous protein disulphide-isomerase in protein disulphide isomerization and in thiol-protein-disulphide oxidoreduction. Biochem. J. 213: 235-43.

[25] Sanger F, Coulson AR. 1975. A rapid method for determining sequences in DNA by primed synthesis with DNA polymerase. J. Mol. Biol. 94: 441-8.

[26] Sanger F, Nicklen S, Coulson AR. 1977. DNA sequencing with chain-terminating inhibitors. Proc. Natl. Acad. Sci. 74: 5463-7.

[27] Saiki R, Scharf S, Faloona F, Mullis K, Horn G, et al. 1985. Enzymatic amplification of beta-globin genomic sequences and restriction site analysis for diagnosis of sickle cell anemia. Science 230: 1350-4.

[28] Bardwell JC, McGovern K, Beckwith J. 1991. Identification of a protein required for disulfide bond formation *in vivo*. Cell 67: 581-9.

[29] Akiyama Y, Kamitani S, Kusukawa N, Ito K. 1992. In vitro catalysis of oxidative folding of disulfide-bonded proteins by the *Escherichia coli dsbA* (*ppfA*) gene product. J. Biol. Chem. 267: 22440-5.

[30] Bardwell JC, Lee JO, Jander G, Martin N, Belin D, Beckwith J. 1993. A pathway for disulfide bond formation *in vivo*. Proc. Natl. Acad. Sci. U. S. A. 90: 1038-42.

[31] Kadokura H, Tian H, Zander T, Bardwell JC, Beckwith J. 2004. Snapshots of DsbA in action: detection of proteins in the process of oxidative folding. Science 303: 534-7.

[32] Missiakas D, Georgopoulos C, Raina S. 1993. Identification and characterization of the *Escherichia coli* gene *dsbB*, whose product is involved in the formation of disulfide bonds in vivo. Proc. Natl. Acad. Sci. U. S. A. 90: 7084-8.

[33] Kishigami S, Kanaya E, Kikuchi M, Ito K. 1995. DsbA-DsbB interaction through their active site cysteines. Evidence from an odd cysteine mutant of DsbA. J. Biol. Chem. 270: 17072-4.

[34] Dutton RJ, Wayman A, Wei JR, Rubin EJ, Beckwith J, Boyd D. 2010. Inhibition of bacterial disulfide bond formation by the anticoagulant warfarin. Proc. Natl. Acad. Sci. U. S. A. 107: 297-301.

[35] Kadokura H, Beckwith J. 2002. Four cysteines of the membrane protein DsbB act in concert to oxidize its substrate DsbA. EMBO J. 21: 2354-63.

[36] Inaba K, Takahashi YH, Fujieda N, Kano K, Miyoshi H, Ito K. 2004. DsbB elicits a red-shift of bound ubiquinone during the catalysis of DsbA oxidation. J. Biol. Chem. 279: 6761-8.

[37] Inaba K, Takahashi YH, Ito K. 2005. Reactivities of quinone-free DsbB from *Escherichia coli*. J. Biol. Chem. 280: 33035-44.

[38] Grauschopf U, Fritz A, Glockshuber R. 2003. Mechanism of the electron transfer catalyst DsbB from *Escherichia coli*. EMBO J. 22: 3503-13.

[39] Zeng H, Snavely I, Zamorano P, Javor GT. 1998. Low ubiquinone content in *Escherichia coli* causes thiol hypersensitivity. J. Bacteriol. 180: 3681-5.

[40] Regeimbal J, Bardwell JC. 2002. DsbB catalyzes disulfide bond formation de novo. J. Biol. Chem. 277: 32706-13.

[41] Regeimbal J, Gleiter S, Trumpower BL, Yu CA, Diwakar M, et al. 2003. Disulfide bond formation involves a quinhydrone-type charge-transfer complex. Proc. Natl. Acad. Sci. U. S. A. 100: 13779-84.

[42] Bader M, Muse W, Ballou DP, Gassner C, Bardwell JC. 1999. Oxidative protein folding is driven by the electron transport system. Cell 98: 217-27.

[43] Bader MW, Xie T, Yu CA, Bardwell JC. 2000. Disulfide bonds are generated by quinone reduction. J. Biol. Chem. 275: 26082-8.

[44] Collet JF, Bardwell JC. 2002. Oxidative protein folding in bacteria. Mol. Microbiol. 44: 1-8.

[45] Kobayashi T, Kishigami S, Sone M, Inokuchi H, Mogi T, Ito K. 1997. Respiratory chain is required to maintain oxidized states of the DsbA-DsbB disulfide bond formation system in aerobically growing *Escherichia coli* cells. Proc. Natl. Acad. Sci. U. S. A. 94: 11857-62.

[46] Kobayashi T, Ito K. 1999. Respiratory chain strongly oxidizes the CXXC motif of DsbB in the *Escherichia coli* disulfide bond formation pathway. EMBO J. 18: 1192-8.

[47] Missiakas D, Georgopoulos C, Raina S. 1994. The *Escherichia coli dsbC* (*xprA*) gene encodes a periplasmic protein involved in disulfide bond formation. EMBO J. 13: 2013-20.

[48] Berkmen M, Boyd D, Beckwith J. 2005. The nonconsecutive disulfide bond of *Escherichia coli* phytase (AppA) renders it dependent on the protein-disulfide isomerase, DsbC. J. Biol. Chem. 280: 11387-94.

[49] Bessette PH, Qiu J, Bardwell JC, Swartz JR, Georgiou G. 2001. Effect of sequences of the active-site dipeptides of DsbA and DsbC on *in vivo* folding of multidisulfide proteins in *Escherichia coli.* J. Bacteriol. 183: 980-8.

[50] Hiniker A, Bardwell JC. 2004. *In vivo* substrate specificity of periplasmic disulfide oxidoreductases. J. Biol. Chem. 279: 12967-73.

[51] Joly JC, Swartz JR. 1997. *In vitro* and *in vivo* redox states of the *Escherichia coli* periplasmic oxidoreductases DsbA and DsbC. Biochemistry 36: 10067-72.

[52] Shouldice SR, Cho SH, Boyd D, Heras B, Eser M, et al. 2010. *In vivo* oxidative protein folding can be facilitated by oxidation-reduction cycling. Mol. Microbiol. 75: 13-28.

[53] Chung J, Chen T, Missiakas D. 2000. Transfer of electrons across the cytoplasmic membrane by DsbD, a membrane protein involved in thiol-disulphide exchange and protein folding in the bacterial periplasm. Mol. Microbiol. 35: 1099-109.

[54] Bessette PH, Cotto JJ, Gilbert HF, Georgiou G. 1999. *In vivo* and *in vitro* function of the *Escherichia coli* periplasmic cysteine oxidoreductase DsbG. J. Biol. Chem. 274: 7784-92.

[55] Missiakas D, Schwager F, Raina S. 1995. Identification and characterization of a new disulfide isomerase-like protein (DsbD) in *Escherichia coli.* EMBO J. 14: 3415-24.

[56] Stewart EJ, Katzen F, Beckwith J. 1999. Six conserved cysteines of the membrane protein DsbD are required for the transfer of electrons from the cytoplasm to the periplasm of *Escherichia coli.* EMBO J. 18: 5963-71.

[57] Rietsch A, Belin D, Martin N, Beckwith J. 1996. An *in vivo* pathway for disulfide bond isomerization in *Escherichia coli.* Proc. Natl. Acad. Sci. U. S. A. 93: 13048-53.

[58] Rietsch A, Bessette P, Georgiou G, Beckwith J. 1997. Reduction of the periplasmic disulfide bond isomerase, DsbC, occurs by passage of electrons from cytoplasmic thioredoxin. J. Bacteriol. 179: 6602-8.

[59] Katzen F, Beckwith J. 2000. Transmembrane electron transfer by the membrane protein DsbD occurs via a disulfide bond cascade. Cell 103: 769-79.

[60] Goldstone D, Haebel PW, Katzen F, Bader MW, Bardwell JC, et al. 2001. DsbC activation by the N-terminal domain of DsbD. Proc. Natl. Acad. Sci. U. S. A. 98: 9551-6.

[61] Haebel PW, Goldstone D, Katzen F, Beckwith J, Metcalf P. 2002. The disulfide bond isomerase DsbC is activated by an immunoglobulin-fold thiol oxidoreductase: crystal structure of the DsbC-DsbDalpha complex. EMBO J. 21: 4774-84.

[62] Goulding CW, Sawaya MR, Parseghian A, Lim V, Eisenberg D, Missiakas D. 2002. Thiol-disulfide exchange in an immunoglobulin-like fold: structure of the N-terminal domain of DsbD. Biochemistry 41: 6920-7.

[63] Rozhkova A, Stirnimann CU, Frei P, Grauschopf U, Brunisholz R, et al. 2004. Structural basis and kinetics of inter- and intramolecular disulfide exchange in the redox catalyst DsbD. EMBO J. 23: 1709-19.

[64] Hayden EC. 2014. Technology: the $1000 genome. Nature 507: 294-5.

[65] Land M, Hauser L, Jun S-R, Nookaew I, Leuze MR, et al. 2015. Insights from 20 years of bacterial genome sequencing. Funct. Integr. Genom. 15: 141-61.

[66] Köser CU, Holden MTG, Ellington MJ, Cartwright EJP, Brown NM, et al. 2012. Rapid whole-genome sequencing for investigation of a neonatal MRSA outbreak. New Engl. J. Med. 366: 2267-75.

[67] Harris SR, Cartwright EJP, Török ME, Holden MTG, Brown NM, et al. 2013. Whole-genome sequencing for analysis of an outbreak of meticillin-resistant *Staphylococcus aureus*: a descriptive study. Lancet Infect. Dis. 13: 130-6.

[68] Jorda J, Yeates TO. 2011. Widespread disulfide bonding in proteins from thermophilic archaea. Archaea 2011: 409156.

[69] Beeby M, O'Connor BD, Ryttersgaard C, Boutz DR, Perry LJ, Yeates TO. 2005. The genomics of disulfide bonding and protein stabilization in thermophiles. PLoS Biol. 3: e309.

[70] Mallick P, Boutz DR, Eisenberg D, Yeates TO. 2002. Genomic evidence that the intracellular proteins of archaeal microbes contain disulfide bonds. Proc. Natl. Acad. Sci. U. S. A. 99: 9679-84.

[71] Heinemann J, Hamerly T, Maaty WS, Movahed N, Steffens JD, et al. 2014. Expanding the paradigm of thiol redox in the thermophilic root of life. Biochim. Biophys. Acta 1840: 80-5.

[72] Boutz DR, Cascio D, Whitelegge J, Perry LJ, Yeates TO. 2007. Discovery of a thermophilic protein complex stabilized by topologically interlinked chains. J. Mol. Biol. 368: 1332-44.

[73] Pedone E, Ren B, Ladenstein R, Rossi M, Bartolucci S. 2004. Functional properties of the protein disulfide oxidoreductase from the archaeon *Pyrococcus furiosus*: a member of a novel protein family related to protein disulfide-isomerase. Eur. J. Biochem. 271: 3437-48.

[74] Pedone E, D'Ambrosio K, De Simone G, Rossi M, Pedone C, Bartolucci S. 2006. Insights on a new PDI-like family: structural and functional analysis of a protein disulfide oxidoreductase from the bacterium Aquifex aeolicus. J. Mol. Biol. 356: 155-64.

[75] D'Ambrosio K, Pedone E, Langella E, De Simone G, Rossi M, et al. 2006. A novel member of the protein disulfide oxidoreductase family from *Aeropyrum pernix* K1: structure, function and electrostatics. J. Mol. Biol. 362: 743-52.

[76] Pedone E, Limauro D, D'Alterio R, Rossi M, Bartolucci S. 2006. Characterization of a multifunctional protein disulfide oxidoreductase from *Sulfolobus solfataricus. FEBS J.* 273: 5407-20.

[77] Dutton RJ, Boyd D, Berkmen M, Beckwith J. 2008. Bacterial species exhibit diversity in their mechanisms and capacity for protein disulfide bond formation. Proc. Natl. Acad. Sci. U. S. A. 105: 11933-8.

[78] Wang X, Dutton RJ, Beckwith J, Boyd D. 2011. Membrane topology and mutational analysis of *Mycobacterium tuberculosis* VKOR, a protein involved in disulfide bond formation and a homologue of human vitamin K epoxide reductase. Antioxid. Redox Signal. 14: 1413-20.

[79] Li W, Schulman S, Dutton RJ, Boyd D, Beckwith J, Rapoport TA. 2010. Structure of a bacterial homolog of vitamin K epoxide reductase. Nature 463: 507-12.

[80] Dailey FE, Berg HC. 1993. Mutants in disulfide bond formation that disrupt flagellar assembly in *Escherichia coli.* Proc. Natl. Acad. Sci. U. S. A. 90: 1043-7.

[81] Masip L, Pan JL, Haldar S, Penner-Hahn JE, DeLisa MP, et al. 2004. An engineered pathway for the formation of protein disulfide bonds. Science 303: 1185-9.

[82] Chng SS, Dutton RJ, Denoncin K, Vertommen D, Collet JF, et al. 2012. Overexpression of the rhodanese PspE, a single cysteine-containing protein, restores disulphide bond formation to an *Escherichia coli* strain lacking DsbA. Mol. Microbiol. 85: 996-1006.

[83] Rensing C, Mitra B, Rosen BP. 1997. Insertional inactivation of *dsbA* produces sensitivity to cadmium and zinc in *Escherichia coli.* J. Bacteriol. 179: 2769-71.

[84] Hiniker A, Ren G, Heras B, Zheng Y, Laurinec S, et al. 2007. Laboratory evolution of one disulfide isomerase to resemble another. Proc. Natl. Acad. Sci. U. S. A. 104: 11670-5.

[85] Pan JL, Sliskovic I, Bardwell JC. 2008. Mutants in DsbB that appear to redirect oxidation through the disulfide isomerization pathway. J. Mol. Biol. 377: 1433-42.

[86] Chatelle C, Kraemer S, Ren G, Chmura H, Marechal N, et al. 2015. Converting a sulfenic acid reductase into a disulfide bond isomerase. Antioxid. Redox Signal. 23: 945-57.

[87] Zhang L, Chou CP, Moo-Young M. 2011. Disulfide bond formation and its impact on the biological activity and stability of recombinant therapeutic proteins produced by *Escherichia coli* expression system. Biotechnol. Adv. 29: 923-9.

[88] Kinch MS. 2015. An overview of FDA-approved biologics medicines. Drug Discov. Today 20: 393-8.

[89] Ecker DM, Jones SD, Levine HL. 2015. The therapeutic monoclonal antibody market mAbs 7: 9-14.

[90] Lawrence S, Lahteenmaki R. 2014. Public biotech 2013[mdash]the numbers. Nat. Biotechnol. 32: 626-32.

[91] Lee YJ, Lee DH, Jeong KJ. 2014. Enhanced production of human full-length immunoglobulin G1 in the periplasm of *Escherichia coli.* Appl. Microbiol. Biotechnol. 98: 1237-46.

[92] Zhou Y, Liu P, Gan Y, Sandoval W, Katakam AK, et al. 2016. Enhancing full-length antibody production by signal peptide engineering. Microb. Cell Fact. 15: 47.

[93] Yoon SH, Kim SK, Kim JF. 2010. Secretory production of recombinant proteins in *Escherichia coli.* Recent Pat. Biotechnol. 4: 23-9.

[94] Lobstein J, Emrich CA, Jeans C, Faulkner M, Riggs P, Berkmen M. 2012. SHuffle, a novel *Escherichia coli* protein expression strain capable of correctly folding disulfide bonded proteins in its cytoplasm. Microb. Cell Fact. 11: 56.

[95] Bessette PH, Aslund F, Beckwith J, Georgiou G. 1999. Efficient folding of proteins with multiple disulfide bonds in the *Escherichia coli* cytoplasm. Proc. Natl. Acad. Sci. U. S. A. 96: 13703-8.

[96] Robinson MP, Ke N, Lobstein J, Peterson C, Szkodny A, et al. 2015. Efficient expression of full-length antibodies in the cytoplasm of engineered bacteria. Nat. Commun. 6: 8072.

[97] Magdelaine-Beuzelin C, Pinault C, Paintaud G, Watier H. 2010. Therapeutic antibodies in ophthalmology: old is new again. mAbs 2: 176-80.

[98] Mazor Y, Van Blarcom T, Mabry R, Iverson BL, Georgiou G. 2007. Isolation of engineered, full-length antibodies from libraries expressed in *Escherichia coli.* Nat. Biotechnol. 25: 563-5.

[99] Burton DR, Barbas CF, 3rd, Persson MA, Koenig S, Chanock RM, Lerner RA. 1991. A large array of human monoclonal antibodies to type 1 human immunodeficiency virus from combinatorial libraries of asymptomatic seropositive individuals. Proc. Natl. Acad. Sci. U. S. A. 88: 10134-7.

[100] Nixon AE, Sexton DJ, Ladner RC. 2014. Drugs derived from phage display: from candidate identification to clinical practice. mAbs 6: 73-85

[101] Dombkowski AA, Sultana KZ, Craig DB. 2014. Protein disulfide engineering. FEBS Lett. 588: 206-12.

[102] Sauer RT, Hehir K, Stearman RS, Weiss MA, Jeitler-Nilsson A, et al. 1986. An engineered intersubunit disulfide enhances the stability and DNA binding of the N-terminal domain of lambda repressor. Biochemistry 25: 5992-8.

[103] Wetzel R, Perry LJ, Baase WA, Becktel WJ. 1988. Disulfide bonds and thermal stability in T4 lysozyme. Proc. Natl. Acad. Sci. U. S. A. 85: 401-5.

[104] Wells JA, Powers DB. 1986. *In vivo* formation and stability of engineered disulfide bonds in subtilisin. J. Biol. Chem. 261: 6564-70.

[105] Hagihara Y, Saerens D. 2014. Engineering disulfide bonds within an antibody. Biochim. Biophys. Acta 1844: 2016-23.

[106] Clarke J, Fersht AR. 1993. Engineered disulfide bonds as probes of the folding pathway of barnase: increasing the stability of proteins against the rate of denaturation. Biochemistry 32: 4322-9.

[107] Heikoop JC, van den Boogaart P, Mulders JW, Grootenhuis PD. 1997. Structure-based design and protein engineering of intersubunit disulfide bonds in gonadotropins. Nat. Biotechnol. 15: 658-62.

[108] Arredondo S, Segatori L, Gilbert HF, Georgiou G. 2008. *De novo* design and evolution of artificial disulfide isomerase enzymes analogous to the bacterial DsbC. J. Biol. Chem. 283: 31469-76.

[109] Peek JA, Taylor RK. 1992. Characterization of a periplasmic thiol: disulfide interchange protein required for the functional maturation of secreted virulence factors of Vibrio cholerae. Proc. Natl. Acad. Sci. U. S. A. 89: 6210-4.

[110] Barbieri JT, Sun J. 2005. In Reviews of Physiology, Biochemistry and Pharmacology, pp. 79-92. Berlin, Heidelberg: Springer Berlin Heidelberg.

[111] Miki T, Okada N, Danbara H. 2004. Two periplasmic disulfide oxidoreductases, DsbA and SrgA, target outer membrane protein SpiA, a component of the Salmonella pathogenicity island 2 type III secretion system. J. Biol. Chem. 279: 34631-42.

[112] Godlewska R, Dzwonek A, Mikuła M, Ostrowski J, Pawłowski M, et al. 2006. *Helicobacter pylori* protein oxidation influences the colonization process. Int. J. Med. Microbiol. 296: 321-4.

[113] Stenson TH, Weiss AA. 2002. DsbA and DsbC are required for secretion of pertussis toxin by *Bordetella pertussis*. Infect. Immun. 70: 2297-303.

[114] Okamoto K, Nomura T, Fujii Y, Yamanaka H. 1998. Contribution of the disulfide bond of the A subunit to the action of *Escherichia coli* heat-labile enterotoxin. J. Bacteriol. 180: 1368-74.

[115] Lasica AM, Jagusztyn-Krynicka EK. 2007. The role of Dsb proteins of Gram-negative bacteria in the process of pathogenesis. FEMS Microbiol. Rev. 31: 626-36.

[116] Wülfing C, Rappuoli R. 1997. Efficient production of heat-labile enterotoxin mutant proteins by overexpression of dsbA in a degP-deficient *Escherichia coli* strain. Arch. Microbiol. 167: 280-3.

[117] Foreman DT, Martinez Y, Coombs G, Torres A, Kupersztoch YM. 1995. TolC and DsbA are needed for the secretion of STB, a heat-stable enterotoxin of *Escherichia coli*. Mol. Microbiol. 18: 237-45.

[118] Agudo D, Mendoza MT, Castañares C, Nombela C, Rotger R. 2004. A proteomic approach to study *Salmonella typhi* periplasmic proteins altered by a lack of the DsbA thiol: disulfide isomerase. Proteomics 4: 355-63.

[119] Zhang H-Z, Donnenberg MS. 1996. DsbA is required for stability of the type IV pilin of enteropathogenic *Escherichia coli*. Mol. Microbiol. 21: 787-97.

[120] Lee Y, Kim Y, Yeom S, Kim S, Park S, et al. 2008. The role of disulfide bond isomerase A (DsbA) of *Escherichia coli* O157: H7 in biofilm formation and virulence. FEMS Microbiol. Lett. 278: 213-22.

[121] Smith RP, Paxman JJ, Scanlon MJ, Heras B. 2016. Targeting bacterial Dsb proteins for the development of anti-virulence agents. Molecules 21: 811-25.

[122] Heras B, Shouldice SR, Totsika M, Scanlon MJ, Schembri MA, Martin JL. 2009. DSB proteins and bacterial pathogenicity. Nat. Rev. Microbiol. 7: 215-25.

[123] Singh AK, Bhattacharyya-Pakrasi M, Pakrasi HB. 2008. Identification of an atypical membrane protein involved in the formation of protein disulfide bonds in oxygenic photosynthetic organisms. J. Biol. Chem. 283: 15762-70.

[124] Früh V, Zhou Y, Chen D, Loch C, Eiso AB, et al. 2010. Application of fragment based drug discovery to membrane proteins: biophysical identification of ligands of the integral membrane enzyme DsbB. Chem. Biol. 17: 881-91.

[125] Halili MA, Bachu P, Lindahl F, Bechara C, Mohanty B, et al. 2015. Small molecule inhibitors of disulfide bond formation by the bacterial DsbA-DsbB dual enzyme system. ACS Chem. Biol. 10: 957-64.

[126] Landeta C, Blazyk JL, Hatahet F, Meehan BM, Eser M, et al. 2015. Compounds targeting disulfide bond forming enzyme DsbB of Gram-negative bacteria. Nat. Chem. Biol. 11: 292-8.

[127] Inaba K, Murakami S, Suzuki M, Nakagawa A, Yamashita E, et al. 2006. Crystal structure of the DsbB-DsbA complex reveals a mechanism of disulfide bond generation. Cell 127: 789-801.

[128] Duprez W, Premkumar L, Halili MA, Lindahl F, Reid RC, et al. 2015. Peptide inhibitors of the *Escherichia coli* DsbA oxidative machinery essential for bacterial virulence. J. Med. Chem. 58: 577-87.

[129] Consortium TU. 2015. UniProt: a hub for protein information. Nucleic Acids Res. 43: D204-12.

[130] Tsirigos KD, Peters C, Shu N, Käll L, Elofsson A. 2015. The TOPCONS web server for consensus prediction of membrane protein topology and signal peptides. Nucleic Acids Res. 43: W401-7.

Chapter 19

Survival Strategy of *Escherichia coli* in Stationary Phase: Involvement of σ^E-Dependent Programmed Cell Death

Tomoyuki Kosaka, Masayuki Murata and
Mamoru Yamada

Additional information is available at the end of the chapter

http://dx.doi.org/10.5772/67672

Abstract

In a natural habitat, microbes respond to alterations in the amounts of nutrients or to stresses such as osmotic stress and stresses caused by low or high pH, salt, heat, and antibiotics by changing their mode for proliferation or survival. Similarly, *Escherichia coli* cells in a test tube change the growth mode according to environmental conditions when they enter a stationary phase. Until a sufficient supply of nutrients, the organism survives under such stressful and nutrient-limited conditions by altering gene expression to be more protective against such conditions. The definite trigger of the onset of stationary phase is still unclear, but several lines of evidence indicate that the regulation mechanism is very complicated and involves several transcriptional factors including alternative sigma factors, σ^E and σ^S. In addition, *E. coli* cells behave as a community of species and give rise to programmed cell death (PCD) for ensuring survival by controlling the cell number and supplying nutrients to sibling cells in long-term stationary phase (LTSP). The main PCD is probably performed by σ^E in *E. coli*. In this chapter, physiological functions of σ^E and PCD are introduced and reviewed and their possible involvement in survival mechanisms in stationary phase, especially LTSP, is shown.

Keywords: survival mechanism, envelop stress, σ^E, programmed cell death, long-term stationary phase

1. Introduction

1.1. Brief introduction of σ^E

Living *Escherichia coli* cells are constantly suffering from various stresses. The bacterium thus possesses mechanisms to sense stresses and deal with them by changing gene expression levels and metabolisms. σ^E, one of the seven sigma factors existing in *E. coli* [1], is associated with the core RNA polymerase complex and initiates transcription by directly recognizing a promoter consisting of specific elements. σ^E was found for the time as a heat shock sigma factor due to reduction in the expression level of heat shock proteins at 50 °C in mutants of *rpoE*, encoding σ^E [2] and it is thought to be one of heat shock sigmas like σ^H. σ^E has been recognized as an envelope stress-responsive sigma factor [3] that senses an abnormality of the outer membrane integrity. Under the control of this sigma, several important genes are governed, for example, σ^H and genes for protein folding and degradation [4]. In addition, σ^E represses the synthesis of outer membrane proteins (OMPs). We show ingenious mechanisms of σ^E management of its molecule and activity and functions of genes under the control of σ^E in Section 2.

1.2. Brief introduction of PCD

PCD is conserved for all genetically encoded processes that lead to cell suicide. This conceptual word was first proposed in 1964 [5]. PCD that is observed in development, aging, and pathology in eukaryotic multicellular organisms is classified into three categories based on morphological characteristics such as apoptosis, autophagy, and necrosis. Among these, apoptosis, first described in 1972 [6], is the most well-characterized PCD. The morphological manifestations associated with apoptosis include chromatin condensation, chromosomal DNA fragmentation, membrane blebbing, cell shrinkage, and disassembly of the cell into membrane-enclosed vesicles. Apoptosis is highly regulated, and proteases called caspases play key roles in the induction of DNA fragmentation in the activation cascade [7]. Autophagy is the process by which a vesicle called an autophagosome is constructed for atrophy of the nucleus but with no DNA fragmentation [7]. Necrosis is triggered by activation of various receptors for loss of cell membrane integrity and uncontrollable release of intracellular contents into the extracellular space [7]. The physiological importance of these PCDs in the development of an animal has been well defined. For example, during embryonic development, the earliest form of the human hand resembles a paddle due to the elimination of excess cells by apoptosis. PCD mechanisms are also responsible for the homeostasis of multicellular organisms by the elimination of damaged cells that may become a source of cancer cells in the body.

It was thought that PCD only exists in eukaryotic cells, but several scientists have considered the possibility of the existence of bacterial PCD resembling eukaryotic PCD mechanisms. Indeed, a growing body of evidence has shown that PCD is indispensable for bacterial development and is closely associated with bacterial survival mechanisms [8, 9]. Bacterial communities utilize PCD for survival of their population when suffering from oxidative stress, nutrient deprivation, phage infections, or other problems. The cell survival mechanism is a response to stresses outside cells and inside cells, but excessive damage turns on the PCD mechanism of some cells to help sibling cells. In the development processes of bacteria, PCD provides nutrients to sibling cells, releases components, and promotes special aspects. Indeed, biofilm formation, sporulation, and other multiple cell-like developments have been shown to bear PCD mechanisms in these processes. In biofilm development, cell death and lysis are required for the release of genomic DNA (known as extracellular DNA), which becomes incorporated into the biofilm matrix and serves as an adherence molecule [10]. For the development of sporulation, sporulating cells produce a killing factor for nonsporulating cells, from which released nutrients support sporulation. Moreover, the mother cell in the sporulating population undergoes PCD to release the mature spore via its autolysis [11]. As other mechanisms, *Fratricide* behavior during its genetic transformation, autolysis in *Myxococcus xanthus* development, developmental cycle in *Streptomyces*, and coccoid formation in *Helicobacter pylori* also include PCD in their processes [9].

Many bacterial PCDs are induced through the toxin-antitoxin (TA) system. Five types of TA systems have been found and characterized [9, 12]. Type I has an antisense RNA that pairs with its corresponding toxin mRNA. The difference in transcription between toxin RNA and antitoxin RNA controls the toxin activity. Type II has a protein antitoxin that detoxifies its corresponding toxin protein by their protein-protein interaction. This type of TA system is most abundant. Type III has an antitoxin RNA that interacts directly with the target toxin protein to form an antitoxin RNA-toxin inactive complex. Type IV has a protein antitoxin that stabilizes the target of the toxin by direct binding. Type V has an endoribonuclease that cleaves the target toxin mRNA. These TA systems play important roles in several cellular processes such as plasmid stabilization, formation of persistent cells, peptidoglycan synthesis, resistance to bacteriophages and antibiotics, and inhibition of macromolecule and biofilm formation [9, 12]. PCD via a TA system is executed by the role of toxin proteins. *mazEF* in the type II TA system in *E. coli* has been the most intensively investigated and it has been shown to play a key role in the PCD process.

It has been suggested that the bacterial strategy for survival against DNA damage resembles the PCD mechanisms in eukaryotes [13]. The PCD mechanisms characterized in both prokaryotic and eukaryotic cells indicate that DNA damage leads to cell death when the damage is irreparable. Bayles reported that the death pathway also leads to apoptosis-like processes or autolysis [13]. The similarity of cell death systems in eukaryotes and bacteria suggests that the common origin of this system is derived from endosymbiotic bacteria [9]. Therefore, PCD is a basic mechanism for organisms in all kingdoms for the maintenance of communities, and this system has been acquired at a very early stage of appearance of life on earth. In Section 3, we summarize PCDs in *E. coli* and show σ^E-dependent cell lysis as one of the PCDs and its physiological roles, which our group has discovered.

1.3. Brief introduction of LTSP

In nutrient-sufficient media in the laboratory, *E. coli* exhibits a typical growth curve consisting of five phases: lag phase, log phase, stationary phase, death phase, and LTSP (**Figure 1**) [14, 15]. Among these phases, characteristics of first three phases have been described in detail elsewhere [15]. It has been thought that cells in the death phase gradually die, and it is known that 99.9% of the cells are not viable in that phase. However, Finkel reported that *E. coli* is able to survive for 5 years in LB medium without any additional nutrients if the volume and osmolarity of the medium are maintained [14]. The transition of viable (colony-forming) cell number from 10^9 cells/ml at the stationary phase to 10^6 CFU/ml at the LTSP [14] is accomplished by a rapid decrease in an exponential fashion in the death phase. Then the viable cell

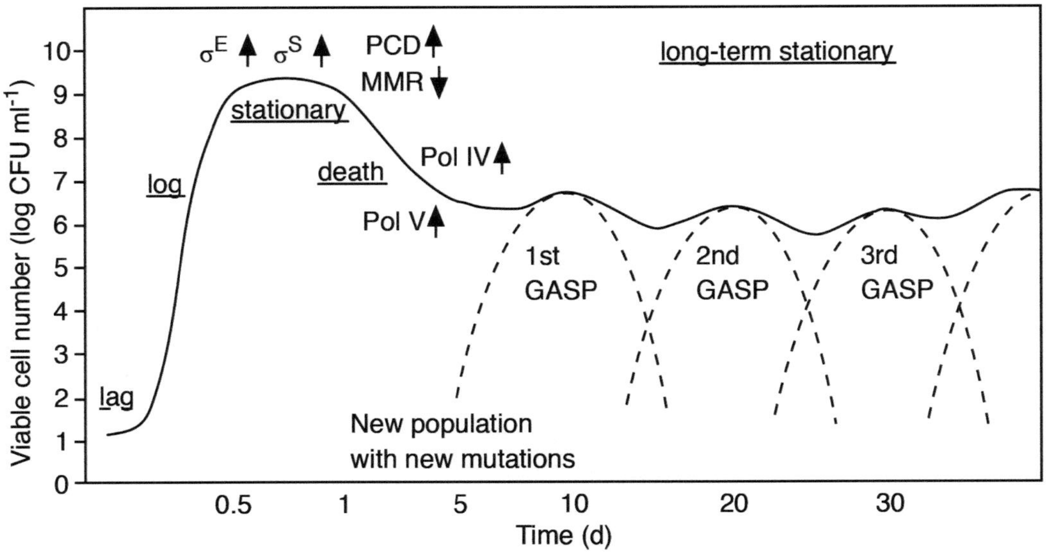

Figure 1. Transition model of viable cells until the LTSP in *E. coli*. The LTSP is created presumably by the sequential alteration of the expression of regulators. The sigma factors σ^E and σ^S are important regulators for onset of the stationary phase and the consequent death phase. PCD and SOS-induced DNA polymerases, Pol II, Pol IV, and Pol V, are thought to be important factors for maintenance of the LTSP. Adapted from Finkel [14].

number is maintained around 10^6 CFU/ml by unknown mechanisms for a very long period. Interestingly, in the LTSP, viable cells show a growth advantage against parent strains [16]. The phenotype of these cells is called growth advantage in stationary phase (GASP). In addition, GASP mutants consecutively occur every 10 days in the same culture [17]. Therefore, cells in the LTSP are not static and a dramatic population change occurs for adapting to the environmental perturbation of nutrients and conditions for survival.

What factors can lead *E. coli* cells from the stationary phase to the LTSP? The onset and course of the stationary phase have been summarized well in other reviews [15, 18]. Briefly, at the beginning of the stationary phase, the abundance of specific sigma factors is known to change: σ^E and σ^S molecules are increased by fivefold and by threefold to fourfold, respectively [19–21]. The physiological roles of σ^E and σ^S suggest that these factors enable cells to adapt to environments in the stationary phase by changing expression of 10% of the genes of *E. coli*. However, it has not been clarified how the death phase and LTSP start. Since protein expression level is kept low for several days in the stationary phase [22], cells may have some activity to accomplish preparation for the coming phases. These activities are probably related to PCD mechanisms [14] as described below. Several factors have been considered for the transition to the LTSP. One of these factors is reactive oxygen species (ROS). Indeed, mutants of genes for NADH dehydrogenase in the respiratory chain, which is a primary source of ROS, exhibited no GASP phenotype [23]. In addition, GASP phenotypes are altered by vessel volume of cultures, probably affecting dissolved oxygen concentrations in the medium [24]. On the other hand, we have revealed that σ^E-dependent PCD is essential for

http://dx.doi.org/10.5772/67672

the GASP phenotype [25], indicating the responsibility of PCDs for the LTSP transition. We describe the possible survival mechanism of *E. coli* in the LTSP and the importance of σ^E-dependent PCD in Section 4.

2. Functions of σ^E

2.1. Mechanisms of membrane stress responses for σ^E activation

Bacteria have mechanisms for rapid responses to environmental stresses, especially on the envelope because cell structure is maintained by integrity of the membrane. There have been many studies on membrane stress responses. In Gram-negative bacteria, such responses are known as envelope stress responses (ESRs). There are five known ESRs, Cpx, σ^E, Bae, Rcs, and Psp ESRs, that are induced by a variety of envelope stresses and alter the expression of adaptive functions to modify the envelope, rid cells of a toxic entity, and/or repair substantial damage [3]. Of these ESRs, σ^E ESR, a subset first found in *E. coli*, is known to respond to stresses such as stresses from heat and alkali due to damage of the outer membrane [26]. The σ^E ESR detects perturbations in biogenesis of the outer membrane or lipopolysaccharide (LPS) due to protein-folding problems in the periplasmic space and outer membrane (**Figure 2**). The key protein in this response is a transmembrane protein of RseA as an anti-σ^E protein capturing σ^E to inactivate it under nonstress conditions. Under stress conditions, σ^E activation is accomplished by the stepped degradation of RseA via three proteases, DegS, RseP (YaeL), and ClpXP. Senescing of the integrity of OMPs, which causes the activation of DegS by binding with unfolded OMPs, is the first key mechanism of σ^E activation [26]. In addition, DegS cleavage of RseA is physiologically inhibited by RseB binding to a conserved region near the C-terminus of the poorly structured RseA domain [27]. Therefore, RseB can negatively regulate the RseA degradation [27, 28]. RseB senses LPS integrity for binding with released LPS, and LPS displaces RseA from RseB due to antagonization of binding [29]. The subsequent intramembrane proteolysis of RseA by RseP is not performed when RseB is bound to RseA due to blockage through the side filtering function of the two PDZ domains of RseP [30]. Under stress conditions, the exposed periplasmic domain of RseA is cleaved by DegS between V148 and S149 [26]. Consequently, specific recognition of cleaved RseA is performed by the PDZ tandem domains of RseP [30], and specific cleavage of the transmembrane region of $RseA^{1-148}$ is also executed at A108 and C109 [31]. Finally, the cleaved cytoplasmic region of $RseA^{1-108}$ is recognized by SspB, and $RseA^{1-108}/\sigma^E$ complex is delivered to cytoplasmic AAA+ proteinases such as ClpXP [32, 33]. Destruction of the RseA fragment allows σ^E liberation and activation to cause the transcription of stress-responsive genes under the control of σ^E [28, 34].

These dual molecular signals (unfolded OMPs and LPS) are key factors for the σ^E ESR to sense outer membrane stresses [29]. For cell formation, OMPs and LPS are transported from the cytoplasm to the outer membrane in *E. coli*. The transport of OMPs as a beta-barrel structure is performed by the Sec-SurA-BAM system [35]. DegS is activated by binding of a peptide bearing a YxF motif at the C-terminus of an OMP, which is exposed by envelope stress,

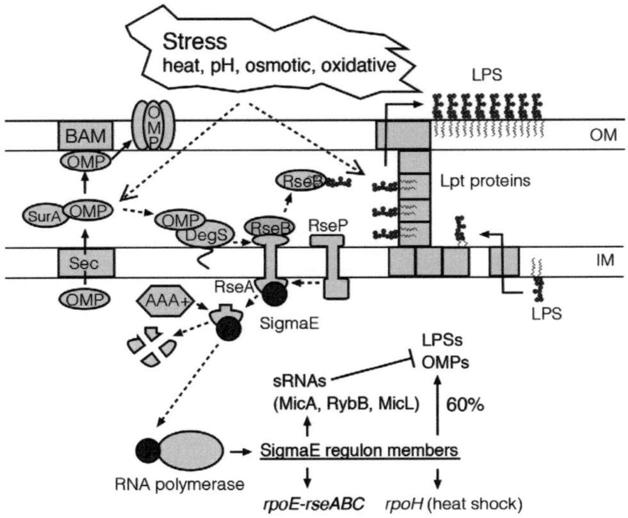

Figure 2. Schematic diagram of the σ^E signaling pathway and the σ^E regulon cascade. RseA is a key protein for σ^E activation. RseA, which is an antisigma factor, captures σ^E and neutralizes its activity. Two types of signaling molecules, OMPs and LPSs, are key activators of the proteinase DegS because the binding of the C-terminus of an OMP is required for DegS activation and the binding of LPS to RseB is required for deblocking of the RseA cleavage by DegS. Consequently, RseA is sequentially digested by RseP, and the RseA-N terminus is degraded by AAA+ proteinase, by which σ^E is released and activated to form a holo-RNA polymerase complex. Expressed σ^E-regulon members consist of LPS- and OMP-related proteins. sRNAs play key roles in the prevention of overproduction of LPSs and OMPs and in elimination of OMPs in σ^E-dependent cell lysis. Adapted from Lima et al. [29].

releasing from SurA or misfolding in BAM [28]. LPS is also transported by the aid of Ltp proteins, and LptA is a key component of the transenvelope complex to shuttle LPS to the outer membrane [36]. LptA less efficiently binds to LPS against RseB at 45°C [29], suggesting that LPS is easily caught by RseB under heat shock conditions. In addition, RseB can sense many mislocalized LPS species [29]. Therefore, both DegS activation and RseB detachment are essential for the initiation of RseA proteolysis for σ^E liberation. However, σ^E activity increases when either OMP or LPS mutations have accumulated [26, 29, 37], suggesting that a crosstalk between OMP and LPS biogeneses might be an additional regulation that can induce σ^E activation [28, 29].

This kind of proteolytic signal transduction and regulator-activating mechanism provides distinctive features for σ^E regulon as a transient expression. In the σ^E ESR, the initial signal-sensing cleavage of RseA is a rate-limiting step but the degradation of cytoplasmically fragmented RseA by AAA+ proteinase is relatively fast. Whereas, RseA is in excess over σ^E under normal conditions and the expression level of *rseA* is higher than that of *rpoE* [38]. Consequently, activated σ^E is rapidly deactivated, resulting in a short-period response to envelope stresses [33].

2.2. σ^E regulon genes

Activated σ^E forms a holo-RNA polymerase with the core RNA polymerase complex to initiate transcription by recognizing consensus sequences located upstream from coding genes

http://dx.doi.org/10.5772/67672

called promoters. Several experiments have been carried out in *E. coli* to find consensus sequences of promoters and σ^E-regulating genes, σ^E regulon genes. Attempts were made to identify consensus sequences for σ^E by several procedures, and genomic information and a search algorithm predicted a conserved −35 motif (GGAACTTTT) and a conserved −10 motif (T/CGGTCAAAA) [39–41]. σ^E regulon members in *E. coli* have been found by proteomics [4, 39], genetic strategies, [39, 40] and microarray analysis [4, 41]. Results of those studies showed that σ^E-holo RNA polymerase transcribes two kinds of RNAs, mRNAs for several genes and antisense sRNAs that repress the expression of several genes. Analysis of σ^E regulon genes showed that the regulon consists of 19 transcription units and 23 proteins. At least 60% of the regulon members are responsible for the synthesis and assembly of LPS and OMPs or regulatory proteins for these two key elements of the outer membrane [41]. The majority of σ^E regulon genes in *E. coli* are genes encoding periplasmic folding factors, periplasmic proteases, OMP assembly proteins, LPS translocation and assembly proteins, proteins for synthesis of phospholipids and lipid A, and a heat shock sigma factor coded by *rpoH* [39, 42]. One of most important operons under the control of σ^E is the *rpoE-rseABC* operon coding σ^E itself, RseA as an anti-σ^E, RseB repressor, and a *soxR*-influencing protein, respectively [43]. This operon is induced by two σ^E promoters, one upstream of *rpoE* and the other upstream of *rseA*. Therefore, σ^E activation causes a negative feedback loop by double transcriptions from the two promoters for rapid repression of σ^E activity. On the other hand, it has been revealed that small RNAs (sRNAs) are controlled by σ^E and work as repressors for gene expression. There are two distinct σ^E-inducible sRNAs, MicA and RybB, that bind to Hfq, an RNA chaperone protein required for the function and/or stabilization of sRNAs, and target mRNAs from 31 genes for major porins, metabolism, ribosome biosynthesis, toxin-antitoxin, and transcriptional factor PhoP [44]. In addition, MicL (SlrA) targets only one mRNA, which encodes the outer membrane lipoprotein Lpp, the most abundant protein of the cell [45]. Taken together, MicA, RybB and MicL allow σ^E to prevent the synthesis of abundant outer membrane proteins in response to stresses.

3. σ^E-dependent PCD

3.1. PCD in *E. coli*

PCD in *E. coli* is also closely associated with the strategy for sensing damage in DNA and the envelope structure. Three PCD mechanisms, a TA system, apoptosis-like death (ALD) and σ^E-dependent cell lysis, have been found in *E. coli* (**Figure 3**). Of these, the most intensively investigated PCD is *mazEF*, a TA system in which *mazF* encodes a stable toxin, sequence-specific endoribonuclease, and *mazE* encodes a labile MazF-antitoxin that is degraded *in vivo* by ATP-dependent ClpPA serine protease [46–48]. Toxicity of MazF is attributable to its endoribonuclease activity, specific for the trinucleotide sequence of ACA in mRNA, including the 3′-end fragment of 16S rRNA, to block protein synthesis and to synthesize specific proteins [49]. Specifically expressed proteins are classified into "survival proteins" and "death proteins" including SlyD, YfiD, YgcR, and ClpX [50]. Death proteins induce the DNA fragmentation and membrane depolarization [48]. In addition, *mazEF*-mediated PCD is regulated by a

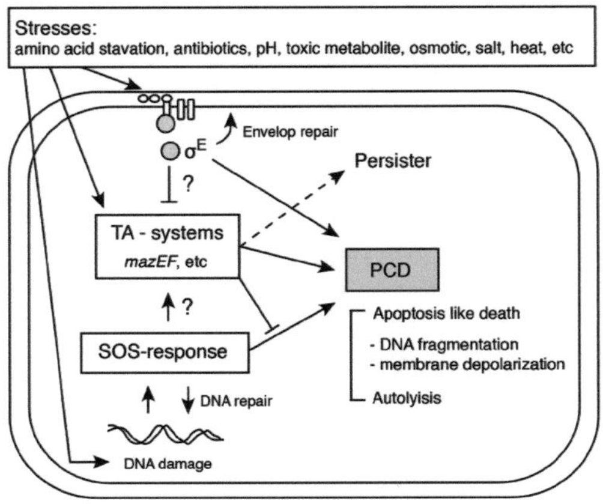

Figure 3. Activation pathways of PCD in *E. coli.* Several stresses affect cellular components including envelopes, DNA, and proteins, and these damaged materials become a signal for each stress response directly or indirectly. If the damage is excessive, PCD is triggered by several mechanisms. In *E. coli,* three mechanisms for PCD including TA systems, SOS-response–dependent cell lysis and σ^E-dependent cell lysis have been reported. SOS mainly responds to DNA damage and σ^E mainly responds to envelope damage. These three responses can directly induce PCD, but they are weakly connected to each other [46, 48].

quorum-sensing factor as a linear pentapeptide Asn-Asn-Trp-Asn-Asn (NNWNN), called an extracellular death factor (EDF) [51]. The EDF directly binds to MazF dimers to release MazF from the MazF–MazE complex, leading to cell death [52]. Moreover, *mazEF*-mediated PCD is activated under various stressful conditions including extreme amino acid starvation, inhibition of transcription and/or translation by antibiotics including rifampicin, chloramphenicol, and spectinomycin, an inhibitor protein of translation, DNA damage caused by thymine starvation as well as by mitomycin C, nalidixic acid and UV irradiation, and oxidative stress [47]. Notably, 28 other putative TA systems including DinJ-DafQ, DinP-YafN, RelB-RelE, and ChpS-ChpB have been identified in the *E. coli* K12 genome [12].

An SOS response-mediated PCD pathway was recently identified in *E. coli* is called apoptosis-like death (ALD) pathway [48]. The ALD pathway is activated by an extreme SOS response under severe DNA damage conditions [53] and follows apoptosis-like characteristics including rRNA degradation by the endoribonuclease YbeY [54], upregulation of a unique set of extensive damage-induced genes, decrease in respiration activity, and formation of high levels of OH^-, resulting in cell death [53]. Analysis of the relationship between *mazEF*-EDF and ALD revealed that the ALD pathway is inhibited by the *mazEF*-EDF–mediated PCD pathway [48].

In addition to DNA damage, envelope damage has been shown to be a trigger of PCD in *E. coli*. Envelope damage is caused by various factors including antibiotics, toxic metabolites, bacteriocins, osmotic, pH, and salt. In Gram-negative bacteria, the damage is sensed and transduced via ESRs. The ESRs alter the expression of specific genes related to functions that modify the envelope, rid cells of the toxic entity and/or repair the envelope damage [3]. σ^E-dependent PCD, which is one of envelope damage related PCDs, was first reported

http://dx.doi.org/10.5772/67672

in 2000 [19]. This PCD occurs as an autolysis mechanism, which is a growth phase-specific cell lysis [19], and removes only viable but nonculturable (VBNC) cells [19]. The molecular mechanism of the PCD is described below in detail. Interestingly, *rpoE* coding σ^E is an essential gene [55] because the absence of σ^E causes a cell death-signaling pathway including *hicB* (*ydcQ*) that encodes for an antitoxin of the HicA toxin proteinase [56, 57].

3.2. Mechanism of σ^E-dependent PCD

At the early stationary phase, *E. coli* cells undergo a decrease in viable cell number and almost all of the cells become VBNC cells [16, 58]. Elevation of the activate intracellular σ^E level, due to disruption of *rseA* for anti-σ^E or *rpoE*-increased expression, causes cell lysis at the beginning of the stationary phase, and this lysis occurs in wild-type cells at a low level [19, 59]. This mechanism may contribute to the removal of VBNC cells that have accumulated at a specific phase probably due to the accumulation of intracellular oxidative stress, and it is called σ^E-dependent PCD. Murata et al. showed that σ^E-dependent PCD is mediated by MicA, RybB, and PpiD [59]. MicA and RybB are transencoded sRNAs, and their expression is positively regulated by σ^E [60–62]. When misfolded OMPs or periplasmic proteins have accumulated, the expression of their sRNAs is induced by active σ^E, and MicA and RybB cause reduction in the levels of mRNAs of *ompA* and both *ompC* and *ompW*, respectively, via interaction between the sRNAs and the corresponding mRNA by assisting Hfq as an RNA chaperon and degradation of the mRNAs by ribonucleases [63]. Some OMPs are known to be physiologically and structurally crucial for cell activity [64]. OmpA as a structure protein is involved in the maintenance of cell shape and the passage of hydrophilic compounds through the outer membrane [65]. OmpC is the major porin protein that functions as a cation-selective porin [66]. However, no physiological function of OmpW has yet been determined [67]. These OMPs are greatly decreased in σ^E-activated cells [4, 19], and *micA*- or *rybB*-disrupted mutants and *micA*- or *rybB*-overexpressed cells repress and induce σ^E-dependent PCD, respectively [59]. Therefore, σ^E-dependent PCD is caused by the reduction of OMPs via posttranscriptional regulation including MicA and RybB. Recently, MicL has been found as the third σ^E-dependent sRNA that targets an mRNA for lipoprotein Lpp [45]. Since Lpp is the most abundant protein in the outer membrane [64], MicL may also be involved in σ^E-dependent PCD.

The level of PpiD is greatly reduced in σ^E-activated cells, though its regulation mechanism is unknown [68]. PpiD is a peptidyl-prolyl *cis-trans* isomerase as a periplasmic folding catalyst that catalyzes the rapid interconversion between the *cis* and *trans* forms of the peptide bond Xaa-Pro [69]. PpiD recognizes the early OMP folding intermediates and suppresses OMP biogenesis defects. Indeed, overexpression of PpiD represses σ^E-dependent cell lysis probably due to the acceleration of OMP folding [68]. Thus, the reduction of PpiD ensures the elimination of OMPs after the degradation of OMP mRNAs by sRNAs.

As shown in the model in **Figure 4**, when cells are exposed to some stresses as signals, mainly oxidative stress [19, 70], unfolded proteins accumulate in the outer membrane or periplasmic space, in turn causing the elevation of active σ^E in the cytoplasm. Active σ^E induces the expression of sRNAs, leading to the reduction of OMPs including Lpp. Furthermore, the reduction of PpiD via active σ^E enhances the disintegration of OMPs, resulting in collapse of the integrity of the outer membrane and finally lysis of cells.

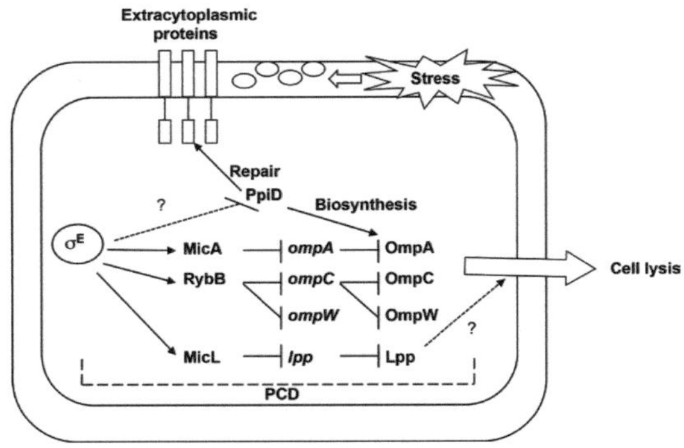

Figure 4. A model of σ^E-dependent PCD. When cells are exposed to stresses such as oxidative stress, σ^E is activated in response to damaged OMPs and increases and decreases the amounts of sRNAs (MicA and RybB) and PpiD as a folding catalyst protein, respectively. The expression of *ppiD* is greatly reduced under the condition of accumulation of active σ^E. The relationship between σ^E and *ppiD*, however, has not been clarified yet. MicA and RybB repress the expression of mRNAs of *ompA* and both *ompC* and *ompW*, respectively. The biosynthesis and repair of damaged OMPs are repressed by reduction in the PpiD level. As a result, the integrity of the outer membrane collapses and cell lysis progresses and finally causes cell death. MicL sRNA, which represses the expression of *lpp* mRNA, may also participate in σ^E-dependent PCD. Adapted from Murata et al. [59].

3.3. Function of σ^E-dependent PCD

Cell lysis in *E. coli* occurs under a general cultivation condition and remarkably increases after the early stationary phase. Most of the lysis seems to be σ^E-dependent because enhanced expression of *rseA* for anti-σ^E diminished the lysis [68]. The lysis level was significantly reduced when plasmid clones of *sodA* and *katE* for superoxide dismutase and catalase, respectively, were introduced [70]. Consistent with the level of lysis, the amounts of ROS are small in the exponential phase and large with a peak at the early stationary phase. The introduction of antioxidative stress genes eliminated about 80% of ROS. These findings suggest that oxidative stress is a trigger for the lysis [70]. The lysis is greatly enhanced in a *katE*-disrupted background, indicating that intracellular oxidative stress is involved in the lysis. Considering the signal transduction cascade to provide active σ^E [28], it is assumed that intracellular oxidative stress causes damage of OMPs by a modification such as carbonylation [71].

The trigger for σ^E-dependent cell lysis seems to be not only oxidative stress but also other stresses. The proposed signal transduction cascade for active σ^E [28] indicates the possibility that extracellular stress evokes σ^E-dependent cell lysis. Indeed, a disrupted mutation of *rpoS* for σ^S enhanced σ^E-dependent cell lysis at the early stationary phase [72]. Consistent with this, extracellular stress like toxic materials increases in a medium at the early stationary phase [14, 18]. Since σ^S functions as a general stress-response sigma factor to protect cells from various stresses [73], *rpoS* mutation results in the elevation of extracellular stress. It is known that σ^E becomes active through the σ^E activation cascade, which is initiated by conformation change of OMPs caused by a high temperature or ethanol as an extracellular stress [26, 29, 61]. Therefore, accumulation of extracellular and/or intracellular stresses beyond the elimination capacity by the stress response mechanism may cause conformation change of outer membrane proteins, which activates σ^E, resulting in σ^E-dependent cell lysis.

http://dx.doi.org/10.5772/67672

As shown in **Figure 4**, active σ^E determines the direction to either the repair or cell lysis pathway, presumably reflecting the level of damage of OMPs. If only a few OMPs are damaged, the number of active σ^E molecules may be not enough to express sRNAs such as *micA* and *rybB*, which may be insufficient to cause cell lysis but can express genes for the repair pathway. On the other hand, damage of OMPs over a certain threshold evokes the cascade of σ^E-dependent cell lysis. The coincidence of the fact that OMPs are monitoring proteins for cell damage and/or σ^E-dependent cell lysis and the fact that σ^E-dependent cell lysis is induced by reduction in the amount of OMPs is highly notable. OMP-damaged cells may be much more sensitive than undamaged cells to σ^E-dependent cell lysis.

σ^E-dependent cell lysis seems to eliminate some of the VBNC cells that have been damaged by some kinds of stress. The amount of cell lysis increases in parallel with increase in VBNC cells in the stationary phase, and most of the lysis was suppressed by enhanced expression of *rseA* [68]. An *rseA*-disrupted mutant that constitutively expresses active σ^E shows a phenotype that is characterized by decrease in cell density without a significant influence on colony-forming unit (CFU) but with protein accumulation in the medium [19]. This phenotype suggests that VBNC cells or some of the VBNC cells are subjected to σ^E-dependent cell lysis. This limited cell lysis might reflect the existence of a mechanism to distinguish damaged and undamaged cells. It is hypothesized that VBNC cells to be lysed have damaged OMPs to some extent and thus are susceptible to σ^E-dependent cell lysis. Notably, sRNAs such as MicA and RybB play crucial roles in σ^E-dependent cell lysis in the LTSP because mutation rate drastically increases in *micA*- and *rybB*-disrupted mutants [25].

Taken together, the findings have shown that *E. coli* has developed an ingenious mechanism for elimination of damaged cells in order to suppress the accumulation of mutated cells, and this mechanism might contribute to the preservation of the species. Since oxidative stress causes damage to DNA molecules in addition to other macromolecules including RNA, protein and phospholipid, it is assumed that the degree of damage of OMPs is consistent with that of DNA and that an abnormality of OMPs is a signal for removal of cells that have damaged DNA molecules from the cell population.

4. Contribution of PCD for LTSP

4.1. Survival mechanisms in LTSP

In the LTSP, *E. coli* cells can survive for several years [14, 17]. For survival, the cells induce specific sets of genes that support maintenance of their viability and protection against environmental stresses such as an oxidative stress [74]. However, there are potentials for genetic alteration in most cells in the LTSP. It was reported that 10-day-old cells, GASP mutants, were able to compete against 1-day-old cells when they were mixed together [14, 16, 17, 75]. It has been proposed that population exchange continuously occurs in the LTSP (**Figure 1**). Interestingly, the GASP phenotype is mediated by stable genomic mutations that provide benefits to cells for survival. The first mutant exhibiting a GASP phenotype was obtained from cells cultured for 10 days in LB medium, and its mutation, which was identified in *rpoS* coding σ^S, causes reduction of σ^S activity [16]. In addition, such σ^S activity-attenuated GASP mutants frequently appeared in nonbuffered media and basic media, but not so many appeared in acid and neutral media [76]. The relationship between the attenuation of σ^S activity and the GASP phenotype has not been clarified yet. The effect of the attenuation might be due to the misregulation of members of σ^S regulon. σ^S competes with other sigma factors to bind to the core RNA polymerase complex, and the attenuation of σ^S activity may change the balance in the competition among sigma factors [16].

Using the *rpoS* mutant as a starting strain, subsequent mutants with GASP phenotypes have been isolated. The additional mutations to the *rpoS* mutation have been mapped to *lrp*, coding the leucine-responsive regulator protein as a global regulator [77], or to the *ybeJ–gltJKL* cluster, encoding a high-affinity aspartate, and glutamate transporter [78]. A mutation in the DNA-binding domain of *lrp* has been shown to cause a GASP phenotype by increase in amino acid catabolism during carbon starvation, and mutants having mutation of *ybeJ–gltJKL* also show GASP phenotypes by increase in amino acid utilization [77]. Therefore, although these mutations are involved in different metabolic processes, it is likely that the enhancement of catabolic activity of amino acids for carbon and energy sources is responsible for these GASP phenotypes. Similarly, *sgaA*, *sgaB*, and *sgaC* mutants have been isolated as GASP mutants but have not been characterized yet [77]. Notably, non-*rpoS* mutation-related GASP mutants have also been reported [79].

The mechanism of GASP acquisition has been investigated and two interesting aspects have been shown. One is the reproducibility of GASP mutants and the other is a relatively high mutation rate in the LTSP. Since the speed of cell proliferation is very low in the LTSP, beneficial mutations for the GASP phenotype can appear only under high mutation conditions. It is thus assumed that there are some molecular mechanisms to generate genetic diversity in the LTSP.

Involvement of the methyl-directed mismatch repair (MMR) system and SOS-induced DNA polymerases has been considered for GASP mutations (**Figure 1**). It is known that when *E. coli* enters the stationary phase, the expression of MMR is reduced [80]. On the other hand, SOS DNA polymerases (Pols II, IV, and V) contribute to the generation of GASP mutations. These polymerases work during DNA replication when DNA polymerase III encounters a lesion and cannot proceed further in DNA synthesis. SOS polymerases are error-prone DNA polymerases and are thus responsible for the generation of adaptive mutations. Pol V Mut is a stand-alone DNA polymerase that is able to perform translesion synthesis, and polymerization of the polymerase is regulated by its intrinsic ATP hydrolase activity [81]. The occurrence of the GASP phenotype is highly related to the presence of SOS polymerases. Indeed, when grown in competition with the wild-type strain, mutants lacking one or more of the SOS polymerases suffer from a severe reduction in fitness to the LTSP. These mutants also fail to express the GASP phenotype as do wild-type strains, instead expressing two additional new types of GASP phenotype [82]. In addition, Pol IV and Pol V confer greater relative fitness than does Pol II during the LTSP, but Pol II can express the GASP phenotype faster than can Pol IV or Pol V [83]. Moreover, genes for the SOS polymerases and other SOS genes, especially genes for Pol IV and Pol V, are induced during the stationary phase [83]. These facts suggest that there are some mechanisms for the expression of these alternative polymerases and that the mechanisms contribute to the relative high mutation rate in the LTSP.

4.2. Importance of σ^E-dependent PCD for survival in the LTSP

E. coli can maintain living cells to some extent for several years (LTSP) in the same medium without supplementation of any nutrients during the cultivation. On the basis of results of recent studies and the discovery of mutants that had gained growth advantages in the beginning of the LTSP [16], it has been proposed that the LTSP consists of a number of distinct populations that continuously appear one after another as shown in **Figure 1** [14]. One of the big questions is how nutrients are supplied to support the formation of each new population in such a closed environment. One possible answer is a simple mechanism by which nutrients are supplied from existing cells. Nagamitsu et al. suggested that σ^E-dependent PCD is involved in the mechanism [25].

σ^E-dependent PCD lyses damaged cells but not undamaged cells or cells with little damage and thus has no influence on viable and culturable (VAC) cells [19]. This PCD is responsible for major cell lysis under general cultivation conditions and is enhanced in the stationary phase due to accumulation of stresses including oxidative stress as described above, and forms ghost cells that discharge cytosolic contents to the outside [59]. This lysis thus appears to be different from explosive cell lysis for the biogenesis of membrane vesicles [84]. As in the stationary phase, it is assumed that cells in the LTSP are exposed to metabolically accumulated stresses including oxidative stress, which trigger σ^E-dependent PCD. Therefore, σ^E-dependent PCD may provide nutrients that are indispensable for the formation and maintenance of new populations in the LTSP.

As mentioned in the previous section, disrupted mutations of *micA* and *rybB*, which are essential factors for σ^E-dependent PCD, caused serious problems such that they were unable to keep VAC cells at the very early period in the LTSP. These mutations give rise to a sudden increase in the mutation rate just before the disappearance of VAC cells [25]. σ^E-dependent PCD thus seems to play an important role in the elimination of DNA-damaged cells in the LTSP in addition to the provision of nutrients. Its role appears to resemble that of PCD, so-called apoptosis in multicellular organisms, by which abnormal cells or DNA-damaged cells are removed.

Although we still have no evidence that dynamic cell population changes continuously occur in the LTSP, results of studies [14, 16, 17] and results of preliminary experiments in its early phase suggest that cells acquiring mutations for GASP become dominant to form a new population and that new GASP mutations constantly appear and displace the preexisting population. σ^E-dependent PCD may contribute to the alteration of populations by the lysis of preexisting populations and the provision of nutrients during the LTSP. For the emergence of GASP mutations, a large number of mutations should be present in addition to them under such nutrient-limited conditions. A hypermutable state might exist in the LTSP as mentioned above [14]. In order for hypermutation and σ^E-dependent PCD to take place, active metabolisms should be maintained in fractions of the cell population. These active metabolisms are thought to lead to the selection of a dominant mutant and generate genetic diversity.

Further analysis of the LTSP *in vitro* seems to be important for understanding the life cycles of bacterial flora or biofilms and for elucidating the mechanisms of bacterial evolution. In addition, fundamental mechanisms for LTSP formation might be targets for drug design.

Acknowledgements

This work was supported by the Japan Society for the Promotion of Science, MEXT/JSPS Kakenhi (25250028) and the Advanced Low Carbon Technology Research and Development Program, Japan Science and Technology Agency (JST). This work was partially performed as collaborative research in the Asian Core Program and in the Core to Core Program, which was supported by the Scientific Cooperation Program agreed by the Japan Society for the Promotion of Science (JSPS), the National Research Council of Thailand (NRCT) and universities involved in the program.

Abbreviations

ALD	apoptosis-like death
CFU	colony-forming unit
ESR	envelope stress response
EDF	extracellular death factor
GASP	growth advantage in stationary phase
LPS	lipopolysaccharide
LTSP	long-term stationary phase
MMR	mismatch repair
OMPs	outer membrane proteins
PCD	programmed cell death
ROS	reactive oxygen species
sRNAs	small RNAs
TA	toxin-antitoxin
VAC	viable and culturable
VBNC	viable but nonculturable

Author details

Tomoyuki Kosaka[1,2], Masayuki Murata[1] and Mamoru Yamada[1,2]*

*Address all correspondence to: m-yamada@yamaguchi-u.ac.jp

1 Department of Biological Chemistry, Faculty of Agriculture and Life Science, Graduate School of Science and Technology for Innovation, Yamaguchi University, Yamaguchi, Japan

2 Research Center for Thermotolerant Microbial Resources, Yamaguchi University, Yamaguchi, Japan

References

[1] Ishihama A. Modulation of the nucleoid, the transcription apparatus, and the translation machinery in bacteria for stationary phase survival. Genes Cells. 1999;**4**:135-143.

[2] Raina S, Missiakas D, Georgopoulos C. The *rpoE* gene encoding the σ^E (σ^{24}) heat shock sigma factor of *Escherichia coli*. EMBO J. 1995;**14**:1043-1055.

[3] Guest RL, Raivio TL. Role of the Gram-negative envelope stress response in the presence of antimicrobial agents. Trends Microbiol. 2016;**24**:377-390. DOI: 10.1016/j.tim.2016.03.001.

[4] Kabir MS, Yamashita D, Koyama S, Oshima T, Kurokawa K, Maeda M, Tsunedomi R, Murata M, Wada C, Mori H, Yamada M. Cell lysis directed by σ^E in early stationary phase and effect of induction of the *rpoE* gene on global gene expression in *Escherichia coli*. Microbiology. 2005;**151**:2721-2735. DOI: 10.1099/mic.0.28004-0.

[5] Lockshin RA. Programmed cell death: history and future of a concept. J Soc Biol. 2005;**199**:169-173.

[6] Kerr JF, Wyllie AH, Currie AR. Apoptosis: a basic biological phenomenon with wide-ranging implications in tissue kinetics. Br J Cancer. 1972;**26**:239-257.

[7] Danial NN, Korsmeyer SJ. Cell death: critical control points. Cell. 2004;**116**:205-219.

[8] Kabir MS, Yamada M. σ^E-dependent programmed cell death in *Escherichia coli*. In: Yamada M, editor. Survival and death in bacteria. Kerala, India: Research Signpost; 2005. pp. 1-13.

[9] Allocati N, Masulli M, Di Ilio C, De Laurenzi V. Die for the community: an overview of programmed cell death in bacteria. Cell Death Dis. 2015;**6**:e1609. DOI: 10.1038/cddis.2014.570.

[10] Bayles KW. The biological role of death and lysis in biofilm development. Nat Rev Microbiol. 2007;**5**:721-726. DOI: 10.1038/nrmicro1743.

[11] González-Pastor JE, Hobbs EC, Losick R. Cannibalism by sporulating bacteria. Science. 2003;**301**:510-513. DOI: 10.1126/science.1086462.

[12] Yamaguchi Y, Inouye M. Regulation of growth and death in *Escherichia coli* by toxin-antitoxin systems. Nat Rev Microbiol. 2011;**9**:779-790. DOI: 10.1038/nrmicro2651.

[13] Bayles KW. Bacterial programmed cell death: making sense of a paradox. Nat Rev Microbiol. 2014;**12**:63-69. DOI: 10.1038/nrmicro3136.

[14] Finkel SE. Long-term survival during stationary phase: evolution and the GASP phenotype. Nat Rev Microbiol. 2006;**4**:113-120. DOI: 10.1038/nrmicro1340.

[15] Navarro Llorens JM, Tormo A, Martínez-García E. Stationary phase in gram-negative bacteria. FEMS Microbiol Rev. 2010;**34**:476-495. DOI: 10.1111/j.1574-6976.2010.00213.x.

[16] Zambrano MM, Siegele DA, Almirón M, Tormo A, Kolter R. Microbial competition: *Escherichia coli* mutants that take over stationary phase cultures. Science. 1993;**259**: 1757-1760.

[17] Finkel SE, Kolter R. Evolution of microbial diversity during prolonged starvation. Proc Natl Acad Sci U S A. 1999;**96**:4023-4027.

[18] Pletnev P, Osterman I, Sergiev P, Bogdanov A, Dontsova O. Survival guide: *Escherichia coli* in the stationary phase. Acta Naturae. 2015;**7**:22-33.

[19] Nitta T, Nagamitsu H, Murata M, Izu H, Yamada M. Function of the σ^E regulon in dead-cell lysis in stationary-phase. J Bacteriol. 2000;**182**:5231-5237.

[20] Costanzo A, Ades SE. Growth phase-dependent regulation of the extracytoplasmic stress factor, σ^E, by guanosine 3′,5′-bispyrophosphate (ppGpp). J Bacteriol. 2006;**188**:4627-4634. DOI: 10.1128/JB.01981-05.

[21] Yuste L, Hervás AB, Canosa I, Tobes R, Jiménez JI, Nogales J, Pérez-Pérez MM, Santero E, Díaz E, Ramos JL, de Lorenzo V, Rojo F. Growth phase-dependent expression of the *Pseudomonas putida* KT2440 transcriptional machinery analysed with a genome-wide DNA microarray. Environ Microbiol. 2006;**8**:165-177. DOI: 10.1111/j.1462-2920.2005.00890.x.

[22] Gefen O, Fridman O, Ronin I, Balaban NQ. Direct observation of single stationary-phase bacteria reveals a surprisingly long period of constant protein production activity. Proc Natl Acad Sci U S A. 2014;**111**:556-561. DOI: 10.1073/pnas.1314114111.

[23] Zambrano MM, Kolter R. *Escherichia coli* mutants lacking NADH dehydrogenase I have a competitive disadvantage in stationary phase. J Bacteriol. 1993;**175**:5642-5647.

[24] Kram KE, Finkel SE. Culture volume and vessel affect long-term survival, mutation frequency, and oxidative stress of *Escherichia coli*. Appl Environ Microbiol. 2014;**80**:1732-1738. DOI: 10.1128/AEM.03150-13.

[25] Nagamitsu H, Murata M, Kosaka T, Kawaguchi J, Mori H, Yamada M. Crucial roles of MicA and RybB as vital factors for σ^E-dependent cell lysis in *Escherichia coli* long-term stationary phase. J Mol Microbiol Biotechnol. 2013;**23**:227-232. DOI: 10.1159/000350370.

[26] Walsh NP, Alba BM, Bose B, Gross CA, Sauer RT. OMP peptide signals initiate the envelope-stress response by activating DegS protease via relief of inhibition mediated by its PDZ domain. Cell. 2003;**113**:61-71.

[27] Cezairliyan BO, Sauer RT. Inhibition of regulated proteolysis by RseB. Proc Natl Acad Sci U S A. 2007;**104**:3771-3776. DOI: 10.1073/pnas 0611567104.

[28] Kim DY. Two stress sensor proteins for the expression of sigmaE regulon: DegS and RseB. J Microbiol. 2015;**53**:306-310. DOI: 10.1007/s12275-015-5112-6.

[29] Lima S, Guo MS, Chaba R, Gross CA, Sauer RT. Dual molecular signals mediate the bacterial response to outer-membrane stress. Science. 2013;**340**:837-841. DOI: 10.1126/science.1235358.

[30] Hizukuri Y, Oda T, Tabata S, Tamura-Kawakami K, Oi R, Sato M, Takagi J, Akiyama Y, Nogi T. A structure-based model of substrate discrimination by a noncanonical PDZ tandem in the intramembrane-cleaving protease RseP. Structure. 2014;**22**:326-336. DOI: 10.1016/j.str.2013.12.003.

[31] Akiyama Y, Kanehara K, Ito K. RseP (YaeL), an *Escherichia coli* RIP protease, cleaves transmembrane sequences. EMBO J. 2004;**23**:4434-4442. DOI: 10.1038/sj.emboj.7600449.

[32] Flynn JM, Levchenko I, Sauer RT, Baker TA. Modulating substrate choice: the SspB adaptor delivers a regulator of the extracytoplasmic-stress response to the AAA+ protease ClpXP for degradation. Genes Dev. 2004;**18** 2292-2301. DOI: 10.1101/gad.1240104.

[33] Chaba R, Grigorova IL, Flynn JM, Baker TA, Gross CA. Design principles of the proteolytic cascade governing the σ^E-mediated envelope stress response in *Escherichia coli*: keys to graded, buffered, and rapid signal transduction. Genes Dev. 2007;**21**:124-136. DOI: 10.1101/gad.1496707.

[34] Hizukuri Y, Akiyama Y. PDZ domains of RseP are not essential for sequential cleavage of RseA or stress-induced σ^E activation *in vivo*. Mol Microbiol. 2012;**86**:1232-1245. DOI: 10.1111/mmi.12053.

[35] Goemans C, Denoncin K, Collet JF. Folding mechanisms of periplasmic proteins. Biochim Biophys Acta. 2014;**1843**:1517-1528. DOI: 10.1016/j.bbamcr.2013.10.014.

[36] Chng SS, Gronenberg LS, Kahne D. Proteins required for lipopolysaccharide assembly in *Escherichia coli* form a transenvelope complex. Biochemistry. 2010;**49**:4565-4567. DOI: 10.1021/bi100493e.

[37] Chaba R, Alba BM, Guo MS, Sohn J, Ahuja N, Sauer RT, Gross CA. Signal integration by DegS and RseB governs the σ^E-mediated envelope stress response in *Escherichia coli*. Proc Natl Acad Sci U S A. 2011;**108**:2106-2111. DOI: 10.1073/pnas.1019277108.

[38] Ades SE, Grigorova IL, Gross CA. Regulation of the alternative sigma factor σ^E during initiation, adaptation, and shutoff of the extracytoplasmic heat shock response in *Escherichia coli*. J Bacteriol. 2003;**185**:2512-2519. DOI: 10.1128/JB.185.8.2512-2519.2003.

[39] Dartigalongue C, Missiakas D, Raina S. Characterization of the *Escherichia coli* σ^E regulon. J Biol Chem. 2001;**276**:20866-20875. DOI: 10.1074/jbc.M100464200.

[40] Rezuchova B, Miticka H, Homerova D, Roberts M, Kormanec J. New members of the *Escherichia coli* σ^E regulon identified by a two-plasmid system. FEMS Microbiol Lett. 2003;**225**:1-7. DOI: 10.1016/S0378-1097(03)00480-4

[41] Rhodius VA, Suh WC, Nonaka G, West J, Gross CA. Conserved and variable functions of the σ^E stress response in related genomes. PLoS Biol. 2006;**4**:e2. DOI: 10.1371/journal.pbio.0040002.

[42] Klein G, Raina S. Regulated control of the assembly and diversity of LPS by noncoding sRNAs. Biomed Res Int. 2015;**2015**:153561. DOI: 10.1155/2015/153561.

[43] Koo MS, Lee JH, Rah SY, Yeo WS, Lee JW, Lee KL, Koh YS, Kang SO, Roe JH. A reducing system of the superoxide sensor SoxR in *Escherichia coli*. EMBO J. 2003;**22**:2614-2622. DOI: 10.1093/emboj/cdg252.

[44] Gogol EB, Rhodius VA, Papenfort K, Vogel J, Gross CA. Small RNAs endow a transcriptional activator with essential repressor functions for single-tier control of a global stress regulon. Proc Natl Acad Sci U S A. 2011;**108**:12875-12880. DOI: 10.1073/pnas.1109379108.

[45] Guo MS, Updegrove TB, Gogol EB, Shabalina SA, Gross CA, Storz G. MicL, a new σ^E-dependent sRNA, combats envelope stress by repressing synthesis of Lpp, the major outer membrane lipoprotein. Genes Dev. 2014;**28**:1620-1634. DOI: 10.1101/gad.243485.114.

[46] Aizenman E, Engelberg-Kulka H, Glaser G. An *Escherichia coli* chromosomal "addiction module" regulated by 3′,5′-bispyrophosphate: a model for programmed bacterial cell death. Proc Natl Acad Sci U S A. 1996;**93**:6059-6063.

[47] Engelberg-Kulka H, Amitai S, Kolodkin-Gal I, Hazan R. Bacterial programmed cell death and multicellular behavior in bacteria. PLoS Genet. 2006;**2**:e135. DOI: 10.1371/journal.pgen.0020135.

[48] Erental A, Sharon I, Engelberg-Kulka H. Two programmed cell death systems in *Escherichia coli*: an apoptotic-like death is inhibited by the *mazEF*-mediated death pathway. Kerala, India: PLoS Biol. 2012;**10**:e1001281. DOI: 10.1371/journal.pbio.1001281.

[49] Zhang Y, Zhang J, Hoeflich KP, Ikura M, Qing G, Inouye M. MazF cleaves cellular mRNAs specifically at ACA to block protein synthesis in *Escherichia coli*. Mol Cell. 2003;**12**:913-923.

[50] Amitai S, Kolodkin-Gal I, Hananya-Meltabashi M, Sacher A, Engelberg-Kulka H. *Escherichia coli* MazF leads to the simultaneous selective synthesis of both "death proteins" and "survival proteins". PLoS Genet. 2009;**5**:e1000390. DOI: 10.1371/journal.pgen.1000390.

[51] Kolodkin-Gal I, Hazan R, Gaathon A, Carmeli S, Engelberg-Kulka H. A linear pentapeptide is a quorum-sensing factor required for *mazEF*-mediated cell death in *Escherichia coli*. Science. 2007;**318**:652-655. DOI: 10.1126/science.1147248.

[52] Belitsky M, Avshalom H, Erental A, Yelin I, Kumar S, London N, Sperber M, Schueler-Furman O, Engelberg-Kulka H. The *Escherichia coli* extracellular death factor EDF induces the endoribonucleolytic activities of the toxins MazF and ChpBK. Mol Cell. 2011;**41**:625-635. DOI: 10.1016/j.molcel.2011.02.023.

[53] Erental A, Kalderon Z, Saada A, Smith Y, Engelberg-Kulka H. Apoptosis-like death, an extreme SOS response in *Escherichia coli*. MBio. 2014;**5**:e01426-14. DOI: 10.1128/mBio.01426-14.

[54] Jacob AI, Köhrer C, Davies BW, RajBhandary UL, Walker GC. Conserved bacterial RNase YbeY plays key roles in 70S ribosome quality control and 16S rRNA maturation. Mol Cell. 2013;**49**:427-438. DOI: 10.1016/j.molcel.2012.11.025.

[55] Hayden JD, Ades SE. The extracytoplasmic stress factor, σ^E, is required to maintain cell envelope integrity in *Escherichia coli*. PLoS One. 2008;**3**:e1573. DOI: 10.1371/journal.pone.0001573.

[56] Button JE, Silhavy TJ, Ruiz N. A suppressor of cell death caused by the loss of σ^E down-regulates extracytoplasmic stress responses and outer membrane vesicle production in *Escherichia coli*. J Bacteriol. 2007;**189**:1523-1530. DOI: 10.1128/JB.01534-06.

[57] Daimon Y, Narita S, Akiyama Y. Activation of toxin-antitoxin system toxins suppresses lethality caused by the loss of σ^E in *Escherichia coli*. J Bacteriol. 2015;**197**:2316-2324. DOI: 10.1128/JB.00079-15.

[58] Desnues B, Cuny C, Grégori G, Dukan S, Aguilaniu H, Nyström T. Differential oxidative damage and expression of stress defence regulons in culturable and non-culturable *Escherichia coli* cells. EMBO Rep. 2003;**4**:400-404. DOI: 10.1038/sj.embor.embor799.

[59] Murata M, Noor R, Nagamitsu H, Tanaka S, Yamada M. Novel pathway directed by σ^E to cause cell lysis in *Escherichia coli*. Genes Cells. 2012;**17**:234-247. DOI: 10.1111/j.1365-2443.2012.01585.x.

[60] Murata M, Kosaka T, Yamada M. Small non-coding RNAs and their involvement in regulation of various biological processes in and other bacteria. In: Yoshito S, Matsumoto K, editors. *Escherichia coli* and *Bacillus subtilis*; the frontiers of molecular microbiology revisited. Research Signpost; 2012. pp. 197-217.

[61] Udekwu KI, Wagner EG. Sigma E controls biogenesis of the antisense RNA MicA. Nucleic Acids Res. 2007;**35**:1279-1288. DOI: 10.1093/nar/gkl1154.

[62] Thompson KM, Rhodius VA, Gottesman S. σ^E regulates and is regulated by a small RNA in *Escherichia coli*. J Bacteriol. 2007;**189**:4243-4256. DOI: 10.1128/JB.00020-07.

[63] Valentin-Hansen P, Johansen J, Rasmussen AA. Small RNAs controlling outer membrane porins. Curr Opin Microbiol. 2007;**10**:152-155. DOI: 10.1016/j.mib.2007.03.001.

[64] Nikaido H. Molecular basis of bacterial outer membrane permeability revisited. Microbiology and Molecular Biology Reviews. 2003;**67**:593-656. DOI: 10.1128/MMBR.67.4.593-656.2003.

[65] Saint N, El Hamel C, Dé E, Molle G. Ion channel formation by N-terminal domain: a common feature of OprFs of *Pseudomonas* and OmpA of *Escherichia coli*. FEMS Microbiol Lett. 2000;**190**:261-265.

[66] Apirakaramwong A, Fukuchi J, Kashiwagi K, Kakinuma Y, Ito E, Ishihama A, Igarashi K. Enhancement of cell death due to decrease in Mg^{2+} uptake by OmpC (cation-selective porin) deficiency in ribosome modulation factor-deficient mutant. Biochem Biophys Res Commun. 1998;**251**:482-487.

[67] Pilsl H, Smajs D, Braun V. Characterization of colicin S4 and its receptor, OmpW, a minor protein of the *Escherichia coli* outer membrane. J Bacteriol. 1999;**181**:3578-3581.

[68] Noor R, Murata M, Nagamitsu H, Klein G, Raina S, Yamada M. Dissection of σ^E-dependent cell lysis in *Escherichia coli*: roles of RpoE regulators RseA, RseB and periplasmic folding catalyst PpiD. Genes Cells. 2009;**14**:885-899. DOI: 10.1111/j.1365-2443.2009.01318.x.

[69] Dartigalongue C, Raina S. A new heat-shock gene, *ppiD*, encodes a peptidyl-prolyl isomerase required for folding of outer membrane proteins in *Escherichia coli*. EMBO J. 1998;**17**:3968-3980. DOI: 10.1093/emboj/17.14.3968.

[70] Noor R, Murata M, Yamada M. Oxidative stress as a trigger for growth phase-specific σ^E-dependent cell lysis in *Escherichia coli*. J Mol Microbiol Biotechnol. 2009;**17**:177-187. DOI: 10.1159/000236029.

[71] Nyström T. Role of oxidative carbonylation in protein quality control and senescence. EMBO J. 2005;**24**:1311-1317. DOI: 10.1038/sj.emboj.7600599.

[72] Kabir MS, Yamashita D, Noor R, Yamada M. Effect of σ^S on σ^E-directed cell lysis in *Escherichia coli* early stationary phase. J Mol Microbiol Biotechnol. 2004;**8**:189-194. DOI: 10.1159/000085791.

[73] Battesti A, Majdalani N, Gottesman S. The RpoS-mediated general stress response in *Escherichia coli*. Annu Rev Microbiol. 2011;**65**:189-213. DOI: 10.1146/annurev-micro-090110-102946.

[74] Hengge-Aronis R, Klein W, Lange R, Rimmele M, Boos W. Trehalose synthesis genes are controlled by the putative sigma factor encoded by *rpoS* and are involved in stationary-phase thermotolerance in *Escherichia coli*. J Bacteriol. 1991;**173**:7918-7924.

[75] Zambrano MM, Kolter R. GASPing for life in stationary phase. Cell. 1996;**86**:181-184.

[76] Farrell MJ, Finkel SE. The growth advantage in stationary-phase phenotype conferred by *rpoS* mutations is dependent on the pH and nutrient environment. J Bacteriol. 2003;**185**:7044-7052. DOI: 10.1128/JB.185.24.7044-7052.2003.

[77] Zinser ER, Kolter R. Prolonged stationary-phase incubation selects for *lrp* mutations in *Escherichia coli* K-12. J Bacteriol. 2000;**182**:4361-4365. DOI: 10.1128/JB.182.15.4361-4365.2000.

[78] Zinser ER, Kolter R. Mutations enhancing amino acid catabolism confer a growth advantage in stationary phase. J Bacteriol. 1999;**181**:5800-5807.

[79] Rozen DE, Philippe N, Arjan de Visser J, Lenski RE, Schneider D. Death and cannibalism in a seasonal environment facilitate bacterial coexistence. Ecol Lett. 2009;**12**:34-44. DOI: 10.1111/j.1461-0248.2008.01257.x.

[80] Saint-Ruf C, Pesut J, Sopta M, Matic I. Causes and consequences of DNA repair activity modulation during stationary phase in *Escherichia coli*. Crit Rev Biochem Mol Biol. 2007;**42**:259-270. DOI: 10.1080/10409230701495599.

[81] Goodman MF. The discovery of error-prone DNA polymerase V and its unique regulation by RecA and ATP. J Biol Chem. 2014;**289**:26772-26782. DOI: 10.1074/jbc.X114.607374.

[82] Yeiser B, Pepper ED, Goodman MF, Finkel SE. SOS-induced DNA polymerases enhance long-term survival and evolutionary fitness. Proc Natl Acad Sci U S A. 2002;**99**:8737-8741. DOI: 10.1073/pnas.092269199.

[83] Corzett CH, Goodman MF, Finkel SE. Competitive fitness during feast and famine: how SOS DNA polymerases influence physiology and evolution in *Escherichia coli*. Genetics. 2013;**194**:409-420. DOI: 10.1534/genetics.113.151837.

[84] Turnbull L, Toyofuku M, Hynen AL, Kurosawa M, Pessi G, Petty NK, Osvath SR, Cárcamo-Oyarce G, Gloag ES, Shimoni R, Omasits U, Ito S, Yap X, Monahan LG, Cavaliere R, Ahrens CH, Charles IG, Nomura N, Eberl L, Whitchurch CB. Explosive cell lysis as a mechanism for the biogenesis of bacterial membrane vesicles and biofilms. Nat Commun. 2016;**7**:11220. DOI: 10.1038/ncomms11220.

Chapter 20

Survival of *Escherichia coli* under Nutrient-Deprived Conditions: Effect on Cell Envelope Subproteome

Maite Orruño, Claudia Parada,

Vladimir R. Kaberdin and Inés Arana

Additional information is available at the end of the chapter

http://dx.doi.org/10.5772/67777

Abstract

In the aquatic ecosystems, microorganisms are exposed to seasonal and circadian cycles. Abiotic factors (e.g. low temperature, nutrient deprivation) can cause morphological and physiological changes in bacteria, thereby facilitating cell survival. While representing the interface between the cells and external environment, the cell envelope plays a major role in bacterial response to stress and characterization of the changes it undergoes can help to understand the adaptation process. In this study, analysis of the morphological and physiological changes as well as variations in protein composition of the Escherichia coli cell envelope was carried out for populations maintained for 21 days under nutrient deprivation and suboptimal temperatures (4°C and 20°C). It was found that the absence of nutrients led to a temperature-dependent reduction of cell culturability but had no effect on cell viability and integrity. The concentration of membrane proteins playing the key roles in cellular transport, maintenance of cell structure or bioenergetics processes remained mainly unchanged. In contrast, the level of several proteins such as the elongation factor EFTu 1, components of Bam complex or proteins implicated in chemotaxis was altered, thus indicating that cells were readily responding and adapting to stress.

Keywords: starvation, suboptimal temperature, cell envelope subproteome

1. Introduction

In their natural environments, including aquatic ecosystems, microorganisms are usually exposed to seasonal and circadian cycles significantly dependent on environmental conditions. Moreover, during transfer from their natural environments to other ecosystems, bacteria can change their status from autochthonous to allochthonous one. This scenario is very typical for enteric bacteria, which are regularly transferred from their hosts to aquatic systems, a process accompanied by changes in the temperature and nutrient content of their habitats.

Escherichia coli (allochthonous, copiotroph, mesophile bacterium) is an indicator of fecal pollution and, therefore, its detection, quantification, as well as assessment of its ability to survive in aquatic environments are important subjects of the study and monitoring pursued by both public administrations and the scientific community.

Many bacteria, including *E. coli*, can cope with adverse conditions and successfully thrive in new environments by adjusting their physiology and metabolism. *E. coli* survival in a hostile aquatic environment depends on both biotic and abiotic factors [1–3]. Several abiotic factors including suboptimal temperature [4, 5], limitation of nutrients [6–8], and exposure to solar radiation [9–11] can lead to the loss of culturability. Barcina and Arana [12], Lothigius et al. [13], and others have demonstrated that, under these conditions, cells still remain physiologically active and intact. Transition from culturable to non-culturable state is known to involve considerable changes in the biochemical content of the cells [14–16].

To learn more about *E. coli* adaptation in aquatic systems, we undertook the present study to focus on adaptation changes affecting the composition of cell envelope and appearance of *E. coli* cells. While representing the interface between the cytoplasm and external environment, the cell envelope plays a major role in how bacteria sense and respond to stress [17] during its adaptation to changing environments [18, 19]. These functions of the cell envelope prompted us to characterize the morphological and physiological changes undertaken by *E. coli* populations during their permanence at suboptimal temperatures and under limitation of nutrients. Moreover, we have analyzed the variations in the subproteome of cell envelopes accompanying this survival process.

2. Materials and methods

To prepare experimental samples, *E. coli* ATCC 27325 cells were cultured aerobically in Tryptone soy broth (TSB) at 37°C with shaking (120 rpm) until they reached the stationary growth phase (24 h). The cells were harvested by centrifugation (4000 g, 4°C, 20 min) and washed three times with sterile saline solution (0.9% NaCl, w/v). All the glass flasks used for handling *E. coli* cultures were cleaned with H_2SO_4 (96%, v/v) beforehand, rinsed with deionized water, and kept at 250°C for 24 h to get rid of residual organic compounds.

Cells were inoculated in Erlenmeyer flasks containing sterile saline solution (absence of nutrients) to obtain a final density of 10^8 cells ml^{-1} and further incubated for 21 days at 4 and 20°C (suboptimal temperatures) with shaking (120 rpm) in darkness.

Subsamples were collected at the beginning of the experiments and after 3, 6, 12, and 21 days of nutrient deprivation to determine the number of total, viable, and culturable cells and to estimate the size of the cells (see below). Subsamples were also collected at 0 (P0), 6 (P1), 12 (P2), and 21 days (P3) to extract membrane proteins further analyzed by mass spectroscopy (see below).

The results from survival experiments are presented as the means of three independent experiments, with coefficient of variation between replicates less than 12%. The one-way analysis of variance (ANOVA) was used to determine the differences between the means. Probabilities less than (or equal to) 0.05 were considered significant.

The total number of bacteria was determined according to the procedure described by Hobbie et al. [20]. Namely, aliquots of cell suspensions from survival assays were filtered throughout 0.22 μm pore size black polycarbonate filters, stained with acridine orange (0.01%, w/v), and examined through epifluorescence microscopy. Viable bacteria, estimated as bacteria with intact cytoplasmic membranes (MEMB+), were counted with Live/Dead BacLight™ kit (Invitrogen) as described by Joux et al. [21]. The bacteria with intact (green fluorescence, MEMB+) and permeabilized (red fluorescence) cytoplasmic membranes were enumerated separately. The number of culturable bacteria was determined by the spread plate method on Tryptone soy agar (TSA) followed by their incubation for 24 h at 37°C.

The length variations of *E. coli* cells during their survival at 4 and 20°C were estimated through image analysis of epifluorescence preparations [22] by using an image analysis system, which included a high-resolution video camera (Hamamatsu 2400). Images of microscopic fields with enough bacteria were selected to be digitized and analyzed by Scion Image 1.62[a] software. For each subsample, 200 bacteria were measured. The values of mean size (x = 1.45 μm) and standard deviation (SD = 0.32) of initial population were used to establish three size categories (≤ x−SD, > x−SD – ≤ x + SD, > x + SD). Therefore, according to their length, the cells fell into one of the following size ranges: ≤ 1.12 μm, >1.12–≤1.77 μm, or >1.77 μm.

Membrane protein preparations were obtained according to the method described by Molloy et al. [23] with minor variations [24]. Subsequent analysis of these proteins was performed by the Proteomics Core Facility-SGIKER at the University of the Basque Country, using the protocol previously described by Gonzalez-Fernandez et al. [25]. Briefly, after protein precipitation by using a 2D Clean-Up Kit (GE Healthcare), the pellet was suspended in RapiGest solution (0.2%) (Waters Corporation) and heated at 85°C for 15 min. Then, the preheated suspension was reduced with DTT (5 mM), alkylated with iodoacetamide (15 mM), and digested with trypsin (2 μg per sample) overnight. MassPREP Enolase Digestion Standard (Waters Corporation) was added to the supernatants collected after centrifugation (16,000 g, 10 min) of HCl-treated samples (inactivation of RapiGest) and was used as a standard for protein absolute quantification. A nanoACQUITY UPLC System coupled to a SYNAPT HDMS (Waters Corporation) was used for data-independent acquisition analyses. Subsamples with tryptic peptides and MassPREP Enolase Digestion Standard were loaded onto a Symmetry300 C18, 180 μm × 20 mm precolumn (Waters Corporation) connected to a BEH130 C18 column (75 μm × 200 mm, 1.7 μm [Waters Corporation]). Peptides were eluted with a linear gradient of acetonitrile (120 min from 3 to 40% and 15 min from 40 to 60% [v/v]). Mass spectra were acquired using a data-independent acquisition mode (MSE) [26] as previously described by

Gonzalez-Fernandez et al. [25] and processed with ProteinLynx Global SERVER v2.4 Build RC7 (Waters Corporation). Protein identification was carried out using the database search algorithm of the program [27] and the parameters specified by Parada et al. [24]. The absolute protein quantification based on peak area intensity of peptide precursors was calculated by the program using enolase peptides as an internal standard [28].

Among proteins confirmed by the presence of at least three protein-derived peptides in the tryptic digests, those detected in two or three of the biological replicates were considered for further analysis. Quantification values of individual proteins were normalized *versus* the total protein in the samples. Only those proteins showing a 1.5-fold increase or a 0.6-fold decrease in their relative abundance (with respect to the previous sampling time) were considered differentially affected by survival conditions.

UniProt and KEGG databases were used to verify the identity and function of proteins. For the prediction of the bacterial protein subcellular localization, the PSORTb 3.0 program [29] was used. According to their main biological functions specified in UniProt database, selected proteins were further grouped to form the categories of proteins that (i) play structural roles involved in (ii) transport, (iii) bioenergetics, (iv) synthesis, degradation, and turnover of protein, (v) stress response, or (vi) have miscellaneous functions.

3. Results and discussion

Consistent with the results of previous studies [4, 11, 30, 31], the total number of *E. coli* cells remained unchanged throughout the experimentation time under nutrient deprivation. The percentages of viable and culturable cells were calculated with respect to the total bacteria for each analyzed time (**Figure 1A** and **C**). Although the viable population did not show significant variations throughout the survival period, the culturable fraction declined progressively. Moreover, the loss of culturability of the cells incubated at 20°C occurred faster (already after 6 days of incubation). This result agrees with those obtained in previous works [4, 32] in which it was established that, in the absence of natural microbiota, the survival of *E. coli* reduces at higher temperatures.

Cellular dwarfing has been described as a typical response of bacteria exposed to adverse conditions. However, our work did not reveal any significant changes in the size of starved *E. coli* cells during 21 days (**Figure 1C** and **D**). For the main fraction of starved *E. coli* cells (63.5–73.5%), the cell length was preserved within the same range (>1.1–≤1.8 μm) during the incubation time. Similar results were obtained by Muela et al. [33], who found no changes in the cell size throughout the long-term survival of *E. coli* in sterile river water.

Thus, analysis of cell physiology and morphology revealed that, although *E. coli* cells remained active and maintained their integrity and size, starvation led to a decrease in the number of culturable cells. Moreover, these changes were temperature dependent. Similar behavior has been previously described for this bacterium [4], and it was attributed to the differences in metabolic activities of cells cultured at low and normal temperatures [34, 35].

http://dx.doi.org/10.5772/67777

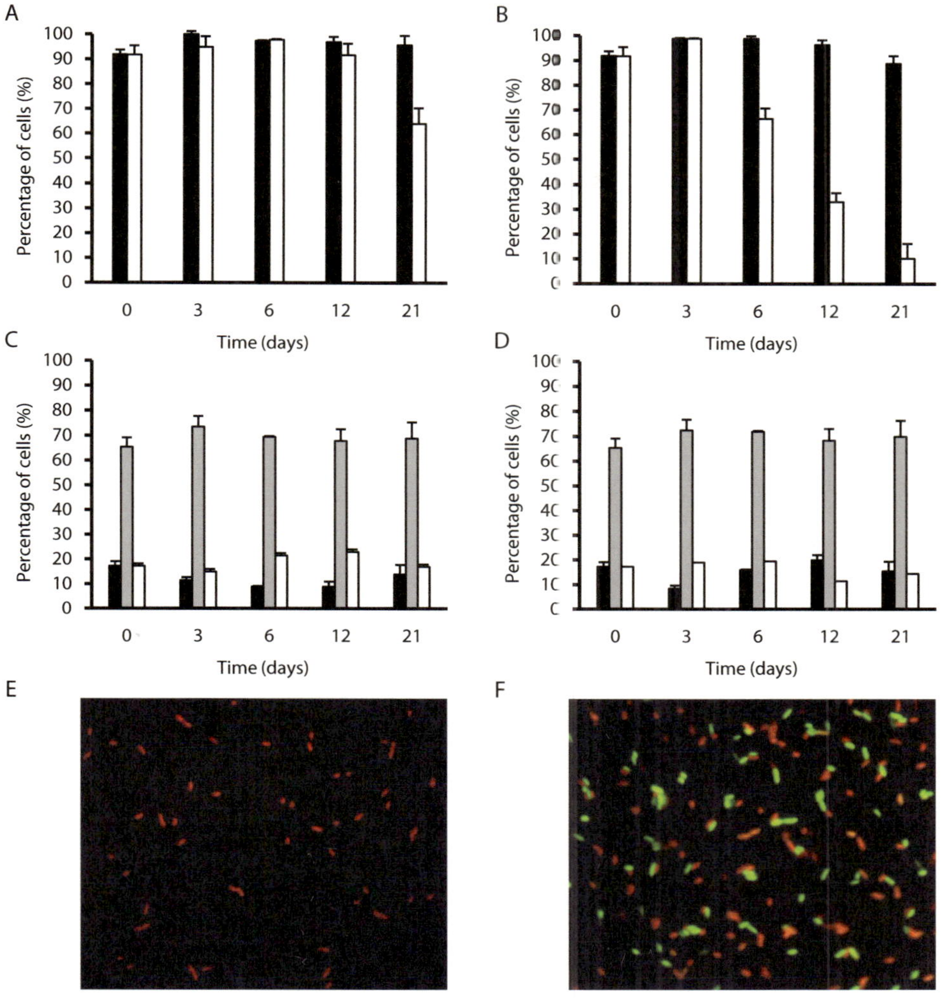

Figure 1. *Escherichia coli* ATCC 27325 survival in the absence of nutrients at 4°C (A, C) and 20°C (B, D). (A and B) Variations in the percentages of viable (■) and culturable (□) bacteria obtained with respect to the total count at each period. (C and D) Variations in cell size distribution (■ ≤ 1.12 μm; ▒ >1.12–≤1.77 μm; □ >1.77 μm). The data are mean values from three independent experiments with error bars representing the standard deviations calculated. Pannels (E and F), images of *E. coli* preparations stained with acridine orange (E) or Live/Dead BacLight™ kit (F) and examined through epifluorescence microscopy.

From survival assays carried out under starvation conditions, the samples for membrane subproteome analysis were collected at different incubation times: 0 (P0), 6 (P1), 12 (P2), and 21 days (P3). Despite the use of membrane fraction for mass spectrometry analysis, the PSORTb 3.0 program revealed that the resulting dataset potentially contained predicted cytosolic proteins (22%), including cytosolic subunits of ATP synthase or proteins that can conditionally be associated with the membrane (**Tables 1** and **2**). The fortuitous presence of cytoplasmic proteins in the membrane fractions was somewhat anticipated, as it was also observed in previous studies [24, 31].

Category	Protein accession number	Location[a]	Protein name
Cell structure	LPP_ECOLI	OM	Major outer membrane lipoprotein Lpp
	PAL_ECOLI	OM	Peptidoglycan-associated lipoprotein
	SLP_ECOLI	OM	Slp
	METQ_ECOLI	CM	D-Methionine-binding lipoprotein MetQ
	DACC_ECOLI	CM	D-Alanyl-D-alanine carboxypeptidase DacC
	SLYB_ECOLI	OM	Outer membrane protein SlyB
	YDGA_ECOLI	CM	YdgA
Transport	OMPA_ECOLI	OM	OmpA
	OMPC_ECOLI	OM	OmpC
	OMPW_ECOLI	OM	OmpW
	OMPX_ECOLI	OM	OmpX
	TOLC_ECOLI	OM	TolC
	GLPT_ECOLI	CM	Glycerol 3 phosphate transporter
	PTNAB_ECOLI	Cyt	PTS system mannose-specific EIIAB component
	PTND_ECOLI	CM	Mannose permease IID component
	COPA_ECOLI	CM	Copper-exporting P-type ATPase A
	ACRA_ECOLI	CM	Multidrug efflux pump subunit AcrA
	YHII_ECOLI	CM	Uncharacterized protein YhiI
	DCUA_ECOLI	CM	Anaerobic C4-dicarboxylate transporter DcuA
Bioenergetics	ATPA_ECOLI	Cyt	ATP synthase, subunit alpha
	ATPB_ECOLI; ATPL_ECOLI	CM	ATP synthase, subunits beta and c
	CYDA_ECOLI; CYDB_ECOLI	CM	Cytochrome bd-I ubiquinol oxidase, subunits 1 and 2
	FRDB_ECOLI; FRDA_ECOLI	CM	Fumarate reductase iron-sulfur subunit and flavoprotein subunit
	DHSA_ECOLI DHSB_ECOLI	CM	Succinate dehydrogenase flavoprotein subunit and iron-sulfur subunit
	NARG_ECOLI	CM	Respiratory nitrate reductase 1 alpha chain
Synthesis, degradation, and turnover of proteins	HFLK_ECOLI	Cyt	Modulator of FtsH protease HflK
	HFLC_ECOLI	CM	Modulator of FtsH protease HflC
Stress responses	YQJD_ECOLI	?	Uncharacterized protein YqjD
	ELAB_ECOLI	?	ElaB
Others	MIND_ECOLI	CM	Septum site-determining protein MinD

[a]OM, outer membrane; CM, cytoplasmic membrane; Cyt, cytosolic protein; ?, unknown.

Table 1. Membrane proteins that did not show significant changes in their level after 0, 6, 12, and 21 days of *E. coli* starvation in saline solution (NaCl 0.9%).

http://dx.doi.org/10.5772/67777

Category	Protein accession number	Location[a]	Protein name	4°C		20°C		
				P1/P0	P3/P1	P1/P0	P2/P1	P3/P2
Cell structure	YBJP_ECOLI	?	Uncharacterized YbjP	NC[b]	NC	0.59[c]	NC	NC
	OSME_ECOLI	?	Osmotically inducible lipoprotein E	1.93	NC	NC	ND	ND
	YIDC_ECOLI	CM	Membrane protein insertase YidC	NC	ND	NC	NC	ND
	BAMA_ECOLI	OM	Outer membrane protein assembly factor BamA	ND	ND	ND	ND	ND
	BAMB_ECOLI	OM	Outer membrane protein assembly factor BamB	ND	ND	ND	ND	ND
Transport	PTW3C_ECOLI	CM	PTS system N-acetylglucosamine-specific EIICBA component	NC	ND	NC	NC	NC
	SECD_ECOLI	CM	Protein translocase subunit SecD	NC	NC	NC	ND	ND
	PTM3C_ECOLI	CM	PTS system mannitol specific EIICBA component	NC	ND	NC	ND	ND
Bioenergetics	NUOCD_ECOLI	Cyt	NADH-quinone oxidoreductase subunits C/D	NC	ND	NC	NC	NC
	DHNA_ECOLI	CM	NADH dehydrogenase	ND	ND	ND	ND	ND
Synthesis, degradation and turnover of proteins	FTSH_ECOLI	CM	ATP-dependent zinc metalloprotease FtsH	NC	NC	NC	0.57	NC
Stress response	BFR_ECOLI	Cyt	Bacterioferritin	NC	NC	ND	ND	ND

Category	Protein accession number	Location[a]	Protein name	4°C		20°C		
				P1/P0	P3/P1	P1/P0	P2/P1	P3/P2
Others	EFTU1_ECOLI	Cyt	Elongation factor Tu 1	2.81	NC	4.22	NC	NC
	HEMX_ECOLI	CM	Putative uroporphyrinogen-III C methyltransferase	NC	NC	0.59	NC	NC
	HEMY_ECOLI	CM	Protein HemY	NC	ND	NC	NC	NC
	QMCA_ECOLI	?	Protein QmcA	NC	NC	NC	ND	ND
	PPID_ECOLI	CM	Peptidyl-prolyl *cis*-trans isomerase D	NC	NC	NC	ND	ND
	FLIC_ECOLI	Ex	Flagellin	NC	ND	NC	NC	ND
	MCP1_ECOLI	CM	Methyl accepting chemotaxis protein I	ND	ND	ND	ND	ND

[a]OM, outer membrane; CM, cytoplasmic membrane; Cyt, cytosolic; ?, unknown; Ex, extracellular.

[b]NC, no significant changes with respect to the previous sample; ND, not detected.

[c]Values higher than 1.5 indicate significant increases, and values lower than 0.6 indicate significant decreases of protein level with respect to the previous time.

Table 2. Membrane proteins that exhibited significant changes in their level at 6 (P1), 12 (P2), and 21 days (P3) of *E. coli* starvation in sterile saline solution (NaCl 0.9%, w/v).

A large group of proteins (**Table 1**) did not show any significant upregulation (>1.5-fold) or downregulation (<0.6-fold) during the survival experiments. This group included proteins related to the maintenance of cell structure (some lipoproteins, YdgA, and other) and/or the transport (porins such as OmpA, OmpW, OmpC, and TolC) (**Table 1**). Noteworthy, some of these proteins (namely, Lpp lipoprotein and OmpA and OmpC porins) belong to the group of the most abundant polypeptides detected in all samples. The above data suggest a role for these proteins in the maintenance of cell integrity observed here and in previous studies [12, 15, 16, 36, 37] upon *E. coli* exposure to adverse conditions. While some of them (e.g., lipoproteins) may be critical for maintaining the lipid bilayer, others (e.g., OmpA and OmpW) are likely involved in sustaining the integrity of the outer membrane [38–40]. No changes in protein level were also observed for different proteases implicated in synthesis, degradation, and turnover of membrane proteins (HflK and HflC) (**Table 1**). It seems that their presence is critical for preservation of cell stability as these proteases might degrade damaged or unnecessary proteins that could potentially accumulate in the lipid bilayer, thus restricting membrane permeability [41, 42], which is one of the fundamental functions of biological membranes [41]. This idea is supported by the results of staining with the Live/Dead BacLight™ kit used to differentiate *live* and *dead* cells (**Figure 1A** and **B**), demonstrating that the membranes of the starved cells remain intact and preserve their selective permeability.

We also observed that the level of numerous proteins implicated in bioenergetics (namely, different subunits of ATP synthase, cytochromes, and reductases) and transport (porins, mannose permease, components of PTS systems, or glycerol 3 phosphate transporter) was nearly the same in the control sample (P0) and samples (P3) mainly containing non-culturable bacteria (**Figure 1** and **Table 1**). Despite the constant presence of these proteins in cell envelope, several studies suggested that starving cells likely preserve a minimal level of metabolic activities. For instance, Ozkanca and Flint [43] indicated that respiration rates greatly decreased to almost undetectable levels in *E. coli* cells exposed to starvation during their incubation in sterile lake water. Likewise, Barcina et al. [44] detected a decrease of glucose uptake for populations maintained in freshwater. Thus, the constant presence of the energy- and sugar metabolism-related proteins seems to indicate that starving cells still stay alarmed and prepared to quickly respond to favorable environmental conditions. Indeed, analysis of glucose uptake by the starving cells revealed a quick response and, as a result, an increase in the respiration rate [44]. Consistently, several authors have demonstrated the function of the electron transport chains in non-culturable bacteria by showing their ability to reduce intracellularly tetrazolium salts [31, 45, 46]. Moreover, in a previous work, Arana et al. [30] found that some *E. coli* cells could release nutrients (mainly monomeric carbohydrates and amino acids) into the surrounding medium under stress conditions. The released nutrients are taken up by other cells, thus could aid in the survival of remaining culturable cells and, therefore, ensure the persistence of the species in adverse environments.

Other constantly present proteins include YqjD and its paralogous protein ElaB, known to be abundant in the stationary growth phase. These proteins seem to be involved in inhibition of ribosomal activity and in localization of ribosomes on the inner membrane during the stationary phase of growth. In cells exposed to some stress conditions (e.g., starvation), both ribosomal biogenesis and protein synthesis are known to be suppressed. Thus, the negative regulation of these processes by YqjD and ElaB could be important for bacterial adaptation and survival in harsh environments [47].

Table 2 shows the membrane proteins (accounted for 17–19% of the total analyzed polypeptides) that became less or more abundant upon starvation of *E. coli* in sterile saline solution. Some of these proteins underwent variations dependent on nutrient status and/or incubation temperature. For example, the level of two proteins (namely, BamA and BamB) belonging to the outer membrane complex Bam (additionally containing BamB, BamC, BamD, and BamE [48, 49]) as well as the membrane protein insertase YidC sharply declined and became undetectable in the starved cells (**Table 2**). Since the β-barrel assembly machinery (BAM) is essential for maintaining the bacterial cell envelope and is involved in OMP recognition, folding, and assembly [48, 50, 51], its depletion with BamA, one of the key components of the *E. coli* Bam complex, after 3 days of incubation under starvation conditions could indicate the reduction in the production and/or active assembly of proteins in the outer membrane. Volokhina et al. [48] suggested that loss of activity of this protein promotes accumulation of proteins in the outer membrane that cannot be inserted therein. This accumulation could be lethal for the bacterium since aggregates would be formed in the periplasmic space. Moreover, this could lead to the incorporation of these OMPs into inner bacterial membranes, which would dissipate the proton-motive force and kill bacteria [52]. However, in this study, we have not detected dead cells (**Figure 1**). This fact could indicate that the Bam complex might become redundant in the nondividing *E. coli* cells due to reduction of production and maturation of OMPs in bacterial cells exposed to starvation.

Similar to BamA and BamB, the membrane protein insertase YidC also was not detectable after 21 days of starvation. This protein has been proposed to mediate the transfer of transmembrane segments of hydrophilic polypeptide chains from the Sec-translocon into the lipid bilayer and can assist folding of inner membrane proteins [53] including ATP synthase subunit c [17]. This finding together with the data obtained for BamA and BamB (see above) suggests that limitation of nutrients leads to the overall reduction of cell envelope biogenesis.

Other proteins that became undetectable in starved cells were the methyl-accepting chemotaxis protein I and the flagellin FLIC_ECOLI. Chen and Chen [54] demonstrated that under starvation, *Vibrio vulnificus* populations exhibited reduced motility. Lemke et al. [55] and Chandrangsu et al. [56] concluded that DksA (protein required for the regulation of certain promoters) and the alarmone ppGpp inhibit expression of the flagellar cascade during cells' entry into the stationary phase or during their starvation. This mechanism could prevent unnecessary waste of energy on synthesis of macromolecular complexes and generation of proton-motive force used to rotate the flagella apparatus [57] and, therefore, would free more energy to sustain the survival process.

Unlike chemotaxis protein I and the flagellin FLIC_ECOLI, the elongation factor Tu 1 became one of the most abundant proteins in populations maintained 6 days at 20°C. This elongation factor is known as a cytoplasmic chaperone implicated in protein synthesis, growth regulation, and stress responses [58, 59]. The high level of this protein in starving cells is consistent with the data presented by Muela et al. [31]. They observed an increase in the level of EFTu in *E. coli* populations under starvation conditions and its subsequent localization on the membrane.

As shown in **Figure 1**, *E. coli* response to starvation was temperature dependent. We identified several proteins whose level was differently affected by temperature. Namely, the protein translocase subunit SecD and bacterioferritin became undetectable in starved cells maintained at 20°C, whereas PTS system N-acetylglucosamine-specific EIICBA component was gradually lost in populations maintained at 4°C (**Table 2**). Unlike above examples, the temperature-dependent regulation of osmotically inducible lipoprotein E (OSME_ECOLI) and ATP-dependent zinc metalloprotease FtsH did not reveal a clear regulation pattern.

Interestingly, the levels of three proteins were below detection at the starting point (P0), but their level was increased afterward. This group of proteins includes the structural protein MreB (MREB_ECOLI), putative porin NmpC, and the cytosolic universal stress protein F (USPF_ECOLI). MreB is a homolog of eukaryotic actin, which has been found to be associated with the membrane in several bacteria [60–62]. Shih et al. [63] stated that the MreB system is required for establishment of the rod shape of cells. MreB proteins form actin-like cables lying beneath the inner cell membrane. The cables are required to guide longitudinal cell wall synthesis. Chiu et al. [64] demonstrated that, in non-culturable *Vibrio parahaemolyticus* populations appeared upon starvation, MreB protein was located near the cytoplasmic membrane. Moreover, these authors reported a reduction in cellular size associated with the increase in the expression of the *mreB* gene. However, Ben Abdallah et al. [65] and Parada et al. [24] described the decline in the expression of the *mreB* gene and MreB protein content, respectively, in *Vibrio* species undergoing morphological changes in response to stress. Kruse et al. [66] demonstrated that a decrease of MreB concentration leads to merodiploid spherical and inflated *E. coli* cells prone to cell lysis. Moreover, Defeu Soufo et al. [67] demonstrated a relationship between MreB and EFTu for *E. coli* and *Bacillus subtilis* cells, and they suggested that EFTu could affect the cellular morphology through interaction with MreB. EFTu improves the ability of MreB to form filaments functioning as a basal structure. Our work suggests that both proteins could interact, as both of them are present during the cell response to stress.

Thus, the present study showed that, although incubation in the absence of nutrients reduced cell culturability in a temperature-dependent manner, the cells still remained active and preserved their integrity and size. In addition, proteome analysis of the cell's envelope revealed that the concentration of membrane proteins playing the key roles in cellular transport, maintenance of cell structure, as well as bioenergetic processes remained almost unchanged, indicating their crucial roles in *E. coli* survival under nutrient-limiting conditions. Moreover, some of the proteins critical for preservation of cell stability and membrane permeability (such as the modulators of FtsH protease, HflK, and HflC) appeared to be steadily present in the populations of mainly non-culturable cells. We also found the continuous increase in the level of elongation factor EFTU1 along the survival process, thus suggesting its essential role in the adaptation process. Interestingly, the level of some proteins (e.g., bacterioferritin) was differently affected by temperature (see above). Finally, the observed depletion of the key components of the Bam complex, insertase YidC, and/or proteins implicated in chemotaxis suggested their redundancy for preserving cell integrity and therefore allowed to save energy during *E. coli* adaptation and survival.

Acknowledgements

The work was supported by the Spanish Ministry of Science and Innovation (CGL2011-26252 and BFU2011-25455), the Basque Government (Spain) (research project IT376-10, grants BFI-2011-85 to C. Parada), and the Basque Foundation for Science, Ikerbasque (Spain). Proteomic analyses were performed at the Proteomics Unit at the University of the Basque Country, UPV/EHU, Spain (SGIker, member of ProteoRed).

Author details

Maite Orruño[1], Claudia Parada[2], Vladimir R. Kaberdin[2,3] and Inés Arana[2*]

*Address all correspondence to: ines.arana@ehu.eus

1 Department of Immunology, Microbiology and Parasitology, Faculty of Pharmacy, University of the Basque Country (UPV/EHU), Spain

2 Department of Immunology, Microbiology and Parasitology, Faculty of Science and Technology, University of the Basque Country (UPV/EHU), Spain

3 IKERBASQUE, Basque Foundation for Science, Bilbao, Spain

References

[1] Barcina I, Lebaron P, Vives-Rego J. Survival of allochthonous bacteria in aquatic systems: A biological approach. FEMS Microbiology Ecology. 1997. 23:1-9. DOI: 10.1016/S0168-6496(97)00016-0.

[2] Noble RT, Lee IM, Schiff KC. Inactivation of indicator microorganisms from various sources of faecal contamination in seawater and freshwater. Journal of Applied Microbiology. 2004. 96:464-472. DOI: 10.1111/j.1365-2672.2004.02155.x.

[3] John DE, Rose JB. Review of factors affecting microbial survival in groundwater. Environmental Science and Technology. 2005. 39:7345-7356. DOI: 10.1021/es047995w.

[4] Arana I, Muela A, Orruño M, Seco C, Garaizabal I, Barcina I. Effect of temperature and starvation upon survival strategies of *Pseudomonas fluorescens* CHA0: Comparison with *Escherichia coli*. FEMS Microbiology Ecology. 2010. 74:500-509. DOI: 10.1111/j.1574-6941.2010.00979.x.

[5] Blaustein RA, Pachepsky Y, Hill RL, Shelton DR, Whelan G. *Escherichia coli* survival in waters: Temperature dependence. Water Research. 2013. 47:569-578. DOI:10.1016/j.watres.2012.10.027.

[6] Ramos JL, Gallegos MT, Marqués S, Ramos-González MI, Espinosa-Urgel M, Segura A. Responses of Gram-negative bacteria to certain environmental stressors. Current Opinion in Microbiology. 2001. 4:166-171. DOI: 10.1016/S1369-5274(00)00183-1.

[7] Ihssen J, Grasselli E, Bassin C, François P, Piffaretti JC, Köster W, Schrenzel J, Egli T. Comparative genomic hybridization and physiological characterization of environmental isolates indicate that significant (eco-)physiological properties are highly conserved in the species *Escherichia coli*. Microbiology. 2007. 153:2052-2066. DOI: 10.1099/mic.0.2006/002006-0.

[8] van Elsas JD, Semenov AV, Costa R, Trevors JT. Survival of *Escherichia coli* in the environment: Fundamental and public health aspects. ISME Journal. 2011. 5:173-183. DOI: 10.1038/ismej.2010.80.

[9] Muela A, García-Bringas JM, Arana I, Barcina I. The effect of simulated solar radiation on *Escherichia coli*. The relative roles of UV-B, UV-A, and photosynthetically active radiation. Microbial Ecology. 2000. 39:65-71. DOI:10.1007/s002489900181.

[10] Whitman RL, Nevers MB, Korinek GC, Byappanahalli MN. Solar and temporal effects on *Escherichia coli* concentration at a Lake Michigan swimming beach. Applied and Environmental Microbiology. 2004. 70:4276-4285. DOI: 10.1128/AEM.70.7.4276-4285.2004.

[11] Arana I, Orruño M, Pérez-Pascual D, Seco C, Muela A, Barcina I. Inability of *Escherichia coli* to resuscitate from the viable but nonculturable state. FEMS Microbiology Ecology. 2007. 62(1):1-11. DOI:10.1111/j.1574-6941.2007.00362.x.

[12] Barcina I, Arana I. The viable but nonculturable phenotype, a crossroad in the live cycle of non differentiating bacteria?. Reviews in Environmental Science and BioTechnology. 2009. 8:245-255. DOI:10.1007/s11157-009-9159-x.

[13] Lothigius Å, Sjöling Å, Svennerholm AM, Bölin I. Survival and gene expression of enterotoxigenic *Escherichia coli* during long-term incubation in sea water and freshwater. Journal of Applied Microbiology. 2010. 108:1441-1449. DOI:10.1111/j.1365-2672.2009.04548.x.

[14] McDougald DM, Rice SA, Kjelleberg S. New perspectives on the viable but nonculturable response. Biologia Bratislava. 1999. 54:617-623.

[15] Oliver JD. Recent findings on the viable but nonculturable state in pathogenic bacteria. FEMS Microbiology Reviews. 2010. 34:415-425. DOI:10.1111/j.1574-6976.2009.00200.x.

[16] Pinto D, Santos MA, Chambel L. Thirty years of viable but nonculturable state research: unsolved molecular mechanisms. Critical Reviews in Microbiology. 2015. 41:61-76. DOI :10.3109/1040841X.2013.794127. Epub 2013 Jul 12.

[17] Silhavy TJ, Kahne D, Walker S. The bacterial cell envelope. Cold Spring Harbor Perspectives in Biology. 2010. 2:a000414. DOI:10.1101/cshperspect.a000414.

[18] Darcan C. Expression of OmpC and OmpF porin proteins and survival of *Escherichia coli* under photooxidative stress in Black Sea water. Aquatic Biology. 2012. 17:97-105. DOI:10.3354/ab00458.

[19] Shimizu K. Regulation systems of bacteria such as *Escherichia coli* in response to nutrient limitation and environmental stresses. Metabolites. 2013. 4:1-35. DOI: 10.3390/metabo4010001.

[20] Hobbie JE, Daley RJ, Jasper S. Use of nucleopore filters for counting bacteria by epifluorescence microscopy. Applied and Environmental Microbiology. 1977. 33:1225-1228.

[21] Joux F, Lebaron P, Troussellier M. Succession of cellular states in *Salmonella typhimurium* population during starvation in artificial seawater microcosms. FEMS Microbiology Ecology. 1997. 22:65-76. DOI:10.1111/j.1574-6941.1997.tb00357.x.

[22] Massana R, Gasol JM, Bjørnsen PK, Blackburn N, Hagström A, Hietanen S, Hygum BH, Kuparinen J, Pedrós-Alió C. Measurement of bacterial size via image analysis of epifluorescence preparations: Description of an inexpensive system and solutions to some of the most common problems. Scientia Marina. 1997. 61:397-407.

[23] Molloy MP, Herbert BR, Slade MB, Rabilloud T, Nouwens AS, Williams KL, Gooley AA. Proteomic analysis of the *Escherichia coli* outer membrane. European Journal of Biochemistry. 2000. 267:2871-2881. DOI:10.1046/j.1432-1327.2000.01296.x.

[24] Parada C, Orruño M, Kaberdin V, Bravo Z, Barcina I, Arana I. Changes in the *Vibrio harveyi* cell envelope subproteome during permanence in cold seawater. Microbial Ecology. 2016. 72:549-558. DOI:10.1007/s00248-016-0802-0.

[25] Gonzalez-Fernandez R, Aloria K, Arizmendi JM, Jorrin-Novo JV. Application of label-free shotgun nUPLC-MS(E) and 2-DE approaches in the study of *Botrytis cinerea* mycelium. Journal of Proteome Research. 2013. 12:3042-3056. DOI: 10.1021/pr3010937.

[26] Silva JC, Denny R, Dorschel CA, Gorenstein M, Kass IJ, Li GZ, McKenna T, Nold MJ, Richardson K, Young P, Geromanos SJ. Quantitative proteomic analysis by accurate mass retention time pairs. Analytical Chemistry. 2005. 77:2187-2200. DOI:10.1021/ac048455k.

[27] Li GZ, Vissers JP, Silva JC, Golick D, Gorenstein MV, Geromanos SJ. Database searching and accounting of multiplexed precursor and product ion spectra from the data independent analysis of simple and complex peptide mixtures. Proteomics. 2009. 9:1696-1719. DOI:10.1002/pmic.200800564.

[28] Silva JC, Gorenstein MV, Li GZ, Vissers JP, Geromanos SJ. Absolute quantification of proteins by LCMSE: A virtue of parallel MS acquisition. Molecular and Cellular Proteomics. 2006. 5:144-156. DOI:10.1074/mcp.M500230-MCP200.

[29] Yu NY, Wagner JR, Laird MR, Melli G, Rey S, Lo R, Dao P, Sahinalp SC, Ester M, Foster LJ, Brinkman FSL. PSORTb 3.0: Improved protein subcellular localization prediction with refined localization subcategories and predictive capabilities for all prokaryotes. Bioinformatics. 2010. 26:1608-1615. DOI:10.1093/bioinformatics/btq249.

[30] Arana I, Seco C, Epelde K, Muela A, Fernández-Astorga A, Barcina I. Relationships between *Escherichia coli* cells and the surrounding medium during survival processes. Antonie Van Leeuwenhoek. 2004. 86:189-199. DOI:10.1023/B:ANTO.0000036146.28808.93.

[31] Muela A, Seco C, Orruño M, Camafeita E, Arana I, López JA, Barcina I. Changes in *Escherichia coli* outer membrane subproteome under environmental conditions inducing the viable but nonculturable state. FEMS Microbiology Ecology. 2008. 64:28-36. DOI: 10.1111/j.1574-6941.2008.00453.x.

[32] Flint KP. The long-term survival of *Escherichia coli* in river water. Journal of Applied Bacteriology. 1987. 63:261-270.

[33] Muela A, Pocino M, Arana I, Justo JI, Iriberri J, Barcina I. Effect of growth phase and parental cell survival in river water on plasmid transfer between *Escherichia coli* strains. Applied and Environmental Microbiology. 1994. 60:4273-4278.

[34] Morita RY. The starvation-survival state of microorganisms in nature and its relationship to the bioavailable energy. Experientia. 1990. 46:813-817.

[35] Semenov AV, van Bruggen AHC, van Overbeek L, Termorshuizen AJ, Semenov AM. Influence of temperature fluctuations on *Escherichia coli* O157:H7 and *Salmonella enterica* serovar Typhimurium in cow manure. FEMS Microbiology Ecology. 2007. 60:419-428. DOI:10.1111/j.1574-6941.2007.00306.x.

[36] Roszak DB, Colwell RR. Survival strategies of bacteria in the natural environment. Microbiological Reviews. 1987. 51:365-379.

[37] Oliver JD. The viable but nonculturable state in bacteria. Journal of Microbiology. 2005. 43:93-100.

[38] Sonntag I, Schwarz H, Hirota Y, Henning U. Cell envelope and shape of *Escherichia coli*: Multiple mutants missing the outer membrane lipoprotein and other major outer membrane proteins. Journal of Bacteriology. 1978. 136 280-285.

[39] Koebnik R, Locher KP, Van Gelder P. Structure and function of bacterial outer membrane proteins: Barrels in a nutshell. Molecular Microbiology. 2000. 37:239-253. DOI:10.1046/j.1365-2958.2000.01983.x.

[40] Asakura H, Kawamoto K, Haishima Y, Igimi S, Yamamoto S, Makino S. Differential expression of the outer membrane protein W (OmpW) stress response in enterohemorrhagic *Escherichia coli* O157:H7 corresponds to the viable but non-culturable state. Research in Microbiology. 2008. 159:709-717. DOI:10.1016/j.resmic.2008.08.005.

[41] Ito K, Akiyama Y. Cellular functions, mechanism of action, and regulation of FtsH protease. Annual Review of Microbiology. 2005. 59:211-231. DOI:10.1146/annurev.micro.59.030804.121316.

[42] Narberhaus F, Obrist M, Führer F, Langklotz S. Degradation of cytoplasmic substrates by FtsH, a membrane-anchored protease with many talents. Research in Microbiology. 2009. 160:652-659. DOI:10.1016/j.resmic.2009.08.011.

[43] Ozkanca R, Flint KP. Relationship between respiratory enzymes and survival of *Escherichia coli* under starvation stress in lake water. Journal of Applied Microbiology. 1997. 82:301-309.

[44] Barcina I, González JM, Iriberri J, Egea L. Survival strategy of *Escherichia coli* and *Enterococcus faecalis* in illuminated fresh and marine systems. Journal of Applied Bacteriology. 1990. 68:189-198.

[45] Besnard V, Federighi M, Declerq E, Jugiau F, Cappelier JM. Environmental and physico-chemical factors induce VBNC state in *Listeria monocytogenes*. Veterinary Research. 2002. 33:359-370. DOI:10.1051/vetres:2002022.

[46] Falcioni T, Papa S, Campana R, Manti A, Battistelli M, Baffone W. State transitions of *Vibrio parahaemolyticus* VBNC cells evaluated by flow cytometry. Cytometry Part B: Clinical Cytometry. 2008. 74:272-281. DOI:10.1002/cyto.b.20427.

[47] Yoshida H, Maki Y, Furuike S, Sakai A, Ueta M, Wada A. YqjD is an inner membrane protein associated with stationary-phase ribosomes in *Escherichia coli*. Journal of Bacteriology. 2012. 194:4178-4183. DOI: 10.1128/JB.00396-12.

[48] Volokhina EB, Grijpstra J, Beckers F, Lindh E, Robert V, Tommassen J, Bos MP. Species-specificity of the BamA component of the bacterial outer membrane protein-assembly machinery. PLoS One. 2013. 8:e85799. DOI:10.1371/journal.pone.0085799.

[49] Wu T, Malinverni J, Ruiz N, Kim S, Silhavy TJ, Kahne D. Identification of a multicomponent complex required for outer membrane biogenesis in *Escherichia coli*. Cell. 2005. 121:235-245. DOI:10.1016/j.cell.2005.02.015.

[50] Hagan CL, Kahne D. The reconstituted *Escherichia coli* Bam complex catalyzes multiple rounds of β-barrel assembly. Biochemistry. 2011. 50:7444-7446. DOI:10.1021/bi2010784.

[51] Albrecht R, Schütz M, Oberhettinger P, Faulstich M, Bermejo I, Rudel T, Diederichs K, Zeth K. Structure of BamA, an essential factor in outer membrane protein biogenesis. Acta Crystallographica Section D. Structural Biology Crystallography. 2014. 70:1779-1789. DOI:10.1107/S1399004714007482.

[52] Gessmann D, Chung YH, Danoff EJ, Plummer AM, Sandlin CW, Zaccai NR, Fleming KG. Outer membrane β-barrel protein folding is physically controlled by periplasmic lipid head groups and BamA. Proceedings of the National Academy of Sciences of the United States of America. 2014. 111:5878-5883. DOI:10.1073/pnas.1322473111.

[53] Luirink J, Yu Z, Wagner S, de Gier W. Biogenesis of inner membrane proteins in *Escherichia coli*. Biochimica et Biophysica Acta. 2012. 1817:965-976. DOI:10.1016/j.bbabio.2011.12.006.

[54] Chen H, Chen CY. Starvation induces phenotypic diversification and convergent evolution in *Vibrio vulnificus*. PLoS One. 2014. 9:e88658. DOI:10.1371/journal.pone.0088658.

[55] Lemke JJ, Durfee T, Gourse RL. DksA and ppGpp directly regulate transcription of the *Escherichia coli* flagellar cascade. Molecular Microbiology. 2009. 74:1368-1379. DOI:10.1111/j.1365-2958.2009.06939.x.

[56] Chandrangsu P, Lemke JJ, Gourse RL. The dksA promoter is negatively feedback regulated by DksA and ppGpp. Molecular Microbiology. 2011. 80:1337-1348. DOI:10.1111/j.1365-2958.2011.07649.x.

[57] Häse CC, Barquera B. Role of sodium bioenergetics in *Vibrio cholerae*. Biochimica et Biophysica Acta (BBA)—Bioenergetics. 2001. 1505:169-178. DOI:10.1016/S0005-2728(00)00286-3.

[58] Yu F, Inouye S, Inouye M. Lipoprotein-28, a cytoplasmic membrane lipoprotein from *Escherichia coli*. Cloning, DNA sequence, and expression of its gene. Journal of Biological Chemistry. 1986. 261:2284-2288.

[59] Caldas TD, El Yaagoubi A, Kohiyama M, Richarme G. Purification of elongation factors EF-Tu and EF-G from *Escherichia coli* by covalent chromatography on thiol-sepharose. Protein Expression and Purification. 1998. 14:65-70. DOI:10.1006/prep.1998.0922.

[60] Wachi M, Doi M, Okada Y, Matsuhashi M. New *mre* genes *mreC* and *mreD*, responsible for formation of the rod shape of *Escherichia coli* cells. Journal of Bacteriology. 1989. 171:6511-6516.

[61] Figge RM, Divakaruni AV, Gober JW. MreB, the cell shape-determining bacterial actin homologue, co-ordinates cell wall morphogenesis in *Caulobacter crescentus*. Molecular Microbiology. 2004. 51:1321-1332. DOI:10.1111/j.1365-2958.2003.03936.x.

[62] Mazza P, Noens EE, Schirner K, Grantcharova N, Mommaas AM, Koerten HK, Muth G, Flärdh K, van Wezel GP, Wohlleben W. MreB of *Streptomyces coelicolor* is not essential for vegetative growth but is required for the integrity of aerial hyphae and spores. Molecular Microbiology. 2006:60:838-852. DOI:10.1111/j.1365-2958.2006.05134.x.

[63] Shih YL, Kawagishi I, Rothfield L. The MreB and Min cytoskeletal-like systems play independent roles in prokaryotic polar differentiation. Molecular Microbiology. 2005. 58:917-928. DOI:10.1111/j.1365-2958.2005.04841.x.

[64] Chiu SW, Chen SY, Wong HC. Dynamic localization of MreB in *Vibrio parahaemolyticus* and in the ectopic host bacterium *Escherichia coli*. Applied and Environmental Microbiology. 2008. 74:6739-6745. DOI:10.1128/AEM.01021-08.

[65] Ben Abdallah F, Ellafi A, Lagha R, Bakhrouf A, Namane A, Rousselle JC, Lenormand P, Kallel H. Identification of outer membrane proteins of *Vibrio parahaemolyticus* and *Vibrio alginolyticus* altered in response to γ-irradiation or long-term starvation. Research in Microbiology. 2010. 161:869-875. DOI:10.1016/j.resmic.2010.10.009.

[66] Kruse T, Bork-Jensen J, Gerdes K. The morphogenetic MreBCD proteins of *Escherichia coli* form an essential membrane-bound complex. Molecular Microbiology. 2005. 55:78-89. DOI:10.1111/j.1365-2958.2004.04367.x.

[67] Defeu Soufo HJ, Reimold C, Breddermann H, Mannherz HG, Graumann PL. Translation elongation factor EF-Tu modulates filament formation of actin-like MreB protein *in vitro*. Journal of Molecular Biology. 2015. 427:1715-1727. DOI:10.1016/j.jmb.2015.01.025.